Chapel and Haeney's Essentials of Clinical Immunology

Chapel and Haeney's Essentials of Clinical Immunology

Seventh Edition

Siraj A. Misbah
MSc, FRCP, FRCPath
Consultant Clinical Immunologist, Honorary Senior Clinical Lecturer in Immunology
Oxford University Hospitals NHS Foundation Trust and University of Oxford
Oxford, UK

Gavin P. Spickett
MA, LLM, DPhil, FRCPath, FRCP, FRCP(E)
Retired Consultant Clinical Immunologist, Royal Victoria Infirmary
Newcastle upon Tyne, UK

Virgil A.S.H. Dalm
MD, PhD
Department of Internal Medicine, Division of Allergy & Clinical Immunology
Department of Immunology, Erasmus University Medical Center Rotterdam
Rotterdam, The Netherlands

WILEY Blackwell

Registered Offices
John Wiley & Sons, Inc., 111 River Street, Hoboken, NJ 07030, USA
John Wiley & Sons Ltd, The Atrium, Southern Gate, Chichester, West Sussex, PO19 8SQ, UK

Editorial Office
9600 Garsington Road, Oxford, OX4 2DQ, UK

For details of our global editorial offices, customer services, and more information about Wiley products visit us at www.wiley.com.

Wiley also publishes its books in a variety of electronic formats and by print-on-demand. Some content that appears in standard print versions of this book may not be available in other formats.

Library of Congress Cataloging-in-Publication Data

Names: Misbah, Siraj A., author. | Spickett, Gavin, author. | Dalm, Virgil
    A. S. H., author.
Title: Chapel and Haeney's essentials of clinical immunology / Siraj
    Misbah, Gavin Spickett, Virgil A.S.H. Dalm.
Other titles: Essentials of clinical immunology
Description: Seventh edition. | Hoboken, NJ : Wiley-Blackwell 2022. |
    Preceded by Essentials of clinical immunology / Helen Chapel, Mansel
    Haeney, Siraj Misbah, Neil Snowden. Sixth edition. 2014. | Includes
    bibliographical references and index.
Identifiers: LCCN 2021061616 (print) | LCCN 2021061617 (ebook) | ISBN
    9781119542384 (paperback) | ISBN 9781119542407 (adobe pdf) | ISBN
    9781119542421 (epub)
Subjects: MESH: Immune System Diseases | Immune System
    Phenomena–physiology
Classification: LCC RC582 (print) | LCC RC582 (ebook) | NLM QW 740 | DDC
    616.07/9–dc23/eng/20220110
LC record available at https://lccn.loc.gov/2021061616
LC ebook record available at https://lccn.loc.gov/2021061617

Cover Design: Wiley
Cover Image: © KATERYNA KON/GETTY IMAGES

Set in 10/12pt AGaramondPro by Straive, Pondicherry, India

Printed in Great Britain by Bell and Bain Ltd, Glasgow

Contents

Preface to the Seventh Edition

The new authors have been honoured to take on the responsibility for this well-respected textbook from Professor Helen Chapel and Dr. Mansel Haeney, who originally created the book and have been heavily involved in the previous six editions. In honour of their contributions both to the textbook and to developing and teaching clinical immunology, the book has now been renamed as Chapel and Haeney's Essentials of Clinical Immunology and we have tried not to deviate too far from their original aims.

The text has been updated as far as possible and all chapters have been revised. The original structure and format have been retained. Many of the illustrations, even though quite old now, are still relevant to illustrate key immunological principles. The Covid pandemic and the additional workload created, particularly for Samras Johnson V, has meant that progress on the book has been slower than anticipated at the initiation meeting pre-pandemic. Covid has also led to significant advances in the clinical immunological field and in particular it has kickstarted the clinical use of mRNA vaccines. Covid has produced its own fascinating immunological problems and unexpected immunological responses to vaccines. Recognition of 'long Covid' has provided new impetus to investigate the causes of post-infectious chronic fatigue. New immunological therapies are being introduced at speed for all immunological diseases and gene manipulation is going to have a huge influence on the management of genetic immunological diseases. Immunology remains an exciting field that is involved in all areas of clinical medicine. We hope that we can convey this excitement to the reader.

As always, the authors are grateful to their families and friends for their forebearance during the writing process and also to many colleagues for direct and indirect help in updating the chapters. In particular, we are most grateful to Dr Martin Barnardo, Consultant Clinical Scientist in Histocompatibility and Immunogenetics for reviewing the chapter on Transplantation. The meticulous work of colleagues at LNS Indexing is also gratefully acknowledged. We are grateful to James Watson, Anne Hunt and the very patient team of editors at Wiley-Blackwell. As most authors, we must apologise to them for being slow to respond to their queries and to return proofs.

Siraj A. Misbah
Gavin P. Spickett
Virgil A.S.H. Dalm

Preface to the First Edition

Immunology is now a well-developed basic science and much is known of the normal physiology of the immune system in both mice and men. The application of this knowledge to human pathology has lagged behind research, and immunologists are often accused of practising a science which has little relevance to clinical medicine. It is hoped that this book will point out to both medical students and practising clinicians that clinical immunology is a subject which is useful for the diagnosis and management of a great number and variety of human disease.

We have written this book from a clinical point of view. Diseases are discussed by organ involvement, and illustrative case histories are used to show the usefulness (or otherwise) of immunological investigations in the management of these patients. While practising clinicians may find the case histories irksome, we hope they will find the application of immunology illuminating and interesting. The student should gain some perspective of clinical immunology from the case histories, which are selected for their relevance to the topic we are discussing, as this is not a textbook of general medicine. We have pointed out those cases in which the disease presented in an unusual way.

Those who have forgotten, or who need some revision of, basic immunological ideas will find them condensed in Chapter 1. This chapter is not intended to supplant longer texts of basic immunology but merely to provide a springboard for chapters which follow. Professor Andrew McMichael kindly contributed to this chapter and ensured that it was up-to-date. It is important that people who use and request immunological tests should have some idea of their complexity, sensitivity, reliability and expense. Students who are unfamiliar with immunological methods will find that Chapter 17 describes the techniques involved.

Helen Chapel
Mansel Haeney
1984

Key to Illustrations

Throughout the illustrations standard forms have been used for commonly-occurring cells and pathways. A key to these is given in the figure below.

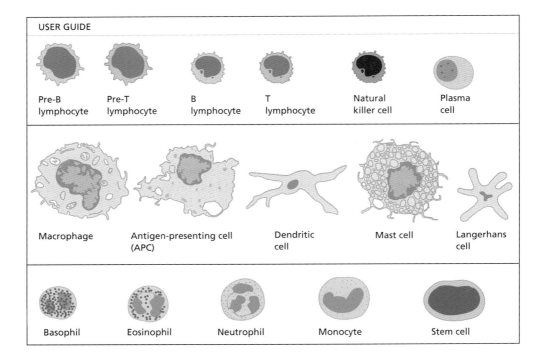

About the Companion Website

The book is accompanied by a website:

 www.wiley.com/go/misbah/immunology

The website contains:
- Interactive multiple-choice questions
- Additional case studies and figures to test your knowledge
- Case studies from the book with additional figures for you to use for revision
- All figures from the book in PowerPoint format
- Useful website links

Scan this QR code to visit the companion website.

CHAPTER 1
Basic Components: Structure and Function

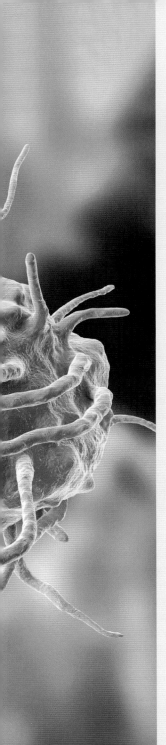

Key topics

 Visit the companion website at **www.wiley.com/go/misbah/immunology** to download cases on these topics.

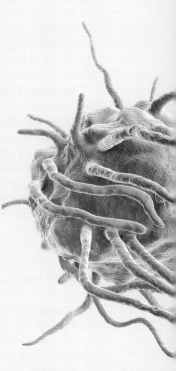

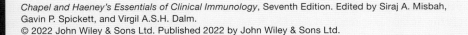

Chapel and Haeney's Essentials of Clinical Immunology, Seventh Edition. Edited by Siraj A. Misbah, Gavin P. Spickett, and Virgil A.S.H. Dalm.

1.1 Introduction

The immune system evolved as a defence against infectious diseases. Individuals with markedly deficient immune responses, if untreated, succumb to infections in early life. There is, therefore, a selective evolutionary pressure for a really efficient immune system. Although innate systems are fast in response to pathogens, the evolution to adaptive responses provided greater efficiency. However, a parallel evolution in pathogens means that all species, plants, insects, fish, birds and mammals have continued to improve their defence mechanisms over millions of years, giving rise to some redundancies as well as resulting in apparent complexity. The aim of this chapter is to provide an initial description of the molecules involved, moving on to the role of each in the immune processes rather than the more traditional sequence of anatomical structure, cellular composition and then molecular components. It is hoped that this gives a sense of their relationship in terms of immediacy and dependency as well as the parallel evolution of the two immune systems. An immune response consists of **five parts**:

- Recognition of material as foreign and dangerous.
- An early innate (non-specific) response to this recognition.
- A slower specific response to a particular antigen, known as an adaptive response.
- Non-specific augmentation of this response.
- A memory of specific immune responses, providing a quicker and larger response when that particular antigen is encountered the second time.

Innate immunity, though phylogenetically older and important in terms of speed of response, is less efficient. Humoral components (soluble molecules in the plasma) and cells in blood and tissues are involved. Such responses are normally accompanied by inflammation and occur within a few hours of stimulation (Table 1.1).

Adaptive immune responses are also divided into humoral and cellular responses. Adaptive humoral responses result in the generation of antibodies reactive with a particular antigen. Antibodies are proteins with similar structures, known collectively as immunoglobulins (Ig). They can be transferred passively to another individual by injection of serum. In contrast, only cells can transfer cellular immunity. Good examples of cellular immune responses are the rejection of a graft by lymphoid cells as well as graft-versus-host disease, where viable transferred cells attack an immunologically compromised recipient that is unable to fight back.

Antibody-producing lymphocytes, which are dependent on the bone marrow, are known as B cells. In response to antigen stimulation, B cells will mature to antibody-secreting plasma cells. Cellular immune responses are dependent on an intact thymus, so the lymphocytes responsible are known as thymus-dependent (T) cells. The developmental pathways of both cell types are fairly well established (Fig. 1.1).

The recognition phase is common to both adaptive and innate immunity. It involves professional cells, known as classical dendritic cells (DCs), that recognize general pathogen features or specific antigenic molecules, process the antigens and present antigen fragments to the other cells of the immune system, as well as initiating non-specific inflammation to the pathogen. In the **effector phase**, neutrophils and macrophages (innate immunity) and antibodies and effector T lymphocytes (adaptive immunity) eliminate the antigen.

In terms of disease, like other organs, the immune system may fail (immunodeficiency), may become malignant (lymphoid malignancies) or may produce aberrant responses (such as in autoimmunity or allergy). This chapter describes the normal immune system in order to lay the basis for discussing these ways in which it can go wrong and so cause disease.

1.2 Key molecules

Many types of molecules play vital roles in both phases of immune responses; some are *shared by both the innate and the adaptive systems*. Antigens are substances that are recognized by immune components. Detection molecules on innate cells recognize general patterns of 'foreignness' on non-mammalian cells, whereas those on adaptive cells are specific for a wide range of very particular molecules or fragments of molecules. Antibodies are not only the surface receptors of B cells (BCRs) that recognize specific antigens, but, once the appropriate B cells are activated and differentiate into plasma cells, antibodies are also secreted into blood and body fluids in large quantities to prevent that antigen from causing damage. T cells have structurally similar receptors for recognizing antigens, known as T-cell receptors (TCRs). Major histocompatibility complex (MHC) molecules provide a means of self-recognition and also play a fundamental role in T lymphocyte effector functions.

Effector mechanisms are often dependent on messages from initiating or regulating cells; soluble mediators, which carry messages between cells, are known as interleukins, cytokines and chemokines.

Table 1.1 Components of innate and adaptive immunity

Features	Innate	Adaptive
Foreign molecules recognized	Structures shared by microbes, recognized as patterns (e.g. repeated glycoproteins), PAMPs	Wide range of very particular molecules or fragments of molecules on all types of extrinsic and modified self-structures
Nature of recognition receptors	Germline encoded – limited PRRs	Somatic mutation results in a wide range of specificities and affinities
Speed of response	Immediate	Time for cell movement and interaction between cell types
Memory	None	Efficient
Humoral components	Complement components	Antibodies
Cellular components	Dendritic cells, neutrophils, macrophages, NK cells, NKT cells, B1 cells, epithelial cells, mast cells	Lymphocytes – T (Th1, Th2, Th17, Tregs), B
iNKT cells, γδ T cells		

NK, natural killer; PAMPs, pathogen-associated molecular patterns; pattern-recognition receptors (PRRs); Tregs, regulatory T cells.

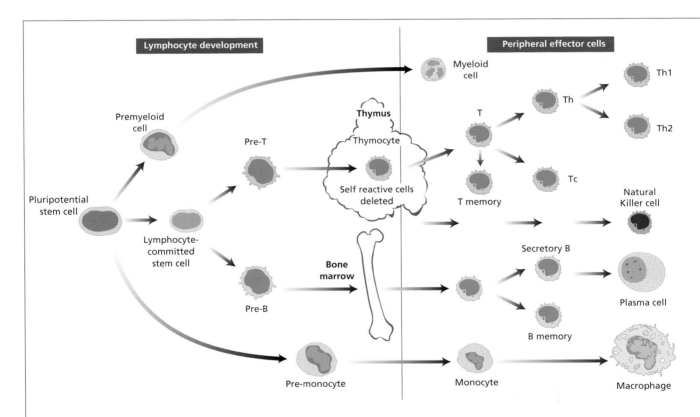

Fig. 1.1 Development of different types of blood cells from a pluripotential stem cell in the bone marrow. The developmental pathway for natural killer (NK) cells is shown separately because it is thought that NK cells may develop in both the thymus and the bone marrow.

1.2.1 Molecules recognized by immune systems

Foreign substances are recognized by both the innate and adaptive systems, but in different ways, using different receptors (see section 1.2.2). The innate system is activated by 'danger signals', due to pattern-recognition receptors on DCs recognizing conserved microbial structures directly, often repeated polysaccharide molecules, known as **pathogen-associated molecular patterns**. Toll-like receptors (receptors that serve a similar function to toll receptors in drosophila) make up a large family of **non-antigen-specific** receptors for a variety of individual bacterial, viral and fungal components such as DNA, lipoproteins and lipopolysaccharides. Activation of DCs by binding to either of these detection receptors leads to inflammation and *subsequently activation of the adaptive system.*

Phagocytic cells also recognize particular patterns associated with potentially damaging materials, such as lipoproteins and other charged molecules or peptides.

Traditionally, **antigens** have been defined as molecules that interact with components of the adaptive system, i.e. T- and B-cell recognition receptors and antibody. *An antigenic molecule may have several antigenic determinants (epitopes)*; each **epitope** can bind with an individual antibody, and a single antigenic molecule can therefore provoke many antibody molecules with different binding sites. Some low-molecular-weight molecules, called **haptens**, are unable to provoke an immune response themselves, although they can react with existing antibodies. Such substances need to be coupled to a carrier molecule in order to have sufficient epitopes to be antigenic. For some chemicals, such as drugs, the carrier may be a host (auto) protein. The tertiary structure, as well as the amino acid sequence, is important in determining antigenicity. Pure lipids and nucleic acids are poor antigens, although they do activate the innate system and can be inflammatory.

Antigens are conventionally divided into thymus-dependent and thymus-independent antigens. **Thymus-dependent antigens** require T-cell participation to provoke the production of antibodies; most proteins are examples. **Thymus-independent antigens** require no T-cell cooperation for antibody production; they directly stimulate specific B lymphocytes by virtue of their ability to cross-link antigen receptors on the B-cell surface, produce predominantly IgM and IgG_2 antibodies and provoke poor immunological memory. Such antigens include bacterial polysaccharides, found in bacterial cell walls. Endotoxin, another thymus-independent antigen, not only causes specific B-cell activation and antibody production, but also acts as a stimulant for all B cells regardless of specificity.

Factors other than the intrinsic properties of the antigen can also influence the quality of the immune response (Table 1.2). Substances that improve an immune response to a separate, often rather weak, antigen are known as **adjuvants**. The use of adjuvants in humans, important in vaccines against infective agents and tumours, is discussed in Chapter 7, section 7.3.2.

Superantigen is the name given to those foreign proteins that are not specifically recognized by the adaptive system but do activate large numbers of T cells regardless of specificity, via direct action with an invariant part of the TCR (see Chapter 2, section 2.4.2).

Self-antigens are not recognized by DCs, so inflammation and co-stimulation of T cells (see section 1.4.1) is not induced. There are mechanisms to control any aberrant adaptive responses to self-antigens, by prevention of the production of specific receptors and regulation of the response if the immune system is fooled into responding (see Chapter 5).

	Table 1.2 Factors influencing the immune response to an antigen, i.e. its immunogenicity
1	Nature of molecule: Protein content Size Solubility
2	Dose: Low doses provoke small amounts of antibody with high affinity and restricted specificity Moderate doses provoke large amounts of antibody but mixed affinity and broad specificity High doses provoke tolerance
3	Route of entry: ID, IM, SC→regional lymph nodes IV→spleen Oral→Peyer's patches Inhalation→bronchial lymphoid tissue
4	Addition of substances with synergistic effects, e.g. adjuvants
5	Genetic factors of recipient animal: Species differences Individual differences

ID, intradermal injection; IM, intramuscular injection; IV, intravenous injection; SC, subcutaneous injection.

1.2.2 Recognition molecules

There are several sets of detection molecules on DCs (Table 1.3): pattern-recognition receptors (PRRs), such as Toll-like receptors, as well as chemotactic receptors and phagocytic receptors. **PRRs** may be soluble or attached to cell membranes. Mannan-binding lectin is a protein that binds sugars on microbial surfaces; if attached to a macrophage, it acts as a trigger for phagocytosis and, if soluble, it activates the complement cascade, resulting in opsonization. Others belonging to this family are less well defined.

Toll-like receptors (TLRs) are part of this family too and are expressed either on the cell surface or intracellularly on endosomal membranes (Table 1.4). These are evolutionarily conserved proteins found on macrophages, DCs and neutrophils. At least ten different TLRs are found in humans, each TLR recognizing a range of particular motifs on pathogens, such as double-stranded RNA of viruses (TLR3), lipopolysaccharides of Gram-negative bacterial cell walls (TLR4), flagellin (TLR5) and bacterial DNA (TLR9), all highly conserved motifs unique to microorganisms. Upon binding to their ligands, TLRs induce signal transduction, via a complex cascade of intracellular adaptor molecules and kinases, culminating in the induction of nuclear factor kappa B transcription factor (NFκB)-dependent gene expression and the induction of proinflammatory cytokines (Fig. 1.2). The clinical consequences of a defective TLR pathway are discussed in Chapter 3, section 3.4.1 (see Box 1.1 in this chapter also).

Inflammasomes are a complex of intracellular proteins that are assembled in response to sensing pathogen-associated

Table 1.3 Markers on dendritic cells

	Immature dendritic cells	Mature myeloid dendritic cells
Function	Antigen capture	Antigen presentation to immature T cells for specific differentiation
Co-stimulatory molecule expression, e.g. CD80, CD86	Absent or low	++
Adhesion molecules, e.g. ICAM-1	Absent or low	++
Cytokine receptors, e.g. IL-12R	Absent or low	++
Pattern-recognition receptors, e.g. mannose receptor	++	–
MHC class II:		
Turnover	Very rapid	Persist >100 h
Density	Reduced (approx. 1×10^6)	Very high (approx. 7×10^6)

ICAM-1, Intercellular adhesion molecule-1; IL, interleukin; MHC, major histocompatibility complex.

Table 1.4 Location and ligands for toll-like receptors (TLRs)

TLR	Location	Ligand
TLR1, TLR2	Cell surface	Bacterial lipopeptides, peptidoglycan
TLR3	Endosomal membrane	ds viral RNA
TLR4	Cell surface	Lipopolysaccharide
TLR6	Cell surface	Bacterial lipopeptides
TLR7	Endosomal membrane	ssRNA
TLR8	Endosomal membrane	ssRNA
TLR9	Endosome	CpG DNA

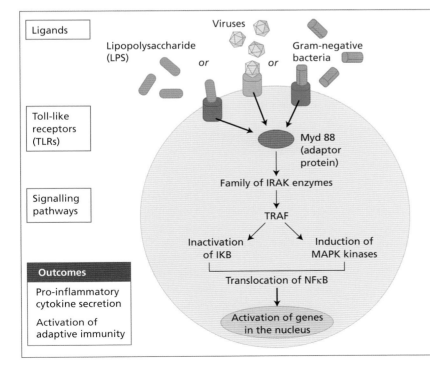

Fig. 1.2 Sequential cellular events induced by engagement of Toll-like receptors on dendritic cells, neutrophils and macrophages by microbial ligands. IKB, inhibitor kappa B; IRAK, interleukin-1 receptor-associated kinase; MAPK, mitogen-activated protein kinase; TRAF, TNF receptor-associated factor.

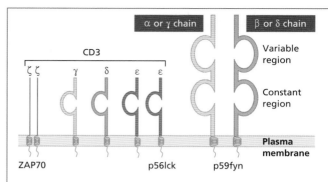

Fig. 1.4 Diagram of the structure of the T-cell receptor (TCR). The variable regions of the alpha (α) and beta (β) chains make up the T idiotype, i.e. antigen/peptide-binding region. The TCR is closely associated on the cell surface with the CD3 protein that is essential for activation.

Box 1.1 Clinical consequences of a defective Toll-like receptor pathway

In humans, deficiency of IRAK-4 (interleukin-1 receptor-associated kinase) or MyDD88, key intracellular molecules responsible for TLR signal transduction (Fig. 1.2), is associated with recurrent pyogenic bacterial infections accompanied by failure to mount an appropriate acute-phase response (see Chapter 3, Case 3.6).

Mice lacking TLR4 are exceptionally susceptible to infection with Gram-negative bacteria.

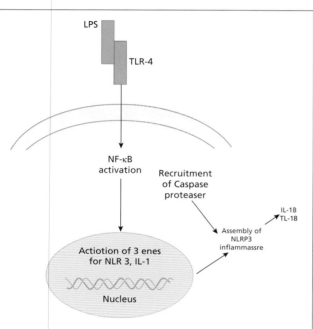

Fig. 1.3 Schematic representation of NLRP3 inflammasome activation.

---

molecular patterns (PAMPs) and danger-associated molecular patterns (DAMPs), derived from external pathogens or damaged host cells (Fig. 1.3). A typical inflammasome is built around a scaffold containing NOD-like receptors (NLRs). An example of a clinically relevant, well-characterized inflammasome is NLRP3, also known as cryopyrin. NLRP3 plays a key role in innate immunity by orchestrating the release of proinflammatory cytokines, in particular interleukin (IL)-1 and IL-18. Mutations in the gene encoding cryopyrin are associated with a number of hereditary periodic fever syndromes (see Chapter 10), which are effectively treated by inhibitors of the IL-1 pathway (e.g. Anakinra).

CD1 molecules are invariant proteins (MHC-like and associated with β_2-microglobulin – see later) that are present on DCs and epithelial cells. CD1 combine with lipids, which are poor antigens and not usually well presented to the adaptive immune system, and so act as recognition molecules for the intestine and other microbial-rich surfaces. CD1 present lipids to the immune cells of the gut in particular, namely non-MHC-restricted natural killer (NK) T cells and γδ T cells in the epithelium.

Antigenic epitopes, having been processed by DCs, are recognized by cells of the adaptive system by means of specific receptors. *Each T cell, like B cells, is pre-committed to a given epitope.* It recognizes this by one of two types of **TCRs**, depending on the cell's lineage and thus its effector function. T cells have either αβTCR – a heterodimer of alpha (α) and beta β) chains – or γδTCR – a heterodimer of gamma γ and delta (δ) chains. αPTCR cells predominate in adults, although 10% of T cells in epithelial structures are of the γδTCR type. In either case, TCRs are associated with several transmembrane proteins that make up the cluster differentiation 3 (CD3) molecule (Fig. 1.4), to make the CD3–TCR complex responsible for taking the antigen recognition signal inside the cell (signal transduction). Signal transduction requires a group of intracellular tyrosine kinases (designated p56 lck, p59 fyn, ZAP 70) to join with the cytosolic tails of the CD3–TCR complex and become phosphorylated. Nearby accessory molecules, CD2, LFA-1, CD4 and CD8, are responsible for increased adhesion (see section 1.2.6), but are not actually involved in recognizing presented antigenic fragments.

The genes for TCR chains are on different chromosomes: β and γ on chromosome α7 and α and δ on chromosome 14. Each of the four chains is made up of a variable and a constant domain. The variable regions are numerous (although less so than immunoglobulin-variable genes); they are joined by D and J region genes to the invariant (constant) gene by recombinases, RAG1 and RAG2, *the same enzymes used for making antigen receptors on B cells and antibodies* (section 1.4.1). The **diversity of T-cell antige0.n receptors** is achieved in a similar way for immunoglobulin, although *TCRs are less diverse since somatic mutation is not involved*; perhaps the risk of 'self-recognition' would be too great. The diversity of antigen binding is dependent on the large number of V genes and the way in which these may be combined with different D and J genes to provide different V domain genes. The similarities between TCRs and BCRs led to the suggestion that the genes evolved from the same parent gene and both are *members of a 'supergene' family*. Unlike immunoglobulin, TCRs are not secreted and are not independent effector molecules.

A particular TCR complex recognizes a processed antigenic peptide in the context of MHC class I or II antigens (section 1.4.1), depending on the type of T cell; helper T cells recognize class II with antigen, and this process is enhanced by the surface accessory protein CD4 (see later) and intracellular signals. Cytotoxic T cells (CTL/Tc) recognize antigens with class I (see section 1.3.1) and use CD8 accessory molecules for increased binding and signalling. Since the number of variable genes available to TCRs is more limited, reactions with antigen might not be sufficient if it were not for the increased binding resulting from these **accessory mechanisms**. Recognition of processed antigen alone is not enough to activate T cells. Additional signals, through soluble cytokines (interleukins), are needed; some of these are generated during 'antigen processing' (see section 1.4.1).

MHC molecules were originally known as 'histocompatibility antigens' because of the vigorous reactions they provoked during mismatched organ transplantation. However, these molecules are known to play a fundamental role in immunity by presenting antigenic peptides to T cells. Histocompatibility antigens in humans (known as human leucocyte antigens, HLAs) are synonymous with the MHC molecules. MHC molecules are cell-surface glycoproteins of two basic types: class I and class II (Fig. 1.5). They exhibit extensive genetic polymorphism with multiple alleles at each locus. As a result, genetic variability between individuals is very great and most unrelated individuals possess different MHC (HLA) molecules. This means that it is very difficult to obtain perfect HLA matches between unrelated persons for transplantation (see Chapter 8). The **extensive polymorphism in MHC molecules** is best explained by the need of the immune system to cope with an ever-increasing range of pathogens adept at evading immune responses (see Chapter 2).

The TCR of an individual T cell will only recognize antigen as a complex of antigenic peptide and self-MHC (Fig. 1.6). This process of dual recognition of peptide and MHC molecule is known as MHC restriction, since the MHC molecule restricts the ability of the T cell to recognize antigen (Fig. 1.6). The importance of MHC restriction in the immune response was recognized by the award of the Nobel Prize in Medicine to Peter Doherty and Rolf Zinkernagel, who found that virus-specific CTLs would only kill cells of the same particular allelic form of MHC molecule.

MHC class I antigens are subdivided into three groups: A, B and C. Each group is controlled by a different gene locus within the MHC region on chromosome 6 (Fig. 1.7) in humans (different in mice). The products of the genes at all three loci are chemically similar. All MHC class I antigens (see Fig. 1.5) are made up of an a heavy chain, controlled by a gene in the relevant MHC locus, associated with a smaller chain called β_2-microglobulin, controlled by a gene on chromosome 12. The differences between individual MHC class I antigens are due to variations in the a chains; the β_2-microglobulin component is constant. The detailed structure of class I antigens was determined by X-ray crystallography. This shows that small antigenic peptides (approx. nine amino acids long) can be tightly bound to a groove produced by the pairing of the two extracellular domains (a_1 and a_2) of the a chain. The *affinity (tightness of binding) of individual peptide binding depends on the nature and shape of the groove*, and accounts for the MHC restriction mentioned earlier.

MHC class II antigens have two heavy chains, α and β, both coded for by genes in the MHC region of chromosome 6. The detailed structure of MHC class II antigens was also

Fig. 1.5 Diagrammatic representation of major histocompatibility complex (MHC) class I and class II antigens. CHO, carbohydrate side chain; β_2m, β_2-microglobulin.

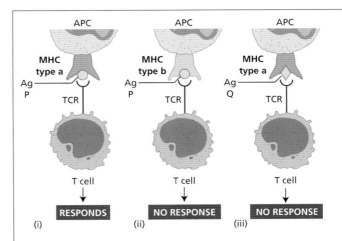

Fig. 1.6 Major histocompatibility complex (MHC) restriction of antigen recognition by T cells. T cells specific for a particular peptide and a particular MHC allele (i) will not respond if the same peptide were to be presented by a different MHC molecule as in (ii) or as in (iii) if the T cell were to encounter a different peptide. APC, antigen-presenting cell; TCR, T-cell receptor.

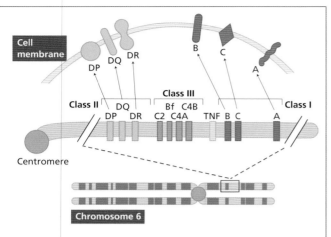

Fig. 1.7 Major histocompatibility complex on chromosome 6; class III antigens are complement components. TNF, tumour necrosis factor.

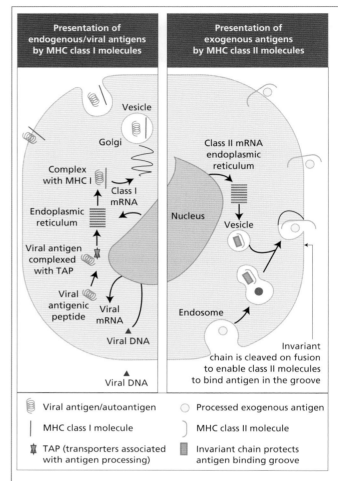

Fig. 1.8 Different routes of antigen presentation, depending on the nature of the antigen. MHC, major histocompatibility complex.

determined by X-ray crystallography. It has a folded structure similar to class I antigens, with the peptide-binding groove found between the α and β chains (see Fig. 1.5). Whereas most nucleated cells express class I molecules, *expression of class II molecules is restricted to a few cell types*: DCs, B lymphocytes, *activated* T cells, macrophages, *inflamed* vascular endothelium and some epithelial cells. However, other cells (e.g. thyroid, pancreas, gut epithelium) can be induced to express class II molecules under the influence of interferon (IFN)-γ released during inflammation. In humans, there are three groups of variable class II antigens: the loci are known as HLA-DP HLA-DQ and HLA-DR.

In practical terms, there are different mechanisms by which antigens in different intracellular compartments can be captured and presented to CD4+ or CD8+ T cells (Fig. 1.8). **Endogenous antigens** (including viral antigens that have infected host cells) are processed by the endoplasmic reticulum and presented by MHC class I-bearing cells exclusively to CD8+ T cells. Prior to presentation on the cell surface, endogenous antigens are broken down into short peptides, which are then actively transported from the cytoplasm to endoplasmic reticulum by proteins. These proteins act as a shuttle and are so named 'transporters associated with antigen processing' (TAP-1 and TAP-2). TAP proteins (also coded in the MHC class II region) deliver peptides to MHC class I molecules in the endoplasmic reticulum, from whence the complex of MHC and peptide is delivered to the cell surface. Mutations that affect function in either TAP gene prevent surface expression of MHC class I molecules.

In contrast, **exogenous antigens** are processed by the lysosomal route and presented by MHC class II antigens to CD4+ T cells (Fig. 1.8). As with MHC class I molecules, newly synthesized MHC class II molecules are held in the endoplasmic reticulum until they are ready to be transported to the cell surface. While in the endoplasmic reticulum, class II molecules are prevented from binding to peptides in the lumen by a protein known as MHC class II-associated invariant chain. The invariant

chain also directs delivery of class II molecules to the endosomal compartment, where exogenous antigens are processed and made available for binding to class II molecules.

The **MHC class III region** (see Fig. 1.7) contains genes encoding proteins that are involved in the complement system (see section 1.4.1): the early components C4 and C2 of the classical pathway and factor B of the alternative pathway. Some inflammatory proteins, e.g. tumour necrosis factor (TNF), are also encoded in adjacent areas. Invariant MHC-like proteins, such as CD1 lipid-recognition receptors (see earlier), are not coded for on chromosome 6, despite being associated with β₂-microglobulin.

In contrast to TCRs, the antigen BCRs are **surface-bound immunoglobulin** molecules that can be secreted as soluble molecules. As with TCRs, they have predetermined specificity for epitopes and are therefore extremely diverse. *The immune system has to be capable of recognizing all pathogens, past and future.* Such diversity is provided by the way in which all three types of molecules, TCR, BCR and antibody, are produced.

The **basic structure of the immunoglobulin** molecule is shown in Fig. 1.9. It has a four-chain structure: two identical

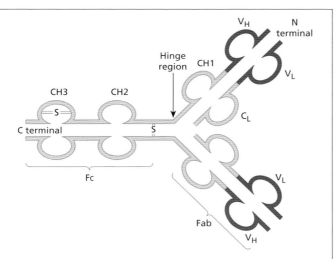

Fig. 1.9 Basic structure of an immunoglobulin molecule. Domains are held in shape by disulfide bonds, though only one is shown. C_{1-3}, constant domain of a heavy chain; C_L, constant domain of a light chain; =S=, disulfide bond; V_H, variable domain of a heavy chain; V_L, variable domain of a light chain.

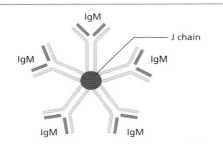

Fig. 1.10 Schematic representation of immunoglobulin (Ig)M pentamer (MW 800 kDA).

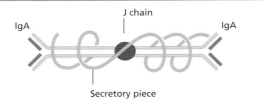

Fig. 1.11 Schematic representation of dimeric secretory immunoglobulin (Ig)A (MW 385 kDA).

heavy (H) chains (mol. wt. 50 kDa) and two identical light (L) chains (mol. wt. 25 kDa). Each chain is made up of domains of about 110 amino acids held together in a loop by a disulphide bond between two cysteine residues in the chain. The domains have the same basic structure and many areas of similarity in their amino acid sequences. The heavy chains determine the isotype of the immunoglobulin, resulting in pentameric IgM (Fig. 1.10), dimeric IgA (Fig. 1.11) or monomeric IgG.

The amino (N) terminal domains of the heavy and light chains include the **antigen-binding site**. The amino acid sequences of these N-terminal domains vary between different antibody molecules and are known as variable (V) regions. Most of these differences reside in three hypervariable areas of the molecule, each only 6–10 amino acid residues long. In the folded molecule, these hypervariable regions in each heavy and light chain come together to form, with their counterparts on the other pair of heavy and light chains, the antigen-binding site (Fig. 1.9). The structure of this part of the antibody molecule is unique to that molecule and is known as the **idiotypic determinant**. In any individual, approximately 10^6–10^7 different antibody molecules could be made up by 10^3 different heavy chain variable regions associating with 10^3 different light chain variable regions, though there are even more epitopes due to further variation during the later processing (see section 1.4.1).

The part of the immunoglobulin chain next to the V region in either heavy or light chains is the constant (C) region; this is made up of one domain in a **light chain** (C_L) and three or four in a **heavy chain** (C_H) (Fig. 1.9). There are two alternative types of C_L chain, known as kappa (κ) and lambda (λ); an antibody molecule has either two κ or two λ light chains, *never one of each*. Of all the antibodies in a human individual, roughly 60% contain κ and 40% contain λ light chains. There are no known differences in the functional properties between κ and λ light chains. In contrast, there are several possible different types of C_H domain, each with important functional differences (Table 1.5). The heavy chains determine the **isotype** of the antibody and the ultimate physiological function of the particular antibody molecule. Once the antigen-binding site has reacted with its antigen, the molecule undergoes a change in the conformation of its heavy chains in order to take part in effector reactions, depending on the isotype of the molecule.

The processes by which the components of this supergene family are produced are identical for TCR and BCR and are known as **recombination.** Immunoglobulin production, whether for BCR or antibody production, is the same initially. As for the TCR, the genes for the different chains in a BCR are carried on different chromosomes (Fig. 1.12). Like those coding for other macromolecules, the genes are broken up into coding segments (exons) with intervening silent segments (introns). The heavy chain gene set on chromosome 14 is made up of small groups of exons representing the constant regions of the heavy chains – e.g. mu (μ) chain – and a very large number of V region genes, perhaps as many as 10^3. Between the V and C genes are two small sets of exons, D and J (Fig. 1.12). In a single B cell, one V region gene is selected, joined to one D and J on the same chromosome; the VDJ product is then joined at the level of RNA processing to Cμ when the B cell is making IgM. The cell can make IgG by omitting the Cμ and joining VDJ to a Cγ. Thus, the cell can make IgM, IgD and IgG/A/E in sequence, while still using the same variable region. *The same enzymes are used for the TCRs, and coded for by two recombination-activating genes controlling VDJ gene recombination: RAG1 and RAG2.* Disruption of the RAG1 or RAG2

Table 1.5 Immunoglobulin classes and their functions

Isotype	Heavy chain	Serum concentration*	Main function	Complement fixation†	Placental passage	Reaction with Fc receptors‡
IgM	μ	0.5–2.0	Neutralization and opsonization	+++	–	L
IgG$_1$	γ1	5.0–12.0	Opsonization	+++	++	M, N, P, L, E
IgG$_2$	γ2	2.0–6.0		+	±	P, L
IgG$_3$	γ3	0.5–1.0	Opsonization	+++	++	M, N, P, L, E
IgG$_4$	γ4	0.1–1.0		–	+	N, L, P
IgA$_1$	α1	0.5–3.0	Neutralization at mucosal surfaces	–	–	M, N
IgA$_2$	α2	0.0–0.2		–	–	–
IgD	δ	Trace	Lymphocyte membrane receptor	–	–	–
IgE	εΣ	Trace	Mast cell attachment	–	–	B, E, L

*Normal adult range in g/L.
†Classical pathway.
‡Fc receptors on: basophils/mast cells, B; eosinophils, E; lymphocytes, L; macrophages, M; neutrophils, N; platelets, P.

function in infants who have mutations in these genes causes profound immune deficiency, characterized by absent mature B and T cells, as neither TCRs or BCRs can be produced. On a different chromosome (either chromosome 22 for λ chains or chromosome 2 for κ chains) in the same cell, a V gene is joined to a J gene (there is no D on the light chain) and then the VJ product is joined at the RNA level to the Cκ or Cλ (Fig. 1.12).

The **wide diversity of antigen binding** is dependent on the large number of V genes and the way in which these may be combined with different D and J genes to provide different rearranged VDJ gene segments. Once V, D and J rearrangement has taken place to produce a functional immunoglobulin molecule, *further V region variations are introduced only at a much later*

stage, when antibodies rather than BCRs are produced by the process of somatic mutation in germinal centres.

Natural killer cells also have recognition molecules. These cells are important in killing virally infected cells and tumour cells. They have to be able to recognize these targets and distinguish them from normal cells. They recognize and kill cells that have reduced or absent MHC class I, using two kinds of receptors – inhibitory (KIR) and activating (KAR) – to estimate the extent of MHC expression. They also have one type of Fc IgG (Fcγ) receptor, that for low-affinity binding of IgG antibodies, and so NK cells are able to kill some cells with large amounts of antibody on their surfaces. Further subsets of NK-like cells that contribute to innate immunity

Fig. 1.12 Immunoglobulin genes (see text for explanation).

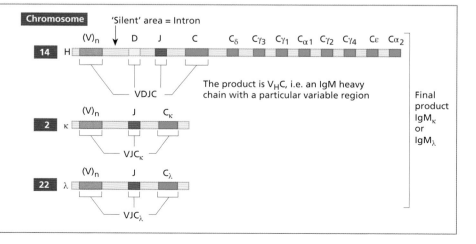

include NKT cells and invariant NKT cells (section 1.3.6); these are thought to be particularly important in tumour immunology (section 1.5.1).

The major purpose of the complement pathways is to provide a means of removing or destroying antigens, regardless of whether or not these are coated with antibody. This requires that *complement components recognize* damaging material such as immune complexes (antigen combined with antibodies) or foreign antigens. The complement pathways are discussed in more detail in section 1.3.5.

1.2.3 Accessory molecules

The binding of a processed antigen–MHC class II complex on an antigen-presenting cell (APC) to the corresponding TCR provides an insufficient signal for T-cell activation; the binding of accessory molecules on the two cell surfaces provides additional stimuli. Accessory molecules are lymphocyte surface proteins, distinct from the antigen-binding complexes, which are necessary for **efficient binding, signalling and homing**. *Accessory molecules are invariant, non-polymorphic proteins.* Each accessory molecule has a particular ligand – a corresponding protein to which it binds. These ligands are present on all cells that require close adhesion for functioning; for example, there are those on T cells for each of the many cell types that can activate or respond to T cells (APCs, endothelial cells, etc.); similar ligands are present on B cells for efficiency of T-cell help as well as stimulation by follicular DCs.

There are several families of accessory molecules, but the most important appear to be the **immunoglobulin supergene family of adhesion molecules**, which derives its name from the fact that its members contain a common immunoglobulin-like structure. Members of the family strengthen the interaction between APCs and T cells (Fig. 1.13); those on T cells include CD4, CD8, CD28, CTLA-4, CD45R, CD2 and lymphocyte function antigen 1 (LFA-1). For interaction with B cells, CD40 ligand and ICOS are important for class switching

(see section 1.4.3). Adhesion molecules, for binding leucocytes (both lymphocytes and polymorphonuclear leucocytes) to endothelial cells and tissue matrix cells, are considered in section 1.2.6. On B cells, such molecules include CD40 (ligand for CD40L, now named CD154; see Chapter 3, Case 3.2), B-7-1 and B7-2 (ligands for CD28).

1.2.4 Effector molecules for immunity

There are humoral and cellular effector molecules in both the innate and the adaptive immune systems (Table 1.6). Several of the same mechanisms are used in both types of immune responses, especially in killing of target cells, suggesting that the evolution of immune responses has been conservative in terms of genes, though with much redundancy to ensure the life-preserving nature of the immune systems in the face of rapid evolution of pathogenic microbes.

Antibodies

Antibodies are the best-described effector mechanisms in adaptive immunity. They are the **effector arm of B cells** and are secreted as soluble molecules by plasma cells in large

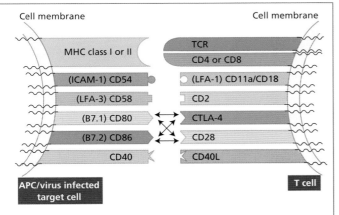

Fig. 1.13 Diagrammatic representation of adhesion molecules on T cells and their ligands on antigen-presenting cells (APCs)/virus-infected target cells. MHC, major histocompatibility complex; TCR, T-cell receptor.

Table 1.6 Effector molecules in immunity		
	Innate	**Adaptive**
Humoral	Complement components for opsonization or lysis	Specific antibodies for opsonization and phagocytosis or lysis with complement
Cellular	Perforin in NK cells creates pores in target cell membranes	Perforin in cytolytic (CD8) T cells creates pores in specific target cell membranes, allowing entry of granzymes to cause apoptosis
		NKT cells induce apoptosis by perforin production
	Granzymes in NK cells induce apoptosis in target cells	
	Lysosomes in phagocytic vacuoles result in death of ingested microbes	
	Preformed histamine and related vasoactive substances as well as leukotrienes in mast cells	

NK, natural killer

quantities, to be carried in the blood and lymph to distant sites. As shown in Table 1.5, there are five major isotypes of antibodies, each with different functions (see also Box 1.2).

IgM is a large molecule whose major physiological role is intravascular neutralization of organisms (especially viruses). **IgM** has five complement-binding sites, resulting in excellent complement activation and subsequent removal of the antigen–antibody–complement complexes by complement receptors on phagocytic cells or complement-mediated lysis of the organism (see section 1.4).

IgG is a smaller immunoglobulin that penetrates tissues easily. Placental transfer is an active process involving specific placental receptors for the Fc portion of the IgG molecule, termed FcRn (Fc receptor of the neonate). The FcRn receptor is also present on epithelial and endothelial cells and is an important regulator of IgG metabolism (see Chapter 7, section 7.4 and Fig. 7.8). Of the four subclasses, IgG_1 and IgG_3 activate complement most efficiently and are responsible for clearing most protein antigens, including the removal of microorganisms by phagocytic cells (see section 1.5). IgG_2 and IgG_4 react predominantly with carbohydrate antigens (in adults) and are relatively poor opsonins (promoters of phagocytosis).

IgA is the major mucosal immunoglobulin. Attachment of the 'secretory piece' prevents digestion of this immunoglobulin

in the intestinal and bronchial secretions. IgA_2 is the predominant subclass in secretions and neutralizes antigens that enter via these mucosal routes. IgA, the monomeric IgA in serum, is capable of neutralizing antigens that enter the circulation, but IgA_1 is sensitive to bacterial proteases and therefore less useful for host defence at mucosal surfaces. IgA has additional functions via its receptor (FcaR or CD89), present on mononuclear cells and neutrophils, for activation of phagocytosis, inflammatory mediator release and antibody-dependent cell-mediated cytotoxicity (ADCC) (see section 1.5).

There is little free **IgD or IgE** in serum or normal body fluids, since these act as surface receptors on mature B cells or mast cells, respectively.

As mentioned previously, mechanisms of recombination in immunoglobulin production, whether for BCR or antibody production, are the same initially (Fig. 1.12). Once V, D and J region rearrangement has taken place, **further variation is introduced when antibodies are made**, by the introduction of point mutations in the V region genes. This process, known as **somatic hypermutation,** occurs in the lymphoid germinal centres and is critically dependent on activation-induced cytidine deaminase (AID), an enzyme responsible for deamination of DNA. Somatic hypermutation helps to increase the possible number of combinations and accounts for the enormous diversity of antibody specificities (10^{14}), which by far exceeds the number of different B cells in the body (10^{10}).

Cytokines and chemokines

Cytokines are soluble mediators secreted by macrophages or monocytes (monokines) or lymphocytes (lymphokines). These mediators act as **stimulatory or inhibitory signals** between cells; those between cells of the immune system were known as interleukins (a phrase that has fallen out of general usage since the range of soluble molecules has widened so tremendously, though the individual names persist to avoid confusion). As a group, cytokines share several common features (see Box 1.3). Among the array of cytokines produced by macrophages and T cells, IL-1 and IL-2 are of particular interest due to their pivotal role in amplifying immune responses. IL-1 acts on a wide range of targets (Table 1.7), including T and B cells. In contrast, the effects of IL-2 are largely restricted to lymphocytes. Although IL-2 was originally identified on account of its ability to promote the growth of T cells, it has similar trophic effects on IL-2 receptor-bearing B and NK cells. The considerable overlap between actions of individual cytokines and interleukins is summarized in Table 1.8.

Cytokines that induce chemotaxis of leucocytes are referred to as **chemokines**, a name derived from chemo + kine, i.e. something chemical to help movement. Some cytokines and interleukins have been redefined as chemokines as their function becomes clearer, e.g. IL-8 = CXCL8. Chemokines are structurally similar proteins of small molecule size (8–10 kDa), which are able to diffuse from the site of production to form a local concentration gradient along which granulocytes and

---

Box 1.2   Immunoglobulin isotypes and their significance

IgM is phylogenetically the oldest class of immunoglobulin. It is a large molecule (Fig. 1.10) and penetrates poorly into tissues. IgM has five complement-binding sites, which results in excellent activation of the classical complement pathway.

IgG is smaller and penetrates tissues easily. It is the only immunoglobulin to provide immune protection to the neonate (Table 1.5) as IgG is actively transported across the placenta. There are four subclasses of IgG, with slightly different functions.

IgA is the major mucosal immunoglobulin – sometimes referred to as 'mucosal antiseptic paint'. IgA in mucosal secretions consists of two basic units joined by a J chain (Fig. 1.11); the addition of a 'secretory piece' prevents digestion of this immunoglobulin in the intestinal and bronchial secretions.

IgD is synthesized by antigen-sensitive B lymphocytes and is not secreted, acting as a cell-surface receptor for activation of these cells by the specific antigen relating to the B-cell receptor; it is essential for activation of antigen-responsive B cells.

IgE is produced by plasma cells, but is taken up by specific IgE receptors on mast cells and basophils. IgE then provides an antigen-sensitive way of expelling intestinal parasites by increasing vascular permeability and inducing chemotactic factors via mast cell degranulation (see section 1.7).

Box 1.3   Common features of cytokines

- Their half-lives are short, so any potential harm due to persistent action is controlled.
- They are rapidly degraded as another method of regulation and thus difficult to measure in the circulation.
- Most act locally within the cell's microenvironment, which confines their action to a particular site.
- Some act on the cell of production itself, promoting self-activation and differentiation through high-affinity cell-surface receptors.
- Many cytokines are pleiotropic in their biological effects, i.e. affecting multiple organs in the body.
- Most exhibit biologically overlapping functions, illustrating the redundancy of the group. For this reason, therapeutic targeting of individual cytokines in disease has had limited success so far (effects of deletion of individual cytokine genes are listed in Table 1.8).

Table 1.7 Actions of interleukin-1

Target cell	Effect
T lymphocytes	Proliferation
	Differentiation
	Lymphokine production
	Induction of IL-2 receptors
B lymphocytes	Proliferation
	Differentiation
Neutrophils	Release from bone marrow
	Chemoattraction
Macrophages	
Fibroblasts	Proliferation/activation
Osteoblasts	
Epithelial cells	
Osteoclasts	Reabsorption of bone
Hepatocytes	Acute-phase protein synthesis
Hypothalamus	Prostaglandin-induced fever
Muscle	Prostaglandin-induced proteolysis

IL, interleukin

lymphocytes can migrate towards the stimulus. There are two types of movement: migration of leucocytes to sites of inflammation and that of differentiating cells moving to a specific activation site (see section 1.2.5); chemokines are involved in both. There are therefore two main types: the **inflammatory**

chemokines (CXC), coded for by genes on chromosome 17 and attractants for granulocytes, and the **homeostatic chemokines**, acting as attractants for lymphocytes (CC) and coded by genes on chromosome 4. The corresponding receptors on inflammatory cells are designated CXCR on neutrophils and CCR on lymphocytes; there are exceptions!

Molecules for lysis and killing

The other major sets of effector molecules are the cytolytic molecules, though less is known about their diversity or mechanisms of action. They include **perforin**, a C9-like molecule present in secretory lysosomes in CD8 T cells and in NK cells that polymerizes to form pores to enable large proteins to enter the cell. These cell types also secrete **granzymes**, enzymes that induce apoptosis in target cells (Table 1.6). Macrophages and polymorphonuclear leucocytes also contain many substances for the destruction of ingested microbes, some of which have multiple actions, such as TNF. The duplication of the functions of this essential phylogenetically ancient protein during evolution underlines the continued development of mammalian immunity to keep up with microbial invaders.

1.2.5 Receptors for effector functions

Without **specific cytokine receptors** on the surface of the target cells, cytokines are ineffective; this has been demonstrated in those primary immune deficiencies in which gene mutations result in absence or non-functional receptors, such as the commonest X-linked form of severe combined immune deficiency (see Chapter 3, Case 3.5), IL-12 receptor or IFN-γ receptor deficiencies (see Chapter 3). Some cytokines may have unique receptors, but many others share a common structural chain, such as the γ-chain in the receptors for IL-2, IL-4, IL-7, IL-9, IL-15 and IL-23, suggesting that *these arose from a common gene originally*. There are other structurally similar cytokine receptors, leading to the classification of these receptors into five families of similar types of receptors, many of which have similar or identical functions, providing a safety net (redundancy) for their functions, which are crucial for both the innate and adaptive immune systems.

Chemokine receptors from a family of G protein-coupled receptors – meaning that they are transmembrane and able to activate internal signalling pathways. These receptors also function as differentiation 'markers', as they become expressed as an immune reaction progresses and cells move in inflammatory responses.

Receptors for the Fc portions of immunoglobulin molecules (FcR) are important for effector functions of phagocytic cells and NK cells. There are at least **three types of Fcγ receptors**: FcRγl are high-affinity receptors on macrophages and neutrophils that bind monomeric IgG for phagocytosis; FcRγII are low-affinity receptors for phagocytosis on macrophages and neutrophils and for feedback inhibition on B cells; and FcRγIII on NK cells as mentioned earlier. There are also FcRn involved in the transfer of IgG across the placenta and these receptors

Table 1.8 Clinically important cytokines grouped by effect on immune or inflammatory responses, to show source and site of action

Cytokines	Action
(a) Promotion of non-specific immunity and inflammation	
Interleukin-17 (IL-17)	Increases chemokine production for inflammatory cells
Interleukin-1 (IL-1)	(See Table 1.7)
Interleukin-6 (IL-6)	Growth and differentiation of T, B and haematopoietic cells
	Production of acute-phase proteins by liver cells
Interleukin-8 (now CXCL8)	Chemotaxis and activation of neutrophils and other leucocytes
Interferon-α (IFN-α)	Antiviral action by activation of NK cells, upregulation of MHC class I antigens on virally infected cells, inhibition of viral replication
Interleukin-5 (IL-5)	Activation of B cells, especially for IgE production
	Activation of eosinophils
Tumour necrosis factor (TNF)	Promotion of inflammation by: activation of neutrophils, endothelial cells, lymphocytes, liver cells (to produce acute-phase proteins)
	Interferes with catabolism in muscle and fat (resulting in cachexia)
Interferon-γ (IFN-γ)	Activation of macrophages, endothelial cells and NK cells. Increased expression of MHC class I and class II molecules in many tissues; inhibits allergic reactions ($\downarrow$IgE production)
(b) Lymphocyte activation, growth and differentiation, i.e. specific immunity	
Interleukin-2 (IL-2)	Proliferation and maturation of T cells, induction of IL-2 receptors and activation of NK cells
Interleukin-4 (IL-4) and interleukin-5 (IL-5)	Induction of MHC class II, Fc receptors and IL-2 receptors on B and T cells
	Induction of isotype switch in B cells Facilitation of IgE production (mainly IL-4) Activation of macrophages Proliferation of bone marrow precursors
Interleukin-12 (IL-12)[†]	Synergism with IL-2; regulates IFN-y production Activation of NK cells
Interleukin-13 (IL-13)	Actions overlap with IL-4, including induction of IgE production
	IL-13 receptor acts as a functional receptor for IL-4
Interleukin-15 (IL-15)	Similar to IL-12
Interleukin-16 (IL-16)	Chemotaxis and activation of CD4 T cells
(c) Colony stimulation of bone marrow precursors	
GM-CSF	Stimulates growth of polymorph and mononuclear progenitors
G-CSF	Stimulates growth of neutrophil progenitors
M-CSF	Stimulates growth of mononuclear progenitors
(d) Regulatory cytokines	
Interleukin-10 (IL-10); also called cytokine synthesis inhibitory factor[‡]	Inhibition of cytokine production Growth of mast cells
Transforming growth factor-ß (TGF-ß)	Antiinflammatory Inhibits cell growth

Table 1.8 (Continued)	
Cytokines	**Action**
(e) Chemokines	
Interleukin-8 (IL-8)	See under section (a)
RANTES (regulated on activation, normal T cell expressed and secreted)	Chemoattractant for eosinophils, monocytes
Monocyte chemotactic protein (MCP 1, 2, 3)	Chemoattractant for monocytes
Exotaxin	Chemoattractant for eosinophils; synergistic with IL-5

Evidence from murine models. See appendix for web address for update on knockout mice.
†IL-12 family of cytokines includes IL-23 and IL-27.
‡IL-10 family includes IL-19, IL-20 and IL-22.
G-CSF, granulocyte colony-stimulating factor; GM-CSF, granulocyte-macrophage colony-stimulating factor; Ig, immunoglobulin; M-CSF, macrophage colony-stimulating factor; MHC, major histocompatibility complex; NK, natural killer.

are involved in IgG recirculation and catabolism. IgE receptors are found on mast cells, basophils and eosinophils for triggering degranulation of these cells. IgA receptors ensure the transport of polymeric IgA across the mucosal cells and other, possibly important functions are slowly being defined.

Complement receptors for fragments of C3 produced during complement activation also provide a mechanism for phagocytosis and are found on macrophages and neutrophils. However, there are several types of **complement receptors**: those on red blood cells for transport of immune complexes for clearance (CR1), those on B cells and follicular DCs in lymph nodes to trap antigen to stimulate a secondary immune response (CR2) (see section 1.4.3), and those on macrophages, neutrophils and NK cells to provide adhesion of these blood cells to endothelium, prior to movement into tissues (CR3).

1.2.6 Adhesion molecules

Adhesion molecules comprise another set of cell surface glycoproteins with a pivotal role, not only in immune responses by **mediating cell-to-cell adhesion**, but also for **adhesion between cells and extracellular matrix proteins**. Adhesion molecules are grouped into two major families: (i) integrins and (ii) selectins (Table 1.9). The migration of leucocytes to sites of inflammation is dependent on three key sequential steps mediated by adhesion molecules (Fig. 1.14): rolling of leucocytes along activated endothelium is selectin dependent; tight adhesion of leucocytes to endothelium is integrin dependent; and transendothelial migration occurs under the influence of chemokines. Cytokines also influence the selectin- and integrin-dependent phases.

Integrins are heterodimers composed of non-covalently associated α and β subunits. Depending on the structure of the β subunit, integrins are subdivided into five families (β_1 to β_5 integrins). β_1 and β_2 integrins play a key role in leucocyte–endothelial interaction. β_1 integrins mediate lymphocyte and monocyte binding to the endothelial adhesion receptor called vascular cell adhesion molecule (VCAM-1). β_2 integrins share a common β chain (CD18) that pairs with a different α chain (CD11a, b, c) to form three separate molecules (CD11a CD18, CD11b CD18, CD11c CD18); they also mediate strong binding of leucocytes to the endothelium. Examples in other systems include β_3 to β_5 integrins mediating cell adhesion to extracellular matrix proteins such as fibronectin and vitronectin in the skin and laminin receptor in muscle.

The **selectin** family is composed of three glycoproteins designated by the prefixes E (endothelial), L (leucocyte) and P (platelet) to denote the cells on which they were first described. Selectins bind avidly to carbohydrate molecules on leucocytes and endothelial cells and regulate the homing of the cells to sites of inflammation (see section 1.6.1, Chapter 11, section 11.1 and Table 1.10).

1.3 Functional basis of innate responses

The aim of an immune response is to destroy foreign antigens, whether these are inert molecules or invading organisms. To reach the site of invasion and destroy the pathogens, the components of the immune systems have to know where to go and to how to breach the normal barriers, such as the endothelial cells of the vascular system. Humoral factors (such as antibodies and complement) are carried in the blood and enter tissues following an increase in permeability associated with **inflammation**. Immune cells (innate and antigen specific) are actively attracted to a site of inflammation and enter the tissues via specific sites using active processes of adhesion.

Table 1.9 Examples of clinically important adhesion molecules

Adhesion molecule	Ligand	Clinical relevance of interaction	Consequences of defective expression
β_1 integrin family			
VLA-4 (CD49d-CD29) expressed on lymphocytes, monocytes	VCAM-1 on activated endothelium	Mediates tight adhesion between lymphocytes, monocytes and endothelium	Impaired migration of lymphocytes and monocytes into tissue. Defective expression of either ß1integrins or VCAM-1 has not yet been described in humans. However, blockade of ß1integrins by natalizumab, a therapeutic monoclonal antibody, is associated with a high risk of progressive multifocal leucoencephalopathy, a severe viral infection of the brain
β_2 integrin family			
CD18/CD11 expressed on leucocytes	ICAM-1 on endothelium	Mediates tight adhesion between all leucocytes and endothelium	Defective expression of CD18/CD11 is associated with severe immunodeficiency, characterized by marked neutrophil leucocytosis, recurrent bacterial and fungal infection, and poor neutrophil migration into sites of infection
β_3 integrin family			
Expressed on platelets	Fibrinogen	Interacts during clotting	Clotting disorder Glanzmann's disease
Selectin family			
E-selectin (CD62E) expressed on activated endothelial cells	Sialyl Lewis X (CD15) on neutrophils, eosinophils	Mediates transient adhesion and rolling of leucocytes on monocytes	Defective expression of CD15 is associated with severe immunodeficiency – clinical features similar to CD18 deficiency. Mice deficient in both E- and P-selectin exhibit a similar clinical phenotype
L-selectin (CD62L) expressed on all leucocytes	CD34, Gly CAM on high endothelial venules	L-selectin mediates transient adhesion and rolling of leucocytes in lymph nodes, and also acts as a homing molecule directing lymphocytes into lymph nodes	L-selectin-deficient mice exhibit reduced leucocyte rolling and impaired lymphocyte homing

ICAM, intercellular adhesion molecule; VCAM, vascular cell adhesion molecule; VLA, very late activation antigen.

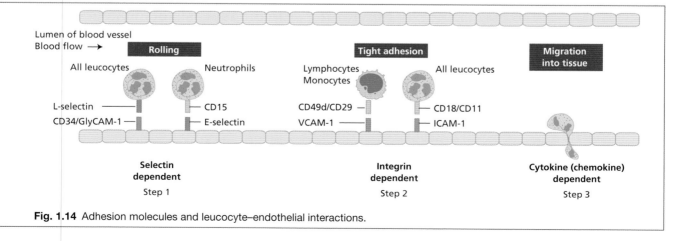

Fig. 1.14 Adhesion molecules and leucocyte–endothelial interactions.

Table 1.10 Proteins controlling classical and alternative complement pathways*

Protein	Function	Clinical consequences of deficiency
Circulating inhibitors		
C1 esterase inhibitor	Binds to activated C1r, C1s, uncoupling it from C1q	Uncontrolled activation of classical pathway leading to hereditary angioneurotic oedema
Factor H	Binds C3b displacing Bb; co-factor for factor I	Total deficiency causes recurrent bacterial infection, glomerulonephritis and renal failure; partial deficiency with familial (atypical) haemolytic uraemic syndrome; a particular allele with adult macular degeneration
Factor I	Serine protease that cleaves C3b; acts synergistically with factor H	As for factor H
Membrane inhibitors		
Complement receptor 1 (CR1; CD35)	Receptor for C3b	Protect mammalian cells. Low CR1 numbers on red cells in SLE is a consequence of fast turnover
Decay accelerating factor (DAF; CD55)	Accelerates decay of C3b Bb by displacing Bb	DAF deficiency alone does not cause disease
Protectin (CD59)	Inhibits formation of lytic pathway complex on homologous cells; widely expressed on cell membranes	In combination with DAF deficiency leads to paroxysmal nocturnal haemoglobinuria (see Chapter 16, section 16.2.4)

*This is not an exhaustive list.
SLE, systemic lupus erythematosus.

Non-specific immunity is older, in evolutionary terms, than antibody production and antigen-specific T cells. The major cells involved in the innate system are phagocytic cells (macrophages and polymorphonuclear leucocytes), which remove antigens including bacteria, and DCs, which are the first cells to react to invaders. The major humoral components of the four complement pathways can either directly destroy an organism or initiate/facilitate its phagocytosis. DCs recognize pathogens in order to provide a rapid initial cytokine response (such as interferon-a in a viral infection by plasmacytoid DCs) and to process antigen for presentation to specific TCRs alongside MHC for activation (classical DCs) (section 1.4.1).

1.3.1 Endothelial cells

The endothelium forms a highly active cell layer lining the inside of blood vessels and thus is present in all tissues. In addition to its critical role in maintaining vasomotor tone, the **endothelium** is closely involved in inflammation, wound healing and the formation of new blood vessels (angiogenesis). Immunologically, endothelial cells are intimately involved in interactions with leucocytes prior to leaving the circulation to enter sites of tissue damage (Fig. 1.14). The endothelium also plays an important role in regulating the turnover of IgG, through the presence of FcRn, a receptor that prevents IgG from undergoing lysosomal degradation (see section 1.2.4 and Chapter 7, section 7.4). The immunological importance of the endothelium is summarized in Box 1.4.

Box 1.4 Immunological importance of the endothelium

- Expresses a wide range of molecules on the cell surface (E-selectin, intercellular adhesion molecule-1 [ICAM-1], vascular cell adhesion molecule [VCAM-1], complement receptors) and thus plays a critical role in leucocyte–endothelial interactions (Fig. 1.14).
- Major site of immunoglobulin (Ig)G turnover due to FcRn (Fc receptor of the neonate).
- Forms an important part of the innate immune response by expressing Toll-like receptors to recognize foreign pathogens.
- Capable of antigen presentation.

1.3.2 Neutrophil polymorphonuclear leucocytes

Neutrophils are short-lived cells that play a major role in the body's defence against acute infection. They synthesize and express adhesion receptors so that they can stick to, and migrate out of, blood vessels into the tissues. Neutrophils move in response to **chemotactic agents** produced at the site of inflammation; substances include CXCL8, complement-derived factors (such as C3a and C5a), kallikrein, cytokines released by THh1 cells and chemotactic factors produced by mast cells.

Neutrophils are **phagocytic** cells. They are at their most efficient when activated after entering the tissues. Morphologically, the process of phagocytosis is similar in both neutrophils and macrophages. Neutrophils are able to kill and degrade the substances that they ingest. This requires a considerable amount of energy and is associated with a 'respiratory burst' of oxygen consumption, increased hexose monophosphate shunt activity and superoxide production. Genetically defective respiratory burst activity is associated with chronic granulomatous disease (see Chapter 3).

1.3.3 Macrophages

Macrophages and monocytes represent the mononuclear phagocytic system, which, along with DCs, forms the cells of the innate system. Lymphoid and myeloid cells are derived from closely related stem cells in the bone marrow (Fig. 1.1); each cell lineage has a different colony-stimulating factor and, once differentiated, they have entirely different functions. Polymorphonuclear leucocytes develop in the bone marrow and emerge only when mature. *Monocytes circulate for only a few hours before entering the tissues, where they may live for weeks or months as mature macrophages or DCs.* **Macrophages differentiate** in the tissues, principally in subepithelial interstitial and lymphatic sinuses in liver, spleen and lymph nodes, sites where antigens gain entry. Tissue macrophages are heterogeneous in appearance, in metabolism and also in function; they include freely mobile alveolar and peritoneal macrophages, fixed Kupffer cells in the liver and those lining the sinusoids of the spleen. When found in other tissues, they are called histiocytes.

A major function of the mononuclear phagocyte system is to phagocytose-invading organisms and other antigens. Macrophages have prominent lysosomal granules containing acid hydrolases and other degradative enzymes with which to destroy phagocytosed material. That material may be an engulfed viable organism, a dead cell, debris, an antigen or an immune complex. In order to carry out their functions effectively, macrophages must be 'activated'; in this state, they show increased **phagocytic and killing** activity. Stimuli include cytokines (see section 1.2.5), substances that bind to other surface receptors (such as IgG: Fc receptors, TLRs for endotoxin and other microbial components, receptors for bacterial polysaccharides and for soluble inflammatory mediators such as C5a; see Fig. 1.15). Activation may result in release of cytokines from monocytes or DCs such as TNF or IL-1, which may cause further damage in already inflamed tissues.

1.3.4 Dendritic cells

Classical or **myeloid dendritic cells** are mononuclear cells derived from bone marrow precursors and closely related to monocytes. There are many subsets, but there are differences between these subsets in mice compared with humans and other primates, particularly in their surface markers. So only those relating to humans are described here, though clearly their corresponding functions have been described in all mammalian species studied so far.

Immature dendritic cells are ubiquitous, particularly in epithelia that serve as a portal of entry for microbes, where they capture antigens as well as reacting to pathogen components quickly, within a few hours of invasion. Subsequently, the activated DCs migrate to draining lymph nodes and mature to present antigen to cells of the adaptive system (Fig. 1.16).

DCs have a range of **functions**: as well as processing antigens (Fig. 1.8), they are able to recognize and respond to pathogens by secreting IFN-α, produce IL-12 and chemokines as well as causing the differentiation of immature T cells to a

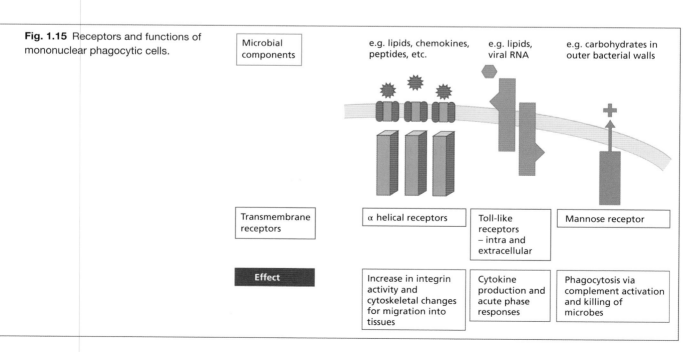

Fig. 1.15 Receptors and functions of mononuclear phagocytic cells.

Microbial components

e.g. lipids, chemokines, peptides, etc.

e.g. lipids, viral RNA

e.g. carbohydrates in outer bacterial walls

Transmembrane receptors

α helical receptors

Toll-like receptors – intra and extracellular

Mannose receptor

Effect

Increase in integrin activity and cytoskeletal changes for migration into tissues

Cytokine production and acute phase responses

Phagocytosis via complement activation and killing of microbes

Cell	Appearance	Site	Mobility	Present to:
Interdigitating dendritic cells	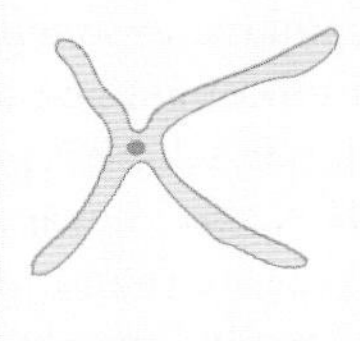	Paracortex of lymph node	Mobile	T cells
Langerhans' cells		Skin	Mobile	T cells
Veiled cells		Lymph	Mobile	T cells
Follicular dendritic cells	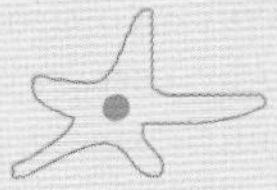	Lymph node follicles	Static	B cells
Macrophages	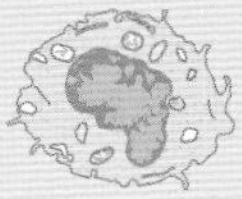	Lymph node medulla Liver (Kupffer cells) Brain (astrocytes)	Mobile Static Static	T and B cells
B cell (especially if activated)	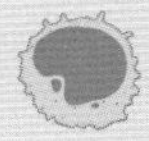	Lymphoid tissue	Mobile	T cells

Fig. 1.16 Antigen-presenting cells and their associated sites.

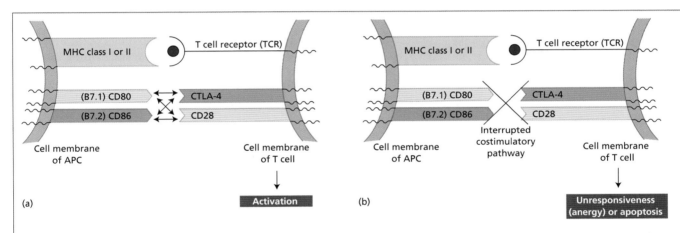

Fig. 1.17 (a, b) Role of co-stimulatory pathway in T-cell activation. APC, antigen-presenting cell; MHC, major histocompatibility complex.

variety of effector T cells. Depending on the environment of the cell, which is not entirely understood, mature DCs can activate CD4⁺ cells to become Th1, Th2, Th17, CTLs and regulatory T cells (Tregs) or to induce apoptosis and so induce tolerance (see section 1.4). Immature and mature DCs have different sets of surface proteins (which act as distinct markers), in keeping with their different functions (see Table 1.3), depending on whether they are immature (for antigen capture/sensing pathogens via PRRs) or mature (for presentation of antigen to T cells).

The interaction between DCs and T cells is strongly influenced by a group of cell surface molecules that function as **co-stimulators**: CD80 (also known as B7-1) and CD86 (B7-2) on the activated DC, each of which engages with counter receptors on the T-cell surface referred to as CD28 and CTLA-4. *A functional co-stimulatory pathway is essential for T-cell activation*. In the absence of a co-stimulatory signal, interaction

between DCs and T cells leads to T-cell unresponsiveness (Fig. 1.17). The importance of the co-stimulatory pathway is underlined by the ability of antagonists to co-stimulatory molecules to interrupt immune responses both *in vitro* and *in vivo*. This observation has been exploited therapeutically in mice with advanced lupus, in which treatment with a CTLA-4 conjugated protein to block CD28 leads to significant improvement in disease activity. Translation to human therapeutic monoclonal antibodies has succeeded despite a rocky start (see Chapter 7, Case 7.3). Abatacept, a CTLA-4 fusion protein, is licensed for the treatment of rheumatoid arthritis. T-cell activation by DCs also depends on cytokines secreted by activated DCs such as IL-12.

Processed antigen is presented to T cells complexed with the MHC class II antigens on the APC surface, since T cells do not recognize processed antigen alone. The most efficient APCs are the **interdigitating dendritic cells** found in the T-cell regions of a lymph node (Figs 1.15 and 1.17). These dendritic cells have high concentrations of MHC class I and II molecules, co-stimulatory molecules (CD80, CD86) as well as adhesion molecules on their surfaces (Table 1.3) and limited enzymatic powers, which enable antigen processing but not complete digestion. Being mobile, they are able to capture antigen in the periphery and migrate to secondary lymphoid organs, where they differentiate into mature dendritic cells and interact with naïve T cells. These cells are known as Langerhans cells when present in the skin.

These cells differ from the **follicular dendritic cells** in the follicular germinal centre (B-cell area) of a lymph node (see Figs 1.15 and 1.17). Follicular dendritic cells have receptors for complement and immunoglobulin components and their function is to trap immune complexes and to feed them to B cells in the germinal centre. This is part of the secondary immune response, since preexisting antibodies are used, accounting for B-cell memory.

Plasmacytoid DCs are found in blood and mucosal-associated lymphoid tissues and can secrete large quantities of type I IFNs in response to viral infections. However, their precise role and repertoire and therefore clinical significance remain unclear.

The few DCs in the blood are typically identified and enumerated in flow cytometry. Three types of DCs have been defined in human blood and these are the $CD11_c^+$ myeloid DCs, the CD141+ myeloid DCs and the CD303+ plasmacy-toid DCs (as per the IUIS Nomenclature committee). Dendritic cells in blood are less mature and have no projections from their surface (dendrites). Still, they can perform complex functions, including chemokine production in $CD11_c^+$ myeloid DCs, cross-presentation of antigen in CD 141+ myeloid DCs and IFN-a production in CD303+ plasmacytoid DCs.

Monocyte-derived DCs, also known as **myeloid** DCs, are activated (mature) DCs that are found in inflammatory sites, from whence they travel to draining lymph nodes. As with other mature DCs, they express co-stimulatory molecules and so can activate T cells. Under certain circumstances they can even secrete TNF-α and nitric oxide. The ability to culture these cells from human blood monocytes has led to the concept of DC vaccines for cancers.

Activated B cells themselves are also able to present antigen (Fig. 1.16).

1.3.5 Complement

The complement system consists of a series of heat-labile serum proteins that are activated in turn. The components normally exist as soluble inactive precursors; once activated, a complement component may then act as an enzyme (Fig. 1.19), which cleaves several molecules of the next component in the sequence (rather like the clotting cascade). Each precursor is cleaved into two or more fragments. The **major fragment** has two biologically active sites: one for

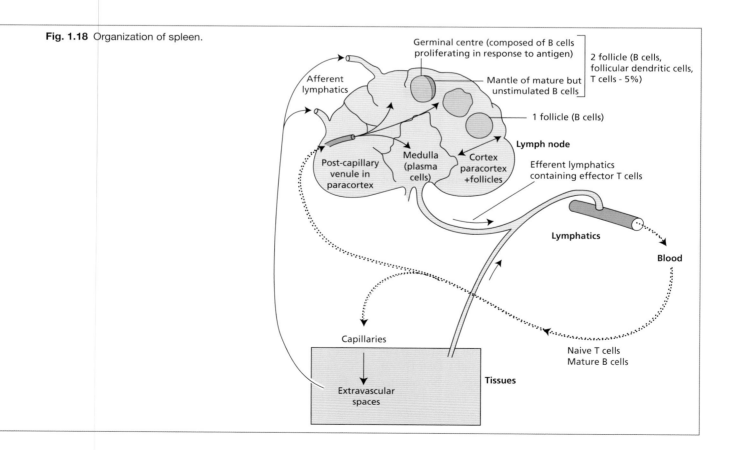

Fig. 1.18 Organization of spleen.

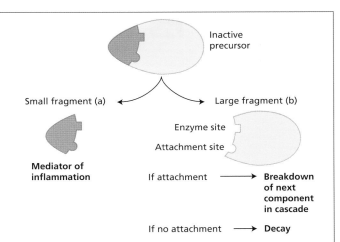

Fig. 1.19 Basic principle underlying the cleavage of complement components.

numerical order; the numbering coincides with the order of their discovery and not with their position in the sequence. Activated components are shown with a bar over the number of the component (e.g. C1 is activated to C$\overline{1}$) and fragments of activated components by letters after the number (e.g. C3 is split initially into two fragments, C3a and C3b).

The major purpose of the complement pathways is to provide a means of removing or destroying antigen, regardless of whether or not it has become coated with antibody (Fig. 1.20). The **lysis** of whole invading microorganisms is a dramatic example of the activity of the complete sequence of complement activation, but that is not necessarily its most important role. The key function of complement is probably the **opsonization** of microorganisms and immune complexes; microorganisms coated (i.e. opsonized) with immunoglobulin and/or complement are more easily recognized by macrophages and more readily bound and phagocytosed through IgG: Fc and C3b receptors.

Similarly, immune complexes are opsonized by their activation of the classical complement pathway (see later); individuals who lack one of the classical pathway components suffer from immune complex diseases (see section 1.6). Soluble complexes are **transported** in the circulation from the inflammatory site by erythrocytes bearing CR1, which bind to the activated C3 (C3b) in the immune complex. Once in the spleen or liver, these complexes are removed from the red cells, which are then recycled (Fig. 1.21).

Minor complement fragments are generated at almost every step in the cascade and contribute to the **inflammatory response**. Some increase vascular permeability (C3a), while others attract neutrophils and macrophages for subsequent

binding to cell membranes or the triggering complex and the other for enzymatic cleavage of the next complement component (Fig. 1.20). Control of the sequence involves spontaneous decay of any exposed attachment sites and specific inactivation by complement inhibitors. **Minor fragments** (usually prefixed 'a') generated by cleavage of components have important biological properties in the fluid phase, such as the chemotactic activity of C5a.

The history of the discovery of the complement pathways has made the terminology confusing. Several of the components have numbers, but they are not necessarily activated in

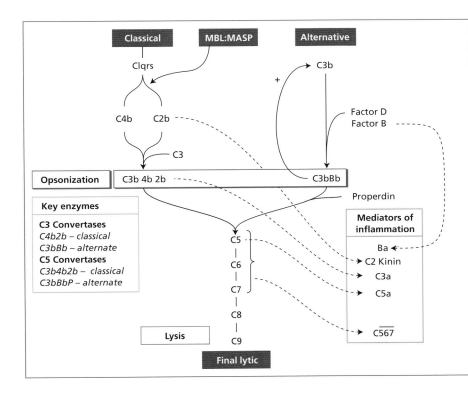

Fig. 1.20 Functions of complement pathways. MASP, MBL-associated serine protease; MBL, mannan-binding lectin.

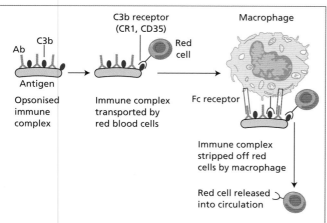

Fig. 1.21 Transport of immune complexes by erythrocytes to macrophages in liver and spleen.

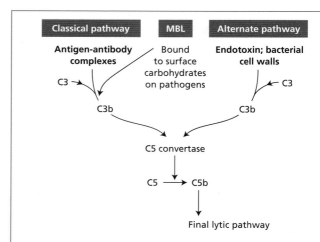

Fig. 1.22 Complement pathways and their initiating factors. MBL, mannan-binding lectin.

opsonization and phagocytosis (C5a) (Fig. 1.20). C5a not only promotes leucocytosis in the bone marrow, but mobilizes and attracts neutrophils to the inflammatory site where it increases their adhesiveness; it also upregulates complement receptors CR1 and CR3 on neutrophils and macrophages to maximize phagocytosis.

Complement **activation** occurs in two phases: activation of the C3 component, followed by activation of the 'attack' or lytic sequence. The critical step is a cleavage of C3 by complement-derived enzymes termed 'C3 convertases'. The cleavage of C3 is achieved by three routes, the classical, alternative and lectin pathways, all of which can generate C3 convertases but in response to different stimuli (Fig. 1.22). The pivotal role of C3 in complement activation is underlined by patients with a deficiency of C3, who cannot opsonize pathogens or immune complexes, predisposing them to bacterial infection as well as immune complex diseases.

The **classical pathway** was the first to be described. It is activated by a number of substances, the most widely recognized being antigen–antibody complexes where the antibody is either IgM or IgG (Fig. 1.22). The reaction of IgM or IgG with its antigen causes a conformational change in the Fc region of the antibody to reveal a binding site for the first component in the classical pathway, C1q. C1q is a remarkable, collagen-like protein composed of six subunits, resembling a 'bunch of tulips' when seen under the electron microscope. C1q reacts with Fc via its globular heads; attachment by two critically spaced binding sites is needed for activation. The Fc regions of pentameric IgM are spaced so that one IgM molecule can activate C1q; in contrast, IgG is relatively inefficient because the chance of two randomly sited IgG molecules being the critical distance apart to activate C1q is relatively low. IgA, IgD and IgE do not activate the classical pathway.

Once C1q is activated, C1r and C1s are **sequentially bound** to generate enzyme activity (C1 esterase) for C4 and C2 (see Fig. 1.20), splitting both molecules into 'a' and 'b' fragments. The complex C4b2b is the classical pathway C3 convertase. Other fragments released are C4a, C2a and a

vasoactive peptide released from C2. C4b2b cleaves C3 into two fragments, C3a possessing anaphylatoxic and chemotactic activity and C3b that binds to the initiating complex and promotes many of the biological properties of complement. The C 4b2b3b complex so generated is an enzyme, C5 convertase, which initiates the final lytic pathway (the 'attack' sequence).

The **alternative pathway** is phylogenetically older than the classical pathway. It is relatively inefficient in the tissues, and high concentrations of the various components are required. The central reaction in this pathway, as in the classical one, is the activation of C3, but the alternative pathway generates a C3 convertase without the need for antibody, C1, C4 or C2. Instead, the most important activators are bacterial cell walls and endotoxin (Fig. 1.22).

The initial **cleavage** of C3 in the alternative pathway happens continuously and **spontaneously** (see Fig. 1.22), generating a low level of C3b. C3b is an unstable substance and, if a suitable acceptor surface is not found, the attachment site in C3b decays rapidly and the molecule becomes inactive. If, however, an acceptor surface (bacterial cell walls and endotoxin) is nearby, the C3b molecules can bind and remain active. C3b is then able to use factors D and B of the alternative pathway to produce the active enzyme 'C3bBb'. This latter substance has two properties. It can break down more C3, providing still more C3b; this is known as the 'positive feedback loop' of the alternative pathway (Fig. 1.20). Alternatively, C3bBb becomes stabilized in the presence of properdin to form the C5 convertase of the alternative pathway.

There are thus two ways of producing **C5 convertase**. In the classical pathway C5 convertase is made up of C3b, C4b and C2b, while in the alternative pathway it is produced by C3b, Bb and properdin (Fig. 1.20).

The third pathway of complement activation is initiated by **mannan-binding lectin** (MBL, also known as mannan-binding protein), a surface receptor (see Fig. 1.20) shed into the circulation, binding avidly to carbohydrates on the surface of microorganisms. MBL is a member of the collectin family of

C-type lectins, which also includes pulmonary surfactant proteins A and D. MBL is structurally related to C1q and activates complement through a serine protease known as MASP (MBL-associated serine protease), similar to C1r and C1s of the classical pathway. Inherited deficiency of MASP-2 has been shown to predispose to recurrent pneumococcal infections and immune complex disease.

All pathways converge on a common **final lytic** pathway ('attack' sequence) of complement involving the sequential attachment of the components C5, C6, C7, C8 and C9 and resulting in lysis of the target cell such as an invading organism or a virally infected cell. The lytic pathway complex binds to the cell membrane and a transmembrane channel is formed. This can be seen by electron microscopy as a hollow, thin-walled cylinder through which salts and water flow, leading to the uptake of water by a cell, swelling and destruction. During the final lytic pathway, complement fragments are broken off. C5a and the activated complex C567 are both potent mediators of inflammation. C5a, along with C3a, are anaphylotoxins, i.e. they cause histamine release from mast cells with a resulting increase in vascular permeability. C5a also has the property of being able to attract neutrophils to the site of complement activation (i.e. it is chemotactic; see Fig. 1.20).

The **control of any cascade sequence** is extremely important, particularly when it results in the production of potentially self-damaging mediators of inflammation. The complement pathway is controlled by three mechanisms (see Box 1.5).

These mechanisms ensure that the potentially harmful effects of complement activation remain confined to the initiating antigen without damaging autologous (host) cells. Table 1.10 lists some of the clinically important complement regulatory proteins. When considering their role in pathology, there are important caveats (see Box 1.5).

1.3.6 Antibody-dependent cell-mediated cytotoxicity

ADCC is a mechanism by which antibody-coated target cells are destroyed by cells bearing **low-affinity FcγRIII receptors** – NK cells (CD16⁺), monocytes, neutrophils (see section 1.2.4 and Fig. 1.23) – without involvement of the MHC. Clustering of several IgG molecules is required to trigger these low-affinity receptors to bind, resulting in secretion of IFN-γ and discharge of granules containing perforin and granzymes, as found in CTLs. The overall importance of ADCC in host defence is unclear, but it represents an additional mechanism by which bacteria and viruses can be eliminated.

1.3.7 Natural killer cells

NK cells look like large granular lymphocytes and are found in blood, liver and secondary lymphoid organs particularly the spleen and mucosal-associated lymphoid tissue (MALT). They can kill target cells, even in the absence of antibody or antigenic stimulation. The name '**natural killer**' reflects the fact that, unlike the adaptive system, they do not need prior activation but have the relevant recognition molecules on their surfaces already. Non-specific agents, such as mitogens, IFN-γ and IL-12, can activate them further. NK cells form an integral part of the early host response to viral infection (Fig. 1.24). The exact mechanism by which NK cells distinguish between infected and non-infected cells is not clear, but is likely to involve **cell-surface receptors** (Fig. 1.25). NK cells express two types of surface receptor (see section 1.2.2). Expression of MHC class I proteins by most normal cells prevents NK cells from killing healthy cells. Interference with this inhibition, by virally induced down-regulation or alteration of MHC class I molecules, results in NK-mediated killing, either directly (secretion of granzymes or perforin), by FcRIII and ADCC or by secretion of IFN-γ and TNF-α.

Box 1.5 Physiological control of complement

- A number of the activated components are inherently unstable; if the next protein in the pathway is not immediately available, the active substance decays.
- There are a number of specific inhibitors, e.g. C1 esterase inhibitor, factor I, factor H.
- There are proteins on cell membranes that block the action of complement:
  - By increasing the rate of breakdown of activated complement components, e.g. DAF (decay accelerating factor, CD55), MCP (monocyte chemotactic protein, CD46).
  - By binding C5b678 and preventing C9 from binding and polymerizing, e.g. CD59.

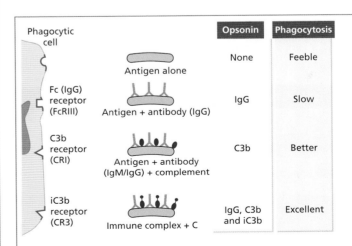

Fig. 1.23 Opsonins and the relationship to phagocytosis.

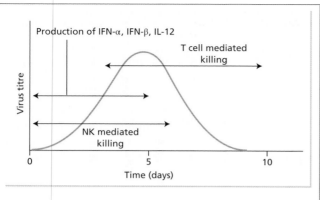

Fig. 1.24 Role of cells in early immune response to virus infection. Early – innate immune cells produce type I interferons (IFN) and interleukin (IL)-12. Late – T-cell-mediated killing by antigen-specific cells: cytotoxic T cells (CTLs). NK, natural killer.

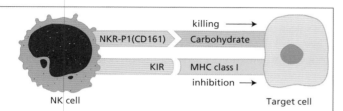

Fig. 1.25 Natural killer (NK) cell recognition of target cells. NK cell killing is mediated by engagement of the receptor NKR-P1 with its carbohydrate ligand on the target cell. This is inhibited by the interaction between the inhibitory receptor (KIR) and major histocompatibility complex (MHC) class I on the target cell.

NK cells are not immune cells in the strictest sense because, like macrophages, they are not clonally restricted; in addition, they show **little specificity** and they have no memory. The range of their potential targets is broad. Animals and rare patients with deficient NK cell function have an increased incidence of certain tumours and viral infections. A subset of NK cells, NKT cells, is therefore important in 'immune' surveillance against tumours (section 1.5.1). The human immunodeficiency X-linked lymphoproliferative syndrome is an example in which Epstein–Barr virus (EBV)-driven tumours are associated with absent NKT cells (see Chapter 2, section 2.3.1).

1.3.8 Innate lymphoid cells

Innate lymphoid cells (ILCs) are tissue-resident lymphocytes that do not express antigen receptors. They are best regarded as innate T cells. Based on their cytokine-secreting profile and functions, three groups of ILCs are recognized (Table 1.11). The cytokine profile of ILC1, ILC2 and ILC3 groups of lymphocytes mirrors that of CD4+ Th1, Th2 and Th17 cells, respectively, with a similar overlap of functions. This classification is not mutually exclusive, with ILCs exhibiting sufficient plasticity to change phenotypes and functional capacities in response to changes in cytokines and transcription factors.

In contrast to adaptive T-cell responses, which take several days, ILCs act promptly in response to cytokine signals during an immune response. Beyond the immune system, ILCs play a key role in metabolic homeostasis and tissue repair. ILCs resident in the intestine and lungs also express receptors for neurotransmitters and neuropeptides, thus playing an important role in cross-talk between mucosal surfaces and the nervous system.

1.4 Functional basis of the adaptive immune responses

Antigen-specific effector lymphocytes are of two types: B cells and T cells. B cells are ultimately responsible for antibody production and act as APCs in secondary immune responses. There are several types of T cells that act as effector cells with several different functional activities (Table 1.12). Some T cells have a regulatory rather than effector role, in terms of assisting maturation of other cell types or regulating immune responses. T-cell functions of help, killing or regulation may depend on different stimuli, resulting in different cytokines being produced with predominantly activating or inhibitory effects.

The factors regulating a normal immune response (see later Box 1.7) are complex and include antigen availability, specific suppression by T cells and the balance of cytokines produced (section 1.4.2).

1.4.1 Antigen processing

The first stage of an antigen-specific immune response involves capture and modification of that antigen by specialized

Table 1.11 Classification of innate lymphoid cells (ILCs)			
	ILC1	**ILC2**	**ILC3**
Key transcription factor required for development	T-bet	GATA-3	RORγt
Secreted cytokine profile	Interferon-γ	Interleukin (IL)-4, IL-5, IL-13	IL-17, IL-22
Function	First line of defence against intracellular pathogens, e.g. viruses, toxoplasma	Defence against parasites	Defence against extracellular bacteria, fungi; regulation of adaptive Th17 cell responses
Key cell surface molecules	CD45, CD127, CD161, IL1R	CD45, CD161, CRTH2 (chemoattractant receptor)	CD45, CD127, CD117, CD161

Table 1.12 Lymphocytes involved in adaptive immune responses

Cell type	Function of cell	Product of cell	Function of product
B	Produce antibody	Antibody	Neutralization
	Antigen presentation		Opsonization
			Cell lysis
Th2	B-cell antibody production Activate T_C	Cytokines IL-3, -4, -5, -10, -13	Help B and T_C cells
Th1	Inflammation: initiation and augmentation	IL-2, IFN-γ, TNF	Inflammatory mediators
TRegs	B-cell antibody production suppress T_C	Suppressor factor(s), e.g. TGF-β	Suppress Th and therefore indirectly B and T_C
Tc	Lysis of antigenic target cells	IFN-γ	Enhances MHC expression
			Activates NK cells
		Perforins	Disrupts target cell membranes
NKT	Target cell killing	IL-4, IFNγ	
Th17	Inflammation	IL-17A, IL-17F and IL-22	Host defence against bacteria and fungi via IL-17s attracting neutrophils

IFN, interferon; IL, interleukin; MHC, major histocompatibility complex; NK, natural killer; T_C, cytotoxic T cell (CTL); TGF, transforming growth factor; Th1 and Th2, helper T-cell types; Th17, effector T cells secreting inflammatory cytokines; TNF, tumour necrosis factor; TRegs, regulatory T cells.

cells, DCs prior to presentation to the immune cells. *This is not an antigen-specific process, unlike the subsequent restricted binding of antigen to lymphocytes predetermined to react with that antigen only.* Antigen is processed, then carried and 'presented' to lymphocytes. T cells cannot recognize antigen without such processing into small peptides and presentation in relation to self-MHC. Since activation of T cells is essential for most immune responses, antigen processing is crucial. The specialized cells involved are dendritic cells (and some monocytes) for a primary immune response and B cells for a secondary immune response when the antigen has been recognized and responded to on a previous occasion.

1.4.2 T-cell-mediated responses

As mentioned earlier, CD4+ T cells have many functions and there are T-cell subsets that reflect this. Furthermore, the function of a particular T cell can change, depending on the environment in which it finds itself. Conventional CD4+ cells that have alpha-beta chains in their TCRs (αβ T cells) are the predominant type in the blood and lymphoid circulations. They can become helper cells, of which there are presently three types: Th0, Th1 and Th2. Th0 are thought to be the precursor naive T cells, as they are able to secrete a wide variety of cytokines. Th1 are proinflammatory T cells and Th2 assist Tc activation and antibody production. CD8+ T cells, which depend on 'help' from CD4+ T cells for antigen specificity, are one of several types of killing (cytotoxic) cells and are particularly important in the control or elimination of viruses. Th17 cells are proinflammatory and are thought to

have evolved to aid in host defence against bacteria and fungi, via their production of inflammatory cytokines IL-17A, IL-17F and IL-22. Tregs control immune responses, particularly aberrant responses such as autoimmunity. In addition, there is a group of more primitive T cells (sometimes called 'unconventional' T cells) that include gamma-delta T cells (γδ T cells), found mainly in relation to the mucosa particularly the gut, and NKT cells, which are important for regulation and recognizing lipid (often tumour) antigens.

T-cell help

T-cell help is always antigen specific. Only helper T cells that have responded to antigen previously presented in the context of MHC class II can subsequently help those CD8+ T cells or CD19+ B cells that are already committed to the same antigen (Burnet's clonal selection theory). **Helper T cells** recognize both antigen and MHC class II antigens as a complex on the presenting cells, via their specific TCR. They then recognize the same combination of antigen and the particular class II antigen on the responding cell. **Co-stimulation** is essential for T-cell activation and accessory molecules are vital (Fig. 1.17).

MHC class II molecules play an important role in the activation of helper T cells. T cells from one individual will not cooperate with the APCs, T cells or B cells from a different person (i.e. of a different HLA type). Certain MHC class II molecules on the presenting cells fail to interact with particular antigens (as a prelude to triggering helper T cells) and so fail to trigger an adaptive immune response to that stimulus. This provides a mechanism for the **genetic regulation of immune responses** (originally attributed to distinct immune response genes). The MHC class II thus helps to determine the responsiveness of an individual to a particular foreign antigen, since they interact with the antigen before T-cell help can be triggered.

When helper T cells meet an antigen for the first time, there is a limited number that can react with that antigen to provide help; these stimulated T cells therefore undergo blast transformation and **proliferation**, providing an increased number of specific helper T cells when the animal is re-exposed, i.e. an expanded clone. In addition, specific memory T cells differentiate.

Memory T cells (which bear the surface marker CD45RO) have increased numbers of adhesion molecules (LFA-1, CD2, LFA-3, ICAM-1; see section 1.2.6) and a higher proportion of high-affinity receptors for the relevant antigen. Memory cells are therefore easily activated and produce high concentrations of IL-2 to recruit more helper T cells of both types, Th1 and Th2 (see later in the chapter). Thus T-cell memory is a combination of an increase of T cells (quantitative) as well as a qualitative change in the efficiency of those T cells, providing a more rapid immune response on second and subsequent exposure as well as a more vigorous response.

Antigen-specific **cell-mediated effector responses** are carried out by T lymphocytes. T cells can lyse cells expressing specific antigens (cytotoxicity), release cytokines that trigger inflammation (delayed-type hypersensitivity), take part in antibody production or regulate immune responses (regulation). **Distinct T-cell populations** mediate these types of T-cell responses: CD8+ Tc cytotoxic cells, CD4+ Th1 cells, CD4+ Th2 and CD4+ Treg cells, respectively.

T-effector cells

CD4+ effector T cells are grouped into four distinct subgroups depending on their cytokine profile. Th1 cells secrete TNF and IFN-γ and consequently mediate inflammation. In contrast, Th2 cells predominantly secrete IL-4, IL-5, IL-10 and IL-13 (Fig. 1.26), stimulate vigorous antibody production and activate Tc. T cells expressing cytokine profiles common to **both Th1 and Th2** cells are designated Th0. It is unclear how a naive T cell selects which cytokine profile to secrete, but there is evidence to suggest that exposure to certain cytokines is an important influence. Exposure to IL-4 and IL-6 stimulates development of Th2 cells, while IL-12 and IFN-γ result in a developing T cell acquiring Th1 properties. Recent evidence suggests that CD8+ T cells are also capable of secreting cytokine profiles typical of these cell types.

In humans, a Th1 cytokine profile is essential for protection against intracellular pathogens, while a Th2 cytokine profile is associated with diseases characterized by overproduction of antibodies including IgE. The clinical consequences of inducing a **particular Th response** are strikingly illustrated in patients with leprosy, an infectious disease caused by Mycobacterium leprae, an intracellular bacterium. Patients who mount a protective Th1

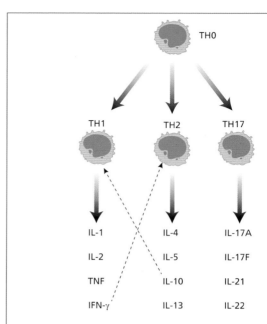

Fig. 1.26 Th1 and Th2 cells and their cytokine profiles; broken arrows indicate inhibition.

response develop only limited disease (tuberculoid leprosy), since their macrophages are able to control M. leprae efficiently. In contrast, patients who produce a predominant Th2 response develop disabling lepromatous leprosy, since without the limitation provided by Th1 inflammation, antibody alone is ineffective in tackling an intracellular pathogen.

T cells for inflammation – Th1 cells and Th17 cells

Both Th1 and Th17 cells are involved in delayed-type hypersensitivity (DTH) reactions to antigens. The tuberculin test (Mantoux test) is a good example of a DTH response. Individuals who have previously been infected with Mycobacterium tuberculosis mount a T-cell response that evolves over 24–72 hours following intradermal injection of tuberculin. This is clinically manifest as local swelling and induration; biopsy of the site reveals both types of T cell as well as macrophage infiltration. The histology of tissue granulomas in tuberculosis, leprosy and sarcoidosis are all examples of DTH. Like the induction of T-cell help, the effector functions in **delayed hypersensitivity** vary with MHC polymorphisms.

Th17 cells are a proinflammatory subset of THCs defined by production of inflammatory cytokines IL-17A, IL-17F and IL-22. Th17 cells are thought to have evolved to aid in host defence against extracellular and intracellular bacteria as well as fungi. IL-17 is important for the recruitment of neutrophils (and possibly eosinophils), but the precise role in inflammation in systemic inflammatory diseases such as rheumatoid arthritis is not yet clear. Th17 cells require the proinflammatory cytokines transforming growth factor (TGF)-β1, IL23 and IL-6, secreted by DCs, for their development, rather than the IL-12 needed for Th1 development.

T-cell lysis

CD8+ CTLs lyse cells infected with virus and possibly those tumour cells with recognizable tumour antigens too. Such cytotoxicity is antigen specific and only cells expressing the relevant viral proteins on their surfaces are killed (see Fig. 1.6), so obeying the rules of the clonal selection theory. Since infected cells express surface viral proteins prior to the assembly of new virus particles and viral budding, **cytotoxic T cells** are important in the recovery phase of an infection, destroying the infected cells before new virus particles are generated. CTLs lyse target cells by means of secretory lysosomes (granules) containing perforin and granzymes (and granulysin capable of antimicrobial activity). The lysosomes fuse with the outer membrane of the target cell and discharge the contents via a synaptic cleft, resulting in death of the target cell. Other methods are used by CTL to cause programmed cell death (apoptosis) that do not involve the secretory lysosomes.

In contrast to CD4+ helper T cells, CD8+ CTLs recognize viral antigens together with MHC class I molecules (rather than MHC class II) on both dendritic cells for activation and target cells for effector function. They show exquisite specificity for self-MHC molecules, in that they can lyse only cells expressing the same MHC class I molecules. MHC class I molecules may affect the **strength of the effector CTL response** to a particular virus, providing further strong evidence for the evolution of a polymorphic MHC system, so that immune responses to pathogens vary to protect the species. All endogenous antigens (including viral antigens) are presented in the context of MHC class I antigens (see Fig. 1.8). This combination on the dendritic cells directly activates CD8+ T cells and provides the appropriate target cells for virally induced T-cell cytotoxicity, as well as mechanisms for graft rejection and tumour surveillance. The relevance of CD8+ T cells to transplantation is discussed in Chapter 8. CD8+ T cells are also involved in autoimmune diseases; the T-cell epitopes of endogenous self-antigens are presented by DCs in the same way and a process known as cross-presentation allows 'B-cell epitopes' of self-antigens to be presented by DCs to T cells to provide T-cell help to B cells.

Regulatory T cells

After initial scepticism in the 1980s regarding the existence of suppressor T cells (renamed regulatory T cells), there is now good evidence to support the presence of several subsets of Tregs with distinct phenotypes that play key roles in immunoregulation by dampening down a wide range of immune responses, including responses to self-antigens, alloantigens and tumour antigens, as well as to pathogens and commensals. A number of immunoregulatory cells have been described, but it is likely that the CD4+ Tregs, identified by high levels of the IL-2 receptor alpha chain (CD25+) and the FOXP3 transcription factor, are the most important for maintaining peripheral tolerance. These **natural regulatory T cells** (natural Tregs) develop in the thymus in response to self-antigens; they maintain peripheral self-tolerance and so prevent autoimmunity. However similar cells, **induced (i) Tregs** (producing IL-10), can be generated from precursors outside the thymus in response to environmental antigens; these cells maintain tolerance to non-self components such as gut flora. Both types seem to be interchangeable with Th17, depending on the cytokines and other mediators such as in inflammation caused by pathogens or CD8+ autoimmune cells.

It is thought that Tregs act by producing immunosuppressive cytokines such as TGFβ and IL-10, as well as direct cell-to-cell contact resulting in apoptosis of the target cell.

The development of Treg cells is under the control of the gene called FOXP3, which encodes a transcription repressor protein specifically in CD4+, CD25+ T cells in the thymus as well as in the periphery. Mutations in the FOXP3 gene result in severe autoimmune disease and allergy (Box 1.6).

Natural killer T cells

A few T cells also express some of the markers of NK cells and are therefore known as NKT cells. These cells form a separate lineage, though they are CD3+. They have α TCR chains, with limited diversity, but are also able to **recognize lipids in conjunction with CD1**, MHC class I-like molecules of equally restricted diversity. They rapidly produce many cytokines after stimulation and thus influence diverse immune responses, such as augmenting the proliferation of

---

Box 1.6   Evidence that CD4+CD25+ T cells are important in immunoregulation

- Depletion of CD4+CD25+ T cells in humans, due to mutations in the FOXP3 gene, is associated with the rare IPEX syndrome – immune dysregulation, polyendocrinopathy, enteropathy, X-linked syndrome – characterized by autoimmune diabetes, inflammatory bowel disease and severe allergy.
- Regulatory T cells (Tregs) determine the disease prognosis in hepatitis B virus (HBV) infection – high levels lead to viral progression and impaired immune response.
- Clinical improvement after allergen immunotherapy for allergic rhinitis and asthma has been associated with the induction of interleukin (IL)-10 and transforming growth factor (TGF)-β producing Foxp3 expressing CD4+CD25+ T cells, resulting in suppression of Th2 cytokines.
- Corticosteroid therapy in asthma acts on Tregs, in part to increase IL-10 production, while vitamin D$_3$ and long-acting beta-agonists enhance IL-10 Treg function.
- The antiinflammatory therapeutic effects of low-dose IL-2 are mediated through an expansion of Tregs.

Tregs in an IL-4-dependent manner. They can also promote cell-mediated immunity to tumours and infectious organisms, while paradoxically they can suppress the T-cell responses associated with autoimmune disease, graft-versus-host disease or allograft rejection. The exact mechanisms by which these cells carry out such contrasting functions are not known. Absence of NKT cells in a particular form of primary immunodeficiency known as X-linked lymphoproliferative disease (XLP) is associated with the development of EBV-driven lymphoma, suggesting an important role in responses to this particular virus and to tumours.

1.4.3 Antibody production

Antibody production involves at least three types of cell: APCs, B cells and helper T cells (Table 1.12).

B cells

Antibodies are synthesized by B cells and their mature progeny, plasma cells. B cells are readily recognized because they express **immunoglobulin on their surface**, which acts as the BCR (see section 1.2.2). During development, B cells first show intracellular μ chains and then surface IgM μ with one light chain – κ or λ. These cells are able to switch from production of IgM to one of the other classes as they mature, so that they later express IgM and IgD and, finally, IgG, IgA or IgE, a process known as isotype switching. The final type of surface immunoglobulin determines the class of antibody secreted; surface and secreted immunoglobulin are identical. This immunoglobulin maturation sequence fits with the kinetics of an antibody response: the primary response is mainly IgM and the secondary response predominantly IgG (Fig. 1.27). **Isotype switching** is mediated by the interaction of several important proteins: for example, CD40 on the B-cell surface engages with its ligand (CD40L) on activated T cells (Fig. 1.28), under the influence of IL-4. Deficiency of either molecule (CD40 or CD40L) in mice and humans leads to a severe immunodeficiency characterized by inability

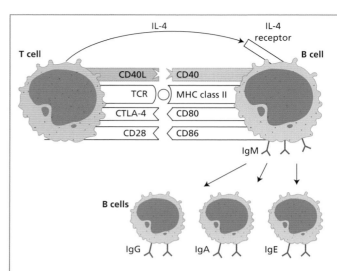

Fig. 1.28 Interaction between CD40L on T cells and CD40 on B cells, under the influence of interleukin (IL)-4, leading to isotype switching. MHC, major histocompatibility complex; TCR, T-cell receptor.

to switch from IgM to IgG production, with consequently low serum concentrations of IgG and IgA for protection against infections but normal or even high serum IgM (hence called a hyper-IgM syndrome), accompanied by poor germinal centre formation and inability to produce memory B cells (see Chapter 3, Case 3.2).

Each B cell is committed to the production of an antibody that has a unique V_H–V_L combination (see section 1.2.4). This uniqueness is the basis of Burnet's clonal selection theory, which states that each B cell expresses a surface immunoglobulin that acts as its antigen-binding site. Contact with antigen and factors released by CD4+ T helper cells (IL-4, -5, -13) stimulates the B cells to divide and differentiate, generating more antibody-producing cells, all of which make the same antibody with the same V_H–V_L pair. Simultaneously, a population of **B memory cells** is produced that expresses the same surface immunoglobulin receptor. The result of these cell divisions is that a greater number of antigen-specific B cells become available when the animal is exposed to the same antigen at a later date; this is known as **clonal expansion** and helps to account for the increased secondary response.

As well as being quicker and more vigorous (Fig. 1.27), secondary responses are more efficient. This is due to the production of antibodies that bind more effectively to the antigen, i.e. have a higher affinity. There are two reasons for this. First, as antigen is removed by the primary response, the remaining antigen (in low concentration) reacts only with those cells that have high-affinity receptors. Second, the **rapid somatic mutation, which accompanies B-cell division in the germinal centre**, provides B cells of higher affinity, a process known as 'affinity maturation'. C3 fragments play a key role in the secondary antibody response by interacting with the co-stimulation receptors on B cells.

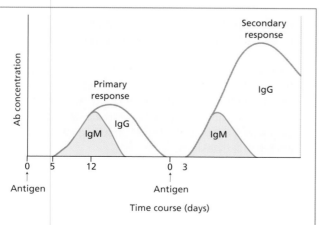

Fig. 1.27 Primary and secondary antibody (Ab) responses following antigenic stimulation.

A minority subset of B cells respond directly to antigens called **T-independent antigens** (see section 1.2.1). These antigens have repeating, identical antigenic determinants and provoke predominantly IgM antibody responses. These responses are relatively short-lived and restricted in specificity and affinity, due to the lack of T-cell involvement. A few T-independent antigens provoke non-specific proliferation of memory B cells and are therefore known as polyclonal B-cell mitogens.

A given B cell produces particular V_H and V_L domains and all the daughter cells of that B cell produce the same V_H and V_L. Initially, the B cell produces intracellular antigen-specific IgM, which then becomes bound to the surface of the cell (surface immunoglobulin) and acts as the antigen receptor for that cell; the B cell is then 'antigen responsive'. On exposure to that antigen, a committed B cell fixes the isotype (or class) of immunoglobulin that it will produce and divides; all the progeny produce identical immunoglobulin molecules (known as monoclonal immunoglobulins). Many of these cells then mature into plasma cells, while others act as APCs (section 1.4.1) or memory B cells.

1.5 Physiological outcomes of immune responses

Once the immune response is initiated, the end result depends on the nature and localization of the antigen, on whether the predominant response has been humoral or cell mediated, on the types of effector T cells and/or antibodies provoked and on whether the augmentation processes have been involved.

1.5.1 Killing of target cells (virally infected/tumour cells)

Target cells killed as a result of an immune response include organisms and cells bearing virally altered or tumour-specific antigens on their surfaces. They may be killed directly by antigen-specific mechanisms such as antibody and complement, ADCC following binding of specific antibody or antigen-specific CTL.

Cytokine production results in activation of NK cells, neutrophils and macrophages and subsequently non-specific killing by mechanisms similar to those in adaptive immunity (see section 1.2.3).

1.5.2 Direct functions of antibody

Although some forms of antibody are good at neutralizing particulate antigens, many other factors, such as the concentration of antigen, the site of antigen entry, the availability of antibody and the speed of the immune response, may influence antigen removal (Box 1.7).

Neutralization is one direct effect of antibody and IgM and IgA are particularly good at this. A number of antigens, including diphtheria toxin, tetanus toxin and many viruses, can be neutralized by antibody. Once neutralized, these substances are no longer able to bind to receptors in the tissues; the resulting antigen–antibody complexes are usually removed from the circulation and destroyed by macrophages.

Box 1.7 Some factors affecting immune responses

Antigen
- Biochemical nature: polysaccharide antigens tend to elicit a predominant immunoglobulin (Ig)M + IgG_2 response in contrast to protein antigens, which elicit both cellular and humoral responses.
- Dose: in experimental animals large doses of antigen induce tolerance.
- Route of administration: polio vaccine administered orally elicits an IgA antibody response than intramuscular injection. Some antigens/allergens given orally can induce tolerance.

Antibody
- Passive administration of antibody can be used to modulate immune responses, e.g. maternal administration of antibodies to the red cell Rh antigen is used to prevent haemolytic disease of the newborn by removing fetal red cells from the maternal circulation.

Cytokines
- Cytokines released by Th1/Th2 lymphocytes influences type of immune response. Th1 cytokines favour development of cellular immunity, while Th2 cytokines favour antibody production.

Genes
- Major histocompatibility complex (MHC) genes help to control immune responses to specific antigens, e.g. studies in mice have identified strains that are high responders to certain antigens but poor responders to others. This is mirrored in humans by the strong link between certain MHC genes and the development of certain autoimmune diseases.
- Non-MHC genes also influence immune responses, e.g. mutations in the recombinase gene responsible for immunoglobulin and T-cell receptor gene rearrangement result in severe combined immunodeficiency in babies.

Although the physiological function of IgE antibody is unknown, it may have a role in the expulsion of parasites from the gastrointestinal tract. IgE antibody is normally bound to tissue mast cells. Attachment of antigen to IgE antibodies results in mast cell triggering, and release of a number of mediators of tissue damage (see Fig. 1.29 and Chapter 4).

1.5.3 Indirect functions of antibody

Opsonization is the process by which an antigen becomes coated with substances (such as antibodies or complement) that make it **more easily engulfed** by phagocytic cells. The coating of soluble or particulate antigens with IgG antibodies renders them

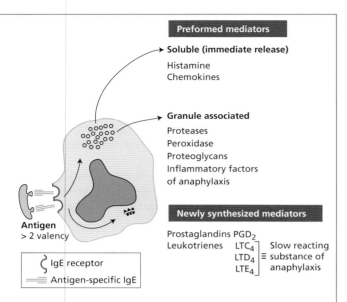

Fig. 1.29 Mechanisms in immunoglobulin (Ig)E-mediated hypersensitivity.

susceptible to cells that have surface receptors for the Fc portions of IgG (FcRIII) (Fig. 1.23). Neutrophils and macrophages both have these Fc receptors and can phagocytose IgG-coated antigens; however, this process is relatively inefficient if only Fc receptors are involved. The activation of complement by antibody (via the classical pathway) or by bacterial cell walls (via the alternative pathway) generates C3b on the surface of microorganisms and makes them susceptible to binding by several types of C3 receptors on macrophages and neutrophils (see Fig. 1.23). C3 receptors are very efficient in triggering phagocytosis.

1.5.4 Regulation

As discussed previously, termination of an ongoing immune response and regulation of the size of the response are crucial if collateral damage is to be prevented. While much is known of the regulation of the complement pathways, the science of cell-mediated regulation is in its infancy (after a false start in the 1980s). Several cell types are thought to have a regulatory function, involving at least three possible mechanisms (cell lysis, induced apoptosis or downregulation via cytokines). Natural and induced T regs (section 1.4.2) seem to be the most important cells at present; absence of these cells, or excess of their counterparts, Th17 cells, results in autoimmune diseases, severe inflammation and allergies. Other cell types involved also include NKT cells.

1.6 Tissue damage caused by the immune system

1.6.1 Inflammation: a brief overview

Inflammation is defined as increased vascular permeability accompanied by an infiltration of 'inflammatory' cells, initially polymorphonuclear leucocytes (usually neutrophils) and

later macrophages, lymphocytes and plasma cells. **Vascular permeability** may be increased (resulting in oedema) by a number of agents, which include complement fragments such as C3a, C5a, factor Ba and C2 kinnin. Some fragments (C3a, C5a and C567) also attract neutrophils and mobilize them from the bone marrow; cytokines generated by activated DCs, T cells and macrophages, such as IL-1, IL-6, TNF and IL-12, have similar properties, as well as activating vasodilation to increase blood flow (resulting in erythema). Inflammatory chemokines also attract a variety of cells to **migrate into tissues**.

The triggering of mast cells via IgE is also a method of causing inflammation, due to release of histamine and leukotrienes (which are quite distinct from cytokines) that increase vascular permeability and attract eosinophilic polymorphonuclear leucocytes too. This is discussed further in Chapter 4.

The inflammatory cytokines (IL-1, IL-6 and TNF) also provoke increased synthesis of particular serum proteins in the liver. The proteins are known as **acute-phase proteins** and include proteins that act as mediators (as in opsonization – C3 and C4 complement components, C-reactive protein [CRP]), enzyme inhibitors (α_1-antitrypsin) or scavengers (haptoglobin); the increased serum concentrations of such proteins are helpful in resolving inflammation. In practical terms, serial measurements of CRP give a useful indication of the extent and persistence of inflammation; since the half-life of CRP is only a few hours, changes in serum levels reflect rapid changes in inflammation (such as after antibiotic therapy) sufficiently quickly to be clinically useful. This is in contrast to fibrinogen (another acute-phase protein and the major factor in the erythrocyte sedimentation rate, ESR), where changes are much slower and therefore not useful clinically.

Unfortunately, the recognition of antigen by antibodies, B cells or T-effector cells can cause incidental tissue damage as well as the intended destruction of the antigen. Reactions resulting in tissue damage are often called **hypersensitivity** reactions; Gell and Coombs defined four types (Table 1.13) and this classification (though arbitrary) is still useful to distinguish types of immunological mechanisms. *Most hypersensitivity reactions are not confined to a single type: they usually involve a mixture of mechanisms.*

Immediate hypersensitivity (type I) reactions are those in which antigen interacts with preformed antigen-specific IgE bound to tissue mast cells or basophils. IgE responses are usually directed against antigens that enter at epithelial surfaces, i.e. inhaled or ingested antigens. Specific IgE production requires helper T cells and is regulated by T-cell-derived cytokines; IL-4 and IL-13 stimulate IgE production, while IFN-y is inhibitory. The balance between help and suppression depends on many variables, including the route of administration of the antigen, its chemical composition, its physical nature, whether or not adjuvants were employed and the genetic background of the animal. Following the interaction of cell-surface IgE and allergen, **activation of the mast cell** causes the release of pharmacologically active substances (see Chapter 4). Type I reactions are rapid; for example, if the antigen is injected into the skin, 'immediate hypersensitivity' can be seen within 5–10 minutes as a 'wheal-and-flare reaction',

Table 1.13 Types of hypersensitivity – mechanism, examples of disease and relevant therapy

Types	Mechanism	Therapy	Disease example
Immediate (type I)	IgE production	Antigen avoidance Neutralization of IgE – e.g. Omalizumab – monoclonal antibody binding free IgE and to B cells with surface IgE	Anaphylaxis Atopic diseases
	Mast cell degranulation	Mast cell stabilizers (disodium cromoglycate)	
	Mediators: histamine	Antihistamines	
	Leukotrienes	Leukotriene receptor antagonists, e.g. Montelukast	
	Granule-associated mediators	Corticosteroids	
Cell-bound antigen (type II)	IgG/IgM autoantibodies		
	Complement lysis	Immune suppression and/or plasma exchange to remove antibodies	Cold autoimmune haemolytic anaemia Myasthenia gravis
	Opsonization leading to neutrophil activation	Plasmapheresis Splenectomy	Goodpasture's syndrome Warm autoimmune haemolytic anaemia Immune thrombocytopenic purpura
	Metabolic stimulation	Correct metabolism	Graves' disease
	Blocking antibodies	Replace factors missing due to atrophy	Pernicious anaemia Myxoedema Infertility (some cases)
Immune complex (type III)	High concentrations of immune complexes, due to persistent antigen and antibody production, leading to complement activation and inflammation	Removal/avoidance of antigen if possible	Serum sickness Extrinsic allergic alveolitis Lepromatous leprosy
		Antiinflammatory drugs: non-steroidals, corticosteroids	Systemic lupus erythematosus
		Immune suppression: cyclophosphamide	Cutaneous vasculitis
Delayed-type hypersensitivity (type IV)	TH1 cytokine production and macrophage activation	Block cytokine production: Ciclosporin Azathioprine	Graft rejection Graft-versus-host disease
		Antiinflammatory: many inflammatory conditions Corticosteroids Reduce macrophage activity: Corticosteroids	Tuberculosis, tuberculoid leprosy Contact dermatitis
		Remove antigen	

Ig, immunoglobulin

where the resulting oedema from increased vascular permeability is seen as a wheal and the increased blood flow as a flare. In humans, there is a familial tendency towards IgE-mediated hypersensitivity, although the genes related to this 'atopic tendency' do not determine the target organ or the disease. Clinical examples of type I reactions include anaphylactic reactions due to insect venoms, peanuts and drugs, as well as the atopic diseases of hay fever and asthma (see Chapter 4).

Type II reactions are initiated by antibody reacting with antigenic determinants that form **part of the cell membrane**. The consequences of this reaction depend on whether or not complement or accessory cells become involved, and whether the metabolism of the cell is affected (Fig. 1.30). IgM and IgG can be involved in type II reactions. The best clinical examples are some organ-specific autoimmune diseases (see Chapter 5) and immune haemolytic anaemias (see Chapter 16 and Table 1.13).

Although type II reactions are mediated by autoantibodies, T cells are also involved. For example, in Graves' disease, which is known to be due to autoantibodies stimulating thyroid-stimulating hormone (TSH) receptors, specific reactive T cells are present also. Although these T cells are instrumental in promoting antibody production (primary effect), they are unlikely to cause tissue damage since the lymphocytic infiltration is mild and consists of B cells too. **Secondary autoantibodies** to antigens are released following tissue damage such as the antibodies to thyroid peroxidase. In contrast, the autoreactive T cells cloned from patients with rheumatoid arthritis and multiple sclerosis have a **primary role** in tissue damage.

Type III reactions result from the presence of immune complexes in the circulation or in the tissues. Localization of **immune complexes** depends on their size, their charge, the nature of the antigen and the local concentration of complement. If they accumulate in the tissues in large quantities, they may activate complement and accessory cells and produce extensive tissue damage. A classic example is the Arthus reaction, where an antigen is injected into the skin of an animal that has been previously sensitized. The reaction of preformed antibody with this antigen results in high concentrations of local immune complexes; these cause complement activation and neutrophil attraction and result in local inflammation 6–24 hours after the injection. Serum sickness is another example: in this condition, urticaria, arthralgia and glomerulonephritis occur about 10 days after initial exposure to the antigen. This is the time when maximum amounts of IgG antibody, produced in response to antigen stimulation, react with remaining antigen to form circulating, soluble immune complexes (Fig. 1.31). As these damaging complexes are formed, the antigen concentration is rapidly lowered; the process only continues as long as the antigen persists and thus is usually self-limiting. Further clinical examples include systemic lupus erythematosus (SLE; see Chapter 5), glomerulonephritis (see Chapter 9) and extrinsic allergic alveolitis (see Chapter 13).

Type IV reactions are initiated by T cells that react with antigen and release **Th1 cytokines**. Cytokines attract other cells, particularly macrophages, which in turn liberate lysosomal enzymes and Th17 cells. The resultant acute lesions consist of **infiltrating lymphocytes**, **macrophages** and occasionally eosinophil polymorphonuclear leucocytes. Chronic lesions show necrosis, fibrosis and, sometimes, granulomatous reactions. An understanding of mechanisms that lead to tissue damage helps to find relevant therapy (Table 1.13).

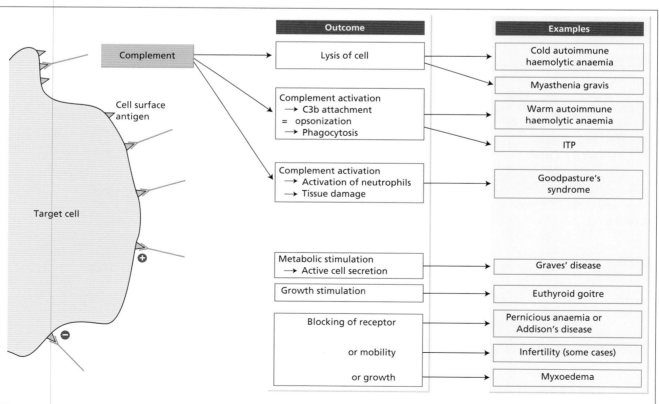

Fig. 1.30 Clinical consequences of cell-bound hypersensitivity. ITP, immune thrombocytopenic purpura.

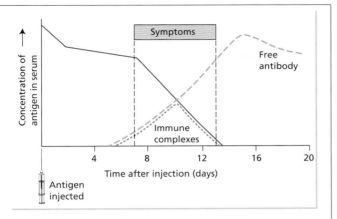

Fig. 1.31 Immune complex formation in acute serum sickness.

1.7 Organization of the immune system: an overview

All lymphoid cells originate in the bone marrow. The exact nature of the uncommitted lymphoid stem cell is unclear (though it is CD34+). An understanding of the developmental pathways is important, not only to clarify the physiology of the normal immune response, but because some immunodeficiency states represent maturation arrest of cells in their early stages of development (see Chapter 3) and some forms of therapy, such as bone marrow transplantation and gene therapy, depend on the identification and use of stem cells.

Lymphoid progenitors destined to become T cells migrate from the bone marrow into the cortex of the **thymus**. Under the influence of stromal cells and Hassalls' corpuscles in the thymic cortex, further differentiation into mature T cells occurs. The passage of T cells from the thymic cortex to medulla is associated with the acquisition of characteristic surface glycoprotein molecules so that medullary thymocytes eventually resemble mature, peripheral T cells. T-cell development in the thymus is characterized by a process of **positive selection** in the thymic cortex; T cells that recognize self-MHC proceed to full maturation. In contrast, T cells that do not recognize self-MHC do not develop any further. **Negative selection** happens in the thymic medulla. Those maturing T cells that recognize and bind to peptides of self-antigens with high affinity are selected out (negative selection) and kill themselves by apoptosis (programmed cell death). Deletion of self-reactive, developing T cells in the thymus is an important mechanism by which autoimmune disease is prevented (Chapter 5). Von Boehmer has succinctly summarized the role of the thymus in T-cell selection: 'the thymus selects the useful, neglects the useless and destroys the harmful' (a reference to autoreactive T cells). The nature of the T cells that survive is variable in terms of final tissue distribution. Those with αβ TCRs have wide-ranging antigen-binding capacity and are distributed to all tissues (including mucosae) as well as circulating according to the nature of their V regions: some to skin, others to the gut or reproductive tract or respiratory mucosa.

In contrast, B-cell development occurs in the **bone marrow** and is closely dependent upon interactions between surface glycoproteins on non-lymphoid stromal cells (such as stem cell factor, SCF) and specific receptors on B-cell precursors (in the case of SCF, Kit tyrosine kinase). Activation of Kit by SCF triggers the early stages of B-cell development; later stages of B-cell development occur under the influence of cytokines secreted by stromal cells, principally IL-7.

The thymus and the bone marrow are **primary lymphoid organs**. They contain cells undergoing a process of maturation from stem cells to antigen sensitivity and restriction. *This process of maturation is independent of antigenic stimulation within the animal.* In contrast, secondary lymphoid organs are those that contain antigen-reactive cells in the process of recirculating through the body. They include lymph nodes, spleen, bone marrow (in part) and mucosal-associated lymphoid tissues. Antigenic stimulation changes the relative proportions of the mature cell types in secondary tissues.

Peripheral T and B cells circulate in a definite pattern through the **secondary lymphoid organs** (Fig. 1.32). Most of the recirculating cells are T cells and the complete cycle takes about 24 hours; some B cells, including long-lived memory B cells, also recirculate. Lymphocyte circulation is strongly influenced by chemokine receptors on the lymphocyte surface that act as homing agents. There are also adhesion molecules directing cells to their respective ligands on high endothelial venules of lymph nodes and mucosal tissue. For instance, L-selectin is a surface glycoprotein on lymphocytes responsible for homing into lymph nodes (see section 1.2.6 and Tables 1.9 and 1.14). Recently, expression of the sphingosine-1-phosphate receptor (S1PR) on lymphocytes and its interaction with its ligand, sphingosine-1-phosphate, has been shown to be a major determinant of lymphocyte trafficking. Inhibition of lymphocyte egress by S1PR agonists has been therapeutically exploited in the treatment of multiple sclerosis.

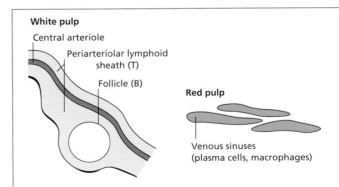

Fig. 1.32 Recirculation pathways of lymphocytes. The majority of naive T cells entering the lymph node cortex from blood will leave the node immediately via efferent lymphatics. Naive T cells that recognize specific antigens differentiate into effector T cells and reenter the circulation. B-cell recirculation follows a similar route: B cells that encounter specific antigens proliferate to form germinal centres; memory B cells form a surrounding marginal zone.

Table 1.14 Key molecular determinants of lymphocyte recirculation

Lymphocyte receptor	Ligand	Function
CD62L (L-selectin)	CD34, glycam	Mediates adhesion and lymphocyte rolling on endothelium
CCR7	CCL21 on lymph node HEV	Lymphocyte homing to lymph nodes
CCR9 (gut tropic)	CCL25 on intestinal HEV	Lymphocyte homing to intestine
Sphingosine-1-phosphate receptor (S1PR)	Sphingosine-1-phosphate	Lymphocyte egress from lymph nodes; S1PR agonists are licensed for the treatment of multiple sclerosis

Lymph node architecture is well adapted to its function (Fig. 1.18). The **lymphatic network**, which drains the extravascular spaces in the tissues, is connected to the lymph nodes by lymphatic vessels; these penetrate the lymph node capsule and drain into the peripheral sinus, from which further sinuses branch to enter the lymph node, passing through the cortex to the medulla and hence to the efferent lymphatic vessel. This sinus network provides an excellent filtration system for antigens entering the lymph node from peripheral tissues (Fig. 1.18).

The **cortex** contains primary follicles of B lymphocytes, surrounded by T cells in the 'paracortex'. There is a meshwork of interdigitating cells throughout the lymph node.

Antigen is filtered and then presented to lymphoid cells by these interdigitating cells. On antigen challenge, the 'primary' follicles of the lymph node develop into 'secondary' follicles. In contrast to primary follicles, secondary follicles contain germinal centres. These comprise mainly B cells with a few helper T cells and a mantle zone of the original primary follicle B cells. B cells in a secondary follicle are antigen activated and more mature; most have IgG on their surfaces, whereas those B cells in the primary follicle and mantle zone are less mature, bearing both IgD and IgM. Activated B cells migrate from the follicle to the medulla, where they develop into plasma cells in the **medullary cords** before releasing antibody into the efferent lymph.

The architecture of the spleen is similar. The white pulp around arterioles is arranged into T- and B-cell areas with primary and secondary follicles (Fig. 1.18). Antigen challenge results in expansion of the white pulp with B-cell activation and the development of secondary follicles. Plasma cells migrate to the red pulp.

1.8 Conclusions

The aim of this chapter is to give an overview of the normal workings of the immune system, so that the pathological processes involved in diseases are easily understood. The subsequent chapters are clinically based, devoted either to the immunological conditions of an organ or a particular type of immunological disease (allergy, autoimmune diseases or immunodeficiency). An understanding of the molecular basis of immunology as well as the cells involved in the four types of immunological mechanisms will assist the reader with the immunopathogenesis of each condition leading to the relevant treatment options.

CHAPTER 2
Infection

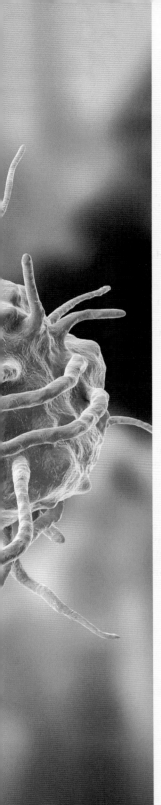

Key topics

 Visit the companion website at **www.wiley.com/go/misbah/immunology** to download cases with additional figures on these topics.

Chapel and Haeney's Essentials of Clinical Immunology, Seventh Edition. Edited by Siraj A. Misbah,
Gavin P. Spickett, and Virgil A.S.H. Dalm.
© 2022 John Wiley & Sons Ltd. Published 2022 by John Wiley & Sons Ltd.

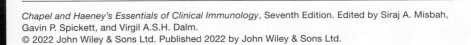

2.1 Introduction

Infectious disease is the major cause of morbidity and mortality worldwide. In Africa alone, the World Health Organization estimated in 2018 that about 200 million people suffer from malaria. New infectious diseases also attract attention in developed countries for several reasons. These include the identification of seemingly 'new' infections, such as Helicobacter pylori (recognized in 1989), new variant Creutzfeldt–Jakob disease (the causative prion was discovered around the same time), the coronavirus causing severe acute respiratory syndrome (SARS, which spread from Hong Kong to infect individuals in 37 countries in early 2003), the H1N1 and H5N1 (bird flu) influenza pandemics and the epidemic of the new coronavirus 2019-SARS-CoV-2 that spread from China in 2019. There are also changes in clinical practice, which have altered patterns of hospital infection, such as antibiotic resistance and the increased spread of Clostridium difficile in hospitals. The growth in numbers of iatrogenically immunosuppressed patients receiving immunosuppression who are at risk from 'opportunistic' infections, as well as an increase in imported diseases accompanying the rising volume of international air travel, provide new challenges. There is also an increasing awareness of diseases resulting from self-damaging host responses to pathogens.

For most infections, a balance is maintained between human defences, including the immune system, and the capacity of the microorganism to overcome or bypass them (Table 2.1). A detailed discussion of **virulence** is outside the scope of this book, but disease will also occur if the host makes an **inadequate** or **inappropriate immune response** to an infection.

Table 2.1 Factors influencing the extent and severity of an infection

Pathogen factors
- Dose (i.e. degree of exposure)
- Virulence of organism
- Route of entry

Host factors
- Integrity of non-specific defences
- Competence of the immune system
- Genetic capacity to respond effectively to a specific organism
- Evidence of previous exposure (natural or acquired)
- Existence of co-infection
- Presence of co-morbidities

2.2 Normal resistance to infection

2.2.1 Non-specific resistance

Non-specific or natural resistance refers to barriers, secretions and the normal flora that make up the external defences (Fig. 2.1), together with the actions of phagocytes and complement.

Mechanical barriers (Fig. 2.1) are highly effective, and their failure often results in infection; for example, defects in the mucociliary lining of the respiratory tract (as in cystic fibrosis) are associated with an increased susceptibility to lung infection. However, many common respiratory pathogens have evolved specific substances on their surfaces (e.g. the haemagglutinin of influenza virus), which help them attach to epithelial cells and so breach physical barriers.

Phagocytic cells ingest invading microorganisms and, in most cases, kill and digest them. There are two types of

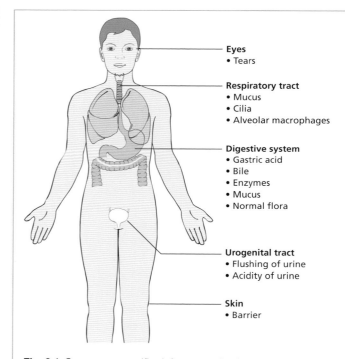

Fig. 2.1 Some non-specific defence mechanisms.

Eyes
- Tears

Respiratory tract
- Mucus
- Cilia
- Alveolar macrophages

Digestive system
- Gastric acid
- Bile
- Enzymes
- Mucus
- Normal flora

Urogenital tract
- Flushing of urine
- Acidity of urine

Skin
- Barrier

phagocyte: monocytes/macrophages and neutrophilic polymorphonuclear leucocytes (neutrophils). A prompt response to infection is achieved by having a population of cells that can be rapidly mobilized during an inflammatory response and being able to concentrate them at likely sites of infection.

Neutrophils form a large circulating pool of phagocytic cells with reserves in the bone marrow. Neutrophils are the body's first line of defence against foreign invaders and constitute the major cell type involved in acute and some forms of chronic inflammation. Invading microorganisms trigger an inflammatory response with the release of cytokines and

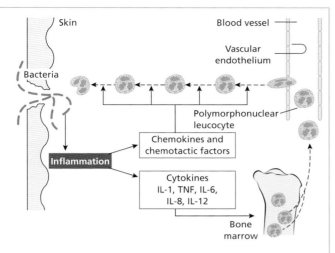

Fig. 2.2 A schematic representation of the mobilization of bone marrow stores of polymorphs following an inflammatory response. IL, interleukin; TNF, tumour necrosis factor.

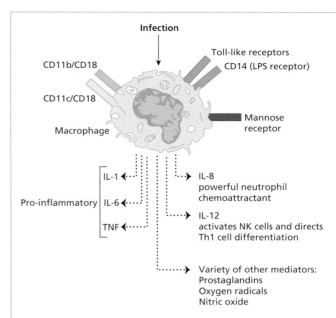

Fig. 2.3 Role of the macrophage in host defence. IL, interleukin; LPS, lipopolysaccharide; NK, natural killer; TNF, tumour necrosis factor.

chemotactic factors; as a result, circulating neutrophils adhere to vascular endothelium, squeeze out of blood vessels and actively migrate towards the focus of infection (Chapter 1, Fig. 1.13, and Fig. 2.2). Phagocytosis then occurs. Severe neutropenia or neutrophil dysfunction is associated with life-threatening infections, usually caused by common organisms such as Staphylococcus aureus, Gram-negative bacteria or fungi (see Chapter 3). Even in normal conditions, neutrophils are short-lived but produced in huge numbers: basal rate of production by the bone marrow of 10^{11} neutrophils/day. In infection, the increased output from the bone marrow results in a neutrophilia, i.e. an excess of neutrophils in the blood. If a particularly rapid response is needed, immature cells may also be released – this was described as 'a shift to the left' on a blood film before C-reactive protein (CRP) was available.

Phagocytosis is promoted and enhanced by serum factors termed **opsonins** (see Chapter 1, Fig. 1.19): IgG antibody, complement and mannan-binding lectin are the best opsonins. Non-opsonized bacteria can still be recognized and bound by phagocyte receptors – **pattern recognition receptors (PRRs)** – particularly those that are specific for sugars present in bacterial cell walls (mannose receptor), but also a variety of other pathogen-associated molecular patterns (PAMPS) (Fig. 2.3). Other receptors include CD14 that acts as a receptor for bacterial lipopolysaccharide (LPS); the integrin molecules CD11b/CD18, CD11c/CD18 that recognize several microbes including Leishmania, Bordetella, Candida and LPS; and Toll-like receptors (TLRs) that recognize a range of pathogens (see Chapter 1, section 1.2.2). Monocytes, dendritic cells and resident macrophages then **initiate inflammation** and also the adaptive immune response (see Chapter 1). **Phagocytic receptors (FcIgRs) and complement receptors (C3R)** are important for removal of bacteria before antigen-specific immune responses (T cells and antibody) have had a chance to develop.

Resident macrophages occur in the subepithelial tissues of the skin and intestine and line the alveoli of the lungs. Organisms that penetrate an epithelial surface will encounter these local tissue macrophages (sometimes referred to as 'histiocytes'). If invasion by microorganisms occurs via blood or lymph, then defence is provided by fixed macrophages lining the blood sinusoids of the liver (Kupffer cells), the spleen and the sinuses of lymph nodes. The interaction of macrophages with certain bacterial components leads to the production of an array of macrophage-derived cytokines, which non-specifically amplify inflammatory reactions (Fig. 2.3). Macrophages are able to engulf opsonized organisms as well as directly bind to certain pathogens by pattern recognition and other receptors.

Most pathogenic microorganisms have evolved methods of resisting phagocytic cells. Staphylococci produce potent extra-cellular toxins that kill phagocytes and lead to the **formation of pus**, so characteristic of these infections. Some microorganisms have substances on their cell surfaces that inhibit direct phagocytosis. Under these circumstances, phagocytosis can proceed effectively only when the bacteria are coated (opsonized) by IgG or IgM antibodies or complement. Other microorganisms, e.g. Mycobacterium tuberculosis, are effectively ingested by phagocytic cells but can resist intracellular killing.

2.2.2 Specific resistance

An antigen-specific immune response is conventionally classified into humoral and cell-mediated immunity (see Chapter 1). The relative importance of humoral versus cell-mediated

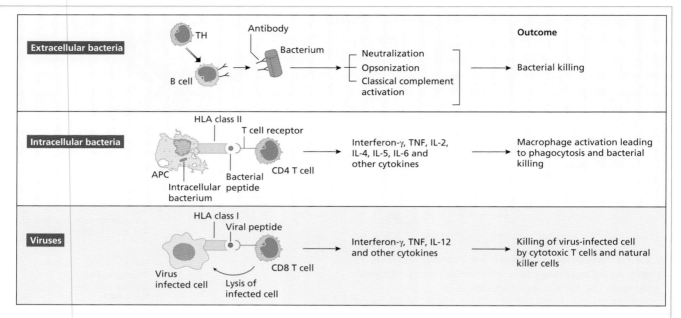

Fig. 2.4 Specific immune responses to microorganisms: an overview. APC, antigen-presenting cells; IL, interleukin; TNF, tumour necrosis factor.

immunity varies from infection to infection. Experimental animal models and naturally occurring immunodeficiencies in humans (see Chapter 3) demonstrate that *certain components of the immune response are essential for controlling particular infections* (Fig. 2.4 and Chapter 2, Fig. 3.2).

Individuals with **antibody deficiency** are prone to repeated infections with pyogenic bacteria (see Chapter 3), but immunoglobulin replacement therapy markedly reduces the frequency of these bacterial infections (Chapter 3, section 3.2.5). The course of infections with many viruses (such as varicella or measles) is normal in these patients.

T-lymphocyte function is more important than humoral immunity in both viral and intracellular bacterial infections. Patients with **impaired cell-mediated immunity** have difficulty in controlling and eradicating infections with viruses such as measles, varicella and herpes. They also show increased susceptibility to mycobacteria, pneumocystis, Listeria monocytogenes and some fungi. *Recurrent viral or fungal infections or infection by an unusual organism suggest the possibility of an underlying T-cell defect, either iatrogenically (as in chemotherapy or immunosuppression) or a (much rarer) primary immunodeficiency.*

Infections are discussed by type of organisms in this chapter. It is impossible to discuss the immune response to all pathogens, so only illustrative examples are given in each section.

2.3 Viral infection

2.3.1 Epstein–Barr virus infection

Infectious mononucleosis is caused by the Epstein–Barr virus (EBV), a member of the herpes group of viruses. By the age of 3 years, 99% of children in developing countries have been

Table 2.2 Patterns of antibodies to Epstein–Barr viral (EBV) antigens

Anti-VCA				
IgM	IgG	Anti-EA	Anti-EBNA	Interpretation
+	+	±	−	Primary infection (with/without symptoms)
−	+	−	+	Past EBV infection (>4 months)

EA, early antigen; EBNA, Epstein–Barr nuclear antigen; VCA, viral capsid antigen.

infected subclinically with EBV. In developed countries, clinically recognizable infection most frequently occurs in the 15–25-year age group; the virus is excreted in oropharyngeal secretions for some months and is responsible for person-to-person transmission.

The pattern of antibody responses to different **EBV antigens** helps to distinguish acute or subclinical infection from past EBV infection (Table 2.2). IgM antibodies to the viral capsid antigen (VCA) appear early in the course of infection; by the time symptoms of infectious mononucleosis develop, IgG antibody titres to VCA are also high; *however, testing of paired sera for a rise in antibody titre, used in the past for diagnosis of many viral infections, is not helpful.* Antibodies to EB nuclear antigen (EBNA) develop about 4 months after infection and remain for life. Antibodies to early antigen (EA) appear during primary infection in about 70% of patients and *were* considered an indicator of active infection until superseded by real-time polymerase chain reaction (RT-PCR) and measurement of EBV-viral load for the early diagnosis of infectious mononucleosis, particularly in cases with inconclusive serological results.

EBV is unique among human viruses in that it produces disease by **infecting and transforming B lymphocytes** via the CD21 molecule on the B-cell surface. Infected B cells proliferate like tumour cells, and small numbers may produce free virus, which can then transform other B lymphocytes. Up to half of the lymphoid cells from the tonsils of EBV-infected patients may be transformed. Primary EBV infection is **stopped by two defences**: a T-cell immune response capable of eliminating almost all virus-infected cells, and virus-neutralizing antibodies that prevent the spread of infection from one target cell to another. The characteristic 'atypical lymphocytes' are predominantly CD8⁺ cytotoxic T lymphocytes, which recognize and destroy EBV-infected B cells (Case 2.1).

The **importance of the immune response** to EBV is illustrated by (i) rare patients with EBV-specific failure of immunity; and (ii) the occurrence of EBV-induced malignant transformation of B cells in patients receiving immunosuppressive therapy (see Chapter 7, Case 7.2). In the first example, the X-linked 'lymphoproliferative syndrome' (XLP) affects males (aged 6 months to >20 years) who are unable to control EBV infection due to mutation in the gene encoding SAP (SLAM-associated protein). *SAP* mutations lead to a failure in signal transduction from the 'signalling lymphocyte activation molecule' (SLAM), which is present on the surface of T and B cells. Many patients with this syndrome die young unless they receive a human stem cell transplant; some die of lymphoma, some of aplastic anaemia, and others of haemophagocytic syndrome as part of their immunodeficiency.

Patients who receive immunosuppressive regimens, such as ciclosporin, antithymocyte globulin or monoclonal anti-T-cell antibodies following transplantation, also develop EBV tumours. These therapeutic agents are associated with **EBV reactivation**. About 1–10% of certain transplants are complicated by EBV-induced lymphoproliferative disease. Similarly, up to 2% of patients infected with human immunodeficiency virus (HIV) (Chapter 3) develop non-Hodgkin's lymphoma, but the incidence may be higher as many tumours are not found till post mortem (see Chapter 3, Case 3.10); EBV has been identified in most acquired immune deficiency syndrome (AIDS)-associated lymphomas.

Burkitt's lymphoma is a highly malignant, extranodal tumour of B lymphocytes also strongly associated with EBV infection. It is endemic in certain African countries, where it represents approximately 30–50% of childhood cancers, in contrast to 3% in developed countries. The link between EBV and Burkitt's lymphoma was substantiated by the demonstration of the EBV genome and EBV antigens in tumour cells. It is likely that Burkitt's lymphoma is due to EBV-induced lymphoproliferation in individuals rendered susceptible by chronic malaria. Proposed mechanisms for this failure to limit EBV infection include the ability of the malaria parasites to activate latently infected B cells with the emergence of a proliferating clone, and exhaustion of EBV-specific T-cell responses after repeated malaria infections in children. EBV infection in this setting leads to chromosomal translocation(s) with consequent activation of the c-myc oncogene, resulting in lymphoma.

2.3.2 Herpes viruses in general

The herpes virus group consists of at least 60 viruses, 8 of which commonly infect humans (Table 2.3). Two features of **pathogenesis** are common to all human herpes viruses. First, close physical contact must occur between infected and uninfected human individuals for transmission of virus and no other species is involved. 'Close contact' between cells, as occurs in blood transfusion or organ transplantation, provides potential routes of transmission for several herpes viruses – most notably cytomegalovirus (CMV). Second, after a primary infection, *herpes viruses persist in the host throughout life*.

To limit virus dissemination and prevent reinfection, the immune response must be able to stop virions entering cells, and to eliminate cells already infected in order to reduce virus shedding. Immunological reactions are thus of two kinds: those directed against the virion and those that act upon the virus-infected cell. In general, immune responses to the virion are predominantly humoral, while T-cell-mediated responses act on virus-infected cells. Antibodies and B cells see different epitopes from those seen by T cells. The major humoral mechanism involved is viral neutralization by antibody, but complement-mediated lysis of virus also occurs.

🔍 Case 2.1   Infectious mononucleosis

A 20-year-old carpet fitter presented with a 1-week history of a sore throat, stiffness and tenderness of his neck, and extreme malaise. On examination, he was mildly pyrexial with posterior cervical lymphadenopathy, palatal petechiae and pharyngeal inflammation without an exudate. Abdominal examination showed mild splenomegaly. There was no evidence of a skin rash or jaundice.

The clinical diagnosis of infectious mononucleosis ('glandular fever') was confirmed on investigation. His white cell count was 13×10^9/l (NR 4–10×10^9/l) with over 50% of the lymphocytes showing atypical morphology ('atypical lymphocytosis'). His serum contained IgM antibodies to Epstein–Barr viral capsid antigen (VCA), a common test for acute infectious mononucleosis (see Table 2.2). Liver function tests were normal.

He was treated symptomatically and was advised to avoid sporting activity until his splenomegaly had completely resolved, because of the danger of splenic rupture. Many patients show clinical or biochemical evidence of liver involvement and are recommended to abstain from alcohol for at least 6 months.

Table 2.3 Clinical aspects of herpes virus infections

	Clinical spectrum	Modes of transmission	Site of latency
Herpes simplex virus type 1 (HSV-1)	Acute gingivostomatitis Herpes labialis Keratoconjunctivitis Encephalitis Disseminated infection	• Oral–respiratory secretions • Skin contact	Trigeminal ganglion
Herpes simplex virus type 2 (HSV-2)	Genital herpes Meningitis Disseminated infection	• Sexual • Intrapartum	Sacral ganglion
Varicella zoster virus (VZV)	Herpes zoster Disseminated Herpes zoster Congenital varicella	• Oral–respiratory secretions • Skin contact • Congenital	Dorsal root ganglion
Cytomegalovirus (CMV)	Glandular fever-like syndrome Retinitis Pneumonia Hepatitis	• Oral–respiratory secretions • Sexual • Congenital • Intrapartum • Iatrogenic, e.g. blood • Transfusion, organ transplant	Leucocytes Epithelial cells of parotid salivary gland, cervix, renal tubules
Epstein–Barr virus (EBV)	Infectious mononucleosis Burkitt's lymphoma Nasopharyngeal carcinoma	• Oral–respiratory secretions	B lymphocytes Epithelial cells of nasopharynx
Human herpes virus type 6 (HHV-6)	Exanthema subitum Glandular fever-type syndrome	• Oral–respiratory secretions	Lymphocytes +/– salivary glands
Human herpes virus type 7 (HHV-7)	Exanthema subitum	• Oral–respiratory secretions	Lymphocytes
Human herpes virus type 8 (HHV-8)	Kaposi's sarcoma	• Via saliva and through sexual intercourse	Lymphocytes +/– salivary glands

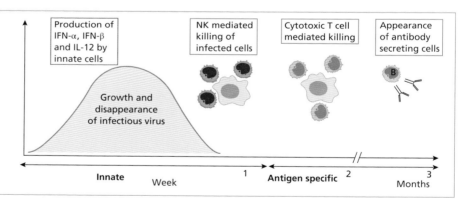

Fig. 2.5 Time sequence of immune response to viral infection. IFN, interferon; IL, interleukin; NK, natural killer.

Production of IFN-α, IFN-β and IL-12 by innate cells

NK mediated killing of infected cells

Cytotoxic T cell mediated killing

Appearance of antibody secreting cells

Growth and disappearance of infectious virus

Innate — Week — 1 — Antigen specific — 2 — 3 — Months

Viral neutralization prevents attachment of virus to target cell and is the function of IgG antibodies in the extracellular fluid, IgM in the blood and secretory IgG antibodies on mucosal surfaces. *Only antibodies to those viral components responsible for attachment are neutralizing.* The generation of antibodies of the correct specificity is therefore essential for an effective viral vaccine; antibodies to inappropriate antigens not only may fail to protect, but may actually provoke immune complex disease (see section 2.3.5).

Cell-mediated immunity is concerned with virus-infected cells rather than free virus. Virus-immune T lymphocytes recognize viral antigens in association with self-major histocompatibility complex (MHC) class I glycoproteins (see Chapter 1). Cytotoxic T (Tc) cells lyse virally modified cells and limit disease by stopping production of infectious progeny, along with natural killer (NK) cells. *T and NK cells are therefore concerned with recovery from virus infections;* containment of the initial infection is mediated by type I interferons (IFN-α and INF-β) (Fig. 2.5).

Most viral infections are self-limiting. Recovery from acute viral infections usually produces specific long-term immunity; secondary attacks by the same virus are uncommon and indicate immunodeficiency.

2.3.3 Direct effects of viruses

The clinical importance of viral infection *depends not only on the number of host cells destroyed, but also on the function of those cells.* Destruction of relatively few cells with highly specialized function, such as neurotransmission or immunoregulation, can be disabling or life threatening. In contrast, destruction of larger numbers of less specialized cells, such as epithelial cells, has less drastic results. In order to gain entry into specialized cells, viruses interact with specific receptors on host cells – **viral tropism**. For example, EBV uses the C3d receptor (CD21), HIV uses multiple receptors (CD4, chemokine receptors: CCR5, CXCR-4) and the SARS-coronavirus (SARS-CoV) uses angiotensin-converting enzyme (ACE)-2 in order to gain entry into target cells.

Once inside a cell, a **virus can kill the cell** in several ways. Some viruses, such as poliovirus or adenovirus or their products, can block enzymes needed for cell replication or metabolism, while others may disrupt intracellular structures, such as lysosomes, releasing lethal enzymes. Some viral proteins inserted into the cell membrane can alter its integrity: measles virus, for instance, possesses fusion activity and causes cells to form syncytia. Some viruses can **alter the specialized function** of a cell without killing it. Usually, such cells belong to the central nervous or endocrine systems; dementia caused by HIV infection is an example of both atrophy and loss of function.

Transformation of host cells may occur with certain viruses that are potentially *oncogenic* (Table 2.4). Mostly, these are viruses that establish latency. Cells from Burkitt's lymphoma, for instance, show a characteristic translocation between the long arms of chromosomes 8 and 14, suggesting that the tumour results from the translocation of the oncogene, c-myc, to an active region of the cellular genome (in this example, the locus for the immunoglobulin heavy chain). Human papilloma virus (HPV) oncogenicity is another example of viral transformation of host cells. The interaction of HPV E6 and E7 with critical cell cycle components is fairly well understood and leads to hyperplastic lesions (warts) or, when coupled with other mutations (e.g. through DNA damage through ultra-violet radiation), results in skin or cervical malignancies (Table 2.4).

Some viruses can **interfere with the immune response** by suppressing it or infecting cells of the immune system (Table 2.5). The best example of this phenomenon is AIDS (see Chapter 3), caused by HIV types 1 and 2 (HIV-1, HIV-2), which selectively infect and deplete CD4$^+$ T lymphocytes and macrophages. The resulting profound immunosuppression leads to the development of the severe, disseminated, opportunistic infections and tumours that characterize AIDS. Measles virus is a less well known but important example. Before widespread measles immunization and treatment for tuberculosis (TB) were available, outbreaks of acute measles infection were associated with the reactivation and dissemination of miliary TB, due to reduced T-cell-mediated immunity.

2.3.4 Viral strategies to evade the immune response

Viruses have evolved ingenious mechanisms for evading or interfering with immune responses. An important viral strategy for evasion is entry into a **latent state**. *All human herpes viruses can remain latent (see Table 2.3),* undergoing periodic cycles of activation and replication. The viral genome remains within the host cell, but no expression of viral antigens occurs. When the equilibrium between virus and host defence is upset, perhaps by other infections, metabolic disturbances, ageing or immunosuppression, the virus is no longer controlled, with subsequent expression of disease.

Table 2.4 Viruses and malignant disease

Malignancy	Virus
Certain T-cell leukaemias	Human T-cell leukaemia virus (HTLV-I)
Carcinoma of cervix	Herpes simplex (type 2) Human papilloma viruses (HPV)
Burkitt's lymphoma Hodgkin's disease Oropharyngeal carcinoma	Epstein–Barr virus (EBV) EBV HPV
Nasopharyngeal carcinoma	EBV
Skin cancer	HPV Merkel cell polyomavirus (MCV)
Hepatocellular carcinoma	Hepatitis B Hepatitis C
Kaposi's sarcoma	Human herpes virus 8 (HHV-8)

Table 2.5 Examples of viruses infecting cells of the immune system

Cell	Virus	Outcome
B lymphocytes	Epstein–Barr virus	Transformation and polyclonal B-cell activation
T lymphocytes	Measles Human T-cell leukaemia virus I	Replication in activated T cells T-cell lymphoma/ leukaemia
	Human immunodeficiency virus 1 and 2	Acquired immune deficiency syndrome
Macrophages	Dengue Lassa Marburg – Ebola	Viral haemorrhagic fevers

Varicella zoster (VZV) is a good example of a disorder caused by a virus that normally lies **latent** in the dorsal root ganglion, but becomes active when host immunity is impaired, to cause shingles as in Case 2.2, following prolonged corticosteroid therapy. Other herpes viruses may remain latent in other anatomically defined sites (see Table 2.3), for instance herpes simplex virus in the trigeminal ganglion (producing 'cold sores') and activated by sunlight, stress or intercurrent infection.

Other mechanisms of evading immune responses are given in Table 2.6. Antigenic variation is best illustrated by influenza A, an RNA virus surrounded by a lipid envelope with two inserted proteins – haemagglutinin and neuraminidase – against which most neutralizing antibodies are directed. The virus can evade antibody responses by modifying the structure of these proteins in two ways: antigenic drift and antigenic shift. **Antigenic drift** is minor structural change caused by point mutations altering an antigenic site on haemagglutinin. Such mutations probably account for the 'minor' epidemics of influenza occurring most winters. **Antigenic shift** is a major change in the whole structure of haemagglutinin or neuraminidase, which has caused periodic influenza pandemics in the past.

Case 2.2   Recurrent herpes zoster

A 72-year-old woman was commenced on oral corticosteroids for giant cell arteritis. Over the next 6 months she had three episodes of a painful, vesicular rash ('shingles') typical of herpes zoster, affecting the ophthalmic division of the right trigeminal nerve. Each episode was successfully treated with oral acyclovir, but she experienced considerable post-herpetic neuralgia. A steady improvement in her arteritic symptoms and inflammatory indices allowed a reduction in steroid dosage over a period of 6 months, with no further episodes of zoster.

Table 2.6 Mechanisms of immune evasion by viruses

Mechanism	Example
Non-expression of viral genome	Herpes simplex virus (latent in neurons)
Production of antigenic variants	Influenza, HIV
Inhibition of MHC expression	Adenovirus, cytomegalovirus
Mimicking MHC	Cytomegalovirus
Suppress NK activity	Cytomegalovirus
Induction of lymphocyte apoptosis	Cytomegalovirus
Production of inhibitory cytokines	EBV and IL-10

EBV, Epstein–Barr virus; HIV, Human immunodeficiency virus; IL-10, interleukin-10; MHC: major histocompatibility complex.

Viral persistence is a feature of certain viral infections. If the provoked immune response does not clear a virus, a low-grade infection with persistent shedding of infectious virus may result. For example, hepatitis C may persist for many months or years with continuous carriage in the liver if treatment is not successful, due to **continuous point mutations** limiting effective immune responses (Chapter 14).

Human cytomegalovirus (CMV) has evolved many mechanisms to evade the human immune system (Table 2.6).

2.3.5 Bystander damage caused by the immune response to viral infection

Although immunological reactions are usually beneficial, they can initiate or aggravate tissue damage (see Chapter 1, section 1.6) and this may be difficult to distinguish from viral damage. Such mechanisms in viral diseases are less well defined than in bacterial infections.

During recovery from some viral infections, such as infectious mononucleosis or hepatitis B, patients may develop circulating autoantibodies. Viral infections upset tolerance to self-antigens in two ways: (i) viruses, such as EBV, are polyclonal B-cell activators and may result in the production of autoantibodies; and (ii) the virus may combine with host antigens to form new antigens (see Chapter 1). Antibodies or activated T cells to these new antigens may recognize healthy host tissue as well as the virus-infected cells. Persistence of a viral infection may eventually cause **autoimmune disease** in susceptible individuals. Some patients, following hepatitis B infection, develop chronic autoimmune liver disease associated with T cells, or immune complex features such as vasculitis, arthropathy or glomerulonephritis associated with continued antibody production (see Chapter 14, section 14.7.2).

Some viruses induce production of **inappropriate antibodies** that facilitate viral entry to host target cells. Dengue virus, for instance, has evolved to infect macrophages efficiently via Fc receptors, and its capacity to enter the target cell is enhanced if it is bound to IgG antibodies. Consequently, a second infection by a different virus serotype may be potentiated by preexisting antibody. This is termed antibody-dependent enhancement of infection (ADEI).

The best example of **damage mediated by T cells** is hepatitis C virus (HCV) infection. Viral persistence is responsible for liver damage in that HCV-specific T cells induce hepatocellular damage during chronic HCV infection. Infiltration of the liver by CD8$^+$ and some CD4$^+$ cells producing interleukin (IL)-17, IL-22 or both results in entry of virus-specific inflammatory cells – Th17 inflammatory cells – into the liver. These T cells have high expression of the homing receptor CD161 and low levels of inhibitory receptors and upregulation of proteins for apoptosis (see Chapter 1, section 1.3.4), resulting in T-cell exhaustion. It has to be confirmed that numbers of specific HCV-Th17 cells correlate with fibrosis severity and intrahepatic inflammatory status, but serum IL-17 levels are high in chronic HCV-infected patients.

2.3.6 Speculative effects of viral infection

Chronic fatigue syndrome (CFS), also known as **myalgic encephalomyelitis (ME)**, is an illness of uncertain cause. CFS describes severe, prolonged, disabling fatigue, often associated with myalgia, and mood and sleep disturbance. The condition mainly affects adults between 20 and 50 years old, and women more frequently than men. A preceding infectious illness, such as EBV, CMV, Coxsackie B or HHV-6, is reported by many patients, but there is no convincing evidence for linkage to any recognized infectious agent. Depression is found in about 50% of patients and frequently precedes the physical symptoms. A similar syndrome ('long Covid') has been seen after SARS CoV2 infection.

The diagnosis of CFS is made entirely on clinical grounds in patients presenting with a characteristic symptom complex dominated by fatigue. While detailed laboratory investigation is unhelpful in most patients, it is important to be aware that patients with unrelated disorders, for example hypothyroidism or systemic lupus erythematosus, may occasionally present with severe fatigue.

A variety of immunological alterations have been reported in a few patients only, are inconsistent and are of uncertain significance. **No treatment**, including intravenous immunoglobulin, has proved reliably effective in the few controlled clinical trials conducted. *A programme of graded exercise significantly improves functional capacity and fatigue* (Case 2.3). The syndrome appears to be a disease of uncertain aetiology, prolonged duration and considerable morbidity, but no mortality.

🔍 Case 2.3 Chronic fatigue syndrome

A 25-year-old woman presented with a 6-month history of extreme lethargy and difficulty in concentration following a flu-like illness. She was unable to work as a physiotherapist and experienced considerable stress as a result of having to give up work. Clinical examination was unremarkable with the exception of globally reduced muscle strength; the rest of the neurological examination was normal. She was assessed by several specialists, who found no other explanation for her extreme lethargy. Investigations were normal. A diagnosis of chronic fatigue syndrome of unknown aetiology was made and a programme of graded exercises and cognitive behavioural therapy was recommended. Over the next 2 years she improved steadily, enabling her to resume employment.

2.4 Bacterial infection

2.4.1 Normal immune responses to bacterial infections

There are two major categories of bacterial antigens that provoke immune responses: **soluble (diffusible) products** of the cell (e.g. toxins) and **structural antigens** that are part of the bacterial cell (such as LPS). Many bacterial antigens contain lipid in association with cell-wall glycoproteins; the presence of lipid appears to potentiate the immunogenicity of associated antigens.

Most bacterial antigens are **T-cell dependent**, requiring helper T lymphocytes for the initiation of humoral and cell-mediated immunity. However, some bacterial antigens, particularly capsule polysaccharides, are relatively **T independent**: these are characterized by their high molecular weight and multiple, repeating antigenic determinants. In children, adequate antibody responses to these antigens can take 2–4 (sometimes even 6) years to develop. Consequently, younger children are susceptible to invasive disease caused by encapsulated bacterial pathogens that include pneumococci, Haemophilus influenza and meningococci (see Chapter 17, Case 17.1).

In the following discussion, streptococci are used as an example, but other bacteria provoke a similar immune response. β-Haemolytic streptococci (especially Group A) most commonly cause localized infection of the upper respiratory tract or skin, but they can, and do, infect almost any organ of the body. There are striking differences in the clinical features of streptococcal infection in patients of different ages, which probably reflect differences in **immune status** to this pathogen. The young infant presents with a mild illness of insidious onset, characterized by low-grade fever and nasal discharge. Pharyngeal signs are usually minimal. This picture contrasts sharply with the acute streptococcal tonsillitis seen in older children (Case 2.4) or adults. This more acute and localized response is probably due to previous exposure to the streptococcus and modification of the response by preformed antibodies to streptococcal toxins and enzymes.

Streptococcal antigens include **specific toxins** (streptolysins O and S and pyrogenic exotoxin), which lyse tissue and circulating cells (including leucocytes), **specific enzymes** (such as hyaluronidase and streptokinase), which promote the spread of infections, and **surface components** of the streptococcal cell wall (M protein and hyaluronic acid). All these proteins are immunogenic, but the M protein is the chief virulence factor.

Specific antibodies are slow to appear (4 days) and are unlikely to play a role in limiting acute primary streptococcal infection. *Antistreptolysin O (ASO) and antistreptococcal deoxyribonuclease B (anti-DNase B) are two streptococcal antibody tests for diagnostic use, but only in post-streptococcal disease to indicate previous infection.* The ASO titre is generally raised after throat infections, but not after skin infections; the anti-DNase B titre is a reliable test for both skin and throat infections and may therefore be useful in the diagnosis of post-streptococcal

Case 2.4 Acute bacterial tonsillitis

A 5-year-old boy presented to his general practitioner with a 36-h history of acute malaise, shivering and vague pains in his legs. For 12 h he had complained of a dry, sore throat and had vomited twice. He was febrile (temperature 40.2 °C) with a tachycardia of 140/min and tender, bilateral, cervical lymphadenopathy. His pharynx, tonsils and buccal mucosa were red and inflamed and his tonsils were studded with white areas of exudate. He was diagnosed as having acute bacterial tonsillitis and treated with phenoxymethyl penicillin for 5 days. A throat swab taken before starting antibiotics grew β-haemolytic streptococci (Group A). After 3 days of treatment, his temperature had returned to normal and he made an uneventful recovery. Haemolytic streptococcal infections illustrate an important point about bacterial infection – namely, that immune defences plus antibiotics cope satisfactorily with most bacterial infections in most people.

Box 2.1 Superantigen-associated diseases

Toxic shock syndrome
- Streptococcal
- Staphylococcal
- Clostridial (Clostridium perfringens)
- Yersinial (Yersinia enterocolitica)

Kawasaki disease
- No organism yet identified (superantigen association based on cytokine profile)
- Covid-induced multisystem inflammatory syndrome (adults and children)

Case 2.5 Streptococcal toxic shock syndrome

A 35-year-old man was admitted to hospital with a 7-day history of high fever, sore throat and a diffuse erythematous rash over the anterior chest wall. Additional findings on examination included hypotension (blood pressure 80/50 mmHg), conjunctival injection and cellulitis of both calves. Over the next 24 h there was increasing pain and swelling of the right calf associated with disappearance of the pedal pulse, necessitating emergency fasciotomies of the anterolateral and posterior compartments of the right leg. At operation, there was marked bulging of muscle in both compartments. Gram stain of the fluid obtained during fasciotomy showed Gram-positive cocci with an abundant growth of Group A β-haemolytic streptococci on muscle culture eventually. The same organism was also isolated from throat and blood cultures. Rapid exotoxin typing with a gene probe revealed pyrogenic exotoxins A and B.

A diagnosis of streptococcal toxic shock syndrome was made on the basis of the above findings. The patient made a full recovery following treatment with intravenous clindamycin.

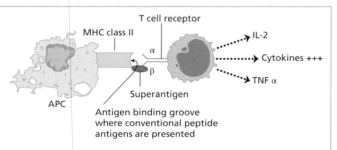

Fig. 2.6 Superantigen-induced T-cell stimulation. APC, antigen-presenting cells; IL, interleukin; MHC, major histocompatibility complex; TNF, tumour necrosis factor.

glomerulonephritis (see Chapter 9, section 9.5.2 for other specific antibodies for diagnosis). However, this assay has been largely superseded by rapid antigen tests and is less frequently used now.

Some products, such as endotoxin, are powerful **stimulators** of the immune response, leading to polyclonal activation of B lymphocytes. A modest rise in serum immunoglobulin levels in some prolonged infections is probably due to this polyclonal stimulation, since *increase in specific antibody forms only a very small proportion of the total immunoglobulin level.*

2.4.2 Bacteria as superantigens

Some streptococcal toxins are potent activators of T cells by virtue of their ability to act as **superantigens**. In contrast to conventional antigens, which are processed intracellularly, superantigens simultaneously activate large numbers of T cells carrying a particular T-cell receptor Vβ gene. They bind directly to MHC class II molecules at a site distinct from but close to the antigen-binding groove and subsequently to the Vβ chain of the T-cell receptor (Fig. 2.6). Since there are 50 different Vβ

genes in humans, a superantigen will react with ≥1: 50 T cells in contrast to a conventional peptide antigen, which will react only with the 1: 10^4 to 1: 10^8 antigen-specific T cells. **Widespread T-cell activation** with selective usage of certain T-cell receptor Vβ genes is a feature of superantigen-associated diseases (Box 2.1). Consequently, these disorders are characterized by marked cytokine release, high fever, hypotension and multisystem involvement (Case 2.5).

2.4.3 Bacterial evasion of immune defences

Bacteria survive in the untreated host only if immune responses kill them at a rate slower than the rate at which they multiply. Complete failure of defences is not needed for infection, only evasion or subversion of the immune response, and bacteria have evolved many mechanisms for achieving this (Table 2.7).

Bacterial capsules are important for long-term survival of pathogens: for instance, polysaccharide antigens of pneumococci and meningococci can inhibit phagocytosis; mucoid secretions prevent activation of the alternate pathway of complement.

Antigenic variation occurs in some bacterial infections. Patients infected by Borrelia recurrentis via a body louse bite experience relapsing fever. After a week or so, antibodies destroy the bacteria and the fever subsides. However, **antigenic variants** are formed that reach bacteraemic proportions 5–7 days later, with consequent relapse of the patient. Antibodies to these variants eliminate the bacteria and fever, but further variants are made again. The cycle recurs 5–10 times without antibiotics.

Some bacteria infecting mucous surfaces possess **proteases** that hydrolyse IgA antibody: these include Neisseria gonorrhoeae, N. meningitidis, Haemophilus influenzae and Streptococcus pneumoniae. Others (e.g. some staphylococci) produce enzymes (e.g. catalase) that prevent the bacteria being killed inside phagocytic cells.

Bacteria may survive by **sequestration** in non-phagocytic cells where they are not exposed to immune factors or some antibiotics. An example is the chronic carriage of Salmonella typhi in scarred, avascular areas of the gall bladder and urinary tract.

2.4.4 Bystander damage caused by the immune response to bacterial infection

It is often difficult to distinguish between the direct toxic effects of bacteria and the damage caused by immune reactions to bacterial antigens. This problem is illustrated by the complications of streptococcal infection (Fig. 2.7).

Rheumatic fever is a systemic illness that occurs 2–4 weeks following Group A β-haemolytic streptococcal pharyngitis, although fewer than 1% of untreated infections result in rheumatic fever. It is rare since the widespread use of antibiotics for bacterial infections. There is evidence of an underlying **genetic susceptibility**. Rheumatic fever clusters in families: 40–60% of patients in the US outbreaks in the 1990s had a family history of the disease. Rheumatic fever is three times more common in monozygotic than dizygotic

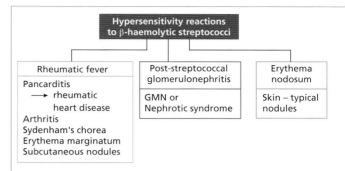

Fig. 2.7 Recognized complications of β-haemolytic streptococcal infection. Gmn, Glomerulonephritis.

twins, and several genome-wide association studies (GWAS) have revealed different alleles associated with an increased risk of disease.

The **pathogenesis of rheumatic fever** has **been** studied intensively. *Immunological mechanisms are important in the pathogenesis* (see Fig. 2.8).

Children with rheumatic fever have a high incidence of **antibodies to extracts of human heart**, suggesting that rheumatic carditis is caused by antibodies to Streptococcal M proteins cross-reacting with cardiac myosin and valvular endothelium (see Case 2.6). Streptococcal components or products probably start the tissue damage, since strains of streptococci that are 'rheumatogenic' show certain characteristics (Box 2.2). However, some patients with streptococcal sore throats develop the cross-reacting antibodies without subsequent cardiac disease, while in animals passive transfer of the antibodies alone has no demonstrable effect on the target organ, suggesting that **prior damage by streptococcal products** is required for antibodies then to cause damage. Rheumatic fever is not confined to the myocardium (see Fig. 2.7) and lesions are found in heart valves, joints, blood vessels, skin and, in the related condition of chorea, in the central nervous system. It is probable that most of the damage is antibody mediated, since cross-reactivity has been demonstrated unequivocally (Box 2.2).

The relationship of streptococcal infection to **acute post-streptococcal glomerulonephritis** differs from that in rheumatic fever in two important respects. Glomerulonephritis seems to occur only after infection with one of the few 'nephritogenic' strains, whereas several but not all serotypes of Group A streptococcus are associated with rheumatic fever. Available evidence suggests that post-streptococcal glomerulonephritis is caused by deposition of circulating immune complexes and not by cross-reacting antibodies (see Chapter 9). The two conditions are only rarely associated with each other in epidemics that are caused by a single strain of a known M serotype, *suggesting individual host susceptibility*.

Table 2.7 Some mechanisms of immune evasion by bacteria

- Capsular polysaccharide – antiphagocytic role
- Mucoid secretions – decreases alternate pathway complement activity
- Antigenic variation – tick-borne relapsing fever due to Borrelia recurrentis
- Proteases – render mucosal IgA ineffective
- Sequestration in non-phagocytic cells – provides shelter from immune response

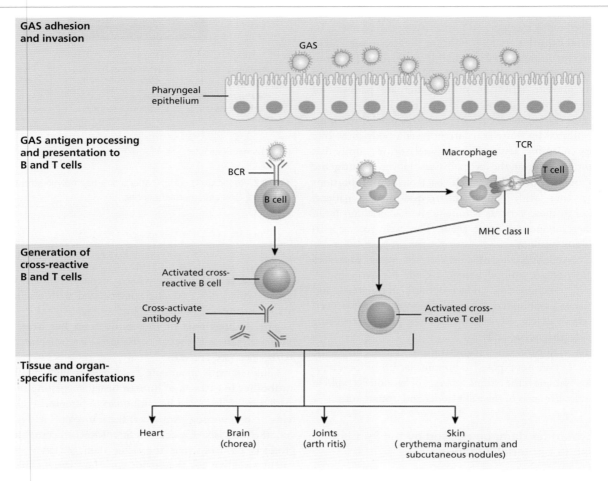

Fig. 2.8 Following Group A Streptococcus (GAS) adhesion to and invasion of the pharyngeal epithelium, GAS antigens activate both B and T cells. Molecular mimicry between GAS group A carbohydrate or serotype-specific M protein and the host heart, brain or joint tissues can lead to an autoimmune response, which causes the major manifestations of acute rheumatic fever (ARF). BCR, B-cell receptor; MHC, major histocompatibility complex; TCR, T-cell receptor. Source: Carapetis, J. R., et al. (2016). Acute rheumatic fever and rheumatic heart disease. *Nature Reviews Disease Primers*, 2(1), 15084. Reproduced with permission of Springer Nature.

Case 2.6   Rheumatic heart disease

A 38-year-old labourer presented with a 3-month history of progressive shortness of breath on effort. Exertion was often associated with central chest pain and irregular palpitations. He had twice woken from sleep with attacks of frightening breathlessness and was unable to lie flat. His general health was good, with no weight loss or anorexia. He had been told that he had suffered from rheumatic fever when he was 9 years old.

On examination, he had the typical physical signs of congestive cardiac failure due to underlying mitral valve stenosis and rheumatic heart disease. There was no evidence of bacterial endocarditis. On treatment with digoxin, diuretics and anticoagulants, his exercise tolerance improved dramatically and cardiac surgery was postponed. Antibiotic cover was provided for any dental or surgical treatment, in order to prevent the development of subacute bacterial endocarditis.

Other examples for diseases in which bacteria can trigger a self-damaging immune response are given in Table 2.8.

2.5 Mycobacterial infection

2.5.1 Mycobacterial infections

Mycobacterium tuberculosis is an *obligate intracellular pathogen* that is responsible for causing 1.5 million deaths each year, and an estimated 10 million new cases annually, so that >2 billion people are estimated to be infected worldwide. How many apparently healthy individuals have latent (post-primary) TB is not known. Only a proportion of infected individuals develop overt disease, underlining the critical role of the host's cellular immune response in successfully containing primary infection, though latent TB remains a future risk. Several risk factors for the development of active disease, including malnutrition, have been identified (Table 2.9). Infection commonly occurs by inhalation,

Box 2.2 Evidence for the involvement of antibodies in the pathogenesis of rheumatic fever

'Rheumatogenic' strains of streptococci:

- are confined to certain M serotypes only
- are heavily encapsulated and form mucoid colonies on culture
- resist phagocytosis by inhibiting alternate complement pathway activation.

'Rheumatogenic' strains of streptococci are cross-reactive between:

- streptococcal Group A carbohydrate and the heart valve glycoprotein
- M protein, cardiac sarcolemma and cardiac myosin
- another cell-wall component and human brain
- a cell-wall glycoprotein and the glomerular basement membrane
- streptococcal hyaluronidase and human synovium

Table 2.8 Examples of diseases caused by immune reactions to bacterial antigens

Immune reactions	Diseases
Cross-reacting antigens (type II hypersensitivity)	
Human heart and Group A streptococci	Rheumatic carditis
Human brain and Group A streptococci	Sydenham's chorea
Association of infective antigen with autoantigens (type II hypersensitivity)	
Mycoplasma antigens and erythrocytes	Autoimmune haemolytic anaemia
Immune complex formation (type III hypersensitivity)	
Subacute bacterial endocarditis Infected ventriculoatrial shunts	Vasculitis, arthritis, glomerulonephritis
Secondary syphilis Gonococcal septicaemia Meningococcal septicaemia	Vasculitis, arthritis
Delayed hypersensitivity reactions (type IV hypersensitivity)	
Tuberculosis	Pulmonary cavitation and fibrosis
Leprosy	Peripheral neuropathy

Table 2.9 Risk factors for the development of tuberculosis

- Impaired cellular immunity
- Human immunodeficiency virus infection
- Immunosuppressive therapy
- Advanced age
- Protein calorie malnutrition
- Alcoholism
- Tobacco smoking
- Intravenous drug abuse

Case 2.7 Tuberculosis

A 25-year-old Asian man was referred to his local chest clinic with a history of a cough and loss of weight over the preceding 6 months. He had lived in the UK for the past 7 years and a chest X-ray taken immediately prior to entry into the UK was reportedly normal.

On examination, left apical crackles were noted on auscultation of his chest and a chest X-ray revealed left apical shadowing with cavitation. His sputum contained Mycobacterium tuberculosis and a skin test with tuberculin was strongly positive. He was promptly treated with standard antituberculous therapy and made a full recovery. The local public health department was notified, who undertook contact tracing.

This patient presented with latent TB, a common form of the disease, which occurs as a result of reactivation of quiescent endogenous primary infection or exogenous reinfection. Since the policy of screening new immigrants in many countries now includes IFN release assays (see section 2.5.2 and Chapter 19), latent TB is detected and individuals treated with 6 months of therapy on arrival.

resulting in pulmonary disease; a few patients develop gastrointestinal disease following ingestion of the bacterium. Dissemination of infection beyond the lungs is uncommon in latent disease, as in Case 2.7, but bacilli may spread systemically to lymph nodes, the genitourinary tract, spine, joints, meninges and pericardium in immunocompromised patients, including those receiving immunosuppressive therapies for autoimmune diseases and HIV patients or malnourished individuals.

The incidence of active TB is high in regions of the world in which HIV is prevalent. The risk of developing TB is estimated to be between 15 and 22 times greater in people infected with HIV than among those without HIV infection. In 2018, 251 000 people are estimated to have died of TB and HIV co-infection. This is due to the immunosuppression by HIV affecting the cells required to contain M. tuberculosis, namely CD4+ cells (see section 3.5.2), as well as the high concordance of both conditions.

TB is a treatable and curable disease. Active, drug-susceptible TB is treated with a standard 6-month course of four antimicrobial drugs, but with the increase in multiresistant strains, there are now concerted efforts by international agencies to tackle this combined problem; not least as the only vaccine against TB, Bacillus Calmette–Guerin (BCG), is not only contraindicated in HIV as a live vaccine, but is not effective against pulmonary TB even if given prior to HIV infection.

Two other mycobacterial species are prominent human pathogens. **Mycobacterium leprae** is currently responsible for 5.5 million cases of leprosy worldwide, causing considerable morbidity in the developing world. The severity and extent of disease in leprosy are closely related to the host immune response. Robust cellular immunity leads to localized tuberculoid leprosy affecting skin and nerves with few bacilli and vigorous granuloma formation. In contrast, patients with poor cellular immunity develop disseminated, bacteraemic lepromatous disease (see later Fig. 2.10). **Mycobacterium avium-intracellulare (MAC)** is an ubiquitous environmental mycobacterium that is handled satisfactorily by immunocompetent individuals, but causes disseminated disease in patients with advanced HIV infection (CD4 T cell count <50/mm^3). MAC is estimated to affect 50% of patients with HIV disease and its increasing prominence is a direct result of the HIV epidemic.

2.5.2 Mycobacteria and the normal immune response

Protection against mycobacterial infection is crucially dependent on **intact macrophage and T-cell function**. On entry into the body, mycobacteria are taken up by alveolar macrophages into phagosomes, but, unlike other extracellular bacteria, the phagosome infected with mycobacteria does not fuse with the lysosome to destroy the pathogen. Mycobacterial epitopes are processed by dendritic cells (activated in the lung via pattern recognition receptors) and transported to local lymph nodes

for presentation to T cells. Once activated, CD4$^+$ and CD8$^+$ cells migrate back to the lung, where IFN-γ secretion activates monocytes and macrophages that have been attracted by the local inflammation. Several pieces of evidence point to the important role played by CD4 and CD8 T cells and the effects of Th1 cytokines – particularly IFN-γ – in controlling mycobacterial infection (Box 2.3).

Presentation of mycobacterial antigens to T cells at the site of infection triggers clonal expansion and cytokine release (Fig. 2.9). The pattern of **cytokine release** is an important determinant in controlling infection. Cellular response with the predominant cytokine profile characterized by interleukin (IL)-12, IL-23, IFN-γ and tumour necrosis factor (TNF) leads to antigen-presenting cell (APC) and T-cell interaction,

---

Box 2.3   Evidence that T cells and Th1 cytokines are crucial in protection against mycobacterial infection

- Patients with HIV infection are particularly prone to Mycobacterium tuberculosis and M. avium-intracellulare (MAC) infection.
- Patients with primary defects in interferon (IFN)-γ receptor or (IFN)-γ/IL-12 production are prone to MAC infection.
- IFN-γ is effective as adjunctive therapy in patients with resistant MAC infection.
- Deletion of the gene for IFN-γ renders mice susceptible to low doses of M. tuberculosis.
- Mice deficient in CD8 T cells, due to deletion of the gene for β$_2$-microglobulin, are unable to control M. tuberculosis infection.
- Patients treated with biological agents that neutralize TNF (anti-TNF, soluble TNF receptor) have a significant risk of developing tuberculosis.

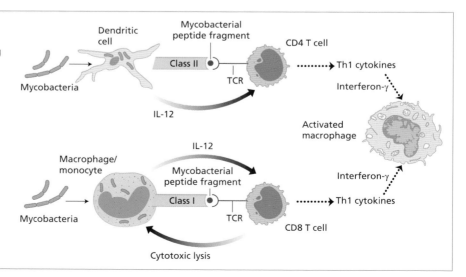

Fig. 2.9 Diagrammatic representation of immune response to mycobacteria resulting in activated macrophages killing intracellular organisms too. IL-12, interleukin-12; TCR, T-cell receptor.

macrophage activation and granuloma formation, enabling immunocompetent individuals to contain disease.

The pivotal role of IFN-γ in the immune response to mycobacteria has been exploited by the development of IFN-γ assays for the **diagnosis of latent TB**. The production of IFN-γ by a patient's T cells on exposure to M. tuberculosis antigen ESAT-6 (Early Secretory Antigenic Target-6) has been shown to be a more reliable marker of latent infection with M. tuberculosis than conventional skin testing with tuberculin.

Not all individuals who are exposed develop TB, but the reasons for this are unclear at present. Although some **genes** are known to play a role in the severity of the immune response – particular TNF alleles are associated with excessive granuloma formation – this was not one of the eight independent loci identified in the GWAS.

2.5.3 Mycobacterial evasion of the immune response

Macrophages fulfil a dual role in the immune response to mycobacteria by acting as **reservoirs of infection**, as well as being fundamental in destruction of the bacteria. The balance between these two opposing functions determines the outcome of infection. Disease-causing strains of mycobacteria are particularly adept at evading the host immune response using a variety of strategies (Table 2.10).

Phagocytes engulf M. leprae and M. tuberculosis via complement receptors; from the microbial perspective, this confers a **survival advantage,** since it avoids triggering the oxidative burst and therefore protects bacteria from exposure to damaging oxygen radicals. Once engulfed, disease-causing mycobacterial strains inhibit macrophage activation by the possession of 'inert' lipoarabinomannan, a cell-wall carbohydrate that inhibits release of IFN-γ and TNF. Additional survival strategies adopted by mycobacteria include inhibition of phagolysosome formation, invasion of the cytoplasm of macrophages and shelter within non-professional phagocytes.

2.5.4 Damage caused by the immune response to mycobacteria

A vigorous immune response to mycobacteria may sometimes have undesirable consequences by way of **tissue damage**. This is well

illustrated by the immune response in patients with leprosy, since the clinical spectrum of disease in leprosy correlates well with the host immune response to M. leprae (Fig. 2.10).

A vigorous cellular immune response characterized by Th1 cytokine release and strong granuloma formation limits spread of M. leprae, but produces tissue damage. For example, patients with tuberculoid leprosy develop disabling neuropathies as a direct result of **granulomatous inflammation**, despite having paucibacillary disease. In patients with disease of intermediate severity (borderline tuberculoid, borderline lepromatous), spontaneous improvement in cellular immunity is associated with perineural and skin inflammation, due to entry of T cells secreting IFN-γ. These so-called reversal reactions require prompt treatment with corticosteroids to avert further nerve damage.

Paradoxically, treatment of patients with a heavy bacillary load, as in lepromatous leprosy, may result in **erythema nodosum leprosum (ENL)**, an immune-complex-mediated reaction (type III hypersensitivity) characterized by high fever, glomerulonephritis, rash, iritis and nerve pain. Release of mycobacterial antigens during antituberculous therapy leads to formation of circulating immune complexes with systemic deposition. Thalidomide is particularly effective at controlling ENL reactions by means of its anti-TNF effect.

2.5.5 Prevention of tuberculosis

BCG has been available since the 1920s and it reduced disseminated TB and TB meningitis in children and infants. It is protective against multiresistant TB (those bacteria resistant to antituberculous drugs), which is rapidly increasing worldwide, as well as to non-tuberculous atypical mycobacteria (such as MAC) because of BCG cross-reactivity. Nevertheless, there are considerable problems associated with BCG. As a live vaccine it is not suitable for immunosuppressed individuals such as HIV+ persons, those taking immunosuppressive drugs for autoimmunity or after transplantation, or infants with severe combined immune deficiencies (SCID). In these individuals, BCG immunization results in disseminated BCG disease, which is difficult to treat and can be fatal. Attempts to make new, more effective, safer vaccines are under intense investigation.

Prevention of TB with drugs, known as **chemoprophylaxis**, can reduce the risk of a first episode of active disease in

Table 2.10 Mechanisms of immune evasion by mycobacteria
• Engulfment via complement receptors – avoids triggering respiratory burst
• Inhibition of macrophage activation by lipoarabinomannan
• Inhibition of phagolysosome formation
• Invasion of macrophage cytoplasm – provides protection from killing by phagolysosome
• Invasion of non-professional phagocytes, e.g. Schwann cells by M. leprae

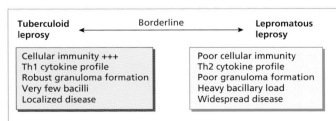

Fig. 2.10 Clinical spectrum of disease in leprosy in relation to immune response.

those exposed to infection or with latent TB. The World Health Organization recommends isoniazid should be taken daily for at least 6 months and preferably 9 months in those at particular risk following exposure (HIV+ patients, infants and children aged less than 4 years old, those on immunosuppression or those with diabetes or chronic renal failure). This policy has been difficult to implement due to failure of compliance by those already taking considerable amounts of medication for their underlying disease (see Chapter 3).

2.6 Fungal infection

2.6.1 Mechanisms of immunity to fungal infections

Fungi cause many diseases, which can be **classified** into superficial, subcutaneous or deep mycoses (Table 2.11). In superficial mycoses, the skin or mucous membranes are the main sites of the attack, while subcutaneous mycoses involve adjacent tissues, such as skin or bone. The term systemic mycosis describes deeper invasion of tissues with involvement of organs such as liver, lung or brain. Fungi causing systemic infections are usually divided into two groups: pathogenic and opportunistic fungi. The term pathogen implies that infection may result from contact with the organism in any individual, *whereas the opportunistic mycoses usually occur only in immunosuppressed hosts.*

Candida infection has been chosen as an example in this discussion, since it is an ubiquitous fungus that frequently causes **superficial infection** in normal hosts. Candida albicans is commonly found in the vagina (see Case 2.8) and in the

gastrointestinal tract from the mouth to the anus. The intact skin and mucous membranes present a formidable barrier to the fungus. Although the pH, temperature and skin-shedding rate are important, the normal bacterial flora probably play the critical role in preventing fungal colonization and subsequent invasion. Disturbances of gastrointestinal ecology, through the use of antibiotics or via traumatic or hormonal changes, are important predisposing factors in many cases of chronic superficial candida infection. Superficial candida is a common infection in otherwise healthy infants, but is severe in those with primary T-cell defects, untreated HIV+ individuals and those patients on immunosuppressive, antibiotic or steroid therapies.

Chronic mucocutaneous candidiasis (CMC) is a disease of repeated or persistent symptomatic mucocutaneous infections caused by C. albicans, affecting the nails, skin and oral mucosae, starting in childhood. Molecular study of these patients has enabled identification of genes involving the **IL-17 pathway**, which indicates that IL-17 cytokines are crucial for mucocutaneous protection against C. albicans. These include IL-17RA deficiency, IL-17F deficiency and gain-of-function variants of STAT1 that result in impairment of IL-17-producing T cells, failure to control candida and ongoing inflammation. Heterozygous gain-of-function variants in STAT1 were recently identified as a cause of CMC; as with STAT3 variants in hyper-IgE syndrome, the associated candidal susceptibility appears secondary to Th17-cell deficiency. The mechanistic link between STAT1 activity and diminished Th17 cells has yet to be clearly defined. Moreover, in these patients autoimmune complications also occur, which are driven by the immunodysregulation in CMC.

Candida infections may be part of a **wider syndromic disease** – such as autosomal dominant hyper-IgE syndrome (AD-HIES; see Chapter 3), and autosomal recessive autoimmune polyendocrinopathy syndrome type I due to AIRE mutations, in which patients also have autoimmunity but are not susceptible to any other infectious disease (see Chapter 5). Variants in STAT3 were identified in 2007 as the cause of AD-HIES, an unusual complex immunodeficiency with marked inflammation

Table 2.11 Some examples of fungal infection in humans

Infection	Clinical presentation
Superficial	
Trichophyton rubrum	Ringworm Athlete's foot
Candida albicans	Vulvo-vaginitis, oral thrush
Subcutaneous	
Sporotrichium schenkii	Ulceration, abscess formation
Systemic	
Histoplasma capsulatum	Pulmonary infection
Coccidioides immitis	Acute pneumonitis
Candida albicans	Bronchopulmonary disease, oesophagitis
Cryptococcus neoformans	Meningitis, solid lung lesions
Aspergillus fumigatus	Aspergilloma, cerebral abscess, eye infections
Pneumocystis jiroveci	Pneumonia

Case 2.8 Acute vulvo-vaginitis

A 27-year-old woman presented with a 4-week history of severe irritation and soreness of her vulva. For 2 weeks she had experienced burning pain on micturition but no frequency. In addition, she had a thick, creamy-white vaginal discharge. Her menstrual periods were regular and she was taking the oral contraceptive pill. On examination, her general condition was good. She had marked erythema of her vulva and vaginal mucosa, with white plaques. The appearances were those of acute vulvo-vaginitis. A vaginal swab showed masses of pseudohyphae, with a profuse growth of Candida albicans on culture. She was treated with oral miconazole with rapid symptomatic relief.

and structural abnormalities. STAT3 is essential for the production of many cytokines, including IL-6, IL-10, IL-11, IL-17, IL-21, IL-22 and IL-23. It therefore has a central role both proinflammatory (e.g. IL-6) and antiinflammatory (e.g. IL-10) processes. STAT3 is also important for particular organ development and this may account for the multiple abnormalities of lungs, teeth, facies, skin and blood vessels seen in **HIES patients**. This is not the whole story, however, as there is no correlation between the genetic findings and the clinical features (genotype–phenotype correlation) in many of the features of HIES, so other genes will be important. Variants in STAT3 lead to failure of Th17 CD4 cell differentiation, a feature of several conditions with low Th17 cells and candidal infection. Understanding this condition has led to the realization that IL-17 signalling is also involved in S. aureus skin infections and that IL-22 and IL-17 play a role in protection against staphylococcal and candidal infections by upregulating human beta-defensin 2 and CC-chemokine ligand 20 (CCL20), both antimicrobial proteins. These proteins are important in atopic dermatitis and gingivitis, also common clinical features in HIES.

Polymorphisms that relate to susceptibility to Candida have also been identified in two other genes, CARD9 and Dectinl, in association with impairment of IL-17 production. A clue to the pathogenesis of some of these conditions was the finding that high levels of **neutralizing autoantibodies** directed against IL-17A, IL-17F and/or IL-22 were found in late presenting patients without AIRE mutations in which CMC is the only major infection.

A *change in systemic immune responses* is the major factor governing **susceptibility to invasive fungal infection**. Colonization of the susceptible host can occur when the fungus gains access via breaks in the skin or mucosae, via indwelling cannulae (especially if hypertonic solutions of glucose and amino acids are being infused) or via urinary catheters. *Cell-mediated immunity appears to be the most important effector mechanism* in these systemic infections, since disseminated fungal infection is a feature only in patients with impaired T cells (primary immune deficiencies or secondary to HIV) or neutrophils, although rare in antibody deficiency.

2.6.2 Bystander damage caused by immune reactions to fungi

There are several possible **outcomes** of fungal infection. Usually, the specific immune response to the fungus, coupled with topical antifungal drugs, eliminates superficial infection. In contrast, *systemic opportunistic fungal infection carries a high mortality rate in the immunosuppressed host,* an outcome only partly improved by the use of newer prophylactic and therapeutic antifungal agents.

There is a third possible outcome. If the fungus is not successfully eliminated, or causes persistent reinfection, then the host's immune response to fungal antigen may trigger a hypersensitivity reaction. For example, Aspergillus fumigatus infection can pre-

sent in a disseminated form or as a persistent aspergilloma, in which the fungus grows in preexisting lung abnormalities (following asthma, successful treatment of pulmonary tuberculosis or bronchiectasis). Allergic bronchopulmonary aspergillosis can occur in those patients who are atopic, as this is due to **IgE-mediated hypersensitivity** to Aspergillus antigens. Bronchi may be obstructed by fragmented mycelia, and there is an inflammatory reaction in the bronchial wall with eosinophilic infiltration. Clinically, the condition usually presents as recurrent episodes of increased wheezing, coughing, fever and pleuritic pain in an asthmatic (see Chapter 13, Case 13.4).

If fungal antigens are inhaled by someone with **preformed precipitating antibodies**, then antigen–antibody complexes may form in the respiratory tract. One example is farmer's lung, a condition resulting from an immune-complex-mediated hypersensitivity response to a fungus (Micropolyspora faeni) present in mouldy hay (see Chapter 13, Case 13.5).

2.7 Parasitic infection

2.7.1 Protozoal infection

Protozoa are a diverse group of parasites. In this section, malaria (Case 2.9), leishmaniasis and trypanosomiasis, which globally constitute a huge burden of parasitic disease, are used to illustrate the immunological interactions between host and parasite.

If parasites **elude** the host's immune response and are sufficiently virulent, they kill the host upon whom their own survival depends; yet, if they are too easily destroyed by the immune response, their own survival is jeopardized. The evolution of humans, in the face of selection pressures associated with parasitic infections, and the evolution of parasites in the face of destruction by host immune responses enable this balance to persist.

Natural selection has enabled **human mutations** in response to malaria to allow survival of infected individuals. The sickle-cell haemoglobin gene confers partial resistance to P. falciparum and limits its multiplication within erythrocytes. Thus, people with the normal haemoglobin genotype (Hb AA) are highly susceptible to falciparum malaria; those with the homozygous sickle-cell genotype (Hb SS) suffer serious and usually lethal sickle-cell anaemia; but those with heterozygous sickle-cell trait (Hb AS) have a survival advantage, particularly in endemic malarial areas. A number of other genetic polymorphisms (rather than disease causing mutations) are associated with resistance to malaria, including HLA-B53 and the absence of the red cell Duffy antigen, which is the receptor for P. vivax.

2.7.2 Normal immune responses to protozoa

Patients react to protozoal infection with a spectrum of responses similar to those evoked by other microbes. An early response is **activation of macrophages** and monocytes with release of cytokines, including TNF, IL-1 and IL-6. Their

Case 2.9 Cerebral malaria

A 44-year-old Nigerian man was admitted as an emergency while visiting relatives in England. His symptoms began 4 days after arrival, and over the following 10 days he deteriorated progressively, with vague upper abdominal pain, sweating, rigors and vomiting. In the past, he had been treated twice for malaria but had never taken malarial prophylaxis. On examination he was ill and jaundiced, with a temperature of 39.2 °C. His blood pressure was 90/70 mmHg but he showed no signs of visceral perforation. The differential diagnosis included occult gastrointestinal bleeding, septicaemia, hepatitis or recurrence of malaria.

Emergency investigations showed a normal haemoglobin (140 g/l) and a white cell count of 6.1 × 10⁹/l. Sickle-cell anaemia was excluded by normal haemoglobin electrophoresis. However, a thick blood film showed a heavy infestation with Plasmodium falciparum. After consultation with a specialist centre, the patient was treated with intravenous artesunate. Unfortunately, his condition rapidly deteriorated over the next 30 h. Terminally, he suffered a cardiac arrest and could not be resuscitated. The post-mortem diagnosis was cerebral malaria.

combined actions cause fever, leucocytosis and production of acute-phase reactants such as CRP. The fever response may itself be a host defence since, for example, certain stages of malarial parasite development are sensitive to elevated temperatures.

Although IgM and IgG **antibodies** are made in response to most adult protozoa, these antibodies are not necessarily protective, making it difficult to produce an effective vaccine. Furthermore, some protozoa penetrate and survive within host cells: examples include the malarial parasite Plasmodium, which invades erythrocytes and hepatocytes, and Leishmania, which survives inside macrophages. Such intracellular protozoa are not accessible to antibodies unless protozoal antigens are also secreted onto the host cell surface.

The role of **cell-mediated immunity** has proved difficult to evaluate in these diseases in humans. In mice, resistance to infection with several intracellular pathogens (mycobacteria, leishmania, salmonella) is controlled by a gene expressed only in reticuloendothelial cells called the natural-resistance-associated macrophage protein 1 gene (Nramp 1). In addition, sensitized T cells and IFN-γ are important determinants of immunity against protozoa that survive within macrophages, e.g. leishmania, as in TB. A predominant Th1 cytokine profile (IFN-γ, IL-2, TNF, IL-12) is associated with localized disease in the form of cutaneous leishmaniasis, while disseminated visceral disease occurs in individuals with a Th2 cytokine profile. In such cases, addition of IFN-γ to conventional antileishmania treatment (still pentavalent antimony compounds first introduced in the 1930s) hastens recovery.

2.7.3 Protozoal evasion of immune responses

There are three main ways in which protozoa can evade or modify the host's immunological attack (Table 2.12): antigenic variation; blunting the attack by immune suppression; or hiding in cells where the immune attack is less effective.

Antigenic variation is the most striking example of successful adaptation and is exemplified by sleeping sickness; this is caused by Trypanosoma brucei and spread by the bite of the tsetse fly. After infection, the number of parasites in the blood fluctuates in a cycle of parasitaemia – remission and recrudescence. This is due to destruction of trypanosomes by host antibody, followed by the emergence of parasites expressing different surface antigens (or variant surface glycoproteins, VSGs). *Antibodies produced after each wave of parasitaemia are specific for that set of VSGs only.* The parasite possesses a number of genes that code for its VSGs and can vary the genes used. The antibodies do not trigger the switch; it occurs spontaneously. By varying the immunodominant antigen, the parasite diverts its host's attack. This type of antigenic variation is known as phenotypic variation and is in contrast to genotypic variation, in which a new genetic strain periodically results in an epidemic, as is the case with influenza virus.

Other protozoa can rapidly change their surface coat to elude the immune response, a process known as **antigenic modulation**.

Table 2.12 Mechanisms of protozoal survival

Mechanism	Examples of disease
Host variation	
• Genetic factors	Malaria
• Suppression of host immunity	Malaria, leishmaniasis, schistosomiasis
• Active induction of IL-10-producing CD25⁺ regulatory T cells to prevent parasite clearance	Leishmaniasis
• Inhibition of IL-12 production	Leishmaniasis
• Inhibition of dendritic cell function	Leishmaniasis, trypanosomiasis, malaria
Parasite variation	
• Antigenic variation	Trypanosomiasis, malaria
• Antigenic modulation	Leishmaniasis
• Antigenic disguise	Schistosomiasis
• Premunition	Schistosomiasis
• Resistance to macrophage killing	Leishmaniasis
	Toxoplasmosis
	Trypanosomiasis
• Resistance to complement-mediated lysis	Leishmaniasis
	Trypanosomiasis

Within minutes of exposure to antibodies, Leishmania parasites can remove ('cap off') their surface antigens, so becoming refractory to the effects of antibodies and complement.

Suppression of the immune response is one of the most obvious adaptive mechanisms for protozoal survival and has been found in all parasitic infections in which it has been sought. The most striking examples occur in malaria and visceral leishmaniasis. Soluble antigens released by the parasite inhibit non-specifically the host's immune response by acting directly on lymphocytes or by saturating the reticuloendothelial system. Leishmania and Trypanosoma have stages that are refractory to complement-mediated lysis. Trypanosoma cruzi, for instance, produces molecules that either inhibit the formation or accelerate the decay of C3 convertases, so blocking complement activation on the parasite surface. Leishmania can downregulate MHC class I expression on parasitized macrophages, reducing the effectiveness of cytotoxic CD8+ T cells.

Some protozoa, including Toxoplasma, Leishmania and T. cruzi, not only easily enter but **survive and grow inside macrophages**, similar to mycobacteria. Infective Leishmania bind C3 actively and these serve as a molecule for binding the parasite to CR3 receptors for entry into macrophages. Monoclonal antibodies to the CR3 receptor inhibit uptake of the parasite into a safe haven. Like mycobacteria, Toxoplasma has evolved mechanisms to prevent fusion of phagocytic vacuoles (with the parasite) with lysosomes. Trypanosomes are also resistant to intracellular killing mechanisms in non-activated macrophages.

2.7.4 Helminth infections

Helminths are **multicellular (metazoan) parasites** that are grouped into three distinct families: nematodes (e.g. Ascaris spp.), trematodes (e.g. Schistosoma spp.) and cestodes (e.g. Taenia spp.). They have complex life cycles with many developmental stages. In the course of a single infection, humans may be repeatedly exposed to larval, adult and egg antigens. For example, free-swimming larval stages (cercariae) of the trematode, S. mansoni, penetrate the skin of humans bathing or swimming in infested water. Following entry, they develop into tissue-stage schistosomula, which migrate via the pulmonary circulation into the liver. In the liver, they trigger a granulomatous inflammatory reaction leading to portal hypertension. Once within the portahepatic system, the schistosomula mature into adult worms and take up their final position in small venules draining the intestine, from where they shed eggs into the intestinal lumen.

Visit the website at **www.wiley.com/go/misbah/immunology** to read the case study on schistosomiasis.

2.7.5 Normal immunity to helminth infection

The immunological characteristics of helminth infection are increased IgE production, eosinophilia and mastocytosis. These responses are regulated by the Th2 subset of CD4+ T lymphocytes (see Chapter 1). People living in tropical or subtropical countries, where helminth infestation is endemic, have grossly raised serum IgE levels but little allergy, additional evidence to support the hygiene hypothesis in terms of types of IgE (Chapter 4). For example, schistosomiasis has been shown to modulate the expression of Toll-like receptor 2 (TLR2) to increase Tregs, suggesting that evolutionary older organisms have evolved to alter our immune systems. The observation of reduced skin test reactivity to allergens, coupled with the inhibition of Th2-associated allergic disease, in schistosome-infected children has led to a reappraisal of the 'hygiene hypothesis'. This states that Th2-associated allergic disease is counteracted by exposure to microorganisms that induce Th1 cells. However, it is now thought that regulatory T cells may play a greater role. This is supported by studies of helminth eradication showing that successful treatment of helminths increases atopic skin sensitization and that treatment against helminths during pregnancy is associated with more infantile eczema.

Parasite-specific IgE antibodies play an important role in protection, for example to S. mansoni. IgE antibodies react with helminth antigens and lead to the release of pharmacologically active mediators from mast cells, eosinophils and basophils that have bound specific IgE and antigen. These mediators cause local accumulation of leucocytes and augment the ability to damage the helminth. They induce local inflammation and act on smooth muscle to aid expulsion of parasites. However, parasite-specific IgE is only a fraction of the massive increase in IgE induced by IL-4 produced by CD4+ TH2 cells (Fig. 2.11). It is possible that the excess polyclonal IgE provoked by helminth infestation may represent a mechanism to saturate IgE receptors on mast cells, thus rendering them refractory to stimulation by parasite antigens.

Eosinophilia is also characteristic of helminth disease and, like IgE responses, is regulated by CD4+ T cells and driven by IL-5. The mediators released from activated mast cells attract eosinophils and even some parasitic material is directly attractant to eosinophils. Eosinophils have an effector role in that they attach to the parasite surface and degranulate, releasing major basic protein; eosinophil cationic protein causes small holes in the tegument of the helminth.

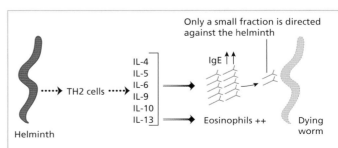

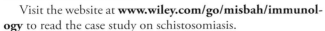

Fig. 2.11 IgE production in helminth infection may be an epiphenomenon. IL, interleukin.

2.7.6 Helminth evasion of immune responses

Antigenic disguise is important in helminth survival. Adult schistosomes 'disguise' their surface antigens (see Table 2.12) by synthesizing host-like antigens, such as β_2-macroglobulin, to mask their own foreignness. Alternatively, they may adsorb host molecules onto their surfaces: red blood cell antigens, immunoglobulins, MHC antigens and complement have all been demonstrated on the outer layer of schistosomes.

Helminth infestation is also associated with **immunosuppression of T- and B-cell responses** through the induction of IL-10. For instance, numerous immune mechanisms are directed against the young schistosomulum as it migrates from the skin to the blood vessels in which it matures. Schistosomes evade such attack by 'disguise', but can also actively protect themselves by releasing peptidases that cleave bound immunoglobulins, and other factors that inhibit either T-cell proliferation, release of IFN-γ or the mast cell signal required for eosinophil activation.

The term 'concomitant immunity' or '**premunition**' is used to describe a form of acquired immunity in which the established infection persists but new infection is prevented by immune mechanisms. Schistosomiasis is again the best example: adult schistosome worms can live in the host for many years, often with little or no evidence of any immune response. However, adult schistosomes do stimulate a response that prevents reinfection of the same animal with immature forms of the parasite, called cercaria.

2.7.7 Bystander damage caused by immune reactions to protozoa and helminths

Many of the clinical features of parasite infection result from the host's immune response to parasite antigens. **Immediate (type I) hypersensitivity** reactions, such as urticaria and angioedema, are found in the acute stages of ascariasis, and in many other helminth infections. Rupture of a hydatid cyst during surgical removal may release vast amounts of antigen and trigger anaphylactic shock.

Type II hypersensitivity reactions are caused by antibodies to cell-surface antigens. Parasite antigens that cross-react with host tissue, or host antigens adsorbed onto the parasite surface, may lead to the development of antibodies that recognize self-antigens. Such autoimmunization is an important factor in the immunopathology of Chagas' disease (see Chapter 13, section 13.7.2).

Circulating immune complexes (type III hypersensitivity) of parasite antigen and host antibodies cause some of the tissue damage seen in malaria, trypanosomiasis and schistosomiasis. In some cases, chronic deposition of immune complexes may lead to glomerulonephritis (see Chapter 9).

Cell-mediated immunity (type IV hypersensitivity) to parasite antigens can also cause severe tissue damage. For example, in schistosomiasis, portal fibrosis and pulmonary hypertension are probably due to cellular responses to schistosome eggs deposited in the tissues.

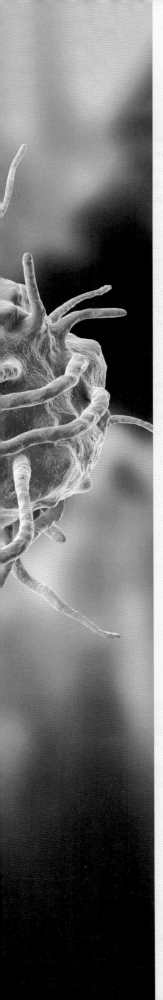

CHAPTER 3
Immunodeficiency

Key topics

 Visit the companion website at **www.wiley.com/go/misbah/immunology** to download cases with additional figures on these topics.

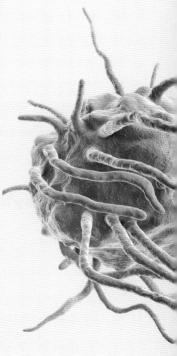

Chapel and Haeney's Essentials of Clinical Immunology, Seventh Edition. Edited by Siraj A. Misbah, Gavin P. Spickett, and Virgil A.S.H. Dalm.
© 2022 John Wiley & Sons Ltd. Published 2022 by John Wiley & Sons Ltd.

3.1 Introduction

Once a newborn infant leaves the sterile intrauterine environment, he or she meets many microorganisms and becomes colonized with 'healthy bacteria'. Most microflora are non-pathogenic, so this colonization does not cause symptoms. When the child is exposed to a pathogen that he or she has not met before, clinical infection may occur, expanding the child's immunological memory and producing long-lasting immunity.

In any encounter with a microorganism, the development of infection depends on the resistance of the host balanced against the **virulence** of the microorganism and the size of the inoculum. Infections with certain organisms, for example Pneumocystis jiroveci, are unknown except in patients with underlying immunodeficiency, and such bugs are therefore known as 'opportunistic'. **Host defence factors** are very variable; increased infection susceptibility can be inherited or acquired, including environmental, dietary or drug induced. Some infective agents, for example human immunodeficiency virus (HIV) or cytomegalovirus (CMV), have potent immunosuppressive effects and can cause serious disease. These causes of secondary immune deficiencies are discussed in this chapter as well as those of primary immune deficiencies.

Underlying immunodeficiency should be suspected in every patient, *irrespective of age*, who has recurrent, persistent, severe or unusual infections. Defects in immunity can be **classified** into primary disorders due to an intrinsic defect in the immune system that may be congenital or late onset, or those secondary to a known condition (Fig. 3.1). They may involve adaptive or innate immune mechanisms and maybe be permanent (genetic) or transient (if due to a viral infection). Furthermore, many defects are subtle and defy classification at present.

The **type of organism** causing the infections may give a clue to the nature of the defect (Fig. 3.2). The speed of the infection is also important. The innate immune system is the first line of defence and, if this fails, an infection will be acute and severe (even overwhelming). Infections due to defects in adaptive immunity are usually identified and treated as they often develop more slowly; in the main, bacterial infections indicate humoral (antibody and/or complement) or phagocytic defects and viral or fungal infections suggest T-cell defects.

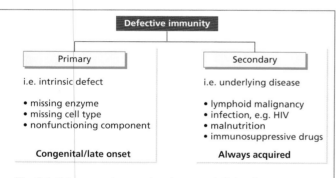

Fig. 3.1 Primary and secondary immune deficiencies.

3.2 Primary immune deficiencies

Primary immune deficiencies, or inborn errors of immunity, manifest as increased susceptibility to infections, autoimmunity, autoinflammatory diseases, allergy and/or malignancy. Primary immune deficiencies are traditionally considered to be rare diseases, affecting approximately 1 in 10 000 to 1 in 50 000 births. However, with ongoing discovery of novel primary immune deficiencies and improved definition of clinical phenotypes, the prevalence is more likely to be at least 1 in 1000 to 1 in 5000. These primary immune deficiencies present with heterogeneous clinical phenotypes based on the cells and/or mechanisms involved in pathogenesis. The introduction of whole exome and

whole genome sequencing in primary immune deficiencies has contributed to a better definition of clinical pictures and currently variants in over 400 genes have been described that give rise to a primary immune deficiency. The identification of underlying genetic variants in primary immune deficiencies results in better understanding of the pathogenesis, but also plays a pivotal role in risk stratification and counselling of family members. Moreover, novel targeted treatment approaches can be developed to improve clinical outcome and patients' quality of life.

3.3 Primary antibody deficiencies

3.3.1 Diagnosis of primary antibody deficiencies

The **commonest** forms of primary immune deficiencies are those due to antibody failure and are discussed first (Table 3.1). These occur in children and adults and may be congenital or late onset. Congenital antibody deficiencies are rarer than late onset; >90% of patients who fail to produce protective antibodies present after 10 years of age (Table 3.2). It is easier, however, to discuss the various forms of antibody deficiencies in relation to the development of B cells, and so the clinical types are given here in this order too – Case 3.1 (lack of B-cell differentiation) to Case 3.4 (failure of T cells to help B cells to immunoglobulin class switch). Regardless of the precise defect, the outcome is failure of production of

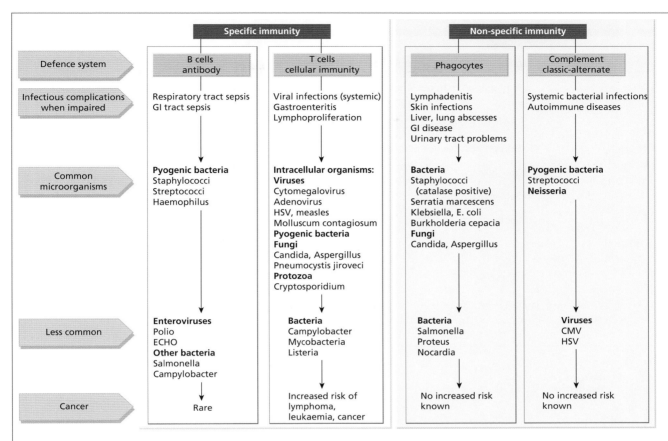

Fig. 3.2 Defects in immunity suggested by infections with certain organisms. CMV, cytomegalovirus; GI, gastrointestinal; HSV, herpes simplex virus.

Table 3.1 Prevalence of primary antibody deficiencies	
Comparison with other diseases	**Per 10⁵ population**
Rheumatoid arthritis	1000
Insulin-dependent diabetes	200
Multiple sclerosis	60
Systemic lupus erythematosus	50
Primary antibody deficiencies	4–6
Scleroderma	1

protective antibodies resulting in increased susceptibility to bacterial infections.

In **genetic forms of antibody deficiency**, recurrent infections usually begin between 4 months and 2 years of age, since maternally transferred IgG affords some passive protection for the first 3–4 months of life (Fig. 3.3). Some forms of primary antibody deficiency (PAD) are inherited as X-linked or autosomal recessive traits; a history of affected relatives, especially boys, is therefore of diagnostic value, although a negative family history does not exclude an inherited condition or a *de novo*

mutation. Primary immune deficiencies are relatively rare. A **detailed history** (Box 3.1) helps to distinguish them from more common causes of recurrent infection; for example, cystic fibrosis or inhaled foreign bodies are more likely causes of recurrent chest infections in childhood. However, *if tests for cystic fibrosis are done, immunoglobulin measurements should always be performed at the same time.*

Clues from the examination are few: there are rarely any diagnostic physical signs of antibody deficiency, although examination often shows evidence of the consequences of previous severe infections, such as a ruptured tympanic membrane, grommets, bronchiectasis or failure to thrive.

Laboratory investigations are essential to the diagnosis (Box 3.2). Measurements of serum immunoglobulin levels will often but not always reveal gross quantitative abnormalities. Complete absence of immunoglobulin, i.e. agammaglobulinaemia, is unusual, and even severely affected patients have very low but detectable IgG and IgM. Defects in antibody synthesis can involve one immunoglobulin isotype alone, such as IgA; groups of isotypes, often IgA and IgG; or all three major isotypes, i.e. panhypogammaglobulinaemia. The ability of a patient to make antibodies is a better guide to susceptibility to infection than total immunoglobulin levels. *Failure to make a specific antibody after immunization or documented exposure is*

Table 3.2 Major causes of primary antibody deficiencies in children and adults

Age (years)	Children	Adults
<4	Transient hypogammaglobulinaemia of infancy	
	X-linked agammaglobulinaemia (XLA)	XLA (late presentation is unusual but does occur)
	Hyper-IgM syndromes	
4–15	Common variable immunodeficiency disorders	
	Hyper-IgM syndromes	
	Selective IgA deficiency	
	Selective/partial antibody deficiencies	
16–60		Common variable immunodeficiency disorders
		Selective/partial antibody deficiencies
		Selective IgA deficiency
		Antibody deficiency with thymoma

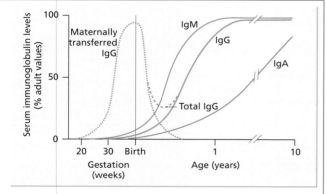

Fig. 3.3 Serum immunoglobulin levels and age. Maternally transferred IgG (· · ·) has mostly disappeared by 6 months. As the neonate synthesizes (—) IgG, the level slowly rises, but a physiological 'trough' of serum IgG is characteristically seen between 3 and 6 months (- - -).

Box 3.1 Clues from the history in primary antibody deficiency

Recurrent sinus/chest infections are common (see Fig. 3.4)

- History of repeated ear, nose and throat (ENT) surgery
- Lobectomy in childhood or adolescence
- Early bronchiectasis

A second system is usually involved
- Skin sepsis (boils, abscesses)
- Gut infections
- Meningitis

Infections are due to common bacteria (Fig. 3.2)
- Streptococcus pneumoniae
- Haemophilus influenzae

Prolonged or repeated use of antibiotic treatment
Non-infectious features are common
- Autoimmune complications, including immune thrombocytopenic purpura and autoimmune haemolytic anaemia
- 'Sarcoid-like' granuloma

Fungal and viral infections are relatively uncommon
Failure to thrive
A family history of primary antibody deficiency

fundamental to the diagnosis. Tests of specific functional antibodies are shown in Table 3.3. Measurements of IgG subclasses are not useful unless backed up by test immunizations and detection of specific IgG responses.

Circulating B cells are identified by monoclonal antibodies to **B-cell antigens** (see Chapter 19). In normal blood, B cells constitute about 5–15% of the total lymphocyte population. The absence of mature B cells in an antibody-deficient individual distinguishes failed B-cell differentiation, such as X-linked agammaglobulinaemia, from other causes of PAD in which non-functional B cells are present. Mutation analysis is essential to confirm a diagnosis of an inherited condition and enables family members to be tested and counselled. Management with replacement immunoglobulin therapy by a clinical immunologist is important (see later in the chapter).

3.3.2 Types of primary antibody deficiency
(see Table 3.2 and Box 3.2)
Transient hypogammaglobulinaemia of infancy

Maternal IgG is actively transported across the placenta to the fetal circulation from the fourth month of gestational life, although maximum transfer takes place during the final

2 months (see section 18.3.2). At birth, the infant has a serum IgG at least equal to that of the mother (see Fig. 3.3), but catabolism of maternal IgG outstrips IgG synthesized by the newborn child, resulting in a phase of **physiological IgG trough**. However, the normal infant is not unduly susceptible to infection because functioning antibodies can be made and T cells can be activated (see section 18.3.2).

Box 3.2 Types of primary antibody deficiencies

- Common variable immunodeficiency disorders
- X-linked agammaglobulinaemia
- Hyper IgM syndromes (e.g. CD40 ligand deficiency)
- IgA and IgG subclass deficiencies
- Selective IgA deficiency
- Specific antibody deficiencies
- Transient hypogammaglobulinaemia of infancy

Table 3.3 Tests for functional antibodies (with examples in brackets)

Detection after natural exposure/infection (chicken pox)

Response to prior or test immunization:

- protein (tetanus toxoid, diphtheria toxoid, measles, etc.)
- carbohydrate (bacterial polysaccharide, e.g. pneumococcal, salmonella)

Caution

Live vaccines (e.g. BCG, MMR) should never be given to children in whom an immunodeficiency is suspected

Normal children under the age of 2 years do not respond to carbohydrate antigens

The trough in IgG is more severe if the child is **premature**, as IgG acquired from the mother is reduced (see Chapter 18, Case 18.2). Improved neonatal care results in more surviving infants born between 26 and 32 weeks of gestation who are at risk of bacterial infections due to reduction of time for placental transfer. However the incidence of such infections is low in the UK, where routine invasive support (e.g. indwelling lines for nutrition, monitoring, etc.) is not used. Low-birthweight babies in countries where such procedures, and the associated severe bacterial infections, are common may benefit from replacement immunoglobulin until they can synthesize their own protective antibodies (see Fig. 3.3).

Transient hypogammaglobulinaemia occurs when the otherwise normal infant is **slow to start to synthesize IgG**. As maternally acquired antibodies fall, the infant becomes susceptible to recurrent pyogenic infections, sometimes for many months, until spontaneous IgG synthesis begins. It is important to distinguish this condition from pathological causes of hypogammaglobulinaemia, because management differs. In most cases, the infant remains well and needs no specific therapy even though immunoglobulin levels remain below the normal range. If infections are severe, then prophylactic antibiotics should prevent further morbidity; these may be needed for 1–2 years or until endogenous IgG synthesis is satisfactory and full immunization responses documented.

X-linked agammaglobulinaemia (Bruton's disease)

Boys with X-linked agammaglobulinaemia (XLA) usually present with **recurrent pyogenic infections** between the ages of 4 months and 2 years (as in Case 3.1). The sites of infection and the organisms involved are similar to other types of antibody deficiency (Figs 3.2 and 3.4), although these young boys are also susceptible to life-threatening enteroviruses.

In almost all patients, **circulating mature B cells are absent** but T cells are normal. There are no plasma cells in the bone

---

Case 3.1 X-linked agammaglobulinaemia (Bruton's disease)

Peter was born after an uneventful pregnancy, weighing 3.1 kg. At 3 months, he developed otitis media; at the ages of 5 months and 11 months, he was admitted to hospital with untypable *Haemophilus influenzae* pneumonia. These infections responded promptly to appropriate antibiotics on each occasion. He is the fourth child of unrelated parents; his three sisters showed no predisposition to infection.

Examination at the age of 18 months showed a pale, thin child whose height and weight were below the third centile. There were no other abnormal features. He had been fully immunized as an infant (at 2, 3 and 4 months) with tetanus and diphtheria toxoids, acellular pertussis, Hib and Mening. C conjugate vaccines and polio (Salk). In addition, he had received measles, mumps and rubella vaccine at 15 months. All immunizations were uneventful.

Immunological investigations (Table 3.4) into the cause of his recurrent infections showed severe reduction in all three classes of serum immunoglobulins and no specific antibody production. Although there was no family history of agammaglobulinaemia, the lack of mature B lymphocytes in his peripheral blood suggested a failure of B-cell differentiation and strongly supported a diagnosis of infantile X-linked agammaglobulinaemia (Bruton's disease). This was confirmed by detection of a disease-causing mutation in the Btk gene. The antibody deficiency was treated by 2-weekly intravenous infusions of human normal IgG in a dose of 400 mg/kg bodyweight/month. Over the following 7 years, his health steadily improved, weight and height are now on the 30th centile, and he has had only one episode of otitis media in the last 4 years. He is now 12 years old and able to treat himself with the same dose of subcutaneous replacement immunoglobulin at home.

Table 3.4 Immunological investigations* in Case 3.1, X-linked agammaglobulinaemia

Quantitative serum immunoglobulins (g/l)		
IgG	0.17	(5.5–10.0)
IgA	Not detected	(0.3–0.8)
IgM	0.07	(0.4–1.8)
Antibody activity		
Immunization responses – no detectable IgG antibodies to		
Tetanus toxoid (post Imx)		
Haemophilus type b polysaccharides (post Imx)		
Polio (post Imx)		
Measles (post Imx)		
Rubella (post Imx)		
Isohaemagglutinins (IgM) not detected (blood group A Rh+)		
Blood lymphocyte subpopulations (×109/l)		
Total lymphocyte count	3.5	NR* (2.5–5.0)
T lymphocytes (CD3)	3.02	NR (1.5–3.0)
B lymphocytes (CD19)	<0.1	NR (0.3–1.0)

*Normal range for age 18 months shown in parentheses. Imx = immunization

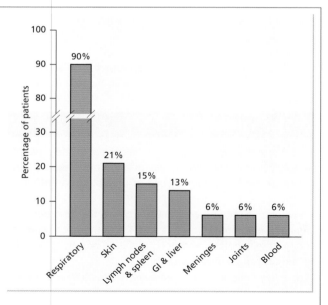

Fig. 3.4 Presenting infections in particular organs in patients with primary antibody deficiencies. GI, gastrointestinal.

membrane clustered around an antigen receptor and is crucial for maturation. The Btk gene is mutated in XLA patients, resulting in either failure to synthesize the Btk protein or an abnormal enzyme that is always non-functional.

The diagnosis of XLA rests on the very low serum levels of all isotypes of immunoglobulin, the absence of circulating mature B lymphocytes and a **mutation in the Btk gene**. The identification of the genetic defect allows asymptomatic female carriers to be identified and counselled, and prenatal diagnosis is now feasible. The gene for Btk is located on the long arm of the X chromosome, resulting in X-linked inheritance. Other defects in the B-cell maturation pathway, though still rare, have autosomal recessive inheritance and occur in girls and boys.

Management consists of high levels of **replacement immunoglobulin** for all affected individuals (see section 3.3.5), to prevent bronchiectasis (Fig. 3.6) and all types of bacterial infections. Complications of XLA include acute and chronic lung disease, but also autoinflammatory conditions, including inflammatory bowel disease, may occur.

Hyper-IgM syndromes

Some children with severe antibody deficiency (including boys with or without affected male relatives) have normal numbers of B cells and normal or raised serum IgM levels at presentation; such syndromes are therefore known as hyper-IgM syndromes, as in Case 3.2. In the **X-linked form**, the boys have

marrow, lymph nodes or gastrointestinal tract. Differentiation of pre-B cells into B cells depends on a tyrosine kinase enzyme, known as Bruton's tyrosine kinase (Btk), normally found in developing B cells, but not mature B cells (Fig. 3.5). This enzyme, like the T-cell counterpart Itk (interleukin-2-inducible T-cell kinase), interacts with lipids on the inner cell surface

Bone Marrow

μ chain/
Igα/Igβ
λ5, E47
BLINK
PIK3R1

BTK

ICOS
BAFF-R, TWEAK
TACI, CD19, CD81
CD20, CD21
LRBA, PIK3CD
NFκB1, NFκB2

Periphery

IgA, AID, CD40L
CD40, UNG, IKK-γ
PIK3CD

Plasma
cell

Lymphoid
lineages

Pro-B cell

Pre-B cell

IgM

Immature
B cell

IgM

Mature
B cell

IgG
IgA
or IgE

HSC

Ikaros

IgD

CXCR4

Memory
B cell

Myeloid
lineages

Fig. 3.5 Gene and protein defects in B-cell development and function. Haematopoietic stem cells (HSCs) give rise to progenitor (pro)-B cells, which then rearrange their immunoglobulin heavy-chain gene segments to generate precursor (pre)-B cells. Pre-B cells subsequently rearrange their immunoglobulin light-chain gene segments to produce a functional cell surface receptor (IgM), composed of heavy and light chains. After the receptor engages with antigen, downstream events lead to the induction of proliferation and differentiation of the B cell. In the periphery, after stimulation with antigen, mature B cells further develop following class-switch recombination and somatic hypermutation and, ultimately, memory B-cell or plasma-cell differentiation. Developmental blocks throughout B-cell maturation and differentiation occur as a result of defects in genes encoding the molecules indicated in boxes. Blocks in the function of mature B cells can also occur. Primary immunodeficiency syndromes that cause these blocks are also listed. AID, activation-induced cytidine deaminase; BAFFR, B-cell-activating-factor receptor; BLNK, B-cell linker; BTK, Bruton's tyrosine kinase; CD40L, CD40 ligand; E47, E47 transcription factor/TCF3 gene; ICOS, inducible T-cell co-stimulator; IgA, selective IgA deficiency; IKK-γ, inhibitor-of-nuclear-factor-κB kinase-γ LRBA, lipopolysaccharide (LPS)-responsive and beige-like anchor protein; NFKB, nuclear factor kappa-light-chain-enhancer of activated B cells; PIK3, phosphatidylinositol 3-kinase; μ chain, μ immunoglobulin heavy chain; TACI, transmembrane activator and calcium-modulating cyclophilin-ligand interactor; TWEAK, TNF-like weak inducer of apoptosis; UNG, uracil-DNA glycosylase. Source: Smith T, Cunningham-Rundles C. (2019). Primary B-cell immunodeficiencies. *Human Immunology*, 80:351–362. Reproduced with permission of Elsevier.

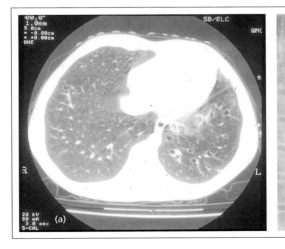

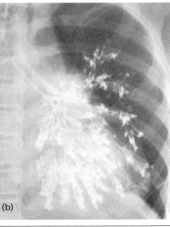

Fig. 3.6 Bronchiectasis – (a) computed tomography scan and (b) bronchogram (no longer performed) show the typical features of damaged terminal bronchioles, leading to structural lung damage.

Case 3.2 CD40 ligand deficiency

Michael was seen in the outpatient department at the age of 4 years with a history of painful mouth ulcers, abdominal pain over 7 weeks but persistent diarrhoea in the last 2 weeks. He had suffered multiple episodes of ear and chest infections, starting with pneumonia at the age of 9 months, when he had been noted to have neutropenia, but this had appeared to be transient. He has three healthy sisters. On examination he had multiple oral ulcers, enlarged tonsils, purulent nasal discharge, scarred tympanic membranes, abdominal distension and hepatomegaly.

He was investigated for an early presentation of inflammatory bowel disease, including stool microscopy. In addition, liver function tests and hepatitis serology were done to determine the cause of the enlarged liver, T-lymphocyte enumeration to exclude severe combined immunodeficiency (SCID) and immunoglobulin levels to exclude a common variable immunodeficiency disorder (CVID). Cryptosporidia were found in the stools and liver enzyme levels were raised. Serum IgG and IgA levels were very low but B and T-cell numbers were normal (see Table 3.5). Since C-reactive protein (CRP) and albumin serum levels were normal, an intestinal biopsy was not indicated. A diagnosis of primary antibody deficiency with cryptosporidiosis was made. Abdominal ultrasound showed a diffusely enlarged liver with a dilated common bile duct.

This was most likely to be due to a hyper-IgM syndrome as the serum IgM was raised and cryptosporidia is a particular feature of this condition. Peripheral blood lymphocytes were separated and stimulated in culture; activation markers, including CD40 ligand, were then detected by flow cytometry. CD69 and CD72 were present but there was no CD40 ligand on activated T lymphocytes. Mutation analysis confirmed a deletion in the CD40 ligand gene on the X chromosome and a substantive diagnosis of CD40 ligand deficiency was made. He was treated initially with replacement immunoglobulin, co-trimoxazole to prevent Pneumocystis infection and specific antibiotics for cryptosporidiosis; if this organism can be controlled, human stem cell transplantation, with or without liver transplantation, will be considered. His mother was tested for carrier status, as will his sisters be when they reach the age of consent.

Table 3.5 Immunological investigations in Case 3.2, CD40 ligand deficiency

Serum proteins				
Albumin		39 g/l		
C-reactive protein		8 mg/l		
Immunoglobulins	IgG	0.9 g/l		NR* (5.8–10.0)
	IgA	<0.07 g/l		NR (0.6–2.0)
	IgM	3.2 g/l		NR (0.5–1.8)

There were no detectable IgG antibodies to immunization or exposure antigens

Blood lymphocyte subpopulations (109/l)				
Total lymphocyte count		2.1		(1.5–3.50)
T lymphocytes				
CD3		1.5		(0.9–2.8)
CD4		0.8		(0.6–1.2)
CD8		0.7		(0.4–1.0)
B lymphocytes				
CD19		0.4		(0.2–0.4)
NK lymphocytes				
CD16: CD56		0.2		(0.2–0.4)

Lymphocyte stimulation assays (with phytohaemagglutinin)

	Pre stimulation**			Post stimulation		
	CD69	**CD71**	**CD40 ligand**	**CD69**	**CD71**	**CD40 ligand**
Control	3%	5%	<1%	73%	49%	62%
Patient	1%	2%	<1%	72%	63%	<1%

*NR Normal range for age 4 years.
**Percentage of CD3 cells with relevant activation marker on surface. NK, natural killer.

an additional susceptibility to Pneumocystis jiroveci infection. Such infection is normally associated with T-cell defects such as HIV or severe combined immune deficiency (see Fig. 3.2). Unlike XLA, this defect is not restricted to B cells, being due to failure of the CD40 ligand accessory molecule on T cells (see Chapter 1, Fig. 1.26). Normally, this ligand reacts with CD40 on B cells to trigger switching in specific antibody production from IgM to IgG or IgA and the formation of germinal centres. Failure of expression or functional activity of this ligand results in failure of switching and poor organization of the germinal centres (Fig. 3.7) and is associated with lack of memory B cells, reduced somatic hypermutation and impaired dendritic cell function to prime naive T cells. The lack of cross-linking of CD40 also results in failure of the B cells to upregulate CD80 and CD86, important co-stimulatory molecules that interact with CD28 and CTLA-4 on T cells for immune regulation and recognition of tumour cells. This accounts for the development of lymphoid and other malignancies in older patients. The lack of CD40 ligand in the thymus results in defective purging of autoreactive thymocytes, hence increased susceptibility to autoimmune diseases including neutropenia (as in Case 3.2).

Management of such patients currently consists of replacement immunoglobulin and genetic testing for potential female carriers. **Human stem cell transplantation** is the only curative approach with improved outcome if performed before organ damage development and is now considered to be the treatment of choice in childhood, since a high proportion of patients develop liver disease or malignancies later in life. Gene therapy for this condition is under study.

Failure of *any part* of the interaction between CD40 ligand and CD40, or of the other essential components of the pathway (including other ligands and intracellular enzymes involved), results in failure in immunoglobulin switch and germinal centre

formation. These **pure B-cell forms of the hyper-IgM syndrome** include defects in the enzymes responsible for repair of DNA in somatic hypermutation in B cells – such as activation-induced cytidine deaminase (AID). Such patients fail to switch and have a limited antibody repertoire; there is an accumulation of immature B cells in abnormal germinal centres and hence clinically enlarged lymph nodes and spleens.

Common variable immunodeficiency disorders

Common variable immunodeficiency disorders (CVIDs) are a heterogeneous group of disorders, making up the **commonest form of primary antibody deficiency**, accounting for about 90% of the symptomatic antibody deficiencies. The variable nature of the conditions is reflected in the name. The several diseases with this type of immunological phenotype have become more distinct in recent years. Although some patients present in childhood, most (> 90%) are not diagnosed until adulthood (see Case 3.3 and Chapter 16, Case 16.7). Most patients with a CVID have **low serum levels of IgG and IgA**, with normal or reduced IgM and normal or low numbers of total B cells and low numbers of memory B cells. A small group of patients have low circulating T cells as well and have been redefined as 'late-onset combined immunodeficiency' many of the patients with complex disease and multiple complications also have abnormal T-cell function, which may reflect an, as yet, undescribed combined immune deficiency (CID). Affected individuals experience the same range of bacterial and viral infections as other patients with antibody deficiencies (see Figs 3.2 and 3.4).

Currently, many patients lead normal lives, provided that they receive replacement immunoglobulin therapy. Complications are very varied (see section 3.3.4), probably due to complication-causing or disease-modifying genes (such as PI3Kδ and TACI), resulting in the different syndromes in this large group of disorders. Inheritance is very rare (approximately 2–10%) and affected women have normal offspring, as in Case 3.3.

Selective or partial antibody deficiencies

So-called IgG subclass deficiencies are controversial, since deletion of IgG subclass genes does not necessarily lead to disease. *Investigation of individual patients should be limited to those with significant recurrent bacterial infections.* In such patients, the total IgG level may appear normal, so selective deficiencies of one or two of the three protective IgG subclasses (IgG$_1$, IgG$_2$ and IgG$_3$) may be missed. However, what really matters is the ability to make specific antibodies against infective organisms to prevent recurrent infections, so reduced IgG subclass levels alone are not always significant. Most clinically relevant deficiencies of **IgG subclasses are those associated with IgA deficiency**. IgG subclass measurements are only needed if there is also a low serum IgA level, the patient suffers from recurrent infections and he or she also fails to make specific antibodies to some antigens (Case 3.4).

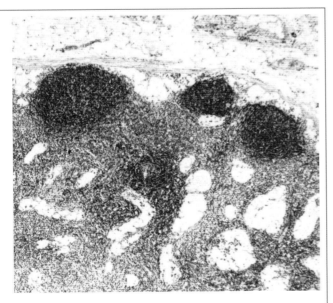

Fig. 3.7 Lymph node from a patient with CD40 ligand deficiency showing impaired germinal centres. Courtesy of F. Fachetti.

Case 3.3 Common variable immunodeficiency disorder (CVID)

A 34-year-old woman developed herpes zoster and lobar pneumonia; over the previous 5 years she had been admitted to hospital with pneumonia on two previous occasions and made a full recovery. There had been no history of recurrent chest infections during childhood. Non-encapsulated Haemophilus influenza and Streptococcus pneumoniae were isolated. At the age of 35, she developed a non-erosive seronegative arthritis. On direct questioning, she gave a history of intermittent diarrhoea since her late teens. These episodes lasted from 2 days to 2 weeks and she passed 5–6 partly formed stools a day. There was no family history of recurrent infections; she had two sons, aged 10 and 7, both of whom were well. Physical examination was normal, although she was thin.

Investigations showed a haemoglobin of 115 g/l, with normal neutrophil and lymphocyte counts. Immunological studies (Table 3.6) showed very low levels of serum immunoglobulins, and no detectable specific antibodies despite culture-proven Streptococcus pneumoniae and a tetanus toxoid boost 1 year earlier. She had normal numbers of circulating T and B lymphocytes. No infective cause of the intermittent diarrhoea was found; barium enema and colonoscopy were normal.

She was diagnosed as having a common variable immunodeficiency disorder, a diagnosis of exclusion, as no underlying cause was found. She was given fortnightly intravenous infusions of human normal IgG (400 mg/kg bodyweight/month) for the antibody deficiency. However three years later she developed pain, bloating and further diarrhoea. Duodenal biopsies showed flat villi without pathogens. A gluten-free diet (to which she adhered rigidly) was not successful in reducing the abdominal symptoms. Ultimately she failed to absorb fat soluble vitamins A, D and E and lost 6 kg in weight. She had the enteropathy associated with CVID, the pathogenesis of which is uncertain. She died suddenly of an unrelated pulmonary embolus.

Table 3.6 Immunological investigations* in Case 3.3, common variable immunodeficiency disorder

Quantitative serum immunoglobulins (g/l)		
IgG	3.15	NR (7.2–19.0)
IgA	0.11	NR (0.8–5.0)
IgM	0.66	NR (0.5–2.0)
Antibody activity		
Post-immunization IgG to		
Tetanus toxoid		Negative (>0.85 IU/ml)
Diphtheria toxoid		Negative (>0.2 IU/ml)
Pneumococcal polysaccharides		Negative (>80 U/ml)
Blood lymphocyte subpopulations ($\times 10^9$/l)		
Total lymphocyte count	1.6	(1.5–3.5)
T lymphocytes		
CD3	1.31	(0.9–2.8)
CD4	0.89	(0.6–1.2)
CD8	0.41	(0.4–1.0)
B lymphocytes		
CD19	0.2	(0.2–0.4)
NK lymphocytes		
CD16: CD56	0.2	(0.2–0.4)

*Normal adult ranges shown in parentheses. NK, natural killer.

👤🔍 Case 3.4 IgA with IgG subclass deficiencies

A 48-year-old man was admitted for investigation of weight loss associated with intermittent diarrhoea; stool examinations had been unhelpful. He had a history of pneumonia as a child and again as a young man working abroad. At the age of 33 he had developed chronic sinusitis, with persistent headaches. On examination, he was thin but had no signs of malignancy. There was no clubbing, lymphadenopathy or hepatosplenomegaly and his chest was clear on auscultation. Haemoglobin, serum albumin, liver function tests and urine electrophoresis were normal. Immunological tests are shown in Table 3.7. Investigations into the cause of the recurrent diarrhoea revealed Giardia lamblia on jejunal biopsy, *even though microscopy was negative*. Endoscopic examination of his maxillary sinuses showed considerable inflammation and hypertrophy of the mucosa.

A diagnosis was made of IgA with IgG subclass deficiencies, with chronic sinusitis and intestinal giardiasis as secondary complications. He was given a course of metronidazole for the Giardia infestation and replacement immunoglobulin was started with weekly infusions initially and subsequently 3-weekly at a dose of 0.4 g/kg per month. The sinusitis gradually improved, the diarrhoea did not return and he remained infection free for many years.

Table 3.7 Immunological investigations* in Case 3.4, IgA with IgG subclass deficiency

Serum immunoglobulins (g/l)			
IgG	7.6		(6.5–12.0)
IgA	<0.1		(0.8–5.0)
IgM	1.2		(0.5–2.0)
IgG1	1.1		(3.6–7.3)
IgG2	3.8		(1.4–4.5)
IgG3	0.1		(0.3–1.1)
IgG4	2.6		(0.1–1.0)
Serum and urine electrophoresis – no monoclonal bands			
Antibody activity – post immunization			
IgG	Tetanus toxoid Diphtheria toxoid Pneumococcal polysaccharides	Negative Negative Negative	(>0.85 IU/ml) (>0.2 IU/ml) (>80 U/ml)
Antibody activity – post exposure			
IgG	Rubella	Not detectable	
	Measles	Not detectable	
	Varicella zoster	Not detectable	
Blood lymphocyte subpopulations (×109/l)			
Total lymphocyte count	2.8		(1.5–3.5)
T lymphocytes			
CD3	2.2		(0.9–2.8)
CD4	1.6		(0.6–1.2)
CD8	0.6		(0.4–1.0)
B lymphocytes			
CD19	0.3		(0.2–0.4)
NK lymphocytes			
CD16:CD56	0.2		(0.2–0.4)

*Normal adult ranges shown in parentheses. NK, natural killer.

Antibodies are produced in different ways to carbohydrate and protein antigens. **Antibodies to polysaccharide capsular antigens** of organisms, such as those of Streptococcus pneumoniae, Salmonella typhi or encapsulated Haemophilus influenzae (see Fig. 3.2), are often transient, low affinity and of the IgG_2 subclass. Those to protein antigens, such as **viral coats** and **toxoids**, are usually persistent, high affinity and of the IgG_1 subclass.

Polysaccharide antigens alone do not stimulate immune responses in children under 2 years of age, explaining why severe infections with encapsulated organisms were relatively common in infants until the advent of conjugated polysaccharide: protein vaccines. *Antibody deficiencies, other than those with a known genetic cause, cannot be diagnosed until children are over 4 years old*, to allow for physiological variation (see the earlier section on transient hypogammaglobulinaemia).

Selective IgA deficiency

This is the commonest primary defect of specific immunity, with an incidence of around 1 in 600 in Europe, Japan and the USA. It can present at any age, although *most patients are diagnosed by an incidental finding* as young adults. It is characterized by undetectable or very low serum IgA levels, with normal concentrations of IgG and IgM and production of normal antibodies to pathogens. So **most individuals are healthy** and do not suffer from recurrent infections.

Nevertheless, selective IgA deficiency **predisposes** the individual to a **variety of disorders** (Fig. 3.8), in particular coeliac disease (gluten sensitivity).

3.3.3 Differential diagnosis

PADs are relatively rare causes of recurrent infections and the differential diagnosis is wide. If **infections recur at a single site**, then a local cause is likely. For example, cases of recurrent meningitis are usually caused by a passage communicating the ear or sinuses with cerebrospinal fluid, while recurrent pneumonia may be due to structural lung damage or aspiration of a foreign body.

Secondary causes of immunoglobulin deficiency (see section 3.6) *are far more common* than primary defects. Many textbooks provide long lists of causes. From the practical viewpoint, however, this is not a particularly helpful approach. For example, although the nephrotic syndrome is relatively common in childhood

(compared with PAD) and certainly causes isolated low serum IgG levels, recurrent infections are rarely a significant problem, since **antibody production** is normal.

It should be remembered that patients with PAD can present at any age and *a search for an underlying cause for antibody deficiency should always be made in patients with recurrent/severe/persistent/unusual infections* (as in Cases 3.1–3.4).

3.3.4 Complications of primary antibody deficiencies

Patients with all forms of PAD suffer from a **wide range of bacterial** infections (Fig. 3.2). Chronic sepsis of the upper and lower respiratory tracts can lead to chronic otitis media, deafness, sinusitis, bronchiectasis, pulmonary fibrosis and ultimately cor pulmonale. Mild infective gastrointestinal disease occurs in up to two-thirds of patients with PADs, and in about 20% it warrants further investigations. Diarrhoea, with or without malabsorption, is most frequently caused by infestation with Giardia lamblia; bacterial overgrowth of the small intestine; or persistent infection with cryptosporidium (in those with CD40 ligand deficiency), salmonella, campylobacter, rotavirus or enteroviruses. Chronic cholangitis may be due to ascending infection of the biliary tract; some cases progress to sclerosing cholangitis or hepatic cirrhosis.

Virus infections are rare, but patients with XLA or a CVID are susceptible to **chronic enterovirus infection**. This can result in severe, persistent meningoencephalitis, sometimes with an associated dermato-myositis-like syndrome. Death often follows, despite high doses of immunoglobulin therapy. **Ureaplasma** may cause genitourinary infections.

Disease-related complications often include autoimmune features. Various autoimmune features can be seen in patients with CVID, but of those autoimmune cytopenias are particularly common, with 15% of CVID patients presenting with autoimmune haemolytic anaemia or immune thrombocytopenia and 40% of CD40 ligand deficiency patients having neutropenia. Autoimmune thyroid disease affects >10% of CVID patients and a pernicious anaemia-like syndrome is also fairly common (but without autoantibodies) in which atrophic gastritis involves the entire stomach without antral sparing. **Autoimmune enteropathy**, resistant to gluten withdrawal, occurs in 5–8% of CVIDs.

In some patients with CVID, benign hyperplasia of gut-associated lymphoid tissue occurs. There is an enlarged spleen in 30% of CVID patients, causing diagnostic confusion with lymphoma (see Chapter 6, section 6.4). Other **non-infective polyclonal lymphoproliferative complications** include granulomata, usually outside lymphoid tissue, and lymphoid infiltration of the lung, known as granulomatous-lymphocytic interstitial lung disease (GL-ILD), which results, when left untreated, in irreversible lung damage and decline in lung function. The association between different complications of CVIDs has led to the definition of four clinical phenotypes: patients with no disease-related complications, those with autoimmune cytopenias, those with polyclonal lymphoproliferation and those with unexplained

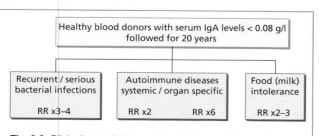

Fig. 3.8 Clinical associations of IgA deficiency. RR, Relative risk.

enteropathy. There is significant reduction of survival in those with the latter three phenotypes (see the next section).

As with other patients with immunodeficiency involving humoral and/or cell-mediated immunity, CVID patients have an increase in incidence of **malignant disease**. Most tumours are lymphoid in origin, although carcinoma of the stomach may follow atrophic gastritis.

3.3.5 Management of antibody deficiencies

Early diagnosis is essential if further infections are to be prevented and the incidence of infective complications reduced.

Prophylactic immunoglobulin replacement therapy is mandatory for children and adults with persistently defective antibody production. Preparations are available for intravenous or subcutaneous use; the choice depends on the severity of failure of antibody production, preexisting complications and venous access, as well as convenience and patient choice. Most patients require 400–600 mg of immunoglobulin/kg per month to prevent further bacterial infections, especially in those patients with chronic lung, eye or gut infections. Intravenous immunoglobulin (IVIG) is usually given at 3- or 4-weekly intervals, the dose and timing being adjusted *to provide maximum reduction in infections for each patient*. Serum immunoglobulin levels are monitored and, once a steady state is reached (usually after about 6 months), trough (pre-infusion) levels are maintained at a level that keeps the patient infection free. Adverse reactions are uncommon with modern, highly purified IVIG preparations. This makes self-infusion by the patient at home by the IV route, as well as subcutaneous immunoglobulin (SCIG), safe provided the patients are trained and registered in a recognized programme.

The **dose per month** of replacement immunoglobulin by the subcutaneous route is equivalent to that given intravenously; most patients receive weekly infusions of 30–60 ml of a more concentrated solution, given into several sites simultaneously. A syringe driver usually controls infusion rates and each site infusion takes about 30 min. Serum levels equivalent to those with IVIG are achieved. Adverse reactions are mostly unusual, enabling this route to be used at home also.

Immunoglobulin is derived from a plasma pool of 6000–10 000 donor units, in order to give the widest possible range of protective antibodies. Transmitted viruses are, therefore, of great concern. Cold ethanol precipitation, the initial process involved in the manufacture of both intravenous and subcutaneous preparations, has been shown to kill retroviruses (such as HIV) and probably kills many other viruses transmitted in blood or blood products (see Chapter 16). **Screenings** of donor units, **viral inactivation** steps and other processes such as ultrafiltration have reduced the risk of hepatitis. However, in the past there were cases of transmission of hepatitis C (see Chapter 16, Case 16.7) and all patients must have **regular monitoring** including liver function tests.

Treatment of autoimmune complications in patients with antibody deficiencies remains challenging, as the use of immunosuppressive agents for these disease manifestations may again result in an increased risk of infectious complications.

General management measures include the early recognition and diagnosis of new infections or complications. Coexistent problems may be mistakenly attributed to the complications of antibody deficiency, e.g. an inhaled foreign body may be overlooked in a child with fresh chest symptoms. Antibody-deficient patients respond promptly to appropriate antibiotics, but it may be necessary to give a course of 10–14 days' therapy. Better use of prophylactic immunoglobulin, physiotherapy and more appropriate use of antibiotics have improved survival hugely. Prognosis in CVIDs depends on the complications, which are not necessarily related to B-cell failure but represent immune dysregulation, such as polyclonal lymphoproliferation, enteropathy or autoimmune cytopenias, as well as preexisting structural damage such as bronchiectasis. In general, patients who suffer from infections only have a very good prognosis, while prognosis of patients with non-infectious complications is much worse, with estimated 40-year survival of around 40% (see Fig. 3.9).

Gene-targeted therapies for PADs have shown some promising results. By the introduction of whole exome sequencing and whole genome sequencing in patients with PADs, genetic variants have been described in patients with CVID that explain the clinical phenotype. Based on the genetic variants found, targeted therapies have been intro-

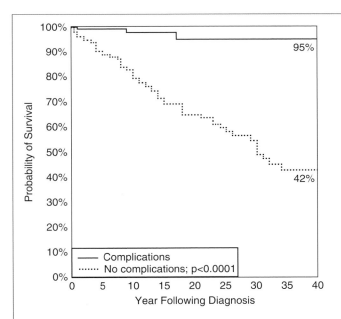

Fig. 3.9 Kaplan-Meier curve for patients with and without non-infectious complications. Patients with non-infectious complications were significantly more likely to die than those with infections only (P <. 0001). Source: Resnick, E. S., et al. (2012). Morbidity and mortality in common variable immune deficiency over 4 decades. *Blood*, 119(7):1650–1657. Reproduced with permission of Elsevier.

duced in clinical practice, for instance mTOR inhibitors and application of CTLA-4-fusion proteins in CTLA-4 deficiency, or in ongoing clinical trials, like selective PI3Kδ inhibition in patients with PI3Kδ gain-of-function variants.

3.4 Combined primary T- and B-cell immunodeficiencies

3.4.1 Types of defects

Depressed or defective T-cell immunity is usually accompanied by variable abnormalities of B-cell function, reflecting the T–B-cell cooperation needed for antibody synthesis to most antigens. Most defects of antigen-specific immunity, other than antibody deficiencies, are therefore combined immune deficiencies of the adaptive system. Some combined defects are associated with failure in other systems as well as the immune system and these are known as complex combined immunodeficiencies. Wiskott–Aldrich syndrome is an example with platelet and vascular defects as well. The severe combined deficiencies (Case 3.5) usually present within the first few months of life (see Box 3.3).

Those infants in whom there is complete failure of T-lymphocyte function have **severe combined immune deficiency (SCID)**, for even though B cells may be present, there is no antibody production as B-cell function fails. Several variants

---

 Case 3.5 Severe combined immunodeficiency (SCID)

David was born at full term after a normal pregnancy; his parents were unrelated. He was not given Bacille Calmette–Guérin (BCG) at birth. He was well until 2 months, when he became 'chesty' and needed antibiotics. Routine immunizations were postponed until he had recovered, but he then developed 'antibiotic-related' diarrhoea, which did not settle after the antibiotics were stopped. After 3 months a further chest infection occurred, his weight fell from the 25th centile to below the 3rd. He was admitted for investigation for failure to thrive and was found to have a silent atypical pneumonia on initial chest X-ray.

On examination, he was a thin, scrawny infant on the 25th centile for length. There were no rashes or lymphadenopathy, but his liver was palpable just below the right costal margin. He had slight tachycardia and tachypnoea; bronchoscopy to obtain a sample for microbiological tests revealed Pneumocystis jiroveci on staining of the fluid. Investigations (Table 3.8) showed a marked deficiency of T cells with normal numbers of B cells, but no immunoglobulin production. He had a T– B++ natural killer (NK)– form of SCID. He was treated with high-dose co-trimoxazole for the Pneumocystis and referred promptly to a specialist unit for human stem cell transplantation, where he was put in isolation and given immunoglobulin therapy to prevent further infections. The diagnosis was investigated further by mutation analysis, starting with the commonest form of this type of SCID, X-linked common γ chain cytokine receptor deficiency, which was positive.

Table 3.8 Immunological investigations* in Case 3.5, severe combined immune deficiency

Full blood count		Immunological results	
Haemoglobin	108 g/l	IgG	0.9 g/l
Neutrophil count	3.5 × 10⁹/l	IgA	<0.1 g/l
Lymphocyte count	0.5 × 10⁹/l – NR for age (4–15)	IgM	0.1 g/l
Microbiology results		**Lymphocytes**	
Blood	Negative for HIV and CMV by PCR	CD3⁺/CD4⁺	0.09 × 10⁹/l
		CD3⁺/CD8⁺	0.04 × 10⁹/l
Urine	Negative for CMV antigen	CD19⁺	0.23 × 10⁹/l
		NK cells	0.08 × 10⁹/l
Nasopharyngeal swab	Rhinovirus		
Stool	Echovirus-22		
Sputum lavage fluid	Negative for bacterial culture Pneumocystis: PCR positive and staining		

*Normal range for 3 months shown in parentheses (see Fig. 3.10). CMV, cytomegalovirus; HIV, human immunodeficiency virus; PCR, polymerase chain reaction.

Box 3.3 Clues in severe combined immune deficiency

- Present in first few weeks/months of life
- Infections are often viral or fungal rather than bacterial
- Chronic diarrhoea is common and often labelled as 'gastroenteritis'
- Respiratory infections and oral thrush are common
- Failure to thrive, even in absence of obvious infections, must be investigated
- Lymphopenia is present in almost all affected infants and is often overlooked (Fig. 3.10)
- Human immunodeficiency virus (HIV) must be excluded

are recognized (Table 3.9), depending on the presence or absence of T, B and natural killer (NK) cells, even though these cells do not function normally. Infants present in the first few weeks of life with chronic or persistent infection and failure to thrive. The condition should be suspected in any sick infant with infection, who should be checked for a low lymphocyte count (Box 3.3 and Fig. 3.10). *Early recognition and differentiation from paediatric HIV are essential.* Since many children die from severe infections before human stem cell transplantation (HSCT) can be completed and yet HSCT (see Chapter 8, section 8.5) is successful in repairing many types of immune defect, newborn screening has been established in Europe and the USA. Using real-time quantitative polymerase chain reaction (PCR) to amplify T-cell receptor excision circles (TRECs) from dried blood spots on Guthrie cards, this has proved cost

Table 3.9 Examples of some of the commonest severe combined immunodeficiencies (SCID) defined by the numbers of T, B and natural killer (NK) cells present in the blood. This list is not intended to be exhaustive, but gives examples of several mechanisms by which SCID can occur

Condition	Pathogenesis	Inheritance	Frequency of type in overall SCID populations
T– B– NK– SCID			
Reticular dysgenesis	No stem cells	Autosomal recessive	Very rare
Adenosine deaminase deficiency (ADA)	Defective ADA genes lead to toxic metabolites in T, B and NK cells	Autosomal recessive	8%
T– B– NK+ SCID			
RAG1/2 defect	RAG1/2 enzymes snip DNA for VDJ rearrangement for T-cell and B-cell receptors – partial defect known as Omenn's syndrome	Autosomal recessive	20%
Artemis deficiency	Failure to repair DNA after RAG1/2 snips	Autosomal recessive	Very rare
T– B+ NK– SCID			
X linked	Absent IL receptors for range of cytokines due to lack of common γ chain	X linked	40%
Jak 3 kinase deficiency	No Jak 3 kinase to follow signal via IL-R binding	Autosomal recessive	8%
T– B+ NK+ SCID			
IL-7 receptor deficiency	No IL-7α chains lead to failure of T cells differentiation	Autosomal recessive	24%
CD3δ chain defect	Defective CD3 molecules, as CD3δ essential for assembly	Autosomal recessive	Very rare
CD3 activation failure	Defective signal transduction, e.g. ZAP-70 deficiency	Autosomal recessive	Very rare
T+ B+ NK+ MHC failure			
MHC class I deficiency ('bare lymphocyte syndrome')	Failure to express MHC class I due to defect in TAP-2 transcription	Autosomal recessive	Very rare
MHC class II deficiency	Defect in transcription of MHC class II proteins	Autosomal recessive	Very rare

IL, interleukin; MHC, major histocompatibility complex; RAG, recombination activation genes; TAP, transporter associated with antigen processing; ZAP-70, an intracellular tyrosine kinase.

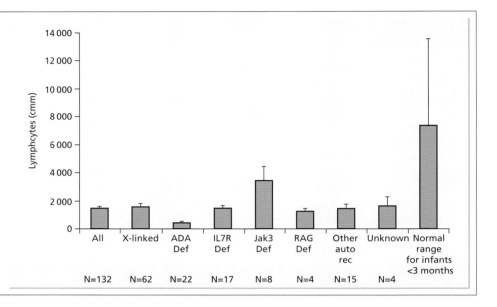

Fig. 3.10 Absolute lymphocyte count (mean +/– SD) in 132 infants with severe combined immune deficiency. Source: Buckley R. (2004). Molecular defects in human severe combined immunodeficiency and approaches to immune reconstitution. *Annual Review of Immunology*, 2004:625–55. Reproduced with permission of Annual Reviews.

effective as well as humanitarian in several countries. Some types of SCID, e.g. cytokine receptor common γ-chain deficiency, are prototypes for gene therapy, but only if a suitable bone marrow donor is not available (see Chapter 7, section 7.4.2). The **variety of different forms of SCID** (Table 3.9) reflects the complexity of the cell surface receptors and the corresponding intracellular signalling enzymes. Recognition of these immune deficiencies in patients has contributed substantially to the further understanding of immune physiology.

As mentioned, some combined immune deficiencies affect other systems as well as the immune system (Table 3.10). Adenosine deaminase (ADA) deficiency is another example in which there are neurological defects too.

The severity, and therefore the **clinical significance**, of the immune defect varies from patient to patient. In the Di George anomaly, which consists of a group of developmental abnormalities resulting in distinctive clinical features (Table 3.10), now known to be due to defects on chromosomes 22 q11 or 4, 7, 8 or 10, the immune defect is usually mild despite the abnormal development of the thymus.

3.4.2 Management of defects in cellular immunity

The management of patients with severe defects in cell-mediated immunity, including SCIDs, involves not only appropriate **antimicrobial therapy** but prophylactic measures also. To **avoid potentially infecting** situations, infants are nursed in positive pressure areas. Immunization with *live vaccines and conventional blood transfusions must be avoided* in patients with proven or suspected T-cell defects: live vaccines (such as Bacillus Calmette–Guérin, BCG) can lead to disseminated infection and blood transfusion and may result in graft-versus-host disease (GVHD; see Chapter 8, section 8.5.3 and Case 8.4) unless irradiated blood is used.

Grafting of viable immunocompetent cells offers the only hope of permanent restoration of immune responsiveness. HSCT (see Chapter 8, section 8.5) is the treatment of choice for all forms of SCID; intrauterine infusion has also been shown to be feasible, though unusual in view of the practical risks. Many SCID babies are now diagnosed at birth (or even antenatally) due to a positive family history. These infants have excellent survival; with good matching, survival post transplant reaches 90% in experienced centres. Replacement of missing factors is a logical approach for enzymes and cytokines, but is temporary and fails to produce a permanent cure. For example, ADA replacement is successful in the short term, provided a chemically modified enzyme with a prolonged *in vivo* life is used, but early stem cell transplantation is preferable.

Gene mapping of many of the defects involved in SCID has led to the relevant genes being cloned. Successful **transfection of genes** into benign retroviral vectors has shown that gene therapy is now practical. However, there is a risk of leukaemia if the vector inserts next to a regulator gene, and a few cases have been reported in children who have been treated in this way. New vectors, or inbuilt auto-destruction of the vector, may resolve this problem. Until now, gene therapy has been reserved for those in whom there is no good match for stem cell transplantation, but clinical studies are evolving. There are a number of prerequisites before gene transfer becomes routine in any human system (Table 3.11), but work in the primary immune deficiencies has led the way. Common γ-chain deficiency, leucocyte adhesion deficiency and chronic granulomatous disease show promising results. ADA-SCID is an example for which gene therapy is now clinically available. This consists of an infusion of autologous gene-corrected haematopoietic stem cells from patients' own bone marrow. These stem cells are genetically modified using a gamma-retroviral vector, thereby inserting a functional copy of the ADA gene.

Table 3.10 Some primary combined immune deficiencies with other non-immunological features, to show the wide range of these associated defects

Condition	Distinctive clinical features	Associated immunological features
DiGeorge anomaly (CATCH 22)	1 Hypoparathyroidism, convulsions, tetany 2 Cardiovascular defects 3 Abnormal facies – low-slung ears, laryngeal dysfunction 4 Recurrent or severe infections are rare	Deletion on chromosome 22 (or rarely other chromosomes) Thymus is abnormal; CD3 cells low but rise with age Complete DiGeorge is rare but if CD3 cells absent, HSCT is urgent
Chronic mucocutaneous candidiasis	1 Candida albicans infections of mucous membrane/nails/skin 2 Associated endocrine abnormalities – hypoparathyroidism, Addison's disease, etc. 3 May be recurrent bacterial infections as well	Gain-of-function mutations in STAT1 genes lead to defects in interferon-γ, IL-17 and IL-22 pathways
Purine nucleoside phosphorylase	1 Recurrent infections, bacterial, fungal and viral 2 Neurological disorders (60%) 3 Autoimmune diseases 4 Failure to thrive	Mutations in PNP gene prevent normal degradation of inosine and guanosine and lead to a build-up of T-cell toxins
Ataxia telangiectasia	1 Cerebellar ataxia with progressive neurological deterioration and radiation sensitivity 2 Oculocutaneous telangiectasia 3 Recurrent viral infections 4 Gonadal dysgenesis 5 Chromosomal abnormalities 6 Malignant disease	Low numbers of CD3 cells that fall with time
Wiskott–Aldrich syndrome	1 Thrombocytopenia 2 Bleeding due to small platelets 3 Eczema 4 Recurrent bacterial infections 5 Malignant disease	Partial antibody deficiency with loss of response to carbohydrate antigens including pneumococcal capsules

HSCT, human stem cell transplantation; IL, interleukin.

Table 3.11 Prerequisites for gene therapy in humans

1 Absence of reasonable present therapy

2 Determination of the precise genetic defect in the patient requiring therapy

3 Single gene disease with mutation known to cause disease (i.e. no complex gene regulation)

4 Cloning of normal gene for the missing product

5 Identification of target cell that will replicate and mature (preferably with survival advantage against defective cells)

6 Transfer of normal gene efficiently to appropriate target cell

7 Synthesis of gene product by that cell

8 Assurance that the transfected gene has no deleterious effects or oncogenic potential (preferably designed with 'off switch' to control replication)

3.5 Primary defects in non-specific immunity

The clinical significance of defects in non-specific immunity has been appreciated for many years; patients with low neutrophil counts have been known to be at risk of overwhelming infection. Furthermore, since **innate immunity** is responsible for host defence very early in infection and adaptive humoral immunity requires non-specific dendritic cells to **initiate antigen-specific responses**, the role of innate immunity is gaining new importance (see Chapter 1). These two systems work in tandem to provide efficient protection against infection. The best-known example is the opsonization of microorganisms, i.e. coating (opsonized) with IgG antibodies and complement; these pathogens are then readily bound, ingested and destroyed by phagocytic cells, such as neutrophils. This interdependence partly explains some similarities between the infectious complications experienced by patients with defects of antibody or complement synthesis and those with neutrophil or macrophage/monocyte dysfunction (see Fig. 3.2).

In terms of missing cell types, monocytopenia is very rare and absence of macrophages would be difficult to detect in humans, though functional defects are known (see Chapter 2, Box 2.3). Neutropenia, however, is common secondarily to therapy or rarely as a primary immune defect.

3.5.1 Functional defects in monocytes and dendritic cells

The major role of the macrophage is to ingest opsonized bacteria and to kill them intracellularly by fusing phagosomes with lysosomes – intracellular structures containing digestive enzymes (see Chapter 1, section 1.3.3). Activation occurs non-specifically via large numbers of germline cellular receptors – **pattern recognition receptors (PRRs)** – that are distinct from the phagocytic receptors. These recognize conserved components of pathogens, known as pathogen-associated molecular patterns (PAMPs) (see Chapter 1, Fig. 1.4). Macrophage PRRs are not specific for individual organisms, unlike T-cell receptors and B-cell receptors, but are communal; they do not undergo gene rearrangement. Macrophages, dendritic cells and monocytes use these to distinguish non-self from self-molecules. Like the adaptive system, defects in the genes for these receptors can lead to absent or non-functional proteins, resulting in excessive or persistent infections, i.e. immune deficiency disorders.

One family of non-phagocytic receptors, known as **Toll-like receptors (TLRs)**, is implicated in such immune deficiencies (see Chapter 1, Fig. 1.2). In the same way as patients with adaptive immune deficiencies suffer from a range of bacterial or viral infections, so in TLR deficiencies patients have a range of pathogens, including intracellular mycobacteria and salmonellae and extracellular streptococci and staphylococci. Many more TLR deficiencies will be found. Already there are similar patients who lack the enzymes in the pathways that activate downstream pathways for killing mechanisms (see Chapter 1, Fig 1.4, and Case 3.6), drawing a parallel with common

γ-chain SCID, in which the clinical disease can result from absence of the enzyme JAK3.

Monocytes and dendritic cells respond to microorganisms very early in infection, to produce cytokines that stimulate the antigen-specific system to produce activated T cells and antibodies. They also trigger **acute-phase responses** to provide additional mechanisms for the limitation of spread of pathogens. These include abnormalities in cytokine receptors for cell activation (IL-15R/IL-17R and IL-1R/TLRs), as well as some intracellular receptors (such as nucleotide-binding oligomerization, NOD) that lead to a common pathway for gene transcription, NF-κB. Since NF-κB regulates the expression of numerous genes controlling the immune and stress responses, inflammatory reactions, cell adhesion and protection against apoptosis, defects in NF-κB result in severe infections with a wide range of organisms. IL-1 receptor-associated kinase (IRAK)-4 deficiency (Case 3.6) is specifically associated with defects affecting the responses to TLRs and IL-1 receptors (IL-1Rs), essential for both the innate and adaptive immune systems. TLRs sense various microbial products (see Chapter 1) and initiate the immune response by leading to the production of key inflammatory cytokines, IL-1 and IL-18, which then amplify the response. IL-1 receptors are responsible for acute-phase responses. Known protein defects in NF-κB activation pathway so far include NEMO, IκB, MyD88 and IRAK-4 (see Chapter 1, Box 1.1) and these are now known to result in primary immune defects in humans and mice. As in the adaptive immune system, defects in either receptors or in the intracellular enzymes of this innate pathway can result in significant immune deficiency (see Table 3.13).

3.5.2 Defects in neutrophil function

The major role of the neutrophil is to ingest, kill and digest invading microorganisms, particularly bacteria and fungi. Failure to fulfil this role leads to infection. Defects in neutrophil function can be quantitative – neutropenia – or qualitative – neutrophil dysfunction. However, irrespective of the basic cause, clinical features are similar and certain generalizations are possible.

🔍 Case 3.6 IRAK-4 deficiency

A 9-year-old girl was admitted with meningitis due to Shigella; previously she had been in hospital with septic arthritis due to Streptococcus pneumoniae as well as several deep-seated abscesses caused by Staphylococci or Streptococcus pyogenes. On each occasion, full blood counts were normal, including lymphocyte and neutrophil counts. Curiously, her C-reactive protein (CRP) had also been low despite severe infections, never higher than 35 mg/l. Other screening tests such as liver function tests, functional complement (CH_{50} and AP_{50}) were normal, as were serum immunoglobulin levels and antibody production (Table 3.12). The only abnormality was failure to reduce dihydrorhodamine on stimulation with lipopolysaccharide *in vitro*, the significance of which was unknown at the time. Years later, when more was known about the innate immune system, peripheral blood mononuclear cells were isolated from her blood and tested *in vitro* for interleukin (IL)-6 production following stimulation with a variety of agents including lipopolysaccharide; poor production of IL-6 was seen. It was thought that she might have a defect in the NF-κB pathway; on sequencing of her IRAK-4 gene, this was found to be the case.

Table 3.12 Immunological investigations in Case 3.6, IRAK-4 deficiency

Investigation	Patient	Normal ranges
Dihydrorhodamine reduction test		
Medium only	2%	8.7 ± 7.3%
Phorbol myristate acid	99%	99.2 ± 0.9%
Lipopolysaccharide	7%	>60%
Serum immunoglobulin concentrations		
IgG *(g/l)*	16.7	6.0–13.0 g/l
IgA *(g/l)*	1.1	0.8–3.0 g/l
IgM *(g/l)*	1.9	0.4–2.5 g/l
IgE (KU/l)	400	<125 kU/l
Post-immunization IgG antibodies to:		
Tetanus	0.06	>0.01 IU/ml
Diphtheria	0.18	>0.01 IU/ml
23 valency Pneumovax	>100	>50 IU/ml
Haemophilus influenzae type b	1.36	>1 µg/ml

Table 3.13 Some parallels between adaptive and innate immune systems: examples of missing immune components leading to immune deficiencies (this is not exhaustive)

	Adaptive defects	Innate defects		
Type of defect	Lymphocytes	Dendritic cells	Neutrophils	Macrophages
Differentiation defect leading to low numbers	Btk for B cells (XLA)		Neutropenia	Unknown at present
	IL-7 for T cells			
Receptors	Cytokine receptor common γ chain (cγR SCID)	Toll-like receptor 2	Leucocyte adhesion molecules	IL-12/IFN-γ receptors
Signalling pathway/ activation defects	JAK 3–tyrosine kinase	IRAK-4/MyD88		
		NEMO		
Effector function defects	Perforin defect in CD8 deficiency		Chronic granulomatous disease – cytochromes for oxidative burst	Chediak–Higashi – failure of fusion of lysosomes

IFN, interferon; IL, interleukin; SCID, severe combined immunodeficiency; XLA, X-linked agammaglobulinaemia.

The circulating neutrophil count normally exceeds 1.5×10^9/l. While mild degrees of **neutropenia** are usually asymptomatic, moderate to severe reductions in numbers are associated with a progressive increase in the risk and severity of infections. Episodes of infection are likely to be life threatening when the neutrophil count falls below 0.5×10^9/l.

Neutropenia is more common than neutrophil dysfunction and *secondary causes of neutropenia are more common than primary ones* (Fig. 3.11); for example, neutropenia is a frequent side effect of chemotherapy for malignant disease. Primary neutropenia is rare; congenital forms range in severity and, if severe, are often fatal. Treatment with recombinant human

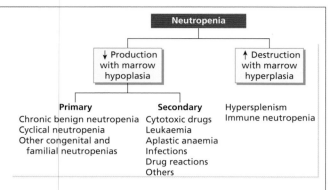

Fig. 3.11 Some causes of neutropenia. Secondary causes are far more common than primary ones.

granulocyte–colony-stimulating factor (G-CSF) stimulates myeloid stem cells, although long-term complications include vasculitis. **Neutrophil function** can be conveniently subdivided into stages: mobilization from bone marrow or spleen; chemotaxis to a site of infection; phagocytosis of pathogen; and fusion with lysosome to release enzymes to kill organism (see Chapter 19, Fig. 19.17). Qualitative defects in these functional steps result in typical infections and some unexplained accompanying features (Table 3.14).

When intracellular killing mechanisms fail, ingested bacteria may survive and proliferate in an intracellular environment free from the effects of antibodies and most antibiotics. One of the most severe types of neutrophil defect occurs in **chronic granulomatous disease** (CGD). CGD is a group of disorders resulting from a failure to produce high concentrations of highly toxic reactive oxygen species during the 'respiratory burst' that accompanies activation of phagocytes. Although it

was originally thought that these toxic oxygen species were directly bactericidal, it is now known that mice deficient in neutrophil-granule proteases, but normal in respect of superoxide production, are also unable to resist staphylococcal and Candida infections. It is the proteases, released by the efflux of potassium ions that follows superoxide production, that are primarily responsible for the destruction of the bacteria.

The **classic type of CGD** is inherited as an X-linked recessive disorder, and typically presents in males in the first two months of life, as in Case 3.7, although the diagnosis may not be made until young adulthood (Box 3.4). The usual **complications** include regional lymphadenopathy, hepatosplenomegaly, hepatic abscesses and osteomyelitis. Affected organs show multiple abscesses caused by Staphylococcus aureus, Gram-negative bacilli or fungi and non-caseating, giant cell granulomas.

The simplest **screening test for CGD** is the nitroblue tetrazolium test (see Chapter 19, section 19.10), which depends on the ability of polymorphs to generate superoxide radicals during phagocytosis. Sensitive assays enable diagnosis of the carrier state in CGD and prenatal diagnosis on cells obtained by fetal blood sampling – the dihydrorhodamine reduction (DHR) test (see Chapter 19, section 19.10). CGD is caused by defects in the phagocyte nicotinamide adenine dinucleotide phosphate (NADPH) oxidase complex, which results in the lack of one specific cytochrome involved in the 'respiratory burst'. Female carriers of the X-linked condition have half the normal amount of this cytochrome and their white cells have about half the normal capacity for generating oxygen radicals. Activation of granulocytes loaded with DHR generates reactive oxygen intermediates that react with DHR, and the resulting increase in fluorescence can be measured by flow cytometry. In the X-linked form of CGD, carriers demonstrate two cell populations, one

Table 3.14 Features of some primary defects of neutrophil function resulting in recurrent infections

Condition	Distinctive clinical features	Functional defect	Inheritance
Leucocyte adhesion deficiency	1 Skin infections and gingivitis 2 Deep abscesses, peritonitis, osteomyelitis	Fail to adhere to endothelial cells and so to traverse into tissues to ingest and kill bacteria	Autosomal recessive
Chediak–Higashi syndrome	1 Giant lysosomal granules in secretory cells 2 Partial oculocutaneous albinism	Abnormal chemotaxis, so fail to reach bacteria, and reduced microbicidal activity as lysosomes fail to fuse with phagosomes	Autosomal recessive
Hyper-IgE: recurrent infection syndrome	1 Coarse facial features 2 Mucocutaneous candidiasis 3 Huge level of serum IgE 4 Lung abscesses and pneumatocoeles 5 Abnormal calcium metabolism 6 Atopic dermatitis	STAT3 defects result in IL-17 and other cytokine defects as well as structural changes	Familial and non-familial cases
Chronic granulomatous disease	1 Abscesses with catalase positive organisms 2 Granuloma formation	↓Oxidative metabolism and fail to kill Staph. and fungi	X-linked or autosomal recessive

IL, interleukin.

Case 3.7 Chronic granulomatous disease

Mark was born by Caesarean section and weighed 3.1 kg. He is the sixth child of unrelated white parents. At the age of 4 weeks, he developed an axillary abscess that healed spontaneously, followed by a staphylococcal abscess of the chest wall, requiring surgical incision and a course of flucloxacillin. He had a total white-cell count of 45 × 10⁹/l, of which 90% were neutrophils, giving an unusually high neutrophil count.

At the ages of 3 months and 7 months, he was readmitted to hospital with large staphylococcal abscesses, first on his face and then on his right buttock; both abscesses were treated by surgical incision and systemic antibiotics for 10 days. By the age of 2 years, he had been admitted to hospital five times with staphylococcal abscesses. The family history was remarkable: three elder brothers had died of infections at ages ranging from 7 months to 3 years, but his parents and two sisters were healthy.

On examination, he was pale and persistently pyrexial. His height and weight were below the third centile. He had bilateral axillary and inguinal lymphadenopathy with marked hepatosplenomegaly.

Laboratory tests showed mild anaemia (Hb 104 g/l) with marked polymorphonuclear leucocytosis. His immunological investigations are summarized in Table 3.15. There was gross polyclonal elevation of all immunoglobulin classes, particularly IgG and IgA. A dihydrorhodamine test on this boy showed that his polymorphs failed to reduce the dye and that his mother had two populations of neutrophils, one normal and one also unable to reduce dihydrorhodamine. These findings, and the X-linked nature of the condition, are diagnostic of chronic granulomatous disease (CGD).

Now aged 7 years, Mark continues to have periodic abscesses despite long-term co-trimoxazole. Since most antibiotics fail to penetrate cells effectively, treatment of acute infections is continued for at least 8 weeks. He has not had a major infection necessitating therapy with interferon (IFN)-γ, but is on a prophylactic antifungal agent. He will be considered for human stem cell transplantation when a matched donor can be found.

Table 3.15 Immunological tests* in Case 3.7, chronic granulomatous disease

Quantitative serum immunoglobulins (g/l)		
IgG	17.8	(5.5–10.0)
IgA	4.8	(0.3–0.8)
IgM	2.0	(0.4–1.8)
Antibody activity		
IgG antibodies: post immunization		
Tetanus toxoid	89	(>1.0 IU/ml)
Diphtheria toxoid	3.0	(>0.6 IU/ml)
Nitroblue tetrazolium (NBT) test†		
Unstimulated	2	(normal <10)
Stimulated	4	(normal >30)
Dihydrorhodamine test‡		
Control		90% cells positive
Patient		0% cells positive

*Normal range for age (or value for healthy control studied in parallel) is shown in parentheses. †Percentage of neutrophils showing reduction of NBT before and after stimulation with endotoxin (see Chapter 19). ‡ See Chapter 19, section 19.8.

> ### Box 3.4 Clues from the history in chronic granulomatous disease
>
> Infections are recurrent and prolonged. Clinical features may be minimal despite severe infection. Infections are:
>
> - poorly responsive to antibiotics
> - commonly staphylococcal
> - in particular caused by catalase-producing microorganisms
> - involve skin and mucous membranes
> - complicated by lymphadenopathy

reacting with DHR and the other not, whereas neutrophils from affected boys are unable to react with DHR.

Treatment of CGD relies on prophylactic antibiotics (usually co-trimoxazole) and antifungal agents when required. Studies with the cytokine IFN-γ have shown some reduction in the numbers of infections without apparently improving the killing capacity of neutrophils. Allogeneic bone marrow transplantation from a human leukocyte antigen (HLA)-matched related donor offers the only long-term hope of cure for patients with CGD. This procedure has a significant mortality rate of about 10%, and it should be reserved for patients with debilitating or life-threatening complications. CGD is well suited for gene therapy, as it results from single gene defects that almost exclusively affect the haemopoietic system.

3.5.3 Defects of effector functions of macrophages

As in SCID, there are also cytokine receptor defects on the surface of macrophages that result in primary immune deficiencies. All species of Mycobacteria enter these cell types to reproduce, but this is normally controlled by the intracellular production of IL-12, which in turn activates T cells to produce IFN-γ. Not surprisingly, **absence of either these cytokines or their receptors** results in susceptibility to both Mycobacterium tuberculosis and atypical (less pathogenic) forms of mycobacteria (Case 3.8).

Structural defects can result in failure of intracellular killing mechanisms in macrophages, though these are very rare indeed. The severe immune deficiency of Chediak–Higashi syndrome is an example, in which the relationship of the mild accompanying defects of partial albinism and defective platelets with the failure to fuse lysosomes and thus kill pathogens remains unexplained (see Tables 3.13 and 3.14).

3.5.4 Complex innate disorders

As in T-cell deficiencies, there are other failures of innate immunity that are associated with abnormalities in non-immune systems. A good example is autosomal dominant **hyper-IgE syndrome (HIES)**; variants in STAT3 cause this unusual complex immunodeficiency with marked inflammation and structural abnormalities (Table 3.14). STAT3 is necessary in embryogenesis

 Case 3.8 IL-12 receptor deficiency

A 3-year-old-girl, Sophia, born to consanguineous parents, came to the outpatient department with a newly enlarged and persistent single lymph node in the supraclavicular region. Her parents were extremely anxious about leukaemia, although the child was well and a full blood count done in advance was normal. She had not been exposed to Mycobacteria tuberculosis, nor had she received Bacille Calmette–Guérin (BCG). She had had a few episodes of otitis media after an upper respiratory tract infection, but no infections elsewhere. Biopsy of the lymph node was performed under general anaesthetic; histology showed a granuloma and the presence of a few acid-fast bacilli; an atypical (environmental) mycobacterium was grown on culture.

In order to be sure that this was not due to human immunodeficiency virus (HIV) disease, the child and her parents were tested after parental consent was given; the results were negative. Analysis of T, B and natural killer (NK) cells was normal, excluding a late presentation of severe combined immunodeficiency (SCID) or another combined defect. Interferon (IFN)-γ and interleukin (IL)-12 production by monocytes and T cells were shown to be normal by Elispot. However a markedly reduced expression of IL-12 receptors on the surface of activated T cells was found and a diagnosis of complete IL-12 receptor deficiency was confirmed on mutation analysis. She has three healthy older siblings who were found to be heterozygous for the defect, as were her healthy parents.

and for the production of many cytokines, including IL-6, IL-10, IL-11, IL-17, IL-21, IL-22 and IL-23. It therefore has a central role, both proinflammatory (e.g. IL-6) and antiinflammatory (e.g. IL-10), as well as in organ development; this may account for the multiple organ abnormalities seen in HIES patients (see Table 3.14). This is not the whole story, however, as there is no correlation between the genetic findings and the clinical features (genotype–phenotype correlation) in many of the features of HIES, so other genes/transcription factors will be found to be important too. Variants in STAT3 also lead to failure of Th17 CD4 cell differentiation, which is STAT3 dependent, and IL-17 signalling is involved in the response to **Staphylococcus aureus** in the skin. IL-22 and IL-17 play a role in protection against staphylococcal and candidal infection by upregulating human beta-defensin 2 and CC-chemokine ligand 20 (CCL20), both antimicrobial proteins. These proteins are also important in atopic dermatitis and gingivitis, common clinical features in HIES.

3.5.5 Complement deficiency

Impaired complement activity is usually secondary to those diseases in which complement is consumed via the classical or alternate pathways. A common example is systemic lupus

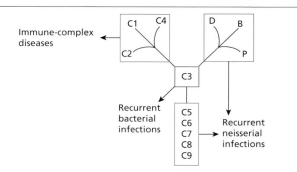

Fig. 3.12 Inherited complement deficiencies: characteristic clinical syndromes are associated with deficiencies of certain groups of components.

erythematosus (SLE; see Chapter 10, section 10.7), in which consumption of the early classical pathway complement components C1, C4 and C2 impairs the ability of complement to solubilize immune complexes, the degree of impairment correlating with disease activity.

In humans, **inherited deficiencies of complement** components are associated with characteristic clinical syndromes (Fig. 3.12). Many patients with C1q, C4 or C2 deficiency have presented with a lupus-like syndrome of malar flush, arthralgia, glomerulonephritis, fever or chronic vasculitis and, in the case of C1q deficiency, with recurrent pyogenic infections. Antinuclear and anti-dsDNA antibodies (see Chapter 10, section 10.7) may be absent. Deficiency of any of these early classical pathway components probably compromises the ability of the host to eliminate immune complexes. Such a defect can be demonstrated by failure to detect haemolytic activity in the classical complement pathway, while the alternate pathway is normal (see Chapter 19).

Patients with **C3 deficiency**, occurring as a primary or secondary defect following deficiencies of C3b inhibitors, i.e. factor I or factor H (see Chapter 1), may have an increased susceptibility to recurrent bacterial infections or other clinical features. For example, total deficiency of Factor H is also associated with glomerulonephritis and renal failure, partial deficiency with familial (atypical) haemolytic uraemic syndrome and the presence of a particular allele with adult macular degeneration (see Chapter 7). Affected individuals with extremely low C3 for whichever reason typically present with life-threatening infections such as pneumonia, septicaemia and meningitis, illustrating the important role of C3 in defence against infection (see Chapter 1). Tests of both haemolytic pathways are abnormal.

There is a striking association between **deficiencies of C5, C6, C7, C8 or properdin** and recurrent neisserial infection. Patients present with recurrent gonococci infection, particularly septicaemia or arthritis, or recurrent meningococcal meningitis, as in Case 3.9. *However, patients should be tested after only one episode of meningitis, as many years may elapse between attacks.*

C1 inhibitor deficiency is the commonest inherited deficiency of the complement system and causes hereditary angioedema (see Chapter 11, section 11.5.1).

3.6 Secondary immunodeficiency

3.6.1 Secondary causes of immunodeficiency

Secondary causes of immunodeficiency are far more common than primary causes. Levels of immune components, as in any system, represent the **net balance** of component

---

Case 3.9 Isolated deficiency of complement component

A 26-year-old West Indian man presented with a 24-h history of occipital headache and vomiting. He was pyrexial (temperature 38.3 °C), confused, irritable and had marked neck stiffness with a positive Kernig's sign. There was no other history of serious infections. His immediate family were healthy.

Lumbar puncture produced turbid cerebrospinal fluid (CSF) with a protein concentration of 4.5 g/l (NR 0.1–0.4), glucose content of <0.1 mmol/l (NR 2.5–4.0) and a leucocyte count of 8000/mm³ (97% neutrophils). Neisseria meningitidis was cultured from the CSF. The patient was treated with intravenous penicillin and oral chloramphenicol and made a rapid recovery over the following 2 weeks.

A search was made for an underlying cause of his meningitis. X-rays of the skull and sinuses showed no abnormal communication with the CSF. The possibility of an underlying immune defect was then considered and the results of immunological tests are shown in Table 3.16. Antibody production to a variety of bacterial and viral antigens was normal. However, total classical pathway haemolytic complement activity (CH$_{50}$) and alternate pathway (AP$_{50}$) were consistently undetectable in his serum during convalescence, indicating a complete functional absence of one or more complement components of the terminal lytic pathway. Eventually, he was shown to have an isolated deficiency of C6, with normal levels of all other components. Half normal levels of C6 were found in the sera of his parents and in three of his four siblings: the other sibling had a normal level.

Unlike immunoglobulin deficiency, long-term replacement of missing complement components is not feasible at present because their half-lives are so short (<1 day). Nasopharyngeal carriage of Neisseria meningitidis by the patient and his close contacts can be eradicated by antibiotics, but at the risk of inducing resistant strains. Prophylactic penicillin is used in those patients with symptomatic complement deficiencies along with immunization to the locally prevalent types of Neisseria for which vaccines are available.

Table 3.16 Immunological investigations* in Case 3.9, complement deficiency

Quantitative serum immunoglobulins (g/l)		
IgG	15.0	(7.2–19.0)
IgA	3.2	(0.8–5.0)
IgM	1.2	(0.5–2.0)
Antibody activity		
Normal titres of antibodies to tetanus toxoid, diphtheria toxoid and pneumococci		
Detectable antibodies to herpes simplex, measles, influenza A and adenovirus		
Complement activity		
CH_{50}		No detectable activity
AP_{50}		No detectable activity

* Normal ranges shown in parentheses.

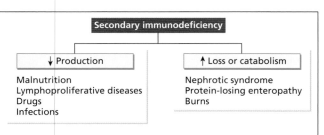

Fig. 3.13 Common causes of secondary immunodeficiency.

synthesis versus consumption, catabolism or loss. Low levels reflect either depressed production or accelerated consumption (Fig. 3.13).

Protein loss severe enough to cause low antibody levels and hypoproteinaemia occurs mainly via the kidney (the nephrotic syndrome) or through the gut (protein-losing enteropathy). The primary diagnosis of nephrotic syndrome usually presents little difficulty; renal loss of immunoglobulin is at least partially selective, so that IgA and IgM levels are maintained despite the fall in serum IgG and albumin. Recurrent infections are rarely a significant problem as specific antibody synthesis is intact. Protein can also be lost from the gut in a variety of active inflammatory diseases such as Crohn's disease, ulcerative colitis or coeliac disease. In intestinal lymphangiectasia, the dilated gut lymphatics leak lymphocytes as well as proteins.

Impaired synthesis is exemplified by malnutrition. Severe protein deficiency causes profound changes in many organs, including the immune system. Malnourished people show an increased incidence of infectious disease but the association is complex, since low-grade infection itself may cause malnourishment. Impaired specific antibody production following immunization, and defects in cell-mediated immunity, phagocyte function and complement

activity, are associated with **extreme poor nutrition**. These reverse after adequate protein and caloric supplementation of the diet.

Patients with **malignant monoclonal lymphoproliferative diseases** are very prone to infection (see Chapter 6, Case 6.2). Untreated chronic lymphocytic leukaemia is often associated with antibody failure and recurrent chest infections, which tend to become more severe as the disease progresses. Non-Hodgkin's lymphoma may be associated with defects of both humoral and cell-mediated immunity. Hodgkin's disease is usually associated with marked impairment of cell-mediated immunity. Chemotherapy for lymphoma, usually with an anti-B-cell agent, often results in secondary antibody deficiency as well as reduced B cells; the B-cell component may not recover and secondary panhypogammaglobulinaemia may ensue.

The infection risk in patients with **multiple myeloma** is five- to tenfold higher than in age-matched controls. Initially, the plasma-cell tumour mass is treated aggressively with chemotherapy (Chapter 6, section 6.5.2). Even before treatment, there is considerable suppression of polyclonal (non-paraprotein) antibody production and chemotherapy results in added suppression of T cells and phagocytic cells. The resultant infections reflect combined B- and T-cell deficiencies and thus may be bacterial, viral or fungal. During remission (plateau phase) the incidence and range of infections decrease; infections at this stage are mainly bacterial, reflecting the dominant polyclonal humoral immune suppression, unless HSTC is done.

The frequency of opportunistic infections in patients with disseminated non-lymphoid malignancies suggests a significant underlying immune defect, although it is difficult to distinguish between the immunosuppressive effects of the disease and those of the treatment. **Immunosuppressive drugs** affect lymphocyte and neutrophil activity, and low antibody levels are unusual (see Chapter 7). Patients on drugs to prevent organ transplant rejection also develop unusual opportunistic infections (see section 3.6.8). Another iatrogenic form of secondary immune deficiency is that associated with splenectomy (see also Chapter 7, Case 7.5). Every year there are deaths from sudden, overwhelming infection due to Streptococcus pneumoniae in patients who have been **splenectomized**, often years before. The overall risk of death from infection following splenectomy is 1–2% over 15 years. All such patients should receive immunization with pneumococcal conjugate vaccine (see Chapter 7, section 7.3.3) as well as prophylactic penicillin and be vaccinated against Haemophilus influenza type b and *N.* meningitides, as these encapsulated organisms can cause significant morbidity and mortality in asplenic patients.

In a number of infections, the **microorganism paradoxically suppresses** rather than stimulates the immune system (see Chapter 2, section 2.3). Severe, though transient, impairment of cell-mediated immunity has been noted in many viral illnesses, particularly cytomegalovirus, measles, rubella, infectious mononucleosis and viral hepatitis. However, the most florid example is infection with HIV (Cases 3.10 and 3.11).

Case 3.10 Acquired immune deficiency syndrome (AIDS): Persistent generalized lymphadenopathy

A 29-year-old man had a history of fatigue, night sweats, diarrhoea and axillary lymphadenopathy for 6 months. Fine-needle lymph-node biopsy suggested a reactive cause rather than malignancy. At a follow-up visit 2 months later he was found to have palpable, non-tender cervical and inguinal nodes and considerable weight loss (8.5 kg) associated with colitis. Further investigations were done to exclude a lymphoma. Computed tomography scan of his chest and abdomen showed no lymph-node enlargement and no organomegaly (Box 3.5).

Immunological investigations are shown in Table 3.17. Full blood counts were normal, as was the C-reactive protein (CRP) level. In view of these findings, he was asked about previous blood transfusions (none) and high-risk activity for human immunodeficiency virus (HIV) infection (three heterosexual partners), counselled and tested for HIV antibody. He was HIV antibody positive. A clinical diagnosis of AIDS was made, on the basis of a positive HIV antibody test and weight loss of more than 10% in 12 months.

Viral load measurement showed 46×10^3 copies of HIV-RNA per millilitre and he was positive for cytomegalovirus infection by PCR. In view of the low CD4 count he was started on prophylactic co-trimoxozole and combination therapy. Cytomegalovirus (CMV) colitis was treated with Ganciclovir. He was initially reviewed at 4-weekly intervals and monitored with regular viral load measurements, but became a poor attender and there was doubt about compliance with therapy. Four years later he complained of headaches, vomiting, a dry cough, sweats and profound breathlessness on minimal exertion. A chest X-ray showed bilateral lower-lobe shadowing and subsequently bronchial washings were positive for Pneumocystis jirovecii; rapid deterioration occurred and he died of respiratory failure.

At post-mortem examination, CMV and Mycobacterium avium-intracellulare were also isolated from the lungs. A particular surprise was the presence of localized, unsuspected central nervous system lymphoma.

Table 3.17 Immunological investigations* in Case 3.10, human immunodeficiency virus (HIV) infection

Quantitative serum immunoglobulins (g/l)		
IgG	16.00	(8.0–18.0)
IgA	7.90	(0.9–4.5)
IgM	1.65	(0.6–2.8)
Peripheral blood lymphocytes (10⁹/l)		
Total lymphocyte count	1.8	(1.5–3.5)
T lymphocytes (CD3)	1.51	(0.9–2.8)
CD4⁺	0.20	(0.6–1.2)
CD8⁺	1.26	(0.4–1.0)
B lymphocytes (CD19)	0.14	(0.2–0.4)

* Normal ranges shown in parentheses.

Case 3.11 Acquired immune deficiency syndrome: Kaposi's sarcoma

A 45-year-old man presented with a skin 'rash' of 2 months' duration. This had started as a single, small spot on his trunk, followed by widespread crops of similar lesions; they were painless and did not itch. He had no other symptoms; in particular, no cough, chest symptoms, fever, weight loss or lymphadenopathy. He was homosexual, with one regular sexual partner over the preceding 2 years, though he participated in casual, unprotected sexual intercourse while on holiday (Box 3.5). He had never used intravenous drugs.

He was apyrexial, with bilateral axillary and inguinal lymphadenopathy. About 20 purplish-red nodules were present on his trunk, face and palate as well as at the anal margin. His nose showed similar discoloration and swelling. White, wart-like projections of 'hairy leucoplakia' were present on the sides of his tongue.

Investigations showed a normal haemoglobin, a normal white-cell count (4.9×10^9/l) and normal absolute lymphocyte count (1.8×10^9/l). After counselling, blood was sent for an human immunodeficiency virus (HIV) antibody test; this was positive by enzyme-linked immunosorbent assay (ELISA) and confirmed by Western blotting (see Chapter 19). A second test was also positive. Immunological studies (Table 3.18) showed a raised serum IgA and analysis of lymphocyte sub-populations showed absolute depletion of $CD4^+$ cells.

Biopsy of one of his skin lesions showed the typical histological features of Kaposi's sarcoma, so the clinical diagnosis was that of the acquired immune deficiency syndrome, caused by HIV-1.

He was started initially on combination therapy and prophylactic co-trimoxazole and undertook regular monitoring. He remains well more than 18 years later, and is religiously compliant with HAART.

Table 3.18 Immunological investigations* in Case 3.11, human immunodeficiency virus (HIV) infection

Serum immunoglobulins (g/l)		
IgG	20.2	(8.0–18.0)
IgA	2.1	(0.9–4.5)
IgM	0.9	(0.6–2.8)
Electrophoresis – hypergammaglobulinaemia		
β_2-microglobulin	3.8 mg/l	(<3.5)
Lymphocyte subpopulations ($\times 10^9$/l)		
Total lymphocyte count	2.80	(1.5–3.5)
T lymphocytes		
$CD3^+$	2.35	(0.9–2.8)
$CD4^+$	0.23	(0.6–1.2)
$CD8^+$	2.04	(0.4–1.0)
B lymphocytes		
$CD19^+$	0.36	(0.2–0.4)

*Normal adult ranges shown in parentheses.

3.6.2 Acquired immune deficiency syndrome

Acquired immune deficiency syndrome (AIDS) is the final stage in the progression of infectious disease caused by HIV. According to a **United Nations report in 2019 (UNAIDS)**, 1.7 million people became newly infected with HIV in 2018 worldwide. Since 2010, new HIV infections have declined by an estimated 16%, from 2.1 million to 1.7 million. AIDS-related deaths have been reduced by more than 56% since the peak in 2004 (1.7 million deaths in 2004 versus 770 000 deaths in 2018). In 2018, there were 38 million people living with HIV worldwide. Sub-Saharan Africa is the region most affected and accounts for 70% of all people living with HIV, with nearly 1 in every 20 adults living with HIV.

HIV produces a **spectrum of disorders** from a transient, acute glandular fever-like illness to life-threatening tumours and opportunistic infections. HIV also causes dementia, auto-immune disorders and atrophy of particular organs (e.g. brain).

Of the global spread of HIV infection, 70% is thought to be by **heterosexual transmission**. In contrast to the USA and

Europe, the African male-to-female ratio of cases is almost 1: 1, with severe implications for the numbers of infants born to HIV-positive mothers. The prognosis was dismal prior to antiviral therapy, but new therapeutic regimens have changed the outlook for HIV-infected individuals. Politicians and drug companies are now finding ways to bring these expensive therapies to patients everywhere.

3.6.3 Transmission of human immunodeficiency virus infection

HIV has been isolated from semen, cervical secretions, lymphocytes, cell-free plasma, cerebrospinal fluid, tears, saliva, urine and breast milk. Not all these fluids transmit infection, since the concentration of virus varies considerably; semen, blood, breast milk and cervical secretions have been proven to be infectious.

Transmission occurs mainly through sexual intercourse, heterosexual or homosexual. To reduce transmission significantly, educational and awareness policies are essential. Many countries in sub-Saharan Africa have introduced voluntary counselling and testing programmes and there is good evidence that these can change HIV-related sexual risk behaviours, thereby reducing HIV-related risk. Epidemics in men who have sex with men are reemerging in many high-income countries and are gaining greater recognition in many low-income and middle-income countries. HIV prevention strategies using preexposure pharmacological prophylaxis (PrEP) using antiretroviral drugs such as emtricitabine have been shown to be effective for this group. Transmission can also occur via blood and blood products. Sharing of contaminated needles and syringes by intravenous drug abusers, and by therapeutic procedures in areas of the world where reuse of contaminated equipment occurs, can result in HIV (and other viral) transmission. There should be no new HIV seroconversions in blood product recipients in countries in which blood is now screened and blood products treated to inactivate any possible virus. **Vertical transmission** from mother to child *in utero* or at delivery is the dominant route of infant infection, although fewer than 20% of children born to HIV-positive mothers become infected. Since maternal antibody to HIV crosses the placenta, *a positive test in an infant does not indicate infection*. Vertical transfer of HIV may also occur after birth through breast milk (see Chapter 18, section 18.3.3). Neonatal diagnosis depends on detection of nucleic acid (by PCR) or viral antigen (by enzyme-linked immunosorbent assay, ELISA) *and the mother must be tested also*. In a previously undiagnosed family it is essential to test both parents: the mother for vertical transmission and the father in case the mother is recently infected but as yet HIV antibody negative due to the window period.

Seroconversion of healthcare workers is still reported after a needle stick injury, but there is no evidence, despite many studies, that the virus is spread by mosquitoes, bed bugs or swimming pools, or by sharing eating utensils or toilets with an infected person.

3.6.4 The clinical spectrum of human immunodeficiency virus infection

HIV produces a spectrum of disorders (Fig. 3.14). A transient, acute glandular fever-like illness occurs first in patients, but this usually goes unsuspected (Box 3.5). Like other viral illnesses, this is accompanied by finding atypical lymphocytes and an increased number of CD8$^+$ T cells in the blood, followed by seroconversion; the time interval between infection and the production of antibodies to HIV (the '**window period**') may be as long as 6 months.

Most HIV-seropositive individuals then remain symptom free for up to 10 years; development of AIDS depends on the contribution of many **co-factors** such as genetic background (those with HLA-B57 or HLA-B27 have a better prognosis), repeated stimulation by foreign antigens (multiple co-infections speed the rate of progression) or pregnancy. Almost all patients developed recurring opportunistic infections in the early stages before antiviral therapy. Some individuals develop asymptomatic persistent generalized lymphadenopathy (Case 3.10), while others suffered from autoimmune diseases (Fig. 3.13). The most important **prognostic factor** for progression to AIDS is the concentration of HIV-RNA in the blood – "viral load" – at diagnosis.

The major clinical manifestations of AIDS are **tumours** and **opportunistic infections**. Kaposi's sarcoma (due to HHV8) is the commonest tumour (Case 3.11), but non-Hodgkin's lymphoma (due to EBV) of B-cell phenotype and often within the central nervous system, and squamous carcinoma of the mouth or anorectum (due to HPV), are also frequent. The many opportunistic infections affect virtually all systems of the body; however, the commonest organs involved are the lung, gut and central nervous system (Fig. 3.13).

HIV is **neurotrophic** as well as lymphotrophic: acute aseptic meningitis, encephalopathy, myelopathy and neuropathy have been reported around the time of seroconversion, while chronic meningitis, lymphoma, encephalopathy and dementia may occur later. Around 70% of AIDS patients suffer from HIV-related dementia, which is probably a direct effect of HIV. Despite the arrival of combination antiretroviral therapy (cART), with reduced incidence and improved survival, the spectrum of central nervous system diseases has remained relatively unchanged. However with long life spans, the incidence of clinical symptoms suggestive of IgE-mediated allergic disease in individuals infected with HIV has become apparent.

Most patients in the USA and Europe present with Pneumocystis jirovecii. pneumonia, other opportunistic infections or Kaposi's sarcoma. The **presentation** in African patients is different: in Africans, AIDS is characterized primarily by a diarrhoea–wasting syndrome ('slim disease'), Kaposi's sarcoma and opportunistic infections such as tuberculosis, cryptococcosis or cryptosporidiosis. **Infants with HIV infection** (<20% of those born to HIV-infected mothers) present at around 6 months, while cases associated with other forms of transmission (e.g. dirty needles for immunization) present later. These children fail to thrive and nearly all have oral candidiasis and recurrent bacterial infections. Chronic interstitial pneumonitis is

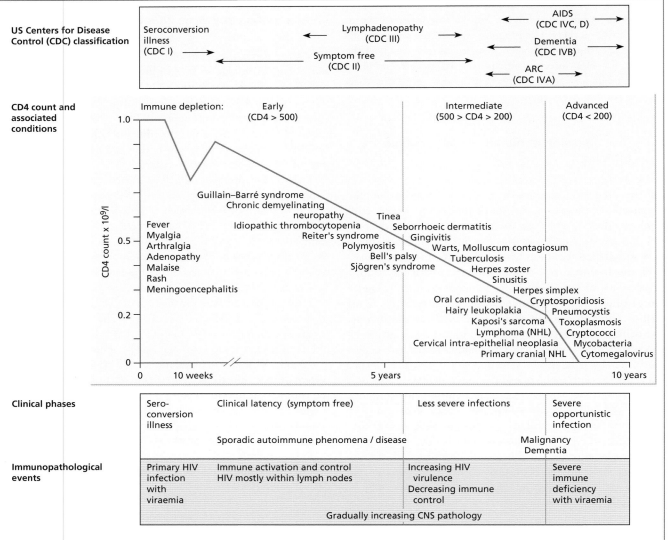

Fig. 3.14 Chronology of human immunodeficiency virus (HIV)-induced disease correlated with time since infection. CD4⁺ T-cell depletion, immunopathology and CDC classification. ARC, acquired immune deficiency syndrome (AIDS)-related complex; CD4, CD4⁺ T lymphocytes; CNS, central nervous system; NHL, non-Hodgkin's lymphoma.

Box 3.5 Important points emphasized by human immunodeficiency virus (HIV) cases

- Not all patients with HIV present with recognizably HIV-related symptoms or signs
- A careful 'high-risk' history is important, but not always helpful
- If there is a possibility of HIV infection, an HIV antibody test should always be done, after appropriate counselling
- If there is still a strong clinical suspicion, HIV-PCR (polymerase chain reaction) testing should be done
- Absolute compliance with therapy is essential to prevent disease progression

characteristic. In the late stage, typical opportunistic infections may occur, but Kaposi's sarcoma and other tumours are rare.

Once AIDS has developed, the **prognosis** is dismal if untreated. Prior to antiviral therapy, survival was about 9–12 months for patients with *P. jirovecii* pneumonia, 6–12 months for other opportunistic infections and 20–30 months for Kaposi's sarcoma. The survival time for patients treated with new therapies will depend on previous treatment (due to viral resistance to the drug), size of the viral load, HLA type of patient and, of course, the virulence and genetic mutation rate of the virus. Rare resistance to HIV in those exposed repeatedly is associated with particular genetic variants of CCR5, a chemokine receptor used for entry of the virus (see section 3.6.7); these resistant patients are known as long-term survivors.

3.6.5 Immunopathogenesis of acquired immune deficiency syndrome

AIDS is a pandemic form of immunodeficiency, caused by several different variants of HIV retroviruses. **Retroviruses** belong to the lentivirus group, so called for the slow development of the disease. They are RNA viruses that possess a unique enzyme, reverse transcriptase, to synthesize virus-specific double-stranded DNA from the viral RNA genome (Fig. 3.15). The new DNA is integrated into the genome of the infected cell and may remain latent in these cells. Once reactivated, viral DNA is used as a template for the RNA required for virus production. Viral release takes place at the cell surface by budding; the envelope of the virus is formed from the host cell membrane, modified by the insertion of viral glycoproteins.

HIV enters susceptible cells either through binding of viral envelope glycoprotein (gp120) to specific receptors on the cell surface or by fusion between the viral lipid envelope and the target cell membrane. The variant of HIV determines the **major route of entry**. Lymphotrophic variants use the CD4 molecule itself, with CXCR4 as a co-factor. Cells, such as macrophages and dendritic cells, with low levels of surface CD4 are infected via the chemokine receptor, CCR5. Other cells, such as glial cells of the central nervous system and epithelial cells in the gut and uterine cervix, have different receptors for HIV and are also susceptible. At mucosal surfaces, where contact with HIV usually occurs, infection occurs predominantly either in the mucosal cells themselves or in intraepithelial dendritic cells; these cell types can then pass the virus to CD4 cells by fusion of the viral lipid envelope and the target cell membrane, bypassing any neutralizing antibodies that may be present.

Since HIV **replicates** at a rate of 10^9–10^{10} new virions per day, resulting in as many as 10^8 new mutants per day, the immune response has an enormous task to limit HIV. In addition, the fast replication results in intrinsically unstable B-cell-binding epitopes and production of high-affinity antibodies for neutralization does not keep up with the mutations. Cytotoxic T cells are less susceptible since, depending on the HLA type, they bind to more stable epitopes.

HIV-associated disease is characterized by major defects in immunity, following the elimination of CD4 cells. When normal CD4 T lymphocytes are stimulated by antigen, they respond by release of lymphokines, including IL-2, interferons and B-cell growth factors (see Chapter 1); these regulate growth, maturation and activation of cytotoxic T cells (antiviral), macrophages (antiintracellular bacteria, protozoa and fungi) and NK cells (involved in tumour surveillance). The most **striking effects of HIV** are therefore on T-lymphocyte-mediated responses. As with other viruses that affect the immune system, autoimmunity and malignancies (both lymphoid and nonlymphoid) reflect loss of immune regulation due to HIV.

3.6.6 Diagnosis of human immunodeficiency virus infection

Primary HIV infection in adults provokes antibodies to the virus envelope and core proteins that are the principal evidence for HIV infection, provided infection with HIV is >6 months prior to testing. These antibodies are directed typically at the envelope glycoproteins (gp120 and gp41) and are detectable throughout most of the life of the infected host. As in other viral infections, **anti-HIV antibodies** only provide indirect evidence of past infection. Absence of antibody, as in the 'window period', does not exclude the presence of the virus, which can be detected by PCR amplification (see Chapter 19).

The hallmark of **disease progression**, in addition to development of new symptoms, is an inexorable fall in the absolute number of CD4$^+$ T cells (Fig. 3.14). As in other virus infections, there may be a rise in the number of CD8$^+$ suppressor/cytotoxic cells within a few weeks of infection but, subsequently, seropositive asymptomatic individuals may have normal numbers of circulating lymphocyte subsets until disease progression begins. Lymph-node biopsies at this stage show many enlarged follicles, often infiltrated by CD8 lymphocytes, with depletion of CD4 cells, and destruction of the normal network structure.

Later, **polyclonal B-cell activation** results in a rise of serum immunoglobulin concentrations in 80–90% of patients with AIDS, including high levels of serum IgE.

3.6.7 Therapeutic options in acquired immune deficiency syndrome

Management of complications involves **early recognition of opportunistic infections**. Responses to new antigens are impaired as a result of dysfunction of CD4$^+$ dendritic cells. Even in patients with widespread opportunistic infections, there may be no detectable antibody response. Consequently, *conventional*

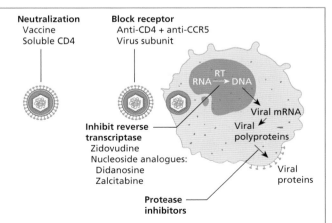

Fig. 3.15 Potential therapies for human immunodeficiency virus (HIV) disease. Reverse transcriptase can be inhibited not only by nucleoside analogues, but also by nucleotide analogues and by non-nucleoside substances. Entry inhibitors include fusion inhibitors (such as enfuvirtide) and receptor blockers (maraviroc, an entry inhibitor that binds to the CCR5 receptor and acts as an allosteric blocker). RT, reverse transcriptase.

serological diagnosis of intercurrent infections is unreliable in those with AIDS; PCR is essential. In infants, the failure of antigen presentation and the subsequent humoral immune defect result in repeated bacterial infections. Immunization with pathogen-specific vaccines, including live vaccines such as measles, mumps and rubella (MMR) and BCG, have been shown to be safe in all but the most immunosuppressed children and are usually recommended in order to give as much protection as possible.

Knowledge of the way in which HIV gains access into cells and its method of replication has led to exploration of **potential therapies** (Fig. 3.15). Attempts to provide antibodies to block binding of receptors on the viral envelope have so far proved fruitless. To be protective, antiviral antibody must also be neutralizing, although, even so, prevention of cell-to-cell spread by syncytium formation is very difficult. Once long-lived memory T cells are infected, patients are difficult to treat; additionally, macrophages and dendritic cells act as **reservoirs of infection** as well as a means of spread to the brain.

Inhibition of viral replication is achieved by inhibiting activity of reverse transcriptase (RT), as this is a unique retroviral enzyme with no mammalian counterpart. Zidovudine is an analogue of thymidine that yields inactive proviral DNA and was the first drug approved to treat HIV. Patients who received zidovudine alone had significantly improved survival due to slowing of viral replication, but this allowed viral resistance to develop and, coupled with significant bone marrow toxicity, it is no longer used alone but in combination therapy called highly active antiretroviral therapy (HAART) (Box 3.6). Zidovudine is included in the Essential Drugs List of the World Health Organization, which is a list of minimum medicinal needs for a basic health care system.

Box 3.6 Highly active antiretroviral therapy, known as HAART

This regime is a combination of drugs (that ultimately will be combined as cART):

- Nucleoside analogues, i.e. reverse transcriptase inhibitors – prevent transcription of viral RNA into cDNA copy, so blocking viral replication
- Non-nucleoside reverse transcriptase inhibitors – also inhibit reverse transcriptase
- Protease inhibitors – prevent the cleavage of viral pro-proteins to prevent formation of structural viral proteins and viral enzymes
- Prevention of viral entry to CD4 cells by fusion inhibitors that prevent syncytium formation between viral envelope and cell membrane
- Prevention of HIV binding by blocking CC5R
- Improved fusion inhibitors to prevent syncytium formation between viral envelope and cell membrane
- Enhanced prevention of viral incorporation into genome by inhibition of HIV integrase by inhibitors of liver enzymes that metabolize other medications used to treat HIV

Other agents have been developed (see Fig. 3.14). Less toxic nucleoside analogues enable lower doses of zidovudine to be used in combination regimens; these have slowed progression significantly in patients with less advanced disease. A major advance was the advent of protease inhibitors, which **prevent the assembly of new infectious viruses**. The efficacy of this type of treatment was demonstrated even in advanced cases. However, resistance to protease inhibitors, as well to some nucleoside analogues, appears after only a few days. By contrast, **resistance** to zidovudine takes months to develop, as it requires three or four mutations in the viral RT, whereas a single mutation can confer resistance to the protease inhibitors and other RT inhibitors. The advent of enfuvirtide, a **fusion inhibitor** that bars the entry of the virus by preventing viral fusion via envelope gp41 with the membrane of the cell, showed improved efficacy. Maraviroc, an entry inhibitor, binds to the CCR5 receptor and acts as an allosteric blocker.

Therapy for HIV infection needs, as do all medicines, to be safe, reliable, avoid the development of resistance and easy to comply with. Once-daily single-tablet regimens represent the ideal. cART aims to meet these requirements and the gold standard of the starting therapy, since approval in 2006, has been efavirenz (a non-nucleoside RT inhibitor) combined with tenofovir disoproxil fumarate or emtricitabine (nucleotide analogue reverse transcriptase inhibitors, NRTIs). Further combination with newer integrase inhibitors and protease inhibitors along with the pharmaco-enhancer cobicistat (see Box 3.6) will promote further ease of compliance and help to optimize regimens that currently may involve up to 20 tablets per day. Combinations of drugs and early treatment are therefore important and reduce the viraemia quickly; monitoring with quantitative measurements of viral load enables tailoring of the dose, resulting in improved compliance and therefore efficacy of drug therapy. Within weeks of starting treatment, the viral load drops below the limit of detection and the CD4 count rises in the blood, due to the mobilization of new CD4 cells from lymphoid tissues and prevention of reinfection of the new T cells, *provided compliance with HAART is complete.*

Monitoring for therapeutic purposes routinely involves regular viral load measurements and frequent measurements of absolute numbers of $CD4^+$ T cells, with serum β_2-microglobulin levels. Prophylaxis against Pneumocystis infection is started when the circulating CD4 count falls below $0.2 \times 10^9/l$. Prophylactic antibiotics and antiviral agents have reduced the risk of opportunistic infections, although these now occur later in the disease rather than being prevented totally. The high rate of replication allows the accumulation of numerous variants of HIV over time and many of these are resistant to antiviral therapy. Considerable mortality from HIV remains. In 2011, 1.7 million AIDS-related deaths occurred worldwide.

The response of $CD8^+$ lymphocytes early in infection and the finding that some individuals have mounted a brisk cytotoxic T-cell response, leading to apparent clearance of HIV, have encouraged **potential vaccine therapy**. Traditional vaccines, using killed or attenuated organisms (see Chapter 7, section 7.7), are unlikely to be of value, since the fragile nature of the HIV envelope makes it a poor immunogen and the high mutation rate poses difficulties of selecting a stable, common epitope to provoke useful immune responses. Since mutation of an attenuated HIV back to its virulent state would be catastrophic, safety concerns are paramount and these exclude live virus vaccines. Despite these challenges, there has been some scientific progress in recent years. In 2009, a large-scale clinical trial known as RV144 demonstrated that an HIV-1 vaccine could modestly reduce the incidence of HIV-1 infection. This trial used a live recombinant viral vector and patients were boosted with protein-based vaccine using HIV gp120, a prime-boost approach, but the reduction was only 31% and the effect was transient. Attempts to make neutralizing monoclonal antibodies (such as VRC01, a human monoclonal antibody capable of neutralizing over 90% of natural HIV-1 isolates *in vitro*) have revealed new opportunities for vaccine design once conserved but important epitopes have been identified. In 2012, RV144 vaccination was shown to induce antibodies that targeted a region that contains conserved epitopes. However, success is elusive and currently *the most effective controls for HIV diseases continue to be education and prevention.*

3.6.8 Infections in the immunosuppressed host

People who are medically immunosuppressed are also **predisposed to infection** (see Chapter 7, Case 7.2, and Chapter 8, Case 8.2). Such immunocompromised patients are at risk from two sources: they can be infected by common pathogens that invade even the immunologically healthy, or by truly 'opportunistic' agents, i.e. those organisms that inflict damage on weakened hosts (Fig. 3.16; see also Cases 7.2 and 8.2). Opportunistic agents account for only one-third of infections, but are responsible for most infective deaths.

This highlights two fundamental points about infections in the compromised host: first, most infections are due to common pathogens – these are usually readily identified and controlled by appropriate therapy; second, difficult problems are those caused by opportunistic organisms, because these are often elusive or impossible to isolate and they may not respond to available drugs. In practical terms, therefore, the clinician needs to know **when to suspect opportunistic infections**.

Several studies have documented diagnostically helpful **patterns of infection** in the immunosuppressed host. The best-studied patients are those who have undergone renal transplantation (see Chapter 8, Fig. 8.10). The major causes of infection in the first month are bacteria related to surgical wounds, indwelling cannulae or postoperative lung infections. After 1–4 months of therapeutic immunosuppression, cytomegalovirus infection dominates a picture that includes various fungal, viral and protozoal infections. Infections occurring beyond 4 months are due either to chronic viral infections, occasional opportunistic infections or infections normally present in the community.

The **major portal of entry of opportunistic** organisms is the oropharynx, so the lung is the commonest site of infection in the compromised host. The clinical picture is non-specific: fever, dyspnoea and an unproductive cough with widespread pulmonary infiltrates on chest X-ray. Unfortunately, sputum, blood cultures and serology are of little help in identifying the organism; more invasive methods such as bronchoalveolar lavage, transbronchial biopsy or open lung biopsy are frequently needed. The importance of early diagnosis and treatment (where feasible) is emphasized by the grim results: the *overall mortality usually exceeds 50%*, largely due to rapid progression in immunocompromised patients combined with lack of effective specific therapies for many opportunistic pathogens. However septicaemia, meningitis and gastrointestinal infections with local spread to the liver are not uncommon (see Case 3.12), though diagnosed more effectively.

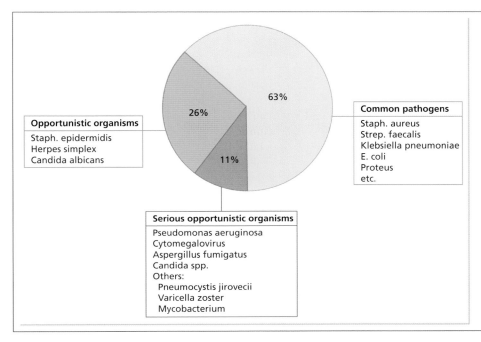

Fig. 3.16 Organisms causing infections in patients on immunosuppressive treatment.

63%

26%

11%

Opportunistic organisms

Staph. epidermidis
Herpes simplex
Candida albicans

Common pathogens

Staph. aureus
Strep. faecalis
Klebsiella pneumoniae
E. coli
Proteus
etc.

Serious opportunistic organisms

Pseudomonas aeruginosa
Cytomegalovirus
Aspergillus fumigatus
Candida spp.
Others:
 Pneumocystis jirovecii
 Varicella zoster
 Mycobacterium

Case 3.12 Listeria monocytogenes meningitis after immunosuppression for systemic lupus erythematosus

A 24-year-old woman presented with a 3-week history of tiredness, a facial rash and progressive swelling of her ankles. There was no past medical or family history of note. On examination, she was pale and pyrexial (temperature 38.2 °C) with a 'butterfly' rash on her face. There was gross oedema to the level of her sacrum and blood pressure was 180/100. Urinalysis showed haematuria (2+) and proteinuria (3+). The clinical diagnosis was nephrotic syndrome, probably due to systemic lupus erythematosus. This was supported by laboratory results: her haemoglobin was 91 g/l with a white-cell count of 3.2×10^9/l and an erythrocyte sedimentation rate (ESR) of 110 mm/h. C-reactive protein (CRP) was normal. Her antinuclear antibody was strongly positive (titre >1/10 000) and she had serum antibodies to dsDNA (98% binding; normal <25%). There was marked complement consumption: C3 was 0.36 g/l (NR 0.8–1.4) and C4 0.08 g/l (NR 0.2–0.4). Her serum albumin was 27 g/l, with proteinuria of 7.5 g per day.

The renal lupus (see Chapter 9, section 9.6.3) was treated aggressively with high-dose methylprednisolone, azathioprine and thrice-weekly plasma exchange. However, 4 weeks later, she suddenly became unusually agitated and disorientated, with mild neck stiffness. Cerebrospinal fluid (CSF) showed a raised protein concentration of 0.85 g/l (NR 0.1–0.4) with 10^4 polymorphs/ mm³. Cultures of blood and CSF grew Listeria monocytogenes. The meningitis was treated with Ampicillin and her mental state rapidly returned to normal.

CHAPTER 4
Anaphylaxis and Allergy

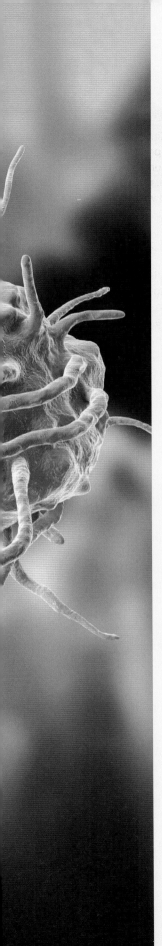

Key topics

Visit the companion website at **www.wiley.com/go/misbah/immunology** to download cases with additional figures on these topics.

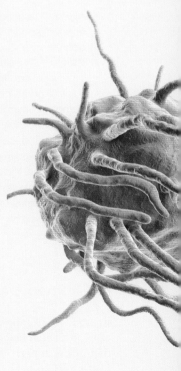

Chapel and Haeney's Essentials of Clinical Immunology, Seventh Edition. Edited by Siraj A. Misbah, Gavin P. Spickett, and Virgil A.S.H. Dalm.
© 2022 John Wiley & Sons Ltd. Published 2022 by John Wiley & Sons Ltd.

4.1 Introduction

'Allergy' is a much-misunderstood term that is used wrongly in general parlance. Unfortunately, the term is often used loosely to describe any intolerance of environmental factors irrespective of any objective evidence of immunological reactivity to an identified antigen. In this chapter, we distinguish those conditions in which immunological reactivity to key antigens is well defined from the rest, since such patients often present to an allergy clinic because of a popular public perception that they are 'allergic' in origin. In order to avoid any confusion, the relationship of these terms is shown in Box 4.1.

Truly allergic diseases are common: about 20% of the population experience some form of allergy and this imposes a substantial physical and economic burden on the individual and society. Some patients have an occasional mild allergic reaction, some suffer life-long debilitating disease, while, more rarely, some react with severe or fatal anaphylactic shock. The prevalence of allergic diseases is increasing. Although not all diagnoses of 'asthma' may be truly immunological (wheeze induced by common childhood viral infections, bronchiolitis in infants), in the USA, UK and many European countries the prevalence of asthma diagnosed in children has risen at a rate of about 5% per year. Multiple factors contribute to the overall risk of developing allergy (Box 4.2), but the decline in family size and a reduced microbial burden during childhood in many countries – the hygiene hypothesis – may partly account for the rising prevalence.

Allergic reactions to antigens that enter the systemic circulation, through an insect sting or intravenous administration of an antibiotic, can produce life-threatening anaphylactic reactions. More commonly, antigens are inhaled or ingested, trigger more local reactions in the upper or lower respiratory tracts (rhinitis or asthma) or in the mouth or upper gastrointestinal tract. However, some ingested (peanut) or inhaled (latex particles) antigens can cause anaphylaxis, a severe systemic reaction.

Box 4.1 To define these mutually exclusive terms

- Allergy – is used to define those conditions in which antigen-specific IgE or sensitized T cells play a definite role
- Atopy – is a state of disordered immunity in which Th2 lymphocytes drive an inherited tendency for hyperproduction of IgE antibodies after exposure to common environmental allergens
- Hypersensitivity – as used in this chapter, refers to the Gell and Coombs classification for immunological diseases (see Chapter 1, section 1.6)
- Intolerance – is used to describe all abnormal but reproducible reactions to food when the causative mechanism is unknown

---

Box 4.2 Risk factors for allergic diseases

- Atopy
- Age – commoner in children than adults
- Sex – commoner in boys than girls
- Family size – less common in large families
- Reduced microbial burden in developed countries (hygiene hypothesis); partly due to use of antibiotics
- Smoking – active or passive
- High levels of antigen exposure
- Dietary factors – poor intrauterine nutrition

4.2 Immediate (type I) hypersensitivity

Recognition of antigen by antibodies and cellular receptors can cause incidental tissue damage as well as the intended destruction of the antigen. Such reactions are called hypersensitivity reactions (Chapter 1, section 1.6) and the term allergy is synonymous with immediate (type I) hypersensitivity, since IgE-mediated reactions occur within a **few minutes of the second antigen exposure**. Antigen-specific IgE plays a key role, being synthesized on first exposure and causing allergy only on subsequent exposures. IgE is only a trace component of normal serum as it is bound, via its Fc regions, to the high-affinity FcΣRI receptor on **mast cells** (Fig. 4.1). Antigen reacts with surface-bound IgE causing cross-linking of receptors, an influx of calcium ions into the cell and explosive degranulation with release of **preformed mediators** (Fig. 4.1); these mediators include histamine, heparin, lysosomal enzymes and proteases, and several chemoattractant cytokines (chemokines) such as interleukin (IL)-8 and RANTES (Chapter 1, Table 1.6). **Other mediators are newly generated** and derived from the metabolism of arachidonic acid via two enzyme pathways: one leads to production of prostaglandins and thromboxane, the other to formation of leukotrienes. Histamine is a dominant mediator in the upper airways and leukotrienes in the lower airways disease.

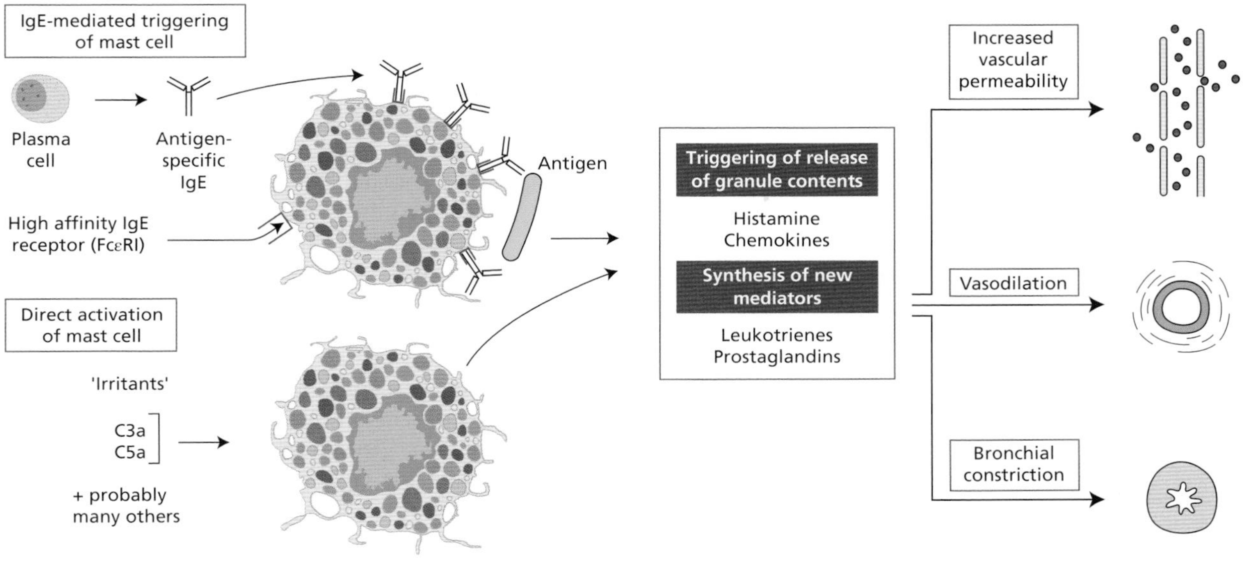

Fig. 4.1 Mast cell triggering and the results of mediator release.

Type I hypersensitivity reactions are rapid; for example, if the antigen is injected into the skin (a skin-prick test), **immediate hypersensitivity can be seen within 5–10 min** as a 'weal-and-flare' response, provided the individual has been exposed previously. IgE-mediated reactions are more commonly directed against antigens that enter at epithelial surfaces – inhaled or ingested antigens – so most allergic reactions occur via mast cells in the upper and lower airways or the gastrointestinal tract. Within the upper airways, this is associated with nasal itch, sneeze and rhinorrhoea, which are neurally mediated, as well as nasal obstruction, which is vascular in origin. In the lower airways, mediator release is associated with bronchoconstriction and mucus hypersecretion, giving rise to symptoms of wheeze, breathlessness, chest tightness and cough. Where allergen exposure is persistent, there is also tissue accumulation of neutrophils and eosinophils. Release of mediators from eosinophils and from activated epithelial cells contributes to symptoms (see section 4.6.2). Reactions to insect venom or drugs cause immediate and systemic symptoms via this mechanism too, presumably with small antigens being transported to sensitized mast cells in vital sites such as the larynx.

Exposure of allergic patients to antigen challenge may trigger both 'immediate' and 'late' phases of bronchoconstriction. This **late-phase response** (LPR) starts 4–6 h after exposure and can last 24 h. The LPR is characterized by accumulation of activated inflammatory cells, including eosinophils and T lymphocytes. Two mechanisms are involved: in one, the LPR is primarily an IgE- and mast cell-dependent reaction, with newly synthesized mediators attracting the cellular infiltration; in the other, it is mainly mediated by IL-4 released by CD4$^+$ T lymphocytes. These mechanisms are not mutually exclusive.

Not all rapid clinical features resulting from mast cell degranulation necessarily involve IgE-mediated sensitivity. **Direct activation of mast cells**, known as **non-immunological**

anaphylaxis, results in release of histamine or other mediators having similar effects (see Fig. 4.1). Tartrazine and preservatives that cause asthma or urticaria in sensitive patients (though rarely true anaphylaxis) probably do so by directly triggering basophils or mast cells. Substances that directly activate complement with the production of C3a and C5a also cause immediate reactions, since C3a and C5a are anaphylatoxins that release histamine from mast cells.

4.3 Atopy

Allergic diseases tend to run in families. **Atopy** defines a state of disordered immunity in which Th2 lymphocytes drive an inherited tendency for hyperproduction of IgE antibodies to common environmental allergens. About 80% of atopic individuals have a family history of 'allergy', compared with only 20% of the normal population. However, this trait is not absolute as there is only 50% concordance in monozygotic twins, so there are strong environment influences. Atopy is a clinical definition involving one or more of the common IgE-mediated diseases, namely atopic eczema, allergic rhinitis, allergic conjunctivitis and extrinsic asthma.

The susceptibility to these atopic disorders is under genetic control, but the evidence suggests that there are many genes with moderate effects (Table 4.1a) rather than one or two major genes. Despite several **genome-wide association studies** identifying potential new genes, there is as yet no consensus let alone confirmatory functional data. That said, it is clear that total serum IgE levels, production of antigen-specific IgE and bronchial hyper-reactivity are all under some degree of **genetic control**, accounting for family clustering. Genes on chromosome 5 (the IL-4 gene cluster) are implicated in the regulation of IgE production and genes on chromosome 11q to the atopic phenotype. Inheritance of the HLA-DR3 haplotype is linked to the development of allergy to rye grass, implicating the role of the major histocompatibility complex (MHC) in presenting the particular epitope.

Although genetic susceptibility to allergic disease is clearly important, environmental risk factors must play a significant role (see Box 4.2). The **epidemiological observation** that allergic sensitization is less common in children with older siblings and in those with early exposure to animals or brought up on farms has given rise to the 'hygiene hypothesis', which argues that different patterns of microbial exposure may render the immune system of children brought up in urban areas more prone to produce allergic responses. This appears to be due to a polarization of T cells towards a Th2, rather than a

Th1, cytokine profile, so posing a greater risk of allergic disease. However, advances in understanding of T-cell biology have revealed important roles for other T-cell populations, indicating that the Th1/Th2 paradigm oversimplifies the complex mechanisms involved and that **T-regulatory cells** have been identified as critical players in maintaining tolerance to environmental antigens and Th17 in persistence of inflammation involved in asthma.

4.4 Anaphylaxis

4.4.1 Anaphylaxis

Systemic anaphylaxis is the most dramatic example of an immediate hypersensitivity reaction. Clinically, the term refers to the sudden, generalized cardiovascular collapse or bronchospasm (Table 4.2) that occurs when a patient reacts to a substance to which he or she is exquisitely sensitive (Box 4.3). Anaphylaxis is a potentially lethal multisystem syndrome resulting from the sudden release of mast cell- and basophil-derived mediators into the circulation. Degranulation of these cells follows antigen exposure and previous sensitization is therefore required. While anaphylaxis is uncommon, it is extremely dangerous, as it is so unexpected, and can be fatal.

When **antigen** is introduced systemically, as in a wasp sting or intravenous antibiotic, *cardiovascular collapse is the predominant clinical feature*. When antigen is absorbed through the skin or mucosa, as in latex rubber anaphylaxis, the reaction develops slightly more slowly (see later Case 4.2). Allergy to latex rubber is increasingly common: several high-risk groups are recognized (Table 4.3) and latex allergy may cross-react

Table 4.1 (a) Some of the candidate genes implicated in development of atopy, asthma and atopic dermatitis

Chromosome	Candidate gene
5q	TH2 cytokine cluster (IL-3, IL-4, IL-5, IL-13 and GM-CSF)
11q	High-affinity IgE receptor β-subunit
16q	IL-4 receptor α-subunit
17q	RANTES
3q	CD80/CD86
20p	ADAM 33 metalloproteinase

Listed in order of likely significance but this will almost certainly change – compare with Table 4.1(b).

Table 4.1 (b) Candidate genes defined so far by genome-wide association studies			
Gene	Chromosome	Brief overview of proposed function/pathway	Number of positive association reports
HLA-DRB1	6p21	Antigen presentation	30
IL-4R	16p12.1-p12.2	Chain of IL-4 and IL-13 receptors	30
IL-13	5q31	T_H2-differentiation and IgE production	26
CD14	5q31.1	PRR involved, with TLR4, in recognizing LPS	24
FcεRI	IIqI3	High-affinity receptor for IgE	21
IL-4	5q31.1	T_H2-differentiation and IgE production	20
IL-10	1q31-q32	Immunoregulatory cytokine	13
HLA-DQB1	6p21	Antigen presentation	12
STAT6	12qI3	IL-4 and IL-13 signalling	12
LTA	6p21.3	Proinflammatory cytokine	11
CTLA4	2q33	T-cell response inhibition	8
IL-18	IIq22.2-q22.3	T_H2-differentiation and IFN-γ and TNF production	8
CCL5	17qII.2-qI2	Monocyte, T-cell and eosinophil chemoattractant	8

GM-CSF, granulocyte–macrophage colony-stimulating factor; IFN, interferon; IL, interleukin; LPS, lipopolysaccharide; PRR, pattern recognition receptor; TLR, Toll-like receptor; TNF, tumour necrosis factor.

Table 4.2 Clinical features of anaphylaxis

Organ	Feature
Cardiovascular system	Vascular collapse
Respiratory system	Bronchospasm
	Laryngeal oedema
Skin	Erythema
	Angioedema
	Urticaria
Gastrointestinal system	Vomiting
	Diarrhoea

Table 4.3 Key features of latex rubber allergy

High-risk groups
- Patients with spina bifida or multiple urological procedures (10–50% risk)
- Healthcare workers (5–10% risk)
  - Operating theatre staff
  - Females
  - Atopics
- Rubber industry workers (5–10% risk)

High-risk latex products
- Surgical latex gloves
- Latex rubber gloves for home use
- Balloons
- Catheters and enema tubes
- Condoms
- Teats and dummies (pacifiers)

Cross-reactivity with food allergies
- Kiwi fruit, banana, avocado, melon, chestnut

Box 4.3 The most common causes of anaphylaxis

- Bee and wasp stings (Case 4.1)
- Foods (Case 4.8)
- Latex rubber (Case 4.2)
- Drugs

with certain foods (Table 4.3). Foods that are absorbed via the oral mucosa seem especially likely to trigger angioedema of the lips, tongue and larynx. In some cases, hypotension and collapse may occur during or after exercise if certain foods are eaten immediately before the exertion – **food-related, exercise-induced anaphylaxis**. This typically occurs after shellfish (Japan) and wheat.

Anaphylaxis can also occur in those **allergic to a particular drug**, such as penicillin. *Penicillin allergy is commonly self-reported, but true anaphylactic reactions are much rarer, with a rate of 25 per 100 000 treated patients.* The risk of a severe reaction is greater following parenteral than oral penicillin, and over six times more likely in a patient with previous reactions to penicillin. However, most serious reactions occur in patients with no previous history of penicillin allergy. Skin-prick testing using major and minor penicilloyl determinants is of limited value, since up to 90% of skin-test-positive patients subsequently tolerate penicillin. On the other hand, a negative skin-prick test usually indicates patients who are not at risk or in whom reactions will be mild.

The only **laboratory test** that is useful at the time of an apparent anaphylactic reaction is blood mast cell tryptase. This is an indicator of mast cell degranulation, but *an elevated level identifies neither the mechanism of mast cell activation nor its cause.* Antigen-specific IgE (RAST) tests are helpful to confirm the nature of the insect venom prior to desensitization, but skin testing is more useful for latex rubber.

As in Cases 4.1 and 4.2, intramuscular epinephrine (adrenaline) is the most important drug in **treating anaphylaxis** and is nearly always effective. It should be followed by parenteral administration of hydrocortisone and chlorpheniramine. Epinephrine (adrenaline) by inhalation is much less effective. A note of caution: a detailed history is vital in distinguishing anaphylaxis from idiopathic angioedema and urticaria (section 4.8.1), with which it is often confused. *While injection of epinephrine (adrenaline) can be lifesaving in anaphylaxis, it can be harmful, even fatal, in elderly arteriosclerotic patients with urticaria and angioedema, who can develop acute coronary ischaemia or ventricular tachycardia.*

Long-term management requires detailed advice on avoidance to prevent further attacks. Preloaded epinephrine (adrenaline) syringes are readily available and effective, but patients must receive training on when and how to use them. Wearing a medical alert bracelet alerts paramedic staff and doctors to the possible cause of collapse. **Hyposensitization, or specific allergen immunotherapy**, is over 90% effective in patients with bee or wasp venom anaphylaxis provided recommended guidelines are followed (Box 4.4). Venom immunotherapy leads to a marked change in cytokine secretion, with a switch from the proallergic Th2 cytokine profile to a Th1 or inducing T-regulatory cells (see Chapter 7).

4.4.2 Non-immunological anaphylaxis

Anaphylaxis should be distinguished from **non-immunological (i.e. anaphylaxis-like) anaphylaxis reactions**. *These are not mediated by IgE antibodies.* Similar pharmacological mediators (such as histamine) are responsible for the clinical features, but the stimulus for their release differs. Substances inducing anaphylactoid reactions do so by a direct action on mast cells or by alternate pathway complement activation (see Fig. 4.1). Since this is not immunologically specific, *the person does not need to have been previously sensitized to the substance.* Collapse following intravenous induction agents for anaesthesia may fall into this category, and expert guidance is required for all patients suffering acute shock during anaesthetic induction to exclude genuine IgE-mediated anaphylaxis. Non-steroidal anti-inflammatory

Case 4.1   Wasp venom anaphylaxis

A 69-year-old woman was fit and well until one August when she was stung on the back of her right hand by a wasp. She had previously been stung on several occasions, the last time 2 weeks earlier. Within 5 min, she felt faint, followed shortly by a pounding sensation in her head and tightness of her chest. She collapsed and lost consciousness and, according to her husband, became grey and made gasping sounds. After 2–3 min, she regained awareness, but lost consciousness immediately when her husband and a friend tried misguidedly to help her to her feet. Fortunately, a doctor neighbour arrived in time to prevent her being propped up in a chair; he laid her flat, administered intramuscular epinephrine (adrenaline) and intravenous antihistamines and ordered a paramedic ambulance. She had recovered fully by the next day.

She had *clinical wasp venom anaphylaxis*. Her total serum IgE was 147 IU/ml (NR <120 IU/ml). Her antigen-specific IgE antibody level to wasp venom was 21 U/ml (radioallergosorbent test [RAST] class 4), but that to bee venom was 0.3 U/ml (RAST class 0). The patient was a candidate for specific allergen injection immunotherapy (hyposensitization). The slight but definite risk of desensitization was explained and balanced against the major risk of anaphylaxis should she be stung again. The first injection consisted of 0.1 ml of 0.0001 µg/ml of wasp venom vaccine given subcutaneously. No reaction occurred. Over the next 12 weeks, gradually increasing doses were given without adverse effects. Over this period, she tolerated injections of 100 µg venom. She then continued on a maintenance regimen of 100 µg of venom per month for 3 years.

At the age of 76 years, she was stung by a wasp that had come into her bathroom. She remained calm, lay down and experienced no significant systemic reaction.

 Case 4.2   Latex-induced anaphylaxis

A 38-year-old woman was referred for investigation following an anaphylactic reaction while visiting a relative in hospital. She gave a 5-year history of recurrent conjunctival oedema and rhinitis when blowing up balloons for her children's birthday parties. In the year prior to admission, three successive visits to her dentist triggered marked angioedema of her face on the side opposite to that requiring dental treatment. The swellings took 48 h to subside.

On the day of admission, she visited a critically ill relative in hospital. The patient was being reverse barrier nursed and visitors were required to wear gown and gloves. About 20 min after putting on the gloves her face and eyes became swollen, she felt wheezy and developed a pounding heart beat and light-headedness. Her tongue started to swell and she was taken to the Emergency Department, where she was given intramuscular epinephrine (adrenaline) and intravenous hydrocortisone (inappropriately as it transpired). She recovered rapidly, but was kept under observation overnight.

She had no history of atopy or other allergies. Ten years earlier she had undergone a series of operations for ureteric reflux and in the preceding 2 years had received colposcopic laser treatment for cervical intra-epithelial neoplasia (CIN-III).

Skin-prick testing to a crude latex extract produced a very strong reaction and her antigen-specific IgE antibody level to latex was significantly elevated at 57 U/ml (RAST class 5).

The diagnosis was that of *latex-induced anaphylaxis*. She was advised to avoid contact with all materials containing latex, and warned that she could react to certain foods (see Table 4.3). It was suggested that she wears a medical alert bracelet, in case she required future emergency surgery, and carry a self-injectable form of epinephrine. The diagnosis has important implications for any further dental, surgical or anaesthetic procedures. Hospitals now have written procedures for latex-free surgery for emergency and planned operations.

drugs (NSAIDs) divert arachidonic acid metabolism towards production of leukotrienes, which are potent inducers of anaphylactoid reactions via their interactions with specific receptors on target tissues.

The **emergency treatment** of a non-immunological anaphylaxis reaction is the same as that of anaphylaxis, but the distinction is important in ensuring the appropriateness and interpretation of investigations and in long-term management of the clinical problem (Case 4.3). In non-immunological reactions, skin-prick tests and measurements of antigen-specific IgE are of no value; the only test available is in vivo challenge. Management requires avoidance of the offending agent, since specific allergen immunotherapy is of no benefit in non-IgE-mediated reactions.

4.5 Allergic conjunctivitis

4.5.1 Seasonal (hay fever) and perennial (vernal) conjunctivitis

Seasonal conjunctivitis is common and mainly affects children and young adults. This is a mild, bilateral disease characterized by itching, redness and excessive tear production (Fig. 4.2). It is associated with the nasal symptoms of hay fever and follows the same seasonal variation each year. Antigen-specific IgE is involved; this has been demonstrated by passive transfer of specific antigen hypersensitivity to a 'volunteer' by serum containing the specific IgE. The IgE is attached to conjunctival mast cells but its site of production is uncertain, and excess free IgE is not necessarily found in the tears. Although pollen-specific IgE is responsible for hay fever conjunctivitis, affected individuals often react to additional antigens when skin tested (as in Case 4.4) since this is one of the 'atopic' diseases, without necessarily developing clinical reactions on exposure. Treatment includes pollen avoidance where possible, sodium cromoglycate eye drops to reduce mast cell sensitivity and topical or systemic antihistamines to block the effects of mediators released from mast cells.

A more severe form of conjunctivitis, persisting throughout the year (with exacerbations in the spring), is known as **vernal conjunctivitis**. It is usually a self-limiting condition of young people (usually lasting 3–5 years) and is characterized by red eyes, photophobia, itching and a mucous discharge. The diagnostic feature is the formation of giant papillae (known as cobblestones) on the upper tarsal conjunctiva. These are due to

---

Box 4.4 Recommended guidelines for specific allergen immunotherapy (hyposensitization)

- Only high-quality standardized allergen extracts may be used
- Administered in hospitals or specialized clinics only
- Medical staff should have appropriate training and experience in immunotherapy
- Epinephrine (adrenaline) should always be immediately available
- Ensure ready access to resuscitative facilities with attendant staff trained in resuscitative techniques
- Patients should be kept under close supervision for 60 min after each injection

---

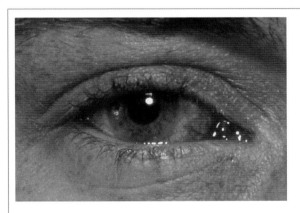

Fig. 4.2 Acute conjunctivitis.

 Case 4.3 Drug-induced reaction

A 77-year-old woman was referred from the Accident and Emergency Department, having been admitted overnight because of sudden onset of massive angioedema of her tongue associated with laryngeal stridor. She was treated with intravenous hydrocortisone only. This was her fifth such episode: an anaphylactoid attack 2 months earlier was severe enough for her to be intubated and ventilated on the Intensive Care Unit.

She had no history of previous allergy and no family history of atopy. A drug history revealed that, in addition to oral prednisolone prescribed in the Accident and Emergency Department, she was taking oral furosemide and ramipiril. Ramipiril is an angiotensin-converting enzyme (ACE) inhibitor and this group of drugs is known to cause severe episodes of angioedema. Ramipiril was discontinued and her mild hypertension was managed with alternative medication. The attacks have not recurred.

 Case 4.4 Seasonal allergic conjunctivitis

A 7-year-old boy developed itchy eyes and swollen lids after playing tennis in the garden. Because his mother had hay fever, the boy's symptoms were also presumed to be an allergy to grass pollen. After several episodes of increasing severity, medical help was sought. He was skin tested; a weal-and-flare reaction appeared 5–15 min after prick testing with extracts of grass pollens, cat fur and house dust mite. The speed and nature of the reaction confirmed *immediate (type I) hypersensitivity* to these antigens, and he was told to try to avoid exposure to high concentrations of grasses in the pollen season. He developed similar reactions the following summer, particularly in June and July; they were sometimes accompanied by sneezing and rhinorrhoea. He was therefore started on prophylactic eye drops containing sodium cromoglicate, which helped control his *seasonal allergic conjunctivitis*.

oedema and hypertrophy of underlying tissue, which contains IgA- and IgE-secreting plasma cells, mast cells and eosinophils. Vernal conjunctivitis is often associated with atopic diseases (eczema and asthma) and most patients have high serum IgE levels, with IgE detectable in their tears. Vernal conjunctivitis probably represents immediate and late-phase reactions. When the conjunctiva over the limbus (corneal–scleral junction) is affected, it is called **limbal vernal conjunctivitis**.

Immediate (type I) reactions in the eye can be **caused by a variety of other antigens,** the commonest being topical agents such as antibiotics or contact lens solutions. In severe cases a cobblestone appearance of the upper tarsal conjunctiva is seen. The development of papillae is not unique to atopy-associated diseases; they are occasionally seen in contact dermatoconjunctivitis (a type IV reaction) and contact lens-associated conjunctivitis (an autoimmune reaction to conjunctival antigens adherent to contact lenses; see Chapter 12). Decisions to treat with anti-inflammatory drugs or steroids/immunosuppressants should only be made in conjunction with an ophthalmologist.

4.6 Respiratory allergy

4.6.1 Allergic rhinitis

Allergic rhinitis may be seasonal or perennial (Fig. 4.3). In the USA, it is the sixth most prevalent chronic disease, outranking heart disease. **Seasonal allergic rhinitis** is often referred to as hay fever and its prevalence is rising. Patients **present** with rhinorrhoea, sneezing and nasal obstruction following antigen exposure. Those with chronic symptoms develop sinusitis, serous otitis media and conjunctivitis, and lose their senses of taste and smell. Many patients also have asthma and, as with asthma, there is an increased susceptibility to irritating fumes, cold or emotional stress. The antigens that cause this condition are usually 'large' and mainly deposited in the nose (Fig. 4.4). However, many particles (10–40 μm diameter), such as grass pollens, release soluble antigenic material while lodged in the nasal mucus. When the causative antigen is present all the year round, for instance house dust mite or animal dander, the patient may suffer **perennial allergic rhinitis** (Case 4.5). Such patients are often misdiagnosed as having a 'permanent cold'.

A careful history is essential if the causative antigen is to be found. Positive **skin tests** help to distinguish allergic rhinitis from non-allergic rhinitis. RAST tests are useful only occasionally, if skin tests are conflicting or contraindicated (in young children, severe disease in which therapy cannot be stopped).

Histopathologically, the nose shows mucosal swelling, with excessive production of nasal fluid containing basophils and eosinophils. The **pathogenesis** is similar to asthma, with mediators of inflammation liberated from mast cells. IgE mechanisms are involved and IgE, IgG and IgA can be detected in nasal secretions. In a few patients with severe chronic hay fever or perennial rhinitis, mucosal hyperplasia may result in the formation of polyps, but only a few cases of nasal polyps are due to an allergic cause (chronic infection is much more likely).

The differential diagnosis of allergic rhinitis is **vasomotor or irritant, non-allergic rhinitis**. This is a non-seasonal condition in which there is no itching, few eosinophils in the nasal fluid and a normal level of serum IgE. In contrast to allergic rhinitis, this responds poorly to nasal sodium cromoglicate. Chronic non-allergic rhinitis is probably the nasal equivalent of idiopathic asthma.

Topical sodium cromoglicate and intranasal corticosteroids are effective prophylactic **treatment** for most patients with allergic rhinitis. Prolonged use of nasal decongestants leads to rebound rhinitis when treatment is stopped – **rhinitis medicamentosa**. Local or oral antihistamines may be needed for relief of troublesome symptoms. In patients with severe symptoms that are not controlled by antiallergic medication, **hyposensitization (antigen-specific immunotherapy)** to grass pollen or cat dander can be effective. Selection of patients is critical and only experienced specialists should carry out immunotherapy, with full resuscitative facilities because of the danger of anaphylaxis (see Box 4.4).

4.6.2 Asthma

Asthma is a syndrome with three cardinal features:

- Generalized but reversible airways obstruction.
- Bronchial hyper-responsiveness.
- Airways inflammation.

It arises as a result of complex interactions between multiple genes and environmental factors (Fig. 4.5) and cannot be explained solely on the basis of IgE-mediated triggering of

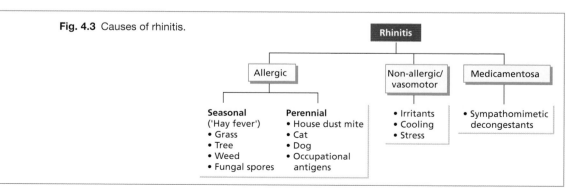

Fig. 4.3 Causes of rhinitis.

mast cells. Although not all cases are allergic in origin (Table 4.4), most cases occur in younger patients who also show immediate hypersensitivity to defined environmental allergens, as in Case 4.6. It is a common condition, affecting 5–10% of the population in the UK. The prevalence and severity of asthma are rising. Despite medical awareness about the dangers of asthma, and an effective range of therapies, *many asthmatics die each year during a severe attack*, although deaths are now less common following decreased use of high-dose formulations of relatively unselective β-agonist drugs.

Asthma is **familial** and many genetic loci predispose to the disease (Table 4.1a). As with atopy in general, asthma is less common in less affluent populations and those who grow up in large families, possibly because transmission of viral or bacterial infections from older siblings leads to preferential stimulation of Th1 lymphocytes over Th2 lymphocytes, so reducing allergic sensitization. While elements of this simple Th1 versus Th2 paradigm remain useful, there is emerging evidence of important roles for other T-lymphocyte subsets – particularly T-regulatory and Th17 cells, which may account for some susceptibility to IgE-mediated conditions.

Like other atopic conditions, the **pathogenesis** of allergic asthma involves initiation of specific IgE to respiratory allergens via the airways and the pathogenesis in such previously sensitized individuals; the pathogenesis can be further subdivided into inflammatory and remodelling components.

The **initiation of asthma** depends on epithelial cells and dendritic cells within the airways. The recent recognition of the role of epithelial cells in response to inhaled allergens is important for new types of therapies in the future. Genomewide association studies have revealed *new asthma susceptibility*

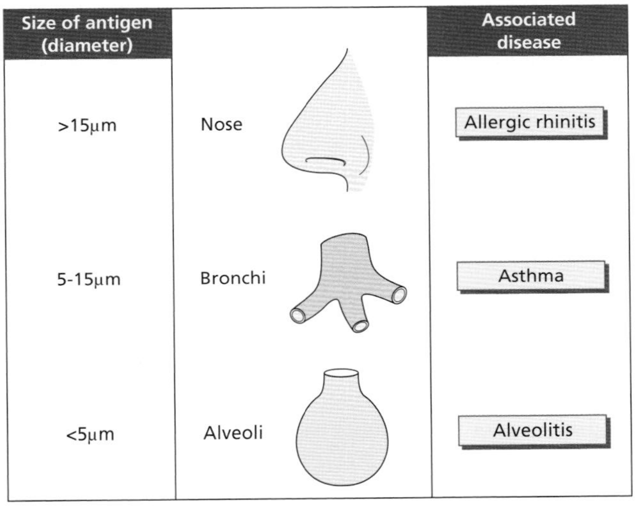

Size of antigen (diameter)		Associated disease
>15μm	Nose	Allergic rhinitis
5–15μm	Bronchi	Asthma
<5μm	Alveoli	Alveolitis

Fig. 4.4 Relationship between antigen size and the site of major symptomatology.

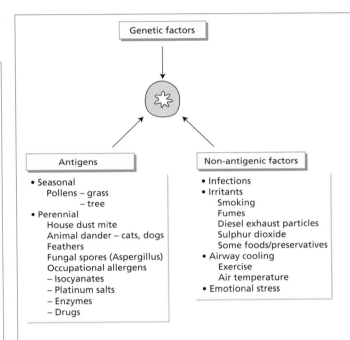

Fig. 4.5 Some precipitating factors in asthma.

Case 4.5 Perennial allergic rhinitis

A 29-year-old doctor developed intense itching of her eyes and nose and a tickling sensation in her ears and palate, followed by sneezing and rhinorrhoea. These symptoms developed within 15 min of visiting an elderly patient who kept four cats. The symptoms settled down over the next 2 h, but started to recur whenever home visits were made to houses where cats were present. Symptoms occurred even though the cats were excluded from the interview room. Each episode took slightly longer to resolve and some were accompanied by a dry cough.

The doctor had suffered from asthma in childhood and her non-atopic parents had a cat. During her years in medical school and in hospital posts, she had no respiratory symptoms. The move into general practice and exposure to cat dander had triggered perennial allergic rhinitis. On investigation, she had strongly positive skin tests to cat dander, house dust mite and grass pollen. She started prophylactic use of a nasal spray and eye drops containing sodium cromoglicate, with abolition of most of her symptoms. Sometimes, she also needed to use a local antihistamine spray to relieve breakthrough attacks of rhinitis. The value of hyposensitization (antigen-specific immunotherapy) to cat dander was discussed because occupational exposure was unavoidable, but not undertaken while her symptoms continued to be controllable. It remains a therapeutic option.

Table 4.4 Features of asthma

	Allergic	Idiopathic	Others
Proportion of total asthmatics	60%	30%	10%
Age of onset	Childhood	>40 years	Variable
Other atopic diseases	Common	Unusual	Unusual
Family history	Yes	No	No
Causes	Seasonal	Unclear	Aspergillus
	Perennial		Carcinoid
	Occupational		Carcinoma, aspirin
			Churg–Strauss syndrome
Prognosis	May persist into adult life (30%)	Many become chronic	Variable
	Deaths do occur particularly in non-compliant patients	Deaths very rare	

Case 4.6 Allergic asthma

A 15-year-old girl presented with a prolonged wheezing attack that had come on suddenly 36 h earlier. She had experienced several episodes of 'wheezy bronchitis' as a child and eczema as an infant. She was a non-smoker. Her father suffered from hay fever, but there was no family history of asthma. On examination, she was tired and unwell, with a rapid respiratory rate and tachycardia (140/min). There were bilateral expiratory wheezes on chest auscultation. Investigations showed a normal haemoglobin but a raised white cell count (14 × 10^9/l). A chest X-ray was normal, but lung function tests showed reversible airways obstruction. The clinical diagnosis was asthma and the family history and skin tests later suggested this was *allergic asthma*. She continues to have periodic attacks of asthma, although they are controlled, in part, by prophylactic inhaled steroids and p$_2$-adrenergic stimulants (salbutamol) as needed.

genes that are mostly expressed in the epithelium and innate immune pathways, including ORMDL3, IL33 and SMAD3 as well as genes associated with atopy and serum IgE production and Th17 cells. In asthma, the epithelium is defective due to incomplete tight junctions that enable penetration of inhaled allergens. In addition, some respiratory allergens (house dust mite, cockroach, animal and fungal allergens) have been shown to disrupt epithelial tight junctions, as can respiratory viruses and some air pollutants. This is similar to the disruption seen in the gut epithelium in food allergy.

Pattern recognition receptors (PRRs) **initially on epithelial cells** (and subsequently on dendritic cells attracted to the airways) then detect and respond to pathogen-associated molecular patterns, and cell damage (cell stress or death) follows rapidly. Activation of epithelial cells can result in the release of chemokines (CCL20, CCL19 and CCL27, the ligands for CCR6, CCR7 and CCR10) that attract immature dendritic cells that then differentiate and activate inflammation and adaptive immunity. Prospective birth cohort studies have identified viral infections in atopic individuals as a particularly potent risk factor for persistent childhood asthma, which fits this hypothesis of genetic susceptibility with early epithelial damage by biologically active allergens.

As discussed, the hygiene hypothesis suggests that some pathogens that stimulate Th1 cells are protective for respiratory allergy, and traditionally it is thought that **Th2 cytokines** drive the production of IgE via IL-4, IL-5, IL-9 and IL-13 only in the absence of a Th1 response. Animal experiments suggest that an additional source of IL-4, to drive activation in favour of a Th2 response, is initially produced by dendritic cells in the respiratory mucosa and then augmented by basophils. However, studies to determine the exact mechanisms of this polarization towards Th2 and the role of Th17 cells are ongoing.

Asthma is **an inflammatory condition** with sensitized CD4 Th2 cells identified readily in bronchial biopsies and bronchoalveolar lavage fluid. These cells release IL-3, IL-4, IL-5, IL-13, tumour necrosis factor (TNF)-α and granulocyte–macrophage colony-stimulating factor (GM-CSF) (Fig. 4.6). IL-3, IL-5 and GM-CSF influence eosinophil development, maturation, activation and survival, while IL-4, IL-5, IL-13 and TNF-α are important in the upregulation of a leucocyte–endothelial cell adhesion molecule, called VCAM-1 (see Chapter 1), which enables neutrophils, monocytes and eosinophils to adhere to vascular endothelium prior to migration into the respiratory mucosa. Recent evidence also implicates the Th17-derived cytokine IL-17A in persistent asthma. Raised levels are found in the serum, sputum and bronchoalveolar lavage fluids and these correlate with asthma severity, and help to account for the inflammation associated with asthma.

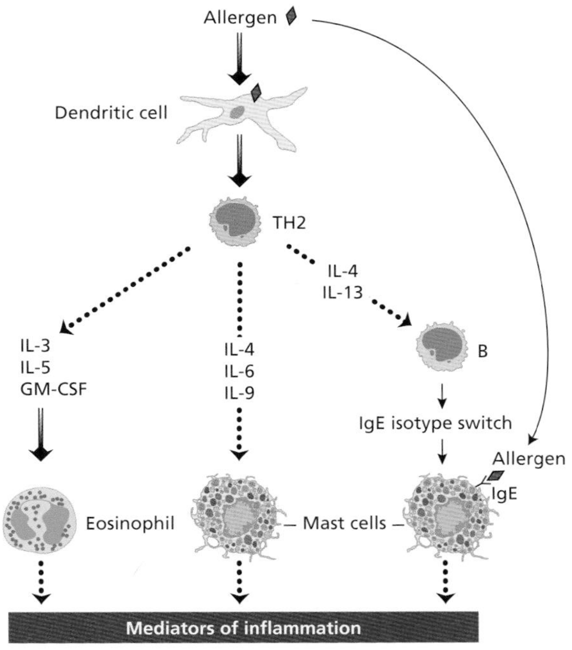

Fig. 4.6 Major cytokines implicated in airways inflammation. *GM-CSF*, granulocyte–macrophage colony-stimulating factor; *IL*, interleukin.

On subsequent exposure, the T-cell receptor on Th2 cells and IgE bound to mast cells react with the allergen (Fig. 4.6). The frequency of antigen exposure determines whether the response is **acute reversible airways obstruction** alone or a chronic allergic response with **bronchial hyper-responsiveness**. In the case of single antigen exposure, the symptoms are due to the release of preformed and newly generated mediators released by mast cells, as described in section 4.2.

Acute inflammation usually resolves as repair processes restore normal structure and function. In chronic asthma, this process is disturbed and inflammation persists that in turn leads to **airways hyper-responsiveness** (Fig. 4.7).

Some patients with chronic asthma have a progressive decline in lung function that reflects the pathological changes of angiogenesis, proliferation of smooth muscle, basement membrane thickening, a cellular infiltrate of eosinophils (see Box 4.5) and mononuclear cells, and fibrosis – changes described as **remodelling**. Epithelial cells release epidermal growth factor, and eosinophils and myofibroblasts produce TGF-β to promote synthesis of extracellular matrix components and collagen; hence the trial with mepolizumab, an antibody that blocks IL-5, that showed the reduction of eosinophils was associated with reduced basement membrane thickening. There is also an increase in the number of goblet cells, resulting in more mucus production and in the non-productive cough that may be a presenting symptom.

The **diagnosis** of asthma is a clinical one, supported by spirometry, as symptoms may not always be obvious. Any sputum can be examined for cells (particularly eosinophils) and pathogens, as many attacks are precipitated by infection; blood eosinophilia may be present. Lung function tests show a reduced forced expiratory volume (FEV$_1$), reversible with bronchodilators – this is the *essential diagnostic test*. Monitoring the response to a trial of treatment with bronchodilators (+/− inhaled corticosteroids) also serves as a useful diagnostic tool. Exhaled nitric oxide (FeNO) is another non-invasive surrogate marker of eosinophilic airway inflammation.

Laboratory tests, such as the total serum IgE level, are unhelpful. There is no evidence that the routine use of RASTs to identify antigens suspected of causing inhalant allergy adds anything to a careful history and the judicious use of skin tests. Bronchial challenge is an important test of occupational asthma, as it not only proves the reversibility of the airways obstruction, but also indicates the inhaled antigens involved. Bronchial challenge results in immediate bronchoconstriction (within 10 min) and a late-phase reaction, and such challenge has definite risks and is performed only in specialized centres. Other tests, such as the difference between metacholine/histamine challenge test spirometry results performed after a week at work, and then after time away from work, give an indication of whether **occupational exposure** is important in the asthma pathogenesis.

Avoidance of precipitating factors (see Fig. 4.5) is important in patients with asthma caused by indoor allergens such as mites, cats and dogs, but these allergens have different aerodynamic characteristics. Mite (faeces) allergens are present as large particles in bedding and soft furnishings, but only become airborne after vigorous disturbance and settle quickly. In contrast, cat and dog allergens are small particles that, following disturbance, remain airborne for long periods. Dust mite-allergic patients experience predominantly low-grade exposure overnight in bed. In contrast, cat or dog-allergic patients develop symptoms within minutes of exposure due to inhalation of large amounts of easily respirable allergens. Even after permanent removal of a cat or dog from the home, it may take 6–12 months before the huge concentration of allergens in the home drops to normal. The value of mattress covers to reduce exposure to house dust mite is controversial: while allergen exposure may fall, there is an inconsistent effect on symptoms or respiratory function.

Treatment, although usually effective, is largely palliative because there is no way to correct permanently the fundamental genetic predisposition. Most asthma treatment guidelines recommend a stepwise approach to drug treatment. **Bronchodilators** (β$_2$-adrenoceptor agonists) are good for relieving bronchospasm only and do not inhibit inflammation. Steroids downregulate proinflammatory cytokine production, especially those released by Th2 cells and activated epithelial cells. The use of potent, topically active, **inhaled steroids** has reduced the need for systemic steroids other than to control a severe attack, or in a few patients with severe, chronic asthma. **Leukotriene receptor antagonists** (such as montelukast) have recently been shown to be effective as prophylaxis in mild to moderate asthma. **Ciclosporin** is also of benefit in some patients with severe, intractable, chronic asthma, illustrating the importance of T cells in pathogenesis. **Omalizumab** is a humanized monoclonal antibody that selectively binds to free

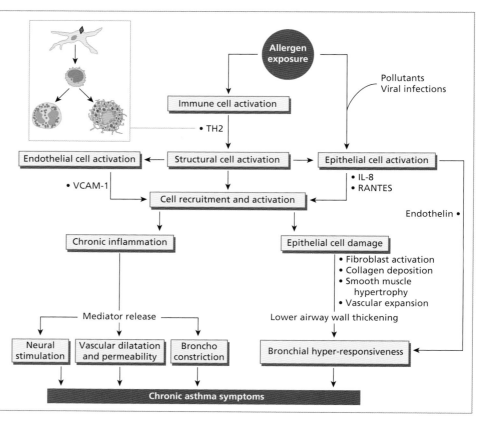

Fig. 4.7 The development of airways inflammation and bronchial hyper-responsiveness in chronic asthma. IL, interleukin.

Box 4.5 Causes of eosinophilic infiltration in chronic allergen exposure

- Upregulation of VCAM-1 enabling eosinophil recruitment
- Maturation and increased survival mediated by interleukin (IL)-3, IL-5 and granulocyte–macrophage colony-stimulating factor (GM-CSF)
- Selective eosinophil migration induced by IL-8 and RANTES (Chapter 1, Table 1.6)

---

human IgE in the blood and interstitial fluid and to B cells expressing surface-bound IgE; omalizumab does not bind to IgE already bound to high-affinity IgE receptor (FcεRI) on the surface of mast cells or basophils.

Treatment guidelines in the UK recommend omalizumab as an add-on option for patients with moderate to severe allergic asthma uncontrolled on high-dose inhaled corticosteroids and long-acting β-agonists. Trials have shown significant improvement in lung function, reduced exacerbations of severe asthma and reduction of usage of inhaled steroids as well as sustained effects up to >5 years of therapy sustained up to 4 years of treatment with omalizumab. Immunotherapy to house dust mite has been shown to be beneficial in moderate asthma, with evidence of house dust mite sensitization.

4.7 Food allergy and intolerance

Food 'allergy' undoubtedly exists, but an extravagant claim that a wide array of symptoms is due to allergies to foods has confused the subject. One cause of confusion lies in poor definition of terms. Several **categories of adverse reactions to foods** – immunological, biochemical (enzyme deficiency) and psychological (food fads and aversion; Case 4.7) – can lead to gastrointestinal, respiratory, skin and even neurological symptoms. An adverse reaction cannot be considered immunological until there is proof of an immune-mediated mechanism. The term **food intolerance** should be used to describe all abnormal but reproducible reactions to food when the causative mechanism is unknown (Table 4.5) or is known to be non-immunological, e.g. a patient with biliary tract disease who cannot tolerate fatty meals is not 'allergic' to fat. The phrase **food allergic disease** should be used only when the abnormal reaction is proved to be immunologically mediated. The public's perception of their illnesses being caused by food has been shown to be over 10 times greater than the proven prevalence of food intolerance.

4.7.1 Food allergy and intolerance

Food intolerance of some sort is a relatively common problem in childhood, especially in the first year of life. Nearly three-quarters of patients present with immediate gastrointestinal symptoms (Fig. 4.8), though the differential diagnosis of such symptoms is wide (Table 4.6). In food intolerance proven by blind challenge, a single food (most commonly cow's milk) is responsible in just under half of the cases. Food intolerance must be considered to be a rare/unproven cause of symptoms that occur remote from the gut (such as attention deficit disorders, arthritis or enuresis); patients apparently benefiting from dietary manipulation have been from highly selected groups. Most reports of proven food intolerance in adults incriminate nuts, milk, eggs, fish, wheat and chocolate, where a direct non-immunological mechanism is suspected (section 4.7.2).

On the other hand, **allergy to peanuts** is IgE mediated and is becoming more common (Box 4.6); most patients are atopic. A minute quantity of peanut antigen can cause a life-threatening reaction, as in Case 4.8. Avoidance is thus vital, but difficult to achieve, because nuts are ubiquitous and often 'hidden' in inadequately labelled foods. There is emerging evidence that early peanut introduction has a role in peanut allergy prevention.

Visit the website at **www.wiley.com/go/misbah/immunology** to read a case study on cow's milk allergy.

Another cause of confusion is the **oral allergy syndrome (pollen–fruit syndrome)**. Some atopic children and adults report itching and swelling of the mouth, tongue and soft palate after eating fresh fruit, typically apples, pears, cherries, plums and peaches (see Case 4.9). This occurs in patients allergic to birch tree pollen because of allergic cross-reactivity between pollen and certain fruits. The allergens are heat-labile and destroyed by cooking, so patients can tolerate cooked fruit or jams. Skin-prick testing with commercial fruit extracts is often negative, as the relevant proteins are destroyed during extraction, but sensitivity to fresh fruit can be demonstrated by 'prick-prick' testing, as in the case. The oral allergy syndrome does not normally progress to cause systemic anaphylaxis.

There are many mechanisms of adverse reactions to food other than immunological ones. These include irritant, toxic, pharmacological or metabolic effects of foods, enzyme deficiencies, or even the release of substances produced by fermentation of food residues in the bowel. For instance, some foods contain pharmacologically active substances (such as tyramine or phenylethylamine) that may act directly on blood vessels in sensitive subjects to produce symptoms such as migraine.

However, traces of drugs or antibiotics (e.g. penicillin in the milk of penicillin-treated cows), foods rich in natural salicylates (e.g. fruits and vegetables), food additives (e.g. monosodium glutamate), colouring agents (e.g. tartrazine) or preservatives (e.g. benzoic acid) can also cause symptoms in susceptible

Table 4.5 Adverse reactions to foods			
	Reproducible reaction on challenge		
	Open challenge	Blind challenge	Immune mediated
Food fad	−	−	−
Psychological aversion	+	−	−
Food intolerance (mechanism unknown)	+	+	?
Food intolerance (mechanism known to be non-immunological)	+	+	−
Food allergy (immune mechanism)	+	+	+

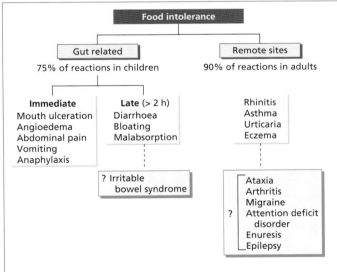

Fig. 4.8 Putative clinical spectrum of food intolerance.

Table 4.6 Differential diagnosis of food intolerance in children			
Common	**Occasionally important**	**Unusual**	**Rare**
Acute angioedema/urticaria in infants under 1 year Perioral erythema Atopic infants with gastrointestinal symptoms Infantile colitis	Atopic eczema in infants under 1 year	Atopic eczema in children over 1 year Chronic urticaria Loose stools Migraine	Asthma

---

Box 4.6   Key points about peanut allergy

- Peanuts are legumes, botanically distinct from nuts
- Peanut allergy is accompanied by increased risk of allergy to tree nuts
- Commonest cause of fatal or near-fatal food-related anaphylaxis in USA and UK
- Affects 1% of children, but is seven times more common in siblings of patients with peanut allergy
- Life-long problem, starting in early childhood (<7 years). Most patients do not 'outgrow' peanut allergy
- T-cell clones from patients produce high levels of IL-4 and low levels of interferon-γ – consistent with a Th2-like profile

---

people by mechanisms that are ill understood, but are probably due to direct effects on mast cells and not to an adaptive immunological mechanism. Salicylates, for instance, inhibit synthesis of prostaglandins and cause release of mast cell mediators.

4.7.2 Diagnosis of food allergy and intolerance

The diagnosis depends on a careful clinical history and thorough examination to exclude other, perhaps more likely, causes of the patient's symptoms such as a food fad or an anxiety state. *Elimination and challenge diets form the basis of the diagnosis of food allergic disease.* A food challenge must be carefully monitored and conducted under double-blind conditions in an expert specialist centre.

 Case 4.7   Is this food allergy?

A 38-year-old woman presented with a 2-year history of abdominal bloating, cramping abdominal pains and loose stools. Attacks occurred every 7–10 days but lasted only 2–3 h. One attack occurred about 8 h after a meal of pasta in a local restaurant and led her to believe her symptoms were food related. She initially eliminated wheat-based products from her diet and then, because the attacks continued, dairy products as well. She was referred to a gastroenterologist and investigated extensively: gastroduodenal endoscopy, duodenal biopsy, barium meal, colonoscopy and pancreatic function tests were all normal.

She continued to believe her symptoms were food related: vague muscular pains, headaches, poor concentration and fatigue were attributed to other foods, which were then eliminated from her diet. She was referred to an allergy clinic for further assessment.

Physical examination showed an undernourished woman with no other abnormal findings. As this was a second opinion, a wide range of tests were done. Her haemoglobin and erythrocyte sedimentation rate were normal. Her serum immunoglobulins were normal and her serum IgE was only 8 IU/ml. She had no detectable antibodies to tissue transglutaminase, endomysium or gliadin (see Chapter 19). While waiting for her outpatient appointment, she had responded to an advertisement in a health food shop and undergone electrodermal or 'Vega' testing. The report listed 24 foods to which she was allergic, many of which she had felt able to tolerate previously. Her diet had become increasingly restricted; expert dietetic assessment showed her diet to be nutritionally unsound, with deficient intake of protein, fat, fat-soluble vitamins and trace elements. The diagnosis was that of *psychological food aversion* and irritable bowel syndrome. She was reluctant to accept this diagnosis and asked her GP for referral to another specialist.

 Case 4.8   Nut allergy

A 15-year-old schoolgirl was admitted to hospital as an emergency while on holiday. Her parents believed her to be allergic to nuts. At the age of 5 years, she vomited about 1 min after eating a bar of chocolate containing nuts. Three years later, she developed marked angioedema of her face, lips and tongue, followed by tightness of her throat and vomiting; this occurred 2–3 min after friends of her brother decided to test her allergic status by pushing peanuts into her mouth and holding her jaws shut. Less severe attacks had followed inadvertent ingestion of hazelnuts and almonds. As a consequence, she avoided peanuts and tree nuts wherever possible.

The emergency admission occurred following a single lick of a vanilla ice cream. Within seconds, she developed angioedema of her lips and tongue, difficulty in breathing, and felt light-headed. Following an emergency call, she was injected with intramuscular adrenaline (and intravenous hydrocortisone inappropriately) by the paramedical service, and admitted to hospital overnight. She made a rapid and uneventful recovery. Her parents later recalled that one ice-cream scoop was used by the vendor to dispense all flavours; the customer immediately before the patient had been served a nut-flavoured ice cream.

On investigation, she had a grade 6 RAST (see Chapter 19) to peanut with significant but lesser (grade 2) reactivity to hazelnut, almonds and brazil nuts. She was also atopic, with strongly positive RASTs to grass pollen (grade 4) and cat dander (grade 3).

The management of her *nut allergy* comprised advice on strict avoidance of peanuts and tree nuts, with particular attention to 'hidden' nuts in food. She was advised to wear a medical alert bracelet as a warning to emergency personnel of a possible cause of sudden collapse, and to carry with her at all times a self-injectable form of epinephrine (adrenaline).

No laboratory test is diagnostic. Immediate-hypersensitivity skin tests and antigen-specific IgE antibodies (RAST) only identify some antigens, even where there is a strongly positive history. Only one-third of patients with a clear history of egg, fish or nut intolerance give positive skin reactions and RAST results and most of those with milk intolerance do not. A negative blood test for IgE antibodies is not proof of lack of food allergic disease; conversely, a RAST result may be positive in a patient who is perfectly able to tolerate the food in question. Testing the blood or skin of a patient clearly does not always reflect what is happening at the level of the gut mucosa.

Other tests are at best misleading, at worst dangerous. A diagnostic procedure used by 'clinical ecologists' is symptom provocation by intradermal or sublingual extracts of test substances. When evaluated under double-blind conditions, this method lacked validity: the high frequency of positive responses to the extracts appeared to be due to suggestion and chance. Other methods, such as hair analysis, are more a matter of gullibility and faith than evidence-based medicine. A double-blind, randomized trial of electrodermal ('Vega') testing found that this method could not distinguish between atopic and non-atopic people. A study of five commercial 'allergy' testing clinics in the UK, conducted by the Consumers' Association, found that these clinics did not reliably identify food allergies in patients known to have them; they gave different results for paired samples from the same patient; and they often gave dubious and risky dietary advice. Be warned, this is still widespread and costly, both financially and for health!

Recognition of the offending food and its elimination from the diet is the cornerstone of treatment of truly allergic patients. Some patients know that a certain food, such as peanuts, regularly produces their symptoms; this food must be avoided – a simple **elimination diet**. Certain foods are eliminated empirically because they are frequently implicated in that form of food 'allergy', e.g. milk and eggs in infant atopic eczema. A very few rare patients who seem intolerant of a wide range of foods may need a very restricted diet – a 'few-food' or 'oligoantigenic' diet – but dietary exclusion has many risks: nutritional deficiency, expense, disruption of lifestyle and psychological consequences.

Coeliac disease involves T cells sensitized to the dietary antigens of gluten and can be considered a type of allergy since an extrinsic antigen is involved, as shown by the clinical improvement following gluten withdrawal. However, since the autoantibodies to tissue transglutaminase and endomysium are also a feature, it is more commonly considered with the autoimmune diseases.

4.8 Skin disease and allergy

4.8.1 Urticaria and angioedema

Urticaria is a physical sign, not a disease. Urticaria refers to transient episodes of demarcated, oedematous, erythematous, pruritic lesions with a raised edge. It has such a distinctive appearance that clinical diagnosis is usually easy; the difficult task is finding the cause, since laboratory tests are unhelpful.

Urticaria results from sudden localized accumulation of fluid in the dermis. Angioedema is a similar process occurring in the deep dermis, subcutaneous tissues or mucous membranes (Fig. 4.9). Urticaria and angioedema commonly co-exist, except in hereditary angioedema in which urticaria plays no part.

Any sudden increase in local vascular permeability in the dermis will cause urticaria. A variety of **mechanisms** may be responsible (Fig. 4.10); some are immune but many are not. Mast cells in the dermis are an important source of the vasoactive mediators and, since a number of mediators are involved in the pathogenesis of urticaria, antihistamines are not always effective.

Spontaneous urticaria can be classified into acute and chronic (Box 4.7). **Acute urticaria** is short-lived, although the cause is identified in only 50% of cases. Episodes caused by an IgE-mediated reaction to extrinsic antigens, such as foods, are usually obvious from the history and can be confirmed by skin-prick testing. Attacks can also be related to drug ingestion (Fig. 4.11) or to acute viral infections.

Chronic urticaria is conventionally defined as the occurrence of widespread urticarial weals on a daily or almost daily basis for at least 6 weeks (Case 4.10). It affects over 1 in 200 of the population at some time during their life and can be very disabling. The term 'chronic spontaneous urticaria' is used when physical urticarias and urticarial vasculitis have been

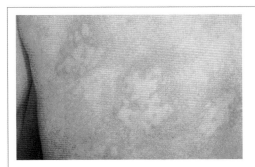

Fig. 4.9 Typical urticaria.

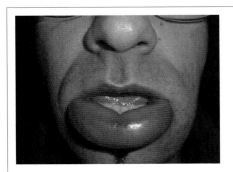

Fig. 4.10 Angioedema of the lower lip.

Box 4.7   Classification of urticaria

- Spontaneous urticaria
- Acute urticaria
- Chronic – spontaneous or autoimmune urticaria
- Physical urticaria
- Contact urticaria
- Urticarial vasculitis

Box 4.8   Clinical identification of urticarial vasculitis

- The weals are usually tender and painful rather than itchy
- They generally last longer than 24 hours
- They fade to leave purpura or bruising
- They are often accompanied by systemic features such as fever and arthralgia

---

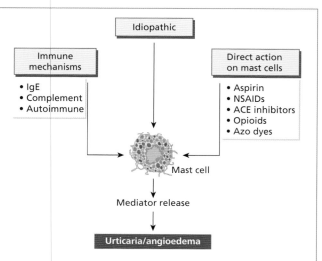

Fig. 4.11 Mechanisms of urticaria production. ACE, angiotensin-converting enzyme; NSAIDs, non-steroidal anti-inflammatory drugs.

excluded. Chronic spontaneous and physical urticarias commonly co-exist in the same patient.

In patients with **physical urticarias**, itching and weals are provoked by physical stimuli such as scratching the skin (dermographism), rapid cooling (cold urticaria), sun exposure (solar urticaria), water (aquagenic urticaria) or exercise, heat or emotion (cholinergic urticaria).

Urticarial vasculitis (Boxes 4.7 and 4.8) is regarded as an immune-complex disease with histological evidence of vasculitis on skin biopsy. The diagnosis is important because patients may have underlying disease, such as systemic lupus erythematosus (SLE), and the treatment differs.

By definition, no cause can be found for **chronic spontaneous urticaria**. Once the physical urticarias and urticarial vasculitis are eliminated, chronic urticaria is divided into autoimmune chronic urticaria (45%) and idiopathic chronic urticaria (55%). Most patients with autoimmune urticaria may involve IgG autoantibodies to high-affinity IgE receptor (FcΣRI) on mast cells and basophils that trigger mediator release. Less commonly, autoantibodies to IgE activate basophils to release histamine. Chronic urticaria can also be triggered directly by food additives, namely azo dyes and preservatives, or by a variety of drugs, including aspirin, other NSAIDs, angiotensin-converting enzyme (ACE) inhibitors and opioids (Fig. 4.11).

Treatment of chronic urticaria is empirical. Avoidance of triggering factors is an obvious step and elimination of Helicobacter pylori infection has been associated with remission of chronic urticaria in some patients. Low-sedation anti-H1 antihistamines, which have a low incidence of adverse effects, are the mainstay of treatment, often in high doses. Reduction of itch and decreases in the frequency and duration of weals are improved more by daily therapy than by intermittent therapy. Montelukast is helpful, but systemic steroids are not indicated in chronic urticaria because of the high doses required, the development of intolerance and the problems of steroid toxicity. For patients with severe autoimmune disease, high-dose ciclosporin therapy is effective. Omalizumab is also used for treatment of patients who do not respond to high-dose H1 antihistamine therapy. European guidelines for the management of urticaria are available. Despite treatment, about 20% of patients still have chronic urticaria 10 years following presentation.

4.8.2 Atopic eczema

Atopic eczema (also referred to as 'atopic dermatitis') is a common, chronic, severely pruritic, eczematous skin disease, usually occurring in individuals with a hereditary predisposition to all atopic disorders (Case 4.11), and often in association with a high serum IgE level.

The **prevalence** of atopic eczema is increasing. It affects about 10–20% of children worldwide and some 2% of adults. Over half of children present during the first year of life. In infants, the dermatitis often appears on the face first, followed by the flexural aspects of the arms and legs (Fig. 4.12). In older children and adults, the flexures are frequently involved, with thickening, lichenification and scaling of the epidermis, which tends to crack and weep. Spontaneous resolution occurs in many patients: about half clear by the age of 7 years and 90% by their late teens but, in the remainder, eczema persists into adult life.

The commonest **complication** is superadded bacterial infection, but some children may develop ocular complications, such as cataracts, psychological problems or side effects from prolonged treatment (particularly with corticosteroids). Although atopic children handle most viruses normally, *superadded infection with herpes simplex virus is life threatening*.

The **diagnosis** of atopic eczema is based on the clinical features, usually with a personal or family history of atopy. There

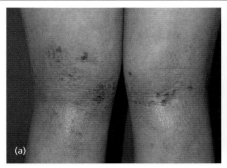 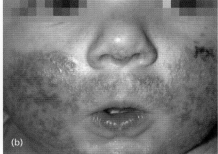

Fig. 4.12 Childhood eczema presents as a rash on the face and in the flexural aspects of arms and legs. Source: Baron SE, Cohen SN, Archer CB. (2012). Guidance on the diagnosis and clinical management of psoriasis. Clinical and Experimental Dermatology, 37(Suppl. 1):7–12. Source: Baron SE, Cohen SN, & Archer CB. (2012). Guidance on the diagnosis and clinical management of atopic eczema. Clinical and Experimental Dermatology, 37, 7–12. doi:10.1111/j.1365-2230.2012.04336.x.

are no pathognomonic clinical or laboratory findings; although a raised IgE and multiple positive prick tests and RASTs are commonly found, *they are unhelpful in management.*

There is a **strong genetic** predisposition to atopic eczema. The concordance rate is up to 85% in monozygotic twins compared with 30% in dizygotic twins. This is in part due to disease causing **mutations in filaggrin**, found in 2006 to be the cause of ichthyosis vulgaris and a strong genetic risk factor for atopic eczema. Since then large-scale genome-wide association studies have confirmed this and identified further susceptibility genes that suggest that changes both in the epidermal barrier and in immunity play a role in the pathogenesis of this disease. Filaggrin is essential for the regulation of homeostasis of epidermal cells. Filaggrin monomers become part of the lipid envelope responsible for skin barrier function as well as assisting positively in water retention.

Mutations that result in loss of functioning filaggrin result in dehydration of the epidermis and defects in the barrier allow exposure to allergens and microbes, resulting in Th2 polarized lymphocyte responses and subsequent chronic skin inflammation. Filaggrin polymorphisms may be involved in other atopic conditions with leaky barriers.

Familial aggregation analysis shows a stronger clustering of atopic eczema between siblings than between siblings and parents, suggesting that **environmental factors** are also important. Exposure to the triggers in atopic eczema is often via the skin, such triggers probably being infections or irritants. House dust mite is one provoking factor and reduction in the house dust mite allergen load in the home may result in significant clinical improvement. The role of food intolerance is controversial: controlled studies of dietary manipulation in children suggest that it is an uncommon trigger, particularly in older children (see Table 4.6). Staphylococcus aureus colonization and infection are found in over 90% of patients with atopic eczema and are the most likely source of exacerbation of the skin inflammation by acting as a superantigen (Chapter 2, section 2.4.2), activating macrophages and particularly T cells expressing the skin homing receptor, cutaneous lymphoid antigen (Chapter 11, section 11.1).

The **pathogenesis** of atopic dermatitis involves these T cells (Box 4.9), which is reflected in the treatment of severe disease. Once the allergen is presented by dendritic cells or Langerhans cells to CD4 T cells, Th0 differentiation to Th2 cells results in secretion of IL-4, IL-5, IL-6 and IL-13, leading to inflammation. IL-4 and IL-13 act as IgE isotype-specific switch factors and induce the expression of VCAM-1 (see Chapter 1), an adhesion molecule involved in the migration of mononuclear cells into sites of allergic tissue inflammation. T lymphocytes migrating into the skin are highly enriched for cutaneous lymphoid antigen-expressing memory Th2 cells.

The most measurable **immunological abnormality** is a raised serum IgE level in up to 90% of patients. The highest levels are found in patients with both eczema and asthma. Since IgE production is under T-cell control, the abnormal regulation of IgE production probably reflects defective T-cell function (Box 4.9) rather than being pathogenic.

Atopic dermatitis is due to an itch that, when scratched, results in a rash, and even bleeding if the scratching is severe. The severe pruritis of atopic eczema serves to exacerbate the condition, as itching has the potential to further disrupt barrier function and mechanical stimulation of keratinocytes and cytokines that sustain the inflammatory process – 'the itch–scratch cycle'. However, the precise initial triggers remain obscure.

Current **management** of atopic eczema is directed at the elimination of exacerbating factors including allergens, infection and irritants, and the reduction of cutaneous inflammation. Bland emollients, which soothe the skin, and rehydration are crucial to provide some symptomatic relief of itching, resulting in an artificial barrier against further triggers. **Topical corticosteroids** suppress inflammation and also help to reduce itching; they are the most successful agents currently available to treat eczema. Long-term use of potent steroids may lead to atrophy of the dermis and epidermis and may even be accompanied by significant systemic absorption if they are applied in excess. Systemic steroids are rarely justified, but may sometimes be used in short bursts to control otherwise intractable eczema, or in an attempt to 'reset' the 'itch–scratch' cycle.

Box 4.9 Evidence that atopic eczema is linked to abnormal T-cell function

Clinical evidence
- Increased susceptibility to skin infections normally controlled by T cells
  - Disseminated vaccinia (eczema vaccinatum)
  - Herpes simplex (eczema herpeticum) or Kaposi's varicelliform eruption
  - Viral warts
  - Dermatophyte fungal infection
- Temporary improvement during measles infection (?Th1 cell response with interferon-γ production)
- Occurrence of eczema in primary immunodeficiency diseases, e.g. Wiskott–Aldrich syndrome; hyper-IgE recurrent infection syndrome; graft-versus-host disease
- Response to T-cell immunomodulatory therapy

Laboratory evidence
- Disappearance of eczema in children with Wiskott–Aldrich syndrome following stem cell transplantation
- Decreased CD8$^+$ T-cell number and function in blood in active disease
- Decreased number of interferon-γ-secreting Th1 cells
- Expansion of interleukin (IL)-4-, IL-5- and IL-13-secreting Th2 cells in the skin and peripheral blood
- Chronic macrophage activation with increased secretion of granulocyte–macrophage colony-stimulating factor (GM-CSF), prostaglandin E$_2$ (PGE$_2$) and IL-10

Animal evidence
- Absence of T cells prevents eczema in mouse model

There is limited and conflicting evidence regarding the efficacy of bed covers impermeable to mite allergens and other measures to reduce any potential triggers.

A number of **therapeutic approaches** are now directed at modulating signal transduction in Th2 lymphocytes. Ciclosporin has proved safe and effective as a short-term treatment for severe, refractory atopic eczema. Controlled trials have shown topical calcineurin inhibitors (Chapter 7, section 7.2), such as **tacrolimus or pimecrolimus**, to be effective in controlling moderate to severe atopic eczema without the atrophic side effects of topical steroids, and are recommended by the National Institute for Clinical Excellence (NICE) for patients who have moderate to severe eczema that is unresponsive to conventional first-line treatment. Dupilumab, a monoclonal antibody that prevents IL-4/IL-3 signalling, is approved for severe eczema. Guidelines for primary care physicians and specialists are widely available.

4.8.3 Contact dermatitis

Contact dermatitis is an inflammatory skin disease caused by T-cell-mediated (type IV) hypersensitivity to external agents that come into contact with the skin rather than an IgE (type I) hypersensitivity. It is an important cause of occupational skin disease. Contact dermatitis is quite distinct from atopic dermatitis, both clinically and in immunopathogenesis, and is discussed fully in Chapter 11, section 11.4.

 Case 4.9 Oral allergy (pollen-fruit) syndrome

A 40-year-old man knew he had longstanding 'hay fever', although his symptoms were worse in March and April each year rather than in summer months. For the previous 4 years he had noticed that eating certain fruits, particularly apples, pears and peaches, produced tingling, burning and swelling of his lips and gums. These symptoms occurred within seconds of starting to eat these fruits and lasted about 30 min, but were never associated with vomiting, urticaria, bronchospasm or circulatory collapse. He found that he could eat cooked or preserved apples without any reactions. He was worried that these reactions heralded an increasing potential to develop anaphylaxis to fruit.

He was skin-prick tested to a variety of allergens: he showed strongly positive reactivity to tree pollen and peach, but a negative reaction to the commercial apple solution. However, when the skin test lancet was first pricked into a fresh apple and then into the patient's skin – so-called 'prick-prick' testing – a strongly positive immediate reaction developed.

He has the oral allergy (pollen-fruit) syndrome.

Case 4.10   Chronic urticaria and angioedema

A 25-year-old joiner presented with a 12-month history of an intensely itchy 'nettle rash' on his chest and back (see Fig. 4.9). The lesions appeared suddenly and lasted from 6 to 12 h, to be replaced by new lesions at other sites. The lesions varied in size from a few millimetres to several centimetres. Attacks occurred two to three times each week. In addition, he had experienced four episodes of sudden swelling of lips that took 48 h to subside. He said he looked as though he had been punched (see Fig. 4.10). He was unaware of any triggering factors and there was no personal or family history of atopy. His general health was excellent and he was not taking any medications. On examination, the lesions consisted of raised, red, irregular patches, some with white centres, and were typically urticarial. General examination was entirely normal.

Laboratory investigations showed a normal haemoglobin and white cell count, with no eosinophilia. His complement C4 and C1 inhibitor levels were normal, excluding hereditary angioedema (see Chapter 11, Case 11.5).

The urticaria was fairly well controlled by a long-acting antihistamine (levocetirizine), but he was reluctant to take these tablets on a long-term basis. Three years later, his urticarial lesions are still present, although less severe; their cause is unknown.

 Case 4.11   Atopic eczema

Sam was born at full term, after a normal pregnancy, and weighed 3.4 kg. He was breast fed. At the age of 4 weeks, he was admitted with a 2-day history of screaming attacks, loose motions and rectal bleeding. He was treated conservatively, but 3 days after discharge his symptoms recurred, together with patches of eczema on his arms and trunk. On detailed questioning, it transpired that a health visitor had told Sam's mother that her breast milk was of 'poor quality' and had advised her to 'top up' each feed with cow's milk. His mother had been following this advice from the time Sam was 2 weeks old. When investigated at the age of 6 weeks, strongly positive IgE-specific antibodies to cow's milk were present on RAST testing. His mother returned to exclusive breast feeding and excluded dairy products from her own diet, to eliminate any possibility that cow's milk antigens might be excreted in her breast milk. Within 2–3 days, the screaming attacks stopped.

At the age of 10 months Sam was referred back to hospital with extensive atopic eczema. It had recurred behind his knees at the age of 7 months, when solids were first introduced into his diet, and steadily worsened. The areas affected were the popliteal and antecubital fossae, arms and abdomen. He scratched the eczematous lesions, especially at night, with the result that his and the family's sleep was badly disturbed. Sam had a strong family history of atopic disease: his mother and maternal grandmother both suffered from asthma. On examination, his height and weight were around the 50th centile. He was covered in extensive eczema, involving 60% of the total skin area.

Laboratory investigations showed a normal haemoglobin (123 g/l) with a raised white cell count (16.0×10^9/l) including an absolute (650/mm³) eosinophilia. His total serum IgE level was markedly raised at 4600 IU/ml (NR for age <50 IU/ml) with strongly positive RASTs to grass pollen, cat epithelium, dog dander, house dust mite, cow's milk, wheat and peas. Skin-prick testing was not considered in the presence of such widespread eczema. Samples of dust from his home showed very high levels of house dust mite in the carpet and on several toys.

He was treated with antihistamines at night and liberal applications of an emollient cream to his skin lesions. Environmental control of antigen exposure was also attempted: the mite count was lowered by changing carpets, and covering the mattress, pillows and duvet with covers impermeable to mite allergens, and the cat was found a new home. Sam was put on a diet free of cow's milk, wheat, oats, peas, beans, nuts, food preservatives and food colourings. Over the following 3 months, there was only partial improvement in the severity of his eczema and topical pimecrolimus was then used, successfully (see Chapter 7).

CHAPTER 5
Autoimmunity

Key topics

 Visit the companion website at **www.wiley.com/go/misbah/immunology** to download cases with additional figures on these topics.

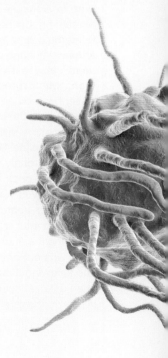

Chapel and Haeney's Essentials of Clinical Immunology, Seventh Edition. Edited by Siraj A. Misbah, Gavin P. Spickett, and Virgil A.S.H. Dalm.
© 2022 John Wiley & Sons Ltd. Published 2022 by John Wiley & Sons Ltd.

5.1 Definition of autoimmunity and autoimmune disease

Autoimmunity is an immune response against a self-antigen or antigens. **Autoimmune disease is tissue damage** or disturbed physiological function due to an autoimmune response. This distinction is important, as autoimmune responses can occur without disease (Case 5.1) or result from diseases caused by other mechanisms (such as infection). Proof that autoimmunity causes a particular disease requires a number of criteria to be met, as in Koch's postulates for microorganisms in infectious diseases (Table 5.1). The best **evidence** for autoimmunity in human disease comes from active transfer of immunoglobulin (Ig)G autoantibodies across the placenta in the last trimester of pregnancy, which may lead to the development of transient autoimmune disease in the fetus and neonate (Table 5.2 and Case 5.2). In contrast, there are diseases that are reliably associated with both T-cell and B-cell autoimmune responses, but where the precise mechanism of disease is unclear. For example, the chronic liver disease primary biliary cirrhosis (Chapter 14, section 14.8.2) is strongly associated with autoantibodies directed against mitochondria (and more specifically against a single isoform of the mitochondrial enzyme pyruvate dehydrogenase); it seems unlikely that these antibodies play any role in liver damage, but are produced secondarily to the damage of unknown aetiology. In another autoimmune disease, myasthenia gravis, transfer of the primary or pathogenic autoantibody causes myasthenic features in a rabbit. **Caution is therefore required in making the assumptions both that autoimmune responses necessarily imply autoimmune disease and that a given autoimmune antibody or T cell plays a role in the pathogenesis.**

 Case 5.1 Is this rheumatoid arthritis?

A 43-year-old woman presented to her general practitioner with sudden onset of acute back pain while gardening, followed by more sustained but less severe pain over the next two weeks. The GP felt that this was mechanical back pain, but performed some 'screening investigations' that included a normal C-reactive protein (CRP) level and a positive test for rheumatoid factor at a titre of 1 in 256. She was negative for antibodies to citrullinated proteins (anti-CCP). She was then referred to her local rheumatology department with a possible diagnosis of 'rheumatoid arthritis'. This caused the patient considerable anxiety as her aunt had had severe rheumatoid arthritis, leading to a very high level of disability. When she was seen in the rheumatology clinic three months later she still had minor back pain, but this was overshadowed by her anxiety. She had no other musculoskeletal symptoms and examination was normal apart from mild restriction of the lumbar spine. The rheumatologist agreed with the initial diagnosis of mechanical back pain and explained that around 5% of healthy normal people have a positive test for rheumatoid factor. The presence of a normal CRP level and negative anti-CCP *was* reassuring and testing for rheumatoid factor *not* useful; it is only used in patients with a clinical diagnosis of rheumatoid arthritis, when it is a helpful prognostic indicator.

5.2 Patterns of autoimmune disease

Autoimmune diseases can affect any organ in the body, although certain systems seem particularly susceptible (e.g. endocrine glands). Autoimmune diseases have been conventionally classified into (i) organ-specific and (ii) non-organ-specific disorders; though this is an arbitrary division, it is useful in thinking about the pathogenesis of each condition.

5.2.1 Organ-specific autoimmune disease

Organ-specific autoimmune disorders (Cases 5.2 and 5.3) usually affect a **single organ** and the autoimmune response is directed against multiple antigens within that organ. Most of the common organ-specific disorders affect one or another endocrine gland. The antigenic targets may be molecules expressed on the surface of cells (particularly hormone receptors) or intracellular molecules, particularly intracellular enzymes (Table 5.3).

Visit the website at **www.wiley.com/go/misbah/immunology** to read case studies on primary autoimmune hypothyroidism and interleukin (IL)-2 treatment in rheumatoid arthritis.

5.2.2 Non-organ-specific autoimmune disease

Non-organ-specific disorders affect **multiple organs** and are usually associated with autoimmune responses against self-molecules that are widely distributed through the body, and particularly with intracellular molecules involved in transcription and translation of the genetic code (Table 5.3). Many of these non-organ-specific disorders fall within the group of multisystem disorders labelled 'connective tissue diseases'; however, even though it is unfortunately still in widespread use, this is a misleading term since the 'connective tissues' are often neither abnormal nor specifically damaged.

Table 5.1 Criteria that confirm that a particular autoimmune response causes a corresponding autoimmune disease

	Criterion	Comment
1	Autoantibodies or autoreactive T cells with specificity for the affected organ are found reliably in the disease	This criterion is met in most endocrine autoimmune diseases. It is more difficult to fulfil where the target antigen (if any) is unknown, as in rheumatoid arthritis. Autoantibodies are much easier to detect than autoreactive T cells, *but autoantibodies can also be detected in some healthy subjects*
2	Autoantibodies and/or T cells are found at the site of tissue damage	True for some haematological and endocrine diseases, systemic lupus erythematosus (SLE) and some forms of glomerulonephritis and muscle or muscle end-plate diseases
3	The levels of autoantibody or T-cell response reflect disease activity	True for some diseases; demonstrable in acute systemic autoimmune diseases with rapidly progressive tissue damage, such as some subjects with renal SLE, systemic vasculitis or antiglomerular basement membrane disease
4	Reduction of the autoimmune response leads to improvement	Benefits of immunosuppression are seen in many disorders, but most immunosuppressive treatments are non-specific and antiinflammatory. Furthermore autoantibodies have a half-life of 3–4 weeks, so reductions in titres are slower than clinical recovery
5	Transfer of antibody or T cells to a second host leads to development of autoimmune disease in the recipient	Easily demonstrated in animal models, such as myasthenia, or in humans, by transplacental transfer of autoreactive IgG antibodies during the last third of pregnancy (see Case 5.2) and by development of autoimmune disease in the recipient of bone marrow transplants when the donor has an autoimmune disease
6	Immunization with autoantigen and consequent induction of an autoimmune response causes disease	Many self-proteins induce an autoimmune response in animals, but only if injected with an appropriate adjuvant. Harder to demonstrate in humans, but in the past rabies immunization involved use of infected (but non-infective) mammalian brain tissue, which induced autoimmune encephalomyelitis

Table 5.2 Immunoglobulin G antibody-mediated diseases capable of placental transfer

Maternal autoantibody to	Disease induced in neonate
Thyroid-stimulating hormone	Neonatal Graves' disease
Epidermal basement membrane cell adhesion molecules	Neonatal pemphigoid
Red blood cells	Haemolytic anaemia
Platelets	Thrombocytopenia
Acetylcholine receptor	Neonatal myasthenia gravis
Ro and La	Neonatal cutaneous lupus and congenital complete heart block

5.2.3 IgG4-related disease

A recently described condition, in which both lymphoproliferation and autoimmunity are significant, is the oddly named 'immuoglobulinG4-related disease (IgG4-RD)'. Originally recognized as autoimmune pancreatitis (acute abdominal pain and gross lymphadenopathy), particularly in middle-aged men in Japan, this syndrome has much wider organ involvement affecting nearly every organ system, such as the gastrointestinal tract, including the salivary glands, and also lymph nodes, retroperitoneum, blood vessels and many other organs. The only common findings are raised serum immunoglobulins due to **excessive levels of IgG4,** positive non-specific autoantibodies (rheumatoid factor, antinuclear antibodies)

and variable increases in serum lactate dehydrogenase levels. Since serum levels of IgG4 are normally extremely low, and many autoantibodies are known to be of the IgG4 isotype, this condition is thought to be largely autoimmune in nature. On biopsy, the **histology** in all tissues is remarkably similar: diffuse plasmacytic infiltrate of IgG4+ plasma cells with variable fibrosis and sometimes with reactive lymphoid follicles that can resemble lymphoma. Unlike the other IgG subclass molecules, the **heavy chains of the IgG4 molecule are unstable** and 50% of IgG4 molecules consist of heavy chains linked weakly by non-covalent forces. This means that the heavy chains can separate and recombine randomly, making new antigen-binding sites but failing to form immune complexes for clearance of antigen. Whether or not this is important in the pathogenesis of this variable condition remains to be seen. Patients have still not been followed long enough to know whether this is a premalignant condition and the long-term outlook is not yet known. Treatment consists of corticosteroids (usually very effective) and rituximab in resistant or recurring disease.

5.3 Who gets autoimmune disease?

The burden of autoimmune diseases is considerable throughout the world; around 3% of the population has an autoimmune disease. Many of the major chronic disabling diseases affecting people of working age are considered to have an autoimmune basis. These include multiple sclerosis (MS), rheumatoid arthritis (RA) and insulin-dependent diabetes mellitus

Case 5.2 Myasthenia gravis and neonatal myasthenia gravis

A 21-year-old woman was referred to a neurology clinic with a one-month history of double vision, difficulty swallowing and weakness in her upper arms. These symptoms were mild or absent in the morning and tended to worsen through the day. When she was seen towards the end of an afternoon neurology clinic, she was found to have a bilateral ptosis and disconjugate eye movements that could not be ascribed to a cranial nerve lesion. Her upper-limb power was initially normal, but deteriorated with repeated testing. An intravenous injection of edrophonium, a short-acting cholinesterase inhibitor, completely abolished the neurological signs, but her eye movements deteriorated again 30 min after the injection. A clinical diagnosis was made of myasthenia gravis. Subsequent blood testing showed the presence of a high level of autoantibodies against the acetylcholine receptor.

She was treated with oral cholinesterase inhibitors with some improvement. However, one month later she deteriorated and corticosteroids were introduced without effect. A computed tomography scan of her thorax showed no evidence of a thymoma, but she was nevertheless referred to a thoracic surgeon for thymectomy, as this can sometimes induce remission in myasthenia even in the absence of a thymoma. A small thymic remnant was removed and she recovered uneventfully and was able to withdraw from all medication without deterioration in her symptoms. Acetylcholine receptor antibody levels fell, but remained detectable. One year later, she became pregnant and after an uneventful 41-week pregnancy she delivered a 4 kg male infant. There were immediate concerns about the baby, who failed to make adequate respiratory efforts and who appeared limp and hypotonic. The baby was intubated and ventilated on the neonatal intensive care unit. In view of the mother's history, a provisional diagnosis of neonatal myasthenia gravis was made, although care was taken to exclude other causes of neonatal respiratory insufficiency such as maternal analgesia with pethidine, hypoglycaemia and sepsis. A cranial ultrasound showed no evidence of bleeding or other pathology. Subsequent testing of a blood sample taken from the umbilical cord showed low levels of acetylcholine receptor antibody. The baby needed ventilation and feeding via a nasogastric tube for three days, after which time the ventilation was successfully withdrawn. There were some initial feeding problems due to difficulty sucking and swallowing, but these resolved over the next 48 h. The child's subsequent development has been entirely normal. The mother also remains well.

 Case 5.3 Fungal infections, fits and hypocalcaemia

A 14-year-old boy presented to a dermatologist with sore, cracked hypertrophic lips, chronic paronychia (tender, swollen nail beds with dystrophic nails) and curious horn-like lesions in the scalp. The dermatologist made a clinical diagnosis of chronic mucocutaneous candidiasis, and subsequently cultured the yeast, Candida albicans, from the boy's mouth and a dermatophyte fungus from the lesions on the scalp. The dermatologist noted a history of epilepsy starting at the age of 5. Subsequent investigation demonstrated profound hypocalcaemia with corrected serum calcium of 1.1 mm/L (normal 2.2–2.6), with undetectable levels of parathyroid hormone. His 4-year-old sister had also recently developed epilepsy and was also found to be severely hypocalcaemic. The classical clinical picture allowed a confident diagnosis of autoimmune hypoparathyroidism (subsequently confirmed by positive autoantibodies against endocrine parathyroid tissue) as a feature of APECED (Autoimmune PolyEndocrinopathy, Candidiasis and Ectodermal Dysplasia). The patient subsequently developed fatigue and vomiting and a short synacthen test revealed adrenal cortical failure as well, and he was found to have autoantibodies to adrenal cortex, confirming autoimmune adrenalitis. As yet there is no evidence of diabetes mellitus. Genetic analysis confirmed a disease-causing mutation in the AIRE gene and the other family members were also screened.

(IDDM). Autoimmune diseases are rare in childhood and the peak years of onset lie between puberty and retirement age, the major exception being the childhood-onset form of diabetes mellitus.

There are striking sex differences in the risk of developing an autoimmune disease. Almost all are **more common in women**, and for some autoimmune diseases the risk of disease is increased eight times in females. There are, however, notable exceptions, such as ankylosing spondylitis, which is rare in women.

The prevalence of autoimmunity tends to be higher in northern latitudes, is probably higher in industrialized societies, and seems to increase progressively as the pattern of social and economic organization develops. It is unclear whether this geographical and socioeconomic variation in autoimmunity reflects differential exposure to pathogens, variations in nutrition, ascertainment of disease or other factors.

Autoimmune diseases also show evidence of **clustering within families** (Case 5.3, Table 5.4) and most show polygenic features that are slowly being unravelled with next-generation sequencing of exomes or genomes. These genetic factors are discussed in more detail in section 5.6.1.

Table 5.3 Some examples of self-antigens and associated diseases. More information can be found in the appropriate organ-based chapters. In general, tissue-specific antigens are associated with organ-specific diseases and those antigens found in all cells are associated with systemic disease

Self-antigen	Disease
Hormone receptors	
TSH receptor	Hyper- or hypothyroidism
Insulin receptor	Hyper- or hypoglycaemia
Neurotransmitter receptor	
Acetylcholine receptor	Myasthenia gravis
Cell adhesion molecules	
Epidermal cell adhesion molecules	Blistering skin diseases
Plasma proteins	
Factor VIII	Acquired haemophilia
β_1-glycoprotein I and other anticoagulant proteins	Antiphospholipid syndrome
Other cell-surface antigens	
Red blood cells (multiple antigens)	Haemolytic anaemia
Platelets	Thrombocytopenic purpura
Intracellular enzymes	
Thyroid peroxidase	Hypothyroidism
Steroid 21-hydroxylase (adrenal cortex)	Adrenocortical failure (Addison's disease)
Glutamate decarboxylase (β-cells of pancreatic islets)	Autoimmune diabetes
Lysosomal enzymes (phagocytic cells)	Systemic vasculitis
Mitochondrial enzymes (particularly pyruvate dehydrogenase)	Primary biliary cirrhosis
Intracellular molecules involved in transcription and translation	
Double-stranded DNA	SLE
Histones	SLE
Topoisomerase I	Diffuse scleroderma
Amino-acyl t-RNA synthases	Polymyositis
Centromere proteins	Limited scleroderma

SLE, systemic lupus erythematosus; TSH, thyroid-stimulating hormone.

5.4 What prevents autoimmunity?

Autoimmune responses are very similar to immune responses to non-self-antigens. Both are driven by antigen, involve the same adaptive immune cell types and produce tissue damage by the same effector mechanisms – both T cells and B cells.

The development of autoimmunity, however, implies a failure of the normal regulatory mechanisms. These regulatory mechanisms are discussed first so that reasons for their breakdown can be examined.

5.4.1 Autoimmunity and self-tolerance

Strong protective mechanisms exist to prevent the development of autoimmune disease. As outlined in Chapter 1, the immune system has the ability to generate a vast diversity of different T-cell antigen receptors and immunoglobulin molecules by differential genetic recombination. This process produces many antigen-specific receptors capable of binding to self-molecules. To avoid autoimmune disease, the T and B cells bearing these self-reactive molecules must be either eliminated or downregulated. Because T cells (in particular CD4⁺ T cells) have a central role in controlling nearly all immune responses, the process of T-cell tolerance seems to be of greater importance in avoiding autoimmunity than B-cell tolerance, since self-reactive B cells require CD4⁺ T cells' help to produce a fully fledged IgG antibody response. However, antigen receptors on B cells undergo somatic mutation as well as recombination events, resulting in additional opportunities for chance cross-reactivity with self-antigens. There are, therefore, several mechanisms to maintain tolerance. These are traditionally divided into **central mechanisms**, such as those that act early in development in the thymus, and **peripheral mechanisms** to eliminate those arising later in adaptive immune responses.

5.4.2 Thymic tolerance

The thymus plays a major role in eliminating T cells capable of recognizing peptides from self-proteins (Fig. 5.1). There are three processes. Developing T cells have antigen receptors (TCRs) that are produced randomly by recombination, but all have the ability to bind to major histocompatibility complex (MHC) molecules; only those that recognize the host MHC in the thymic cortex survive; >90% of the developing T cells die from 'neglect'. T cells with TCRs that fail to bind the host MHC molecules in the thymic cortex die through apoptosis. T cells that survive this process move to the thymic medulla and bind, with a variety of affinities, to the MHC molecules and self-peptide complexes presented on medullary epithelial cells, from whom they also receive survival signals. Those T cells that bind with low affinity are allowed to survive and have the potential to bind to MHC plus a foreign peptide with high affinity, and so initiate protective immune responses at a later time. This is the process known as **positive selection**. In a further process known as **negative selection**, T cells that bind to MHC plus self-peptides with very high affinity in the thymus, and so have clear potential for self-recognition elsewhere in the body with consequent induction of autoimmunity, are eliminated on the basis of their high-affinity binding. This elimination

Table 5.4 Single-gene defects that provide an insight into autoimmune diseases

Gene defect or experimental genetic manipulation	Autoimmune disease seen as consequence of gene defect	Implications for autoimmunity
Deficiency of early classical complement pathway components, C1 q, C2, C4 in humans and knockout mice. Defects in autophagy genes in humans and knockout mice	Systemic lupus erythematosus	Early classical complement pathway important in immune-complex clearance and autophagy provides recycling of cell components and disposal of intracellular debris
Chronic granulomatous disease (defect in NADPH oxidase enzyme complex) in human female carriers	Discoid lupus erythematosus	Phagocytes scavenge and destroy cell debris, preventing activation by self-antigens
Fas (CD95) deficiency. (Binding of cell surface Fas triggers apoptosis.) Other defects in FAS:FASL pathways	Mice: lupus-like disorder Humans: lymphoproliferation and organ-specific autoimmunity, especially cytopenias	Apoptosis deletes potentially autoreactive lymphocytes, particularly B cells
Bcl-2 deficiency in knockout mice (Bcl-2 is intracellular molecule that inhibits apoptosis)	Lupus-like disorder	Apoptosis deletes potentially autoreactive lymphocytes, particularly B cells
Overexpression of tumour necrosis factor (TNF)-α in TNF-α transgenic mice	Destructive joint disease resembling rheumatoid arthritis	Key role of TNF in joint inflammation
Overexpression of human HLA-B27 in transgenic mice	Multisystem disease with some similarity to ankylosing spondylitis (AS): development critically dependent upon bowel flora	Direct link between this HLA molecule and pattern of inflammation found in AS. Implicates infection as trigger, especially in the gut
Absence of CTLA-4 (T-cell molecule involved in negative second signal) in CTLA-4 knockout mice	Lupus-like disorder with lymphoproliferation	Negative second signal is important in switching off autoreactive cells
Absence of transforming growth factor (TGF)-β (a cytokine with potent inhibitory effects on T cells) in TGF-β knockout mouse	Florid multisystem autoimmune disorder	Negative regulation of T cells is important in limiting autoimmunity
Abnormal or absent expression of transcription factor, AIRE in humans and knockout mice (Case 5.3)	Autoimmunity in multiple endocrine organs	AIRE controls expression of self-molecules in the thymus, thus influences thymic tolerance
Absent FOXP3 transcription factor results in lack of regulatory T cells (Tregs)	IPEX – Immune dysregulation, Polyendocrinopathy (usually neonatal diabetes), Enteropathy in males – X-linked	Lack of Tregs causes breakdown of peripheral tolerance

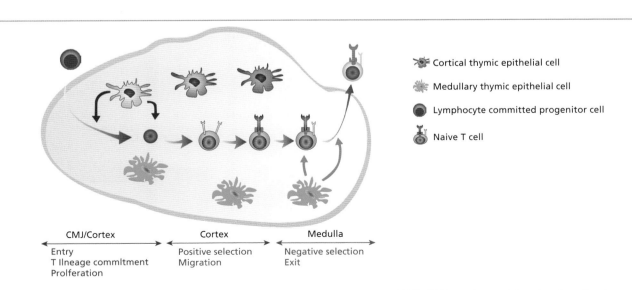

Fig. 5.1 Representation of T-cell selection in the thymus by thymic epithelial cells (TEC). CMJ, corticomedullary junction. Courtesy of Georg Hollander.

of self-reactive cells is known as **negative (deletional) selection** (see Fig. 5.1).

This process of **thymic education** is only partially successful, as autoreactive T cells can be detected in healthy persons. The most important reason for failure of thymic tolerance is that many self-peptides are not expressed at a sufficient level in the thymus to induce negative selection. Many peptides found bound to MHC molecules in the thymus are from either ubiquitous intracellular or membrane-bound proteins or proteins present in the extracellular fluid, expression of which is controlled by a transcription factor known as AIRE (section 5.6.1). The negative selection of self-reactive thymocytes depends on the expression of tissue-specific antigens by medullary thymic epithelial cells. The AIRE protein plays an important role in presenting these antigens, and the absence of even one AIRE-induced tissue-specific antigen in the thymus can lead to autoimmunity in the antigen-expressing target organ.

The vast number of self-antigens, and the need to present them all to each developing T lymphocyte, renders thymic tolerance imperfect. Tolerance is induced to some, but not all, tissue-specific proteins. It is not surprising therefore that T cells responsive to tissue-specific proteins – for example, cartilage collagens or some central nervous system (CNS) antigens – can

be detected in healthy people under certain laboratory conditions. A second level of control is needed to control these potentially autoreactive cells and this is known as peripheral tolerance.

5.4.3 Peripheral tolerance

There are several mechanisms by which peripheral tolerance is maintained. These are outlined here.

Ignorance

A restricted form of peripheral tolerance exists because the antigen is effectively invisible to the immune system. This is known as immunological ignorance (Fig. 5.2). Immunological ignorance can occur because the antigen is sequestered in an **avascular organ** such as the intact vitreous humour of the eye, although when limited amounts of antigen do escape from these sites due to inflammation this will break down. More importantly, immunological ignorance occurs because CD4+ T cells (which are required to initiate most immune responses) will only recognize antigens presented in association with MHC class II

Fig. 5.2 How peripheral T-cell tolerance is maintained. IL, interleukin; TCR, T-cell receptor; TGF, transforming growth factor.

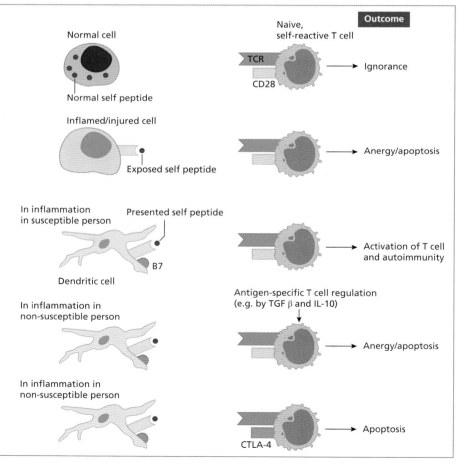

molecules. The **limited distribution of MHC class II molecules in healthy tissues** means that most organ-specific molecules are not expressed alongside MHC class II in health and so are not able to be presented at levels high enough to induce T-cell activation. However, in inflamed tissues MHC II is expressed as part of the inflammation, so additional processes are required to prevent or control self-reactivity.

Separation of autoreactive T cells and autoantigens

Self-antigens and lymphocytes are also kept separate by the **restricted routes of lymphocyte circulation** that limit naive lymphocytes to secondary lymphoid tissue and the blood (Fig. 5.3). Since antigens, including self-antigens, drain via afferent lymphatics to local lymph nodes, and the naive T cells in normal nodes do not express co-stimulatory molecules, no activation occurs in the absence of inflammation (see the next section), i.e. activation of dendritic cells via Toll-like receptors (Fig. 5.2).

To prevent large amounts of self-antigen from gaining access to dendritic cells, debris from self-tissue breakdown needs to be cleared rapidly and destroyed. This is achieved by cell death through **apoptosis**, preventing widespread spilling of cell contents, or **autophagy** to recycle cellular components. A variety of **scavenger mechanisms** help to clear cell debris, including the complement systems, certain acute-phase proteins (such as serum amyloid P and C-reactive protein) and a number of receptors found upon phagocytes. Defects of complement or phagocytes are associated with the development of autoimmunity against intracellular molecules (Table 5.4).

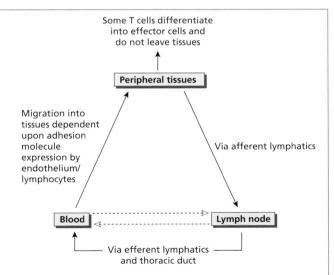

Fig. 5.3 Diagrammatic representation of the different recirculation pathways taken by naive T cells (dotted line) and T cells that have been previously exposed to antigen (solid line).

Anergy, apoptosis and autophagy

The pattern of stimulation through the TCR may also be important in determining whether a cell becomes activated or anergic: continuous low-level stimulation of a small number of T-cell antigen receptors (as might occur with a self-antigen) tends to produce **anergy**, while strong and rapidly increasing stimulation (as in infection) favours activation.

More active mechanisms of peripheral tolerance also operate after antigen recognition (see Fig. 5.2). These involve either deletion of self-reactive cells by apoptosis or induction of a state of unresponsiveness, **anergy**. Naive CD4⁺ T cells need two signals to become activated and initiate an immune response: an antigen-specific signal through the T-cell antigen receptor and a second, non-specific co-stimulatory signal, usually signalled by CD28 (on the T cell) binding to one of the B7 family (CD80 or CD86) on the dendritic or specialized B cell (see Chapter 1, Figure 1.16). If the T cell receives both signals, then it will become activated and proliferate and produce cytokines. If **no co-stimulatory molecules are engaged**, then stimulation through the TCR alone leads to longstanding anergy or death of the T cell by apoptosis. The expression of these co-stimulatory molecules is tightly controlled. Constitutive expression is confined to specialized antigen-presenting cells such as dendritic cells; given their distribution and patterns of recirculation, interaction between **CD4** cells and dendritic cells is likely to happen only in secondary lymphoid tissues such as lymph nodes. The restricted expression of co-stimulatory molecules means that, even if a T cell recognizes a tissue-specific peptide/MHC molecule complex (e.g. an antigen derived from a pancreatic islet cell), then anergy rather than activation is likely to follow, as no antigen-presenting cell (and therefore co-stimulatory signal) will be available in healthy tissue. Expression of co-stimulatory molecules can be induced upon other cells by a variety of stimuli, usually in association with inflammation or cell damage. However, because of the restricted pattern of lymphocyte recirculation, only previously activated cells will gain access to these peripheral sites and these peripheral co-stimulatory molecules are more likely to sustain than initiate an autoimmune response.

Two types of external signals can initiate **apoptosis (programmed cell death)**. Tumour necrosis factor alpha (**TNFα**), the inflammatory cytokine secreted mainly by macrophages, is a major process since almost all cells in the human body have receptors for TNF. The other major external apoptotic pathway involves the expression of **FAS ligand (FASL) on T cells** following activation. This protein then binds to FAS on adjacent cells and results in activation-induced cell death (AICD). This process is needed to prevent excessive immune responses and to eliminate autoreactive T cells (see Chapter 1). There is a third, intrinsic pathway and possibly more, since these are important regulatory processes. There are also inhibitors of apoptosis, the absence of which can result in excessive cell death such as in inflammatory diseases like in the gut.

Autophagy is a basic mechanism conserved in evolution, which is essential for maintaining cellular components in the face of cellular stress (such as nutrient starvation). Damaged proteins and organelles are recognized and recycled, preventing initiation of an immune response. The role of defective autophagy is gradually being appreciated in many inflammatory and neurodegenerative conditions.

Regulation and suppression

Suppression of unwanted immune responses is so important that there are several other mechanisms for peripheral tolerance, including active suppression of self-reactive T cells by regulatory populations of T cells (**Tregs**). There are both antigen-specific induced Tregs, which recognize the same antigen as T-effector cells, and natural Tregs, which are non-antigen specific. Both are formed in the thymus and are generally defined by the markers CD4, CD25 and forkhead box protein P3 (FoxP3). CD4⁺CD25⁺FoxP3⁺ cells exert their regulatory effects either through secretion of immunosuppressive cytokines such as IL-10 and TGF-β or through cell contact-dependent mechanisms, such as CTLA-4 expression.

Activated T cells can also express cell-surface molecules similar in structure to co-stimulatory molecules, but which exert a **negative effect upon T-cell activation**; in particular, CTLA-4 has a similar structure to CD28 and binds to the same ligands to prevent or limit activation. Binding of CTLA-4 to CD80 or CD86 induces anergy or death by apoptosis, as a negative counterpart to co-stimulation that may be important in terminating an immune response (see Chapter 1, section 1.3.4). The importance of apoptotic death of autoreactive lymphocytes in preventing autoimmune disease is emphasized by the development of autoimmunity in patients with immune-genetic defects in the control of apoptosis (see Table 5.4). This has also been exploited in the development of a therapeutic monoclonal antibody that blocks the CTLA4 regulatory signal, which allows cytotoxic T cells to destroy malignant melanoma cells. However, removal of regulatory T-cell inhibition is associated with the induction of iatrogenic autoimmunity in a range of organs (see Table 5.4 and Fig. 5.4). There is also evidence in mice of a variety of specific CD8⁺ T-regulatory cells (known as CD8⁺ Ti) that contribute to peripheral tolerance and such cells have particular features (interferon and apoptosis gene activation) to suggest a protective phenotype. However, their role in humans has yet to be defined.

5.4.4 B-cell tolerance

B-cell tolerance is less complete than T-cell tolerance since there is no organ equivalent of the thymus in mammalian B-cell development. So B-cell tolerance operates at a peripheral rather than central level, and multiple mechanisms exist to limit B-cell autoreactivity: clonal deletion, clonal anergy, receptor editing and maturation arrest.

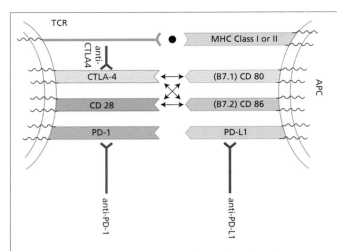

Fig. 5.4 Schematic representation of sites of action of checkpoint inhibitors.

The production of self-reactive antibodies is limited mainly by the lack of T-cell help for self-antigens. New B cells are being produced continuously from bone marrow precursors and many of these are autoreactive. The process of somatic hypermutation of immunoglobulin genes in mature B cells in the germinal centres of lymph nodes also has the potential for the generation of autoantibodies. However, B cells are able to undergo **receptor editing** in the bone marrow – a process that allows new light-chain rearrangement if an autoreactive B cell is produced, to enable new non-self-specificities. In addition, if a newly developed or recently hypermutated B cell binds to the self-antigen, then in the absence of specific antigen T-cell help, that B cell will undergo **apoptosis or anergy**. Thus, there are some similarities between T- and B-cell activation and tolerance, in that two signals are required for activation and the presence of an antigen-specific signal alone leads to death or anergy. As with T cells, low-level chronic stimulation via the antigen receptor favours anergy, and rapidly increasing amounts of antigen favour activation.

5.5 How does tolerance break down?

Our understanding of the breakdown of tolerance is incomplete; many separate mechanisms may be involved. Overcoming T-cell peripheral tolerance seems likely to be the major hurdle and this may involve reversal of active mechanisms or overcoming protective processes. Situations in which transient breakdown of tolerance and autoimmunity can occur include **infections and other non-specific tissue damage**, particularly since **MHC class II** is expressed on inflamed tissues. Autoimmune disease is easy to induce in experimental animals, usually by combining immunization with a self-protein together with a powerful non-specific immune stimulant (**adjuvant** – as used in vaccines, see Chapter 7). Sustained production of autoantibodies occurs in some people without disease, particularly the close relatives of patients with autoimmune disease and with advancing age. Reversal of anergy can occur on exposure to certain cytokines, particularly IL-2 or interferon-α. Development or worsening of autoimmune disease has been seen following treatment with these drugs.

The potential importance of suppression in preventing autoimmunity is seen in animal models, where **loss of regulatory control** leads to widespread autoimmunity (see Table 5.4). Paradoxically, **Tregs** seem to be unusually sensitive to cytotoxic drugs such as cyclophosphamide in animal models, though this has been harder to demonstrate in humans. However, some patients receiving immunosuppression, for example some patients receiving the anti-T-cell monoclonal antibody (Campath-1H) for the treatment of MS, have subsequently developed autoimmune hyperthyroidism (Case 5.4).

Other mechanisms of breakdown of peripheral tolerance include induction of MHC class II expression in inflammation/ infection (Fig. 5.5) or increased activity of proteolytic enzymes or alteration of peptides by viruses or free radicals in such sites, leading to high concentrations of novel peptides (**cryptic epitopes**) being presented to responsive T cells (see Fig. 5.1). Once tolerance has broken down to a particular peptide, the resulting process of inflammation may allow presentation of further peptides. The immune response broadens and local tissue damage accelerates. This domino-like process is known as **epitope spreading** (see Fig. 5.5). This is best demonstrated in experimental models where immunization with a single peptide from a protein found in myelinated nerve sheaths (known as myelin basic protein or MBP) can lead to widespread inflammation in the CNS, with an immune response against many peptides found in both MBP and other CNS proteins.

The requirements for co-stimulation for T-cell activation vary with the differentiation of the T cell: T cells not previously exposed to antigen (naive T cells) require co-stimulation via CD28 in order to take part in an immune response. However, *previously activated T cells can be induced to proliferate and produce cytokines by a much wider variety of co-stimulatory signals*, triggered through adhesion molecules expressed in increased amounts upon these cells. This means that previously activated autoreactive memory T cells will not only recirculate more freely to inflamed tissues (because of their increased expression of adhesion molecules), but will also be much easier to activate once they arrive in the tissue containing the appropriate self-peptide/MHC complex. *This implies that once the barrier of tolerance is broken down, autoimmune responses may be relatively easy to sustain.*

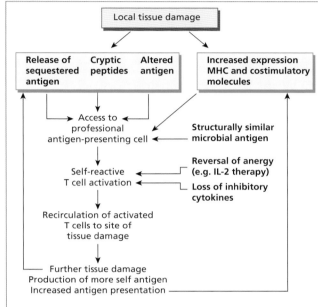

Fig. 5.5 A conceptual demonstration of how breakdown of tolerance leads to autoimmune disease and spreading of responses to epitopes. IL, interleukin; MHC, major histocompatibility complex.

Case 5.4 Lymphocyte-depleting monoclonal antibody treatment for multiple sclerosis (MS) results in Graves' disease

A 38-year-old woman with progressive MS underwent treatment with the monoclonal antibody Campath-1H (alemtuzumab) as part of a clinical trial. The treatment did not seem to slow the progress of her neurological disease, although she developed no new lesions on magnetic resonance imaging scanning of her brain over a three-year period. About two years after treatment with Campath-1H she developed a fine tremor, 5 kg weight loss and heat intolerance. Examination revealed a tachycardia and mild exophthalmos. The clinical impression of thyrotoxicosis was confirmed by a low level of thyroid-stimulating hormone (TSH) at <0.03 mU/L (normal range 0.4–4 mU/L) and raised free T4 elevated at 76 pmol/L (normal range 5–20). Antibodies binding to the TSH receptor were found in the patient's blood; a diagnosis of Graves' disease (autoimmune hyperthyroidism) was made.

Campath-1H targets the CD52 antigen, which is expressed on both T and B cells. Treatment with Campath-1H produces prolonged suppression of peripheral blood lymphocyte numbers. Clinical trials suggest that this form of treatment may slow clinical and radiological progression of MS. However, around 30% of patients treated for MS with Campath-1H subsequently develop Graves' disease or more rarely an autoimmune cytopenia. The precise mechanisms are unclear, though high levels of interleukin (IL)-21 were associated with the development of these autoimmune diseases. Alternatively, Campath-1H depletes all circulating lymphocytes, including regulatory T cells (Tregs), which would otherwise prevent the development of antithyroid autoimmunity.

So we can see how a state of local inflammation, particularly in the presence of a pathogen that has some structural similarity to a self-antigen present at the site of inflammation (see Molecular mimicry in section 5.6.2), could potentially induce a self-sustaining autoreactive process (see Fig. 5.5). What is equally clear, however, is that while **transient autoimmune responses occur commonly after infection** or other forms of tissue damage, the development of sustained immunity is relatively rare. Our knowledge of the factors curtailing autoimmune responses is poor, but is important for understanding both pathogenesis and treatment of autoimmune disease. *It seems likely that genetic and acquired defects in normal immune control mechanisms can combine to allow failure to switch off an autoimmune process.*

5.6 What triggers autoimmunity?

As with most complex chronic illnesses, interactions between genetic and environmental factors are critically important in the causation of autoimmune disease, although it is simpler to deal with these factors separately.

5.6.1 Genetic factors

The use of twin and family studies has confirmed genetic contributions in all autoimmune diseases studied (Table 5.5). *Multiple autoimmune diseases may cluster within the same family* (see Case 5.3) and subclinical autoimmunity is more common among family members than overt disease. *The genetic contribution to most autoimmune diseases, particularly those presenting after the first year of life, almost always involves multiple genes (polygenicity).*

There are, however, a few single-gene defects in both humans and laboratory animals that lead to autoimmunity (see Table 5.4). Rare conditions of endocrine autoimmunity

affecting multiple organs are inherited in an autosomal dominant fashion (see Chapter 15, Figure 15.8). In some of these families this is caused by mutations in a gene on chromosome 21 known as **AIRE** (AutoImmune REgulator). Affected subjects in families expressing disease-causing mutations in the AIRE gene also have chronic mucocutaneous candidiasis and skin/tooth changes; this syndrome is known as **APECED** (Autoimmune PolyEndocrinopathy Candidiasis Ectodermal Dysplasia – see Case 5.3). The AIRE gene is expressed in the thymus, where it is believed to control the normal transcription of genes for non-thymic self-proteins' central tolerance, and hence these mutations result in the failure of central tolerance to these self-proteins. There are other single-gene defects, such as IPEX (Immune dysregulation, Polyendocrinopathy, Enteropathy, X-linked), where disease-causing mutations in the FOXP3 gene results in absence of Tregs, allowing multiple organ-specific autoimmunity. Also multiple autoimmune diseases are classical features in patients with defects in proteins involved in apoptosis, such as in the FAS:FASL pathways (see Table 5.4).

These single-gene human disorders give useful insights into ways in which **multiple genetic differences (polymorphisms) in several genes**, each in themselves incapable of producing autoimmunity on their own, and environmental factors could interact to allow polygenic autoimmune disease to develop. **Genome-wide association studies (GWAS)** have provided insights into the roles of a whole range of genes, with more than 200 loci associated with one or more diseases. A hierarchy of genes is involved in the development of autoimmunity: MHC genes are the most important, but many other genes also participate, their functions ranging from control of the immune response to factors affecting the functioning of the relevant target organ. Now our understanding of the relationship between MHC variants and autoimmunity (Table 5.6) is developing rapidly with exome and genome sequencing, which enable exploration of the functional roles

Table 5.5 The genetic contribution to autoimmune disease as shown by increased risk in family members

	Frequency of the disease in the population (prevalence) (%)	Frequency of the disease in individuals with an affected sibling (%)	Increase in risk with an affected sibling	Frequency of the disease in individuals with an affected identical twin (%)	Increase in risk with an affected identical twin compared with a non-twin sibling*
Rheumatoid arthritis	1	8	×8	30	×3.5
Insulin-dependent diabetes mellitus	0.4	6	×15	34	×5.7
Ankylosing spondylitis	0.13	7	×54	50	×7.1
Multiple sclerosis	0.1	2	×20	26	×13
Systemic lupus erythematosus	0.1	2	×20	24	×12

* Even though the risks of disease are massively increased in identical twins, the diseases still affect only a minority of those with an affected twin, emphasizing that environmental factors have some role to play.

Table 5.6 Possible mechanistic associations between some common autoimmune diseases and certain human leukocyte antigen (HLA) alleles

Disease	HLA association	Molecular specificity	Relationship to pathogenesis
Rheumatoid arthritis	DR4 + DR1	Sequence of five amino acids lying in the peptide-binding groove of HLA-DR	Analysis of the 'shared epitope' in rheumatoid arthritis patients reveals the ability of this HLA to bind 'arthritogenic peptides' – frequently citrullinated proteins. This modification of proteins may partly explain the relationship to environmental factors such as smoking
Insulin-dependent diabetes mellitus	DR3 + DR4	Single amino acid at position 57 in the β chain of HLA-DQ	As above
Organ-specific autoimmune disease: type 1 diabetes, Addison's disease, pernicious anaemia	DR1 *03 (in association with A1 B8 DR3 DQ2 haplotype)	Unknown, but this haplotype is associated with promoter polymorphism in tumour necrosis factor (TNF)-α gene	Unclear but this haplotype is associated with high levels of TNF and vigorous antibody responses

of particular genetic alleles in these polygenic diseases. Genes such as PTPN22, CTLA-4, IL-23R and STAT-4 are shared among multiple autoimmune diseases, raising the possibility that a combination of risk loci may influence an individual's susceptibility to disease. Their relevance, in terms of disease complications and even responses to therapy, will provide exciting studies for the next several years if not decades. For example, patients with CTLA-4 mutations who develop an immune dysregulation syndrome characterized by multiple autoimmune diseases, extensive T-cell organ infiltration and B-cell immunodeficiency are treated with abatacept, a CTLA-4 fusion protein (Chapter 7, Fig. 7.7).

5.6.2 Environmental factors

Environmental factors identified as possible triggers in autoimmunity include hormones, infection, therapeutic drugs and miscellaneous other agents such as ultra-violet radiation.

Hormones

One of the most striking epidemiological observations regarding autoimmune diseases is that **females are far more likely to be affected than males** (see section 5.3). While this may be due to protection from the genes on the Y chromosome, hormones themselves appear to play a major role in the increased prevalence in females; since these can be externally manipulated, they are perhaps best considered with other environmental factors. Most autoimmune diseases have their peak age of onset within the reproductive years, implicating oestrogens as triggering factors. Removal of the ovaries inhibits the onset of spontaneous autoimmunity in animal models, particularly in models of systemic lupus erythematosus (SLE), and administration of oestrogen accelerates the onset of disease. The mechanism is unclear. The pituitary hormone prolactin also has immunostimulatory actions, particularly on T cells; prolactin levels surge immediately after pregnancy and this may be linked with the tendency of some autoimmune diseases, particularly RA, to present at this time.

Infection

The relationship between infection and autoimmunity is clearest in molecular mimicry, as discussed later (Table 5.7), but other possible links exist. Infection of a target organ plays a key role in local **upregulation of co-stimulatory molecules** and also in inducing altered patterns of antigen breakdown and presentation, thus leading to autoimmunity even without molecular mimicry. Attempts have been made repeatedly in some 'autoimmune' diseases, particularly RA and MS, to identify triggering infections, but so far without success.

Infection may also exert a completely different influence upon autoimmune disease. As noted in section 5.3, autoimmune diseases tend to be less common in parts of the world that carry a high burden of parasitic diseases and other infections. Intriguingly, in some animal models of autoimmunity (e.g. the NOD mouse), the development of disease can be dramatically inhibited by keeping the animals in a laboratory environment with a high prevalence of infection. Keeping the same animals in germ-free conditions promotes the development of autoimmunity. The mechanisms behind non-specific protection from autoimmunity by infection (and possibly other environmental factors) are unclear.

Molecular mimicry

Structural similarity between self-proteins and those from microorganisms may also trigger an autoimmune response. A self-peptide in low concentration and with no access to

Table 5.7 Molecular mimicry: microbial antigens and self-antigens potentially involved in this process

Microbial antigen	Self-antigen with similar structure	Disease in which consequent molecular mimicry may play a role*
Group A streptococcal M protein	Antigen found in cardiac muscle	Rheumatic fever
Bacterial heat shock proteins	Self-heat shock proteins	Links suggested with several autoimmune diseases, but not proven as yet
Coxsackie B4 nuclear protein	Pancreatic islet cell glutamate decarboxylase (GAD)	Insulin-dependent diabetes mellitus and Stiff Man syndrome
Campylobacter jejuni glycoproteins	Myelin-associated gangliosides and glycolipids	Guillain–Barré syndrome

*In general, it has been much easier to demonstrate structural similarity between microbial and self-antigens than to prove that this similarity plays any role in disease pathogenesis.

 Case 5.5 Guillain–Barré syndrome

A 23-year-old man developed flu-like symptoms, severe diarrhoea and abdominal pain four days after attending a dinner party at which he had eaten a chicken casserole. Three other guests at the same party developed gastrointestinal symptoms. These symptoms settled within a few days. Stool cultures taken from all four individuals grew Campylobacter jejuni. 10 days later, the man developed diffuse aching around his shoulders and buttocks and pins and needles in his hands and feet. Over the next week the sensory changes worsened and spread to involve his arms and legs. His limbs became progressively weaker and eight days after the onset of neurological symptoms, he could not hold a cup or stand unaided.

He was admitted to hospital and found to have severe symmetrical distal limb weakness and 'glove and stocking' sensory loss to the elbows and knees. Nerve conduction studies showed evidence of a mixed motor and sensory neuropathy and examination of his cerebrospinal fluid (CSF) showed a very high total protein level at 4 g/L, but no increase in the number of cells in the CSF. High titres of immunoglobulin (Ig)M and IgG antibodies to Campylobacter jejuni were found in his peripheral blood. A diagnosis was made of the Guillain–Barré syndrome (acute inflammatory polyneuropathy), probably triggered by Campylobacter jejuni infection.

He was treated with high-dose intravenous immunoglobulin, but his condition deteriorated with respiratory muscle weakness and he required mechanical ventilation. His condition slowly improved and he was able to breathe spontaneously after two weeks. His strength and sensory symptoms slowly improved with vigorous physiotherapy, but one year after the initial illness he still had significant weakness in his hands and feet.

appropriate antigen-presenting cells may cross-react with a structurally similar microbial peptide. In systemic infection, this cross-reactivity will cause expansion of the responsive T-cell population. These T cells may then recognize the self-peptide if local conditions (such as tissue damage) allow presentation of that peptide in the presence of ectopic MHC class II expression and access of the specific T cell to the tissue. This process is known as **molecular mimicry** (Case 5.5 and Table 5.7).

Drugs

Many drugs are associated with idiosyncratic side effects that may have an autoimmune pathogenesis. It is important to distinguish between an immunological response to the drug, either in its native form, a metabolite or complexed with a host molecule, and a true autoimmune process induced by the drug. The former mechanism of **drug hypersensitivity** is usually reversible on drug withdrawal, whereas the second process

may progress initially independently of drug withdrawal and require some form of immunosuppressive treatment (Table 5.8); sometimes patients do eventually respond (Case 5.6).

The **autoimmune mechanisms** underlying drug-induced autoimmunity may involve mechanisms comparable to molecular mimicry, or depend on the drug's ability to bind directly to the peptide-containing groove in MHC molecules, and hence induce abnormal T-cell responses (such as with penicillamine) directly.

Drug-mediated autoimmunity (and drug hypersensitivity in general) affects only a small proportion of those treated. This differential susceptibility is probably largely genetically determined. Genetic variation within the MHC potentially influences recognition of drug–self-complexes by T cells. For example, human leukocyte antigen (HLA)-DR2 is associated with penicillamine-induced myasthenia gravis, whereas DR3 is associated with penicillamine-induced nephritis. Genetic variation in drug metabolism is also important, the best-characterized example being the relationship

Table 5.8 Syndromes of probable autoimmune aetiology triggered by therapeutic drugs

Syndrome	Drug
Chronic active hepatitis	Halothane (*general anaesthetic*)
Haemolytic anaemia	Methyl-dopa (an original *antihypertensive*)
Antiglomerular basement membrane	D-penicillamine (*rheumatoid arthritis*)
Myasthenia gravis	D-penicillamine
Pemphigus	D-penicillamine
Systemic lupus erythematosus	Hydralazine (*antihypertensive*)
	Procainamide (*antiarrhythmic*)
	D-penicillamine
Glomerulonephritis	D-penicillamine
Scleroderma-like syndrome	Tryptophan (*antidepressant*)

NB: Many of these drugs such as D-penicillamine and hydralazine are now only rarely used therapeutically, in part due to the risk of this type of reaction.

between drug-induced SLE and the rate of acetylation of the triggering drug: slow acetylators are prone to SLE. It seems likely that this partial defect in metabolism may allow the formation of immunogenic conjugates between drug and self-molecules.

Drugs may also have unexpected **intrinsic adjuvant or immunomodulatory** effects that disturb normal tolerance mechanisms, for example thyroid autoimmunity may follow interferon-α treatment. More importantly in recent years, with the use of biologics directed towards immune system manipulation, the range of diseases and the patterns of autoantibody profiles have increased. TNF antagonists are associated with features of arthralgia (90%), myalgia (50%) and systemic symptoms of malaise, fever or anorexia are increasingly common, as are serositis, hepatitis or lymphadenopathy, and even relapses of MS. National databases and post-marketing surveillance are essential to capture these side effects.

Autoimmune disease triggered by immune check-point inhibitors

Therapeutic monoclonal antibodies targeted at key T-cell inhibitory molecules such as CTLA-4, PD-1 and PD-L1 are known as immune check-point inhibitors (ICI). They have proven to be transformative in the treatment of many cancers. While removing these physiological brakes on T-cell function has been key to the success of these agents in the treatment of cancer, it has also simultaneously led to the development of a range of autoimmune diseases in these patients (Table 5.9 and Fig. 5.4). Similarly, the use of ICI in organ transplant recipients runs the risk of triggering graft rejection. Because of the risk of autoimmunity, cancer patients with preexisting autoimmune diseases have generally been excluded from clinical trials of ICI, though increasing post-licensing experience has enabled some patients to be treated while being closely monitored.

Other physical agents

Exposure to ultra-violet radiation (usually in the form of sunlight) is a well-defined trigger for skin inflammation and even systemic involvement in SLE in those with preexisting disease. Ultra-violet radiation causes worsening of SLE by a number of mechanisms. It can cause free radical–mediated structural

---

👤 Case 5.6 Minocycline-induced systemic lupus erythematosus (SLE)

A previously healthy 23-year-old woman was referred to a rheumatology clinic with a four-month history of pain and swelling in the small joints of her hands, associated with a blotchy rash over the bridge of her nose and over her knuckles. Examination revealed mild symmetrical synovitis in the hands and red scaly patches over her knuckles and face consistent with a photosensitive rash. Her blood pressure was normal and dipstick testing of her urine showed no blood or protein. Investigations showed a normal full blood count, urea and creatinine. Her erythrocyte sedimentation rate was significantly elevated at 43 mm/h. Antinuclear antibodies were present at a titre of 1/1000 with a homogeneous pattern. Antibodies to double-stranded DNA and extractable nuclear antigens were absent. A diagnosis of mild SLE was made and she was treated with non-steroidal antiinflammatory drugs and hydroxychloroquine. She was also given advice on protection from ultra-violet light.

Her symptoms failed to improve over the next six months and treatment with low-dose corticosteroids was considered. However, she refused to consider steroid treatment, as she had read about side effects and was concerned that this drug would cause her previously troublesome acne to return. At this point it transpired that she had been receiving treatment with daily low doses of the antibiotic minocycline for the last four years because of previously severe acne. She had not mentioned this previously as she had been taking this form of treatment for so long that she did not feel it could be relevant to her more recent problems. The minocycline was discontinued and the clinical and laboratory features of SLE disappeared over the next six months, confirming the revised diagnosis of minocycline-induced SLE. Her acne remained in remission without treatment.

Table 5.9 Selected examples of immune checkpoint inhibitors and autoimmune disease

Monoclonal antibody	Immunological target	Indications	Autoimmune complications – common to all checkpoint inhibitors
Ipilimumab	CTLA-4	Melanoma, renal cell carcinoma	Colitis, hepatitis, pneumonitis, toxic epidermal necrolysis, hypothyroidism, hyperthyroidism, hypophysitis, adrenal insufficiency, myocarditis, insulin-dependent diabetes, myasthenia gravis, encephalitis, Guillain–Barré syndrome
Nivolumab	PD-1	Melanoma, NSCLC, Hodgkin's lymphoma, urothelial carcinoma	
Pembrolizumab	PD-1	Melanoma, NSCLC, Hodgkin's lymphoma, renal cell carcinoma	
Atezolizumab	PD-L1	Urothelial carcinoma, NSCLC, SCLC	

NSCLC, SCLC

modification to self-antigens, thus enhancing their immunogenicity. More subtly, it can also lead to apoptotic death of cells within the skin. This process is associated with cell-surface expression of lupus autoantigens that are associated with photosensitivity (known as Ro and La), usually only found within cells. Surface Ro and La are then able to bind appropriate autoantibodies and trigger tissue damage.

Other forms of physical damage may alter the immunogenicity of self-antigens, particularly damage to self-molecules by oxygen free radicals produced as part of inflammation.

5.7 Mechanisms of tissue damage

Tissue damage in autoimmune disease is mediated by antibody (types II and III hypersensitivity) or by CD4+ T-cell activation of macrophages or CD8+ T cells (type IV hypersensitivity) (Tables 5.3 and 5.10; see also Chapter 1). Most autoimmune diseases involve a predominance of one or another form of hypersensitivity, but there is often considerable overlap between antibody and T-cell-mediated damage.

Apart from organ damage mediated by mechanisms of hypersensitivity, autoantibodies may cause disease by **binding to functional sites** such as hormone receptors, neurotransmitter receptors or plasma proteins. These autoantibodies may either mimic or block the action of the endogenous ligand for the self-protein, and thus cause *abnormalities in function without necessarily causing inflammation or tissue damage*. This phenomenon is best characterized in thyroid autoimmunity, where autoantibodies can mimic or block the action of thyroid-stimulating hormone and hence induce over- or underactivity of the thyroid (see Table 5.10).

Antibody-mediated damage in autoimmunity is usually considered to occur only when the autoantibody recognizes an antigen that is either free in the extracellular fluid or expressed upon the cell surface. However, there is some *in vitro* evidence that some autoantibodies against intracellular antigens can enter living cells and perturb their function. The importance of this phenomenon to autoimmune disease is unclear.

Many of the late and irreversible consequences of autoimmune disease are caused by deposition of extracellular matrix

Table 5.10 Mechanisms of hypersensitivity that predominate in autoimmune diseases*

Type II hypersensitivity†

Type IIA

  Idiopathic thrombocytopenic purpura

  Autoimmune haemolytic anaemia

  Myasthenia gravis

  Antiglomerular basement membrane disease

Type IIB

  Graves' disease

  Insulin receptor antibody syndrome

  Myasthenia gravis

Type III hypersensitivity

  Systemic lupus erythematosus

  Mixed cryoglobulinaemia

  Some forms of vasculitis (e.g. rheumatoid vasculitis)

Type IV hypersensitivity

  Insulin-dependent diabetes mellitus

  Hashimoto's thyroiditis

  Rheumatoid arthritis

  Multiple sclerosis

* Different aspects of the same disease (e.g. rheumatoid disease) can have different pathogenic mechanisms.
† Type II sensitivity has been subdivided as to whether antibody induces cell damage (IIa) or receptor stimulation or blockade (IIb). In some diseases both mechanisms occur.

proteins (such as fibrin) in the affected organ. This process of fibrosis leads to impairment of function in, for example, the lungs (pulmonary fibrosis), liver (cirrhosis), skin (systemic sclerosis) and kidney (interstitial and glomerular fibrosis). *No effective treatments exist for the treatment of established fibrosis.* Historically, an assumption has been made that fibrosis is the consequence of previous chronic inflammation and that treatment with antiinflammatory and immunosuppressive drugs will ameliorate the fibrotic process. However, there is now evidence that **some tissue injury can lead to fibrosis** without any significant intervening inflammation. This might explain the lack of obvious inflammation preceding systemic sclerosis and idiopathic pulmonary fibrosis.

5.8 Treatment of autoimmune disease

Despite recent advances in therapeutic immunomodulation, the treatment of many autoimmune diseases is currently unsatisfactory. The two principal strategies are either to suppress the immune response or to replace the function of the damaged organ.

Replacement of function is the usual treatment in endocrinological autoimmune diseases, which present with irreversible failure of the affected organ (such as insulin-dependent diabetes or thyroid failure). Replacement hormones provide satisfactory treatment for endocrine failure, such as hypothyroidism. However, when the need for a hormone varies considerably over time (such as insulin), failure of replacement therapy to match physiological changes in hormone output can lead to major metabolic problems.

In many autoimmune diseases, such as SLE, RA and autoimmune kidney disease, immunosuppression or immunomodulation is the only means of preventing severe disability or death, short of organ transplantation. As discussed in Chapter 7, however, all currently used modes of immunosuppression are complicated by their lack of specificity and the risk of infection. In contrast, targeted treatment with biologics and small molecule inhibitors offers a greater degree of disease control associated with a narrower spectrum of infectious complications.

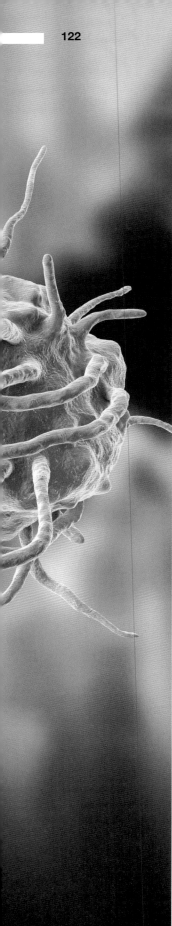

CHAPTER 6
Lymphoproliferative Disorders

Key topics

Visit the companion website at **www.wiley.com/go/misbah/immunology** to download cases with additional figures on these topics.

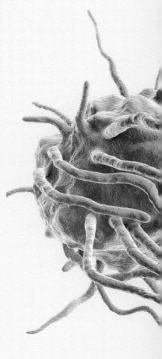

Chapel and Haeney's Essentials of Clinical Immunology, Seventh Edition. Edited by Siraj A. Misbah, Gavin P. Spickett, and Virgil A.S.H. Dalm.
© 2022 John Wiley & Sons Ltd. Published 2022 by John Wiley & Sons Ltd.

6.1 Introduction

The cells involved in immune responses undergo 'reactive' *polyclonal* proliferation as a normal response to infection or inflammation. However, *monoclonal* expansion can give rise to leukaemias, lymphomas or myeloma.

Leukaemia is the malignant proliferation of haematopoietic stem/progenitor cells and may involve cells of lymphoid, myeloid or monocytic lineages. The **clone** of malignant cells originates in the bone marrow. Leukaemic 'blasts' or other less obvious but still malignant cells may then be seen circulating in peripheral blood and may infiltrate other organs such as lymph nodes and the central nervous system.

Tumours of lymphoid cells originating in peripheral lymph tissue constitute the lymphomas. Dissemination of these malignant cells may result in infiltration of other organs, including spleen, liver, brain, bone marrow or lungs. The classification of lymphomas is complex. It is important to distinguish different types of lymphoma in order (i) to provide a reliable diagnosis and prognosis for a given patient, and hence (ii) to choose the most effective form of therapy.

Each leukaemia or lymphoma is thought to arise from a single cell, perhaps a stem cell, which undergoes a **malignant transformation** that enables uncontrolled division of this cell into a 'clone' of identical cells. Mutations in many genes that are involved in normal differentiation from stem cell to mature blood cell have been shown to be present in leukaemias and lymphomas. Many classifications have evolved to take into account such molecular abnormalities, although the leukaemia cell morphology, molecular genetics lineage-specific markers that are identified by flow cytometry, remains the keystone of diagnosis.

The immunological techniques that can be used to identify the phenotype of the malignant clone and to classify these lymphoid malignancies are shown in Table 6.1. These techniques are discussed fully in Chapter 19. Molecular genetics to determine translocations and chromosomal abnormalities and mutation analysis are now used routinely to guide treatment and for prognosis.

Table 6.1 Techniques used to identify lymphoid malignancies*

1 Morphology – how the cell and its nucleus look by light microscopy
2 Special cytochemical stains – to identify characteristic surface markers, enzymes, carbohydrates or lipids
3 Immunophenotyping – use of monoclonal antibodies (MAbs) to identify cell lineage (myeloid/B or T lymphocytic) and stage of differentiation by surface and intracellular antigens using flow cytometry
4 Cytogenetic analysis – to identify characteristic abnormal translocations and deletions on chromosomes by visualization, banding and molecular genetics
5 Gene rearrangement studies – can be used to identify or confirm monoclonality, in T-cell malignancies

*Not all these techniques are needed for every diagnosis of lymphoid malignancy.

6.2 Biology of malignant transformation in haematopoietic cells

In most types of leukaemia and lymphoma, as for solid tumours, the precise stimulus for initiation of the malignant clone is not known. The majority of tumours in humans arise spontaneously. Inherited genetic mutations have been identified for a minority of cancers, for example BRCA genes in breast cancer. However, most cancers involve acquired **gene mutations** (Fig. 6.1). Such mutations commonly arise in genes responsible for cell proliferation, apoptosis (programmed cell death) or DNA repair. Viruses known to be involved in the pathogenesis of lymphoid tumours include the Epstein–Barr virus (EBV) in Burkitt's lymphoma and the retrovirus human T-cell leukaemia virus I (HTLV-I) in adult T-cell leukaemia/lymphoma. It is believed that in neither case does infection alone cause the tumour, since only 1% or less of infected individuals in endemic areas develop the malignancy. Additional instigating factors are needed, which may include other genetic abnormalities, such as DNA repair gene defects as in ataxia telangiectasia, or environmental factors, such as radiation or infection with other microorganisms.

Protooncogenes (see Box 6.1) are genes that encode proteins involved in cell growth, differentiation and division. Mutation of these genes to oncogenes can lead to malignancy. Such mutations can result in constitutively (permanently) active proteins, proteins with abnormal function or increased protein concentrations resulting in heightened activity. An example of a translocation resulting in a new cell proliferation enzyme is given in Fig. 6.1. **Tumour suppressor genes** regulate cell proliferation, DNA repair and apoptosis. Failure of these genes is involved in tumours in general.

6.3 Leukaemia

Leukaemias may be lymphoid, myeloid, monocytic or megakaryocytic in origin (Fig. 6.2). The cells may retain some of their original characteristics; however, some are poorly differentiated and the precise lineage can be difficult to identify by morphology alone. This chapter focuses on lymphoblastic leukaemias – both acute lymphoblastic leukaemia (ALL) and chronic lymphocytic leukaemia (CLL); readers are referred to the *Essentials of Haematology* edition for details on other leukaemias.

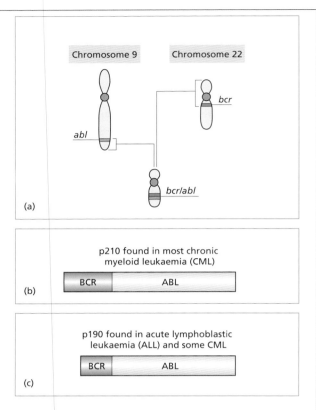

(a)

p210 found in most chronic
myeloid leukaemia (CML)

| BCR | ABL |

(b)

p190 found in acute lymphoblastic
leukaemia (ALL) and some CML

| BCR | ABL |

(c)

Fig. 6.1 A malignant translocation: Abl is an oncogene on chromosome 9; Bcr is a similar oncogene on chromosome 22. When these two are joined by translocation between the two chromosomes, activation of the fused gene produces a new tyrosine kinase, which enables uncontrolled proliferation of the cells. This translocation is visualized as the Philadelphia chromosome in almost all patients with chronic myeloid leukaemia and some with acute lymphoblastic leukaemia. Source: Axford J & O'Callaghan C (eds) *Medicine*, 2e (2004). Reproduced with permission of John Wiley & Sons Ltd.

6.3.1 Acute lymphoblastic leukaemia

ALL is largely a disease of children and young people; it is less common over the age of 20 years (Fig. 6.3). It is five times more common than acute myeloid leukaemia (AML). Patients with ALL often **present** with complications of bone marrow failure, including bleeding, infection and anaemia (as in Case 6.1). Other signs/symptoms include sweats and meningeal irritation. Patients may have palpable lymphadenopathy and a small proportion (10%) have a mediastinal mass apparent on chest X-ray. Over 80% of patients are thrombocytopenic and in some this is severe and results in petechiae. Many (60%) have low haemoglobin levels below 80 g/L. The white cell count is usually low (leucopenia), but a minority of patients present with an apparently high white cell count due to circulating blasts and this indicates a poorer prognosis.

The **diagnosis** of leukaemia is confirmed by performing a bone marrow aspirate and trephine biopsy and finding that >20% of cells are leukaemic blast cells (see Case 6.1). The blasts in the marrow and peripheral blood are

---

Box 6.1 When integration of DNA can result in malignancy

- Activation of a positive regulator gene if the DNA is inserted next to a promoter gene, e.g. 'insertional mutagenesis'
- Inactivation of a negative gene if the DNA is inserted next to an apoptosis or apoptosis promoter gene, e.g. 'insertional mutagenesis of apoptosis'
- Activation of a growth factor production gene if the DNA is inserted next to a growth factor gene, resulting in unregulated cell division
- Inactivation of a DNA repair gene if the DNA is inserted next to a DNA repair gene or promoter gene
- Inactivation of a differentiation gene if the DNA is inserted next to a differentiation gene or promoter gene
- Recombination between host cell genes and viral DNA can result in host genes becoming replicating and therefore oncogenic
- Silent 'protooncogenes' (c-onc genes), incorporated into mammalian cells eons ago, are inherited in a Mendelian fashion, and normally used for growth factor receptors or signal transducers – these can be activated by mutagenesis
- Loss of function if tumour suppression gene inactivated

---

immunophenotyped using flow cytometry (Table 6.2) and immunohistology.

ALL may be of B- or T-cell origin. In B-ALL, the malignant cells have the B-cell **surface markers**, CD10+, CD19+, CD24+ and cytoplasmic CD79+, as well as terminal deoxynucleotidyl transferase (TdT). There is variable expression of lymphoid lineage CD45, and confusingly some cells may have aberrant expression of myeloid lineage surface markers such as CD13 and CD33.

The malignant cells in T-ALL express T-cell markers such as CD2, CD3, CD4, CD5, CD7 and CD8, reflecting transformation of intrathymic T-cell development (Fig. 6.4).

In addition to flow cytometry and histology, cytogenetic studies are performed to identify genetic mutations that correlate with prognosis. For example, in B-ALL, poor prognostic indicators include presence of the BCR-ABL fusion protein caused by the t (9;22) translocation and rearrangements of the MLL gene. The TEL-AML1 or t (12;21) translocation is associated with a good prognosis. Chromosomal translocations involving T-cell receptors are seen in about a third of T-ALL cases; these include NOTCH1, FBW7, MYB, LMO1/2 and CALM-AF10, as well as TCR γ/δ. Better prognosis in T-ALL patients occurs with some HOX rearrangements and some TAL1/SCL mutations.

Other factors used as **prognostic** criteria in ALL include the white cell count and age at presentation. Children under 1 year old or over 10 years and those with a high blast cell count at presentation (>50 × 10⁹/L) are considered high risk.

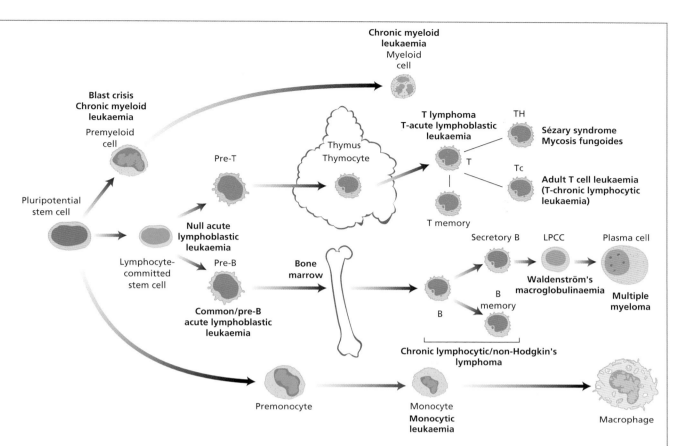

Fig. 6.2 Malignant counterparts at each step in the leucocyte differentiation pathway. B, B cell; LPCC, lymphoplasma cytoid cell; T, T cell; Tc, T cytotoxic cell; TH, T helper cell.

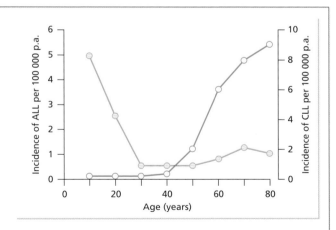

Fig. 6.3 Decade of onset in acute lymphoblastic leukaemia (ALL; yellow line) and chronic lymphocytic leukaemia (CLL; green line).

Complications of ALL include anaemia and thrombocytopenia, resulting in bleeding due to marrow infiltration (Table 6.3). Concentrated red cells are given to correct anaemia, and platelet concentrates to prevent and treat bleeding. Infection is a common complication of ALL and preventive measures, such as barrier nursing and prophylactic antifungal and antiviral agents, are important.

ALL is a fatal condition if untreated, but aggressive chemotherapy may eliminate the clone of malignant cells and induce a cure (see Box 6.2). B-ALL has an excellent outcome in children. A complete remission is achieved with initial **high-dose 'induction' chemotherapy** in around 95% of children and 60–85% of adults. Further treatment is then required to 'consolidate' and 'maintain' the remission. The intensity of the consolidation therapy depends on prognostic factors at presentation and on the initial response to chemotherapy, in particular whether there is any residual disease following induction chemotherapy. For higher-risk patients, an allogeneic **human stem cell transplant (HSCT)** may be performed if a suitably matched donor is identified. A recent major advance in the treatment of end-stage B-ALL refractory to conventional chemotherapy is the use of autologous chimeric antigen receptor T-cell (CAR-T) therapy targeting B-cell antigens such as CD19 (tisagenlecleucel; see Chapter 7). This is licensed for the treatment of children and young adults with B-ALL and adults with refractory diffuse large B-cell lymphoma. Because of its mode of action, CD-19-directed CAR-T cell therapy causes unavoidable B-cell aplasia associated with hypogammaglobulinaemia. Immunoglobulin replacement therapy in the

Case 6.1 Acute leukaemia (common type)

A 7-year-old boy presented with malaise and lethargy of six days' duration. He had become inattentive at school, anorexic and had lost 3 kg in weight. On examination he was thin, anxious and clinically anaemic. There was mild, bilateral, cervical lymphadenopathy and moderate splenomegaly.

On investigation, he was pancytopenic with a low haemoglobin (80 g/L), platelet count (30 × 10⁹/L) and white cell count (1.2 × 10⁹/L). The blood film showed that most leucocytes were blasts; the red cells were normochromic and normocytic. Bone marrow examination showed an overgrowth of primitive white cells with diminished numbers of normal erythroid and myeloid precursors. Acute leukaemia was diagnosed.

The circulating blast cells were typed by immunological methods: they did not react with monoclonal antibodies to human T-cell precursor antigens (CD2, CD7), but they were positive for major histocompatibility complex class II (DR), common acute lymphoblastic leukaemia (CD10) and B-cell precursor (CD19) antigens, and contained the enzyme terminal deoxynucleotidyl transferase (TdT) (see Table 6.2). The phenotype of the blasts was that of acute leukaemia of early precursor B cells (see Fig. 6.2), and the prognosis in this child was relatively good. Cytogenetics confirmed ETV6-RUNX1 mutation or t(12;21) translocation, indicating a good prognosis.

Table 6.2 Panel of antibodies for the diagnosis of acute leukaemias

	B lymphoid	T lymphoid	Myeloid	Non-lineage-restricted
First line	CD19, CD10 (early B cells), CD79a (BCR), CD24	CD2, CD3, CD4, CD5, CD8	CD117 (stem cell growth factor receptor), CD13 Anti-myeloperoxidase	TdT
Second line	CD138	CD7	CD33, CD41, CD42, CD61	CD45

CD antigens are defined by monoclonal antibodies (see Chapters 1 and 19).

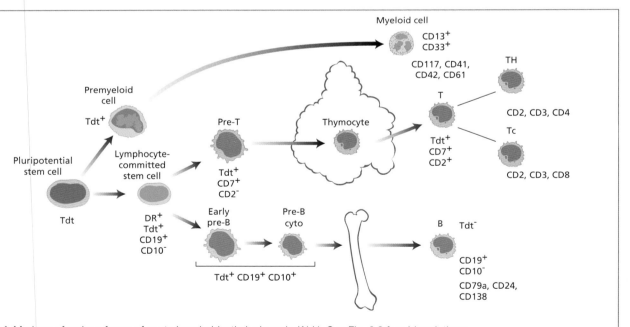

Fig. 6.4 Markers of various forms of acute lymphoblastic leukaemia (ALL). See Fig. 6.2 for abbreviations.

medium term is, therefore, required until B-cell reconstitution occurs.

There are **complications associated with therapy**, both with initial chemotherapy and HSCT (Table 6.3). Severe infection secondary to the profound neutropenia that results from intensive therapy is the major cause of mortality and morbidity in ALL. Barrier nursing and prompt and aggressive treatment of neutropenic fever according to standardized protocols can reduce

Table 6.3 Complications of acute lymphoblastic leukaemia associated with disease or its treatment with chemotherapy and human stem cell transplantation

Due to disease	Due to treatment
Anaemia – bone marrow suppression or hypersplenism Infection – neutropenia due to bone marrow suppression Bleeding – low platelets	Infection – poor neutrophil function and severe neutropenia as a result of chemotherapy Low platelets as result of chemotherapy Graft-versus-host disease secondary to allogeneic transplant
Leukaemic infiltrates, e.g. meninges, testis, skin	Poor growth Intellectual impairment (especially if cranial irradiation is performed in patients with central nervous system disease) Cardiac dysfunction

---

Box 6.2 Objectives of treatment in acute lymphoblastic leukaemia

1 Induction – to induce remission of the disease
2 Consolidation – to eradicate all leukaemic cells and their precursors
3 Maintenance – to prevent relapse. This involves further chemotherapy and in young, high-risk patients with suitably matched donors, an allogeneic bone marrow transplant may be performed
4 Central nervous system (CNS)-directed therapy – to prevent or treat infiltration of the meninges and brain. All patients receive intrathecal chemotherapy (methotrexate) and cranial irradiation is performed in those with CNS disease at presentation

---

the risk of death from sepsis in neutropenic patients, similar to the protocols used after HSCT for primary immunodeficiencies (see Chapter 3 for immunodeficiencies and Chapter 8 for transplantation).

Graft-versus-host disease (GvHD) may occur after allogeneic stem cell transplantation, although some graft-versus-leukaemia effect is helpful for the antileukaemic effect. **Long-term complications of survivors** such as organ damage, infertility and psychological issues must also be considered.

6.3.2 Chronic lymphocytic leukaemia

CLL is a relatively common disease of elderly patients (20 per 10^5 prevalence in those >60 years old). It is uncommon in people under 50 years of age (see Fig. 6.3) and usually runs a relatively benign course, although speed of progression varies enormously. Excessive numbers of small lymphocytes are found in the peripheral blood (Fig. 6.5); in over 90% of cases of CLL, the neoplastic cells are B cells (Fig. 6.6). They have the **characteristic cell-surface markers** of circulating B cells (Case 6.2 and Table 6.4). The cells represent a malignant proliferation of a *single clone of a B cell* and are therefore, as in acute leukaemias, 'monoclonal'. Normally 'reactive' lymphocytic proliferation is polyclonal and therefore the ratio of cells with κ or λ is 3 : 2. In contrast, in a monoclonal B-cell proliferation, this ratio is changed in favour of the malignant clone, as *all the malignant cells express the same light-chain type*. These cells accumulate progressively in the blood, lymph nodes, spleen, liver and bone marrow.

Although most elderly patients with CLL usually have a relatively benign illness and survive for over 8–10 years, the **prognosis is variable**. A combination of genomic, cytogenetic and cellular changes provides useful prognostic information. Chromosomal deletion at 17p and/or TP53 mutations predict poor responses to treatment. Chemotherapy is not necessary in the early stages, although some untreated CLL patients have severe recurrent bacterial infections due to low serum immunoglobulin levels and reduced antibodies (as in Case 6.2). In these cases, immunoglobulin replacement therapy should be considered. **Treatment** with cytotoxic chemotherapy is considered when a patient becomes symptomatic either because of splenomegaly or constitutional symptoms such as sweats and weight loss, or if **autoimmune complications** develop such as autoimmune thrombocytopenia or haemolytic anaemia. The most common chemotherapy regimen used in the UK combines fludarabine (an adenosine deaminase inhibitor), cyclophosphamide (an alkylating agent) and rituximab (a monoclonal antibody to the B-cell marker CD20). Newer therapies include ofatumumab, a humanized monoclonal antibody to another part of the CD20 antigen that appears to be expressed more on malignant B cells than normal B cells. Upregulation of Bruton tyrosine kinase (BTK) on malignant B cells has led to BTK inhibitors such as ibrutinib being successfully adopted as a licensed therapy in CLL.

6.3.3 Other chronic lymphoid leukaemias

Sézary syndrome is part of a spectrum of T-cell malignancies that often involve the skin. The skin is infiltrated with the large, cleaved, mononuclear cells diagnostic of the condition. Immunological markers on peripheral blood have shown these cells to be CD4+ T cells in origin (see Table 6.4). Many patients die within 10 years of diagnosis, often as a result of infections.

Other T-cell malignancies include **adult T-cell leukaemia/ lymphoma** (ATL), which occurs in geographical clusters, particularly in Japan and the Caribbean, where the associated retrovirus (HTLV-I) is endemic. ATL is an aggressive systemic disorder, often with skin and neurological involvement.

Hairy cell leukaemia is a malignancy of late-stage B cells. It is a rare condition of middle-aged males, which although

Case 6.2 Chronic lymphocytic leukaemia

A 62-year-old man presented with general lethargy, night sweats and loss of weight. He had suffered five chest infections during the previous winter, despite being a non-smoker. On examination, there was moderate, bilateral cervical lymphadenopathy and left inguinal lymph node enlargement. The spleen and liver were enlarged 5 cm below the costal margins. There was no bone tenderness and there were no lesions in the skin. On investigation, his haemoglobin was slightly low (10.2 g/L), the platelet count (251 × 10⁹/L) was normal, but his white cell count was increased to 150 × 10⁹/L; the film showed that 98% of these were small lymphocytes.

The features on the blood film were suggestive of chronic lymphocytic leukaemia and immunophenotyping confirmed this diagnosis. Of the cells 90% were B cells (CD 19⁺); they all expressed CD 19 and CD5, confirming the diagnosis (Table 6.4). The serum immunoglobulins were low: IgG 2.2 g/L (NR 7.2–19.0 g/L); IgA 0.6 g/L (NR 0.8–5.0 g/L) and IgM 0.4 g/L (NR 0.5–2.0 g/L). There was no monoclonal immunoglobulin in the serum or the urine.

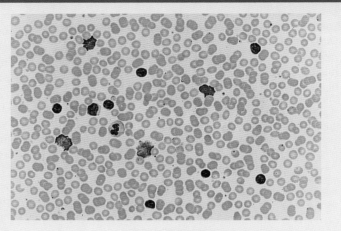

Fig. 6.5 Chronic lymphocytic leukaemia (CLL) blood film. Source: Axford J & O'Callaghan C (Eds) *Medicine*, 2nd Ed (2004). Reproduced with permission of John Wiley & Sons Ltd.

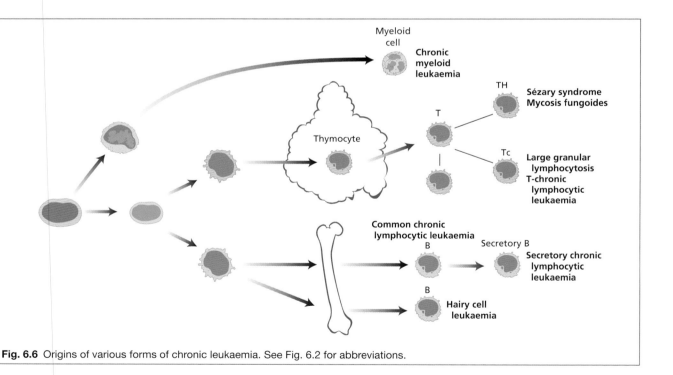

Fig. 6.6 Origins of various forms of chronic leukaemia. See Fig. 6.2 for abbreviations.

termed a 'leukaemia' is not necessarily associated with a high number of leukaemic cells circulating in the peripheral blood and is actually part of the World Health Organization (WHO) classification of lymphomas (see section 6.4.2). Pancytopenia, leading to an increased risk of infection, is common. Two-thirds of the patients have splenomegaly. The abnormal cells are often diagnosed as 'atypical lymphocytes' as they do have a peripheral fringe of spiky projections; close inspection and the use of enzymatic and immunological markers confirm the diagnosis (see Table 6.4). The identity of the 'hairy cell' as a late-stage B cell can be confirmed by flow cytometry using monoclonal antibodies to B-cell-restricted antigens, as well as

Table 6.4 Immunophenotyping in differential diagnosis of chronic lymphocytic leukaemias

Disease	Lymphocyte markers*			
	CD3	CD19	CD5	CD11c
Normal pattern	75	12	2	0
Chronic lymphocytic leukaemia	10	90	90	0
Sézary syndrome	92	2	0	0
Hairy cell leukaemia	10	60	0	60

*Results expressed as percentage of peripheral blood lymphocytes positive for marker.

the integrin CD11c. Interferon (IFN) and cladribine induce remission in a high proportion of patients, with 75% achieving complete remission for >5 years. Splenectomy may be considered in those with large splenomegaly causing discomfort or severe cytopenias. Visit the website at **www.wiley.com/go/misbah/immunology** to read case studies on Sézary syndrome and hairy cell leukaemia.

6.4 Lymphomas

'Lymphoma' is the malignant proliferation of lymphoid cells in **lymph node or spleen**. There are two broad classifications: Hodgkin's disease and non-Hodgkin's lymphoma (NHL). Although the clinical phenotypes and treatments differ, presenting symptoms may be similar. Patients may **present** with painless lymphadenopathy, or with so-called 'B' symptoms (unexplained fever, night sweats, weight loss), itching or increased/severe infections with opportunistic pathogens such as herpes simplex virus (severe cold sores) or varicella zoster virus (shingles, see Fig. 6.7).

The majority of cases of lymphoma occur with no identifiable precipitating factor. As with many other malignancies,

the pathogenesis of lymphomas is complex and involves the accumulation of multiple genetic mutations affecting protooncogenes and tumour suppressor genes. The exact molecular events that occur during malignant transformation are not completely understood. Activation of oncogenes by **translocation** during proliferation, such as that seen in **response to a viral infection**, provides a possible mechanism (Fig. 6.8). Genetic material of oncogenic viruses can be found in malignant cells of certain lymphoma subtypes, implicating viruses such as Epstein–Barr virus, human herpes virus 8, and human T-lymphotropic virus 1 more directly. Two clear examples are Helicobacter pylori–associated gastric malt lymphoma and the EBV-provoked lymphoma seen in transplanted patients receiving aggressive antirejection therapy (Chapter 7, Case 7.2), e.g. ciclosporin or anti-CD3 monoclonal antibodies. Reduction in immunosuppression is associated with tumour regression, indicating a role for T cells in controlling this type of proliferation.

Thus, there may be three phases in the development of the tumour (Fig. 6.8): an early reversible stage with polyclonal proliferation, a later reversible phase associated with oligoclonality and an irreversible late phase, probably associated with translocation of genetic material, when progression is inevitable.

In addition to infective agents, autoimmune disorders and immunosuppressive treatments have been associated with an increased risk of developing lymphomas. For example, there is a 13–15-fold increased risk of either Hodgkin's disease or NHL after alkylating agents used to treat rheumatoid arthritis. However, those treated with gold or penicillamine in the past also had increased rates of either type of lymphoma (particularly Hodgkin's disease), so the risk is partially associated with the underlying dysregulation of immunity, as in primary immunodeficiencies.

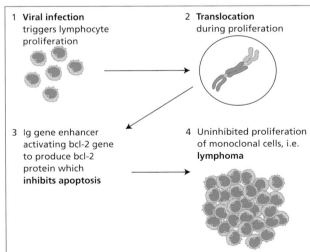

1 **Viral infection**
triggers lymphocyte proliferation

2 **Translocation**
during proliferation

3 Ig gene enhancer activating bcl-2 gene to produce bcl-2 protein which **inhibits apoptosis**

4 Uninhibited proliferation of monoclonal cells, i.e. **lymphoma**

Fig. 6.8 Immunopathogenesis in lymphoma. Source: Axford J & O'Callaghan C (Eds) *Medicine*, 2nd Ed (2004). Reproduced with permission of John Wiley & Sons Ltd.

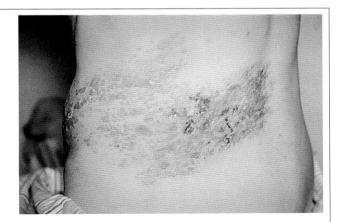

Fig. 6.7 Zoster infection. Source: Axford J & O'Callaghan C (Eds) *Medicine*, 2nd Ed (2004). Reproduced with permission of John Wiley & Sons Ltd.

6.4.1 Hodgkin's disease

Hodgkin's lymphoma is typically a disease affecting young people, often under 30 years of age. Painless lymphadenopathy, especially in the neck or mediastinal region, is a common **initial feature**, as in Case 6.3. While Hodgkin's disease primarily involves the lymph nodes, spleen and liver, involvement of lung, bone and central nervous system may be seen.

Hodgkin's lymphoma is recognized by the classical **histological appearance of** binucleate Reed–Sternberg cells, although mononuclear variants of Hodgkin cells may occur too (Case 6.3). These cells have the markers CD15, CD30 on their surface, with CD30 being exploited as a therapeutic target. How or why they gain their particular morphology remains unknown.

Staging is important for prognosis and therapy; the Ann Arbor stage (Cotswolds modification) of the disease is determined by **positron emission tomography (PET)/computed tomography (CT) scanning** (Table 6.5) and the presence or absence of 'B' symptoms.

Treatment usually consists of cycles of combination chemotherapy, usually with radiotherapy for those with localized disease. The regimen most often employed in the UK is referred to as 'ABVD' (adriamycin, bleomycin, vinblastine and dacarbazine). The intensity of the treatment depends on the

Table 6.5 Simplified staging of Hodgkin's disease

- Stage I – Involvement of a single lymph node region (I) or of a single extra lymphatic organ
- Stage II – Involvement of two or more lymph node regions on the same side of the diaphragm alone (II) or with limited involvement of adjacent extralymphatic organ
- Stage III – Involvement of lymph node regions or lymphoid structures on both sides of the diaphragm (III) which may include the spleen (IIIs) or limited involvement of adjacent tissue
- Stage IV – Diffuse or disseminated disease involving one or more extralymphatic organs
- All cases are subclassified to indicate the absence (A) or presence (B) of one or more of the following three systemic symptoms: significant unexplained fever, night sweats, or unexplained weight loss exceeding 10% of body weight during the six months prior to diagnosis

The subscript 'X' is used if bulky disease is present.

prognosis as determined by disease stage at presentation. Those with only localized disease (i.e. Stages I–IIA) typically receive two to four cycles of ABVD and radiotherapy. Those with Stage IIB or higher are treated with four cycles of ABVD. Treatment may be escalated to more intensive chemotherapy regimens and in some cases an autologous bone marrow transplant if they are not responding to initial therapy. Hodgkin's disease is curable in around 80% of cases. For patients with refractory disease, an antibody drug conjugate targeting CD30 (Brentuximab vedotin) has recently been licensed.

Hodgkin's disease is associated with marked depression of cell-mediated immunity and patients are prone to bacterial, fungal and viral infections (see Chapter 3), both prior to and during therapy. Long-term **complications** of the chemotherapy and radiotherapy include heart disease, lung toxicity (due to bleomycin), secondary tumours and thyroid failure after irradiation to the neck.

Case 6.3 Hodgkin's disease

A 23-year-old man presented with malaise, night sweats, loss of weight and intermittent fever dating from a flu-like illness three months previously. On examination, he had bilateral cervical and axillary lymphadenopathy; the glands were 2–5 cm in diameter, firm, rubbery, discrete and fairly mobile. His liver and spleen were not enlarged. Investigation showed that his haemoglobin was low (113 g/L) and the white cell count was normal (4.2 × 10^9/L), but his erythrocyte sedimentation rate (ESR) was raised at 78 mm/h; the blood film did not show any abnormal cells. No enlargement of the hilar glands was seen on chest X-ray. A cervical lymph node was removed for histology. The gross architecture of the node was destroyed; the tissue consisted of histiocytes, eosinophils, lymphocytes and giant cells known as Reed–Sternberg cells. These large binucleate cells are characteristic of Hodgkin's disease. Bone marrow examination was normal apart from a reactive eosinophilia, and computed tomography (CT-PET) showed no involvement of other lymph nodes. This patient had stage 2 Hodgkin's disease, because, although only lymphoid tissue above the diaphragm was involved, his ESR was above 40 mm/h. In view of his symptoms, the suffix 'B' was added to the stage, suggesting a poorer prognosis associated with systemic symptoms. He was given cytotoxic chemotherapy with ABVD (adriamycin, bleomycin, vinblastine and dacarbazine).

6.4.2 Non-Hodgkin's lymphoma

NHL is the broad group of all lymphomas that do not have the typical histological features of Hodgkin's disease; they may be of either B- or T-cell origin.

Patients **present** with a variety of symptoms, *many similar to those in Hodgkin's disease*, i.e. weight loss, unexplained fever, night sweats and lymphadenopathy or lymphoid infiltration of other organs such as liver, skin, brain or lungs (Fig. 6.9 and Case 6.4). Those with advanced disease may have evidence of bone marrow suppression, i.e. anaemia or bruising due to thrombocytopenia, although these are rarely presenting features.

The **diagnosis** of NHL (as for Hodgkin's disease) is best achieved with an excision biopsy of an intact node to obtain sufficient tissue for assessment of node architecture and constituent cells by histology, immunological, cytogenetic and molecular assessment. Obtaining a whole lymph node as opposed to a needle core biopsy is particularly important in the

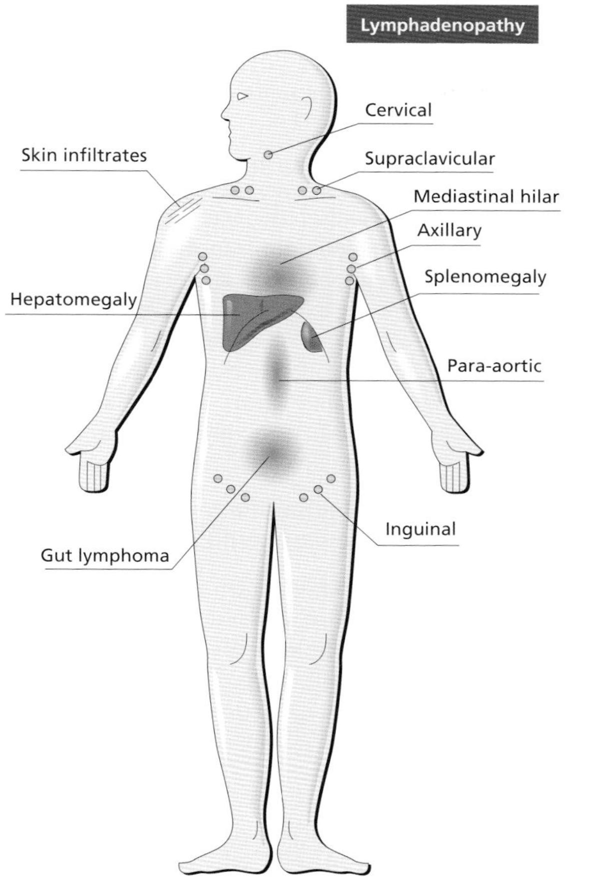

Lymphadenopathy

Fig. 6.9 Distribution of lymph nodes in lymphoma. Source: Axford J & O'Callaghan C (Eds) *Medicine*, 2nd Ed (2004). Reproduced with permission of John Wiley & Sons Ltd.

Case 6.4 Non-Hodgkin's lymphoma

A 59-year-old man presented with a gradually increasing lump in his right groin of six months' duration, which he thought was a 'hernia'. This was a large inguinal lymph node. He had suffered repeated urethritis in the past. He had no other symptoms, but was found on examination to have splenomegaly (7 cm below the costal margin) without hepatomegaly.

On investigation, his haemoglobin was low (118 g/L), but his white cell count and differential were normal. His erythrocyte sedimentation rate (ESR) was 58 mm/h and the lactate dehydrogenase level was also high. His serum immunoglobulins were all reduced: his IgG was 5.2 g/L (NR 7.2–19.0 g/L); IgA 0.3 g/L (NR 0.8–5.0 g/L); and IgM 0.3 g/L (NR 0.5–2.0 g/L). Serum electrophoresis showed no monoclonal bands. The lymph node was excised; light microscopy showed irregular follicles with mixtures of small and large cells throughout, but no organized germinal centres. Reactive follicular hyperplasia was a possibility, but immunophenotyping of tissue sections showed monoclonality, with strong cellular staining of the cells in the multiple follicles with anti-IgG and anti-κ monoclonal antibodies. Normal interfollicular T-cell staining was present. This patient had a follicular type of non-Hodgkin's lymphoma and cytogenetic analysis of the lymph node revealed chromosomal translocations associated with aggressive disease.

Box 6.3 Different types of B-cell lymphoma

- Most NHLs are of B-cell lineage
- Malignancies of immature B cells include chronic lymphocytic leukaemia and small lymphoid cell lymphomas
- Tumours of antigen-stimulated B cells may be follicular or large cell lymphomas
- More mature B cells give rise to more aggressive lymphomas (e.g. Burkitt's lymphoma). Exceptions are well-differentiated tumours of lymphoplasmacytoid cells in Waldenström's macroglobulinaemia

---

diagnosis of low-grade lymphomas and Hodgkin's disease, which may be difficult to differentiate from benign reactive lymphoid reactions. Aggressive lymphomas are more often clearly apparent and so needle core biopsies can suffice, though *this is not known at the onset of investigations.*

The area of the lymph node in which the clonal malignant cells are seen does not indicate the type of lymphoma but can be helpful, with the caveat that predominantly B-cell germinal centres and follicular areas do contain some T lymphocytes and the paracortex (T-cell area) has some B cells. Precise cell lineage is achieved by staining tissue sections with labelled monoclonal antibodies (MAbs) to different surface antigens. The panel of MAbs used for immunostaining of tissue biopsies is designed to confirm that the **abnormal clonal cells are lymphoid** (leucocyte common antigen, CD45) and their lineage (T or B). Reactive lymphoproliferation due to infection or inflammation is, in contrast, polyclonal.

The natural history of NHL is enormously variable. Assessing the **extent of disease** is helpful. Contrast-enhanced CT scanning (neck, thorax, abdomen and pelvis) and PET scanning are used. Bone marrow trephine examination is an important investigation in NHL, as marrow involvement is associated with a poor prognosis and indicates a need for more intensive treatment.

Complications of NHL include autoimmune haemolytic anaemia and thrombocytopenia. Low serum immunoglobulin levels, often resulting in recurrent bacterial infections, are seen in about half the patients.

The aim of a **classification** is to break up a heterogeneous group of diseases in order to provide prognosis so that the most effective form of treatment can be given. To be useful, a classification must distinguish between aggressive and indolent tumours – general principles are outlined in Box 6.3. The Revised European American (REAL) classification, based on clinical features similar to those in Table 6.3 for Hodgkin's disease, did have prognostic value, but this has now been incorporated into the WHO classification. Currently the WHO criteria include information based on immunophenotype and gene expression (see www.lymphomas.org.uk).

Treatment of NHL is primarily determined by (i) whether the lymphoma type is high grade or low grade, (ii) bulk, site of disease and clinical stage and (iii) patient-related factors including age, performance score and co-morbidities. Combination chemotherapy, rituximab (anti-CD20 monoclonal antibody) to specifically target all B cells with cytotoxic chemotherapy agents, provides the mainstay of treatment. This is administered as repeated cycles (usually six) over the course of several months. Ongoing treatment with monthly rituximab for two years as 'maintenance' has been shown to be effective in preventing relapse following completion of primary treatment for some subtypes, in particular follicular lymphoma, that are associated with slow but inevitable progression otherwise. For selected patients with refractory B-NHL, CAR-T cell therapy directed against CD19 has recently been licensed (see section 6.3.1 and Chapter 7) Supportive measures are key to ensuring good outcomes and minimizing treatment-related morbidity and mortality. Antifungal and antiviral prophylaxes, to protect against the inevitable immune suppression and the transient antibody deficiency resulting from rituximab, have improved survival. Prompt treatment of neutropenic sepsis with intravenous antibiotics is essential, as this is a haematological emergency with a high mortality rate if untreated. Recovery of neutrophil counts can be expedited by administering granulocyte colony-stimulating factor (G-CSF) treatment. Transfusions of red cells and platelets may be necessary.

Autologous stem cell transplantation may be used in relapsed or refractory disease or occasionally as part of initial therapy for patients with aggressive lymphoma subtypes known to carry a high rate of relapse. Usually this is performed once remission (or near remission) has been achieved using combination chemotherapy. CD34⁺ stem cells are then collected from the patient following stem cell 'mobilization' treatment, usually G-CSF. High-dose ablative therapy is then combined with 'rescue' of bone marrow function with the harvested CD34⁺ cells. Allogeneic (sibling or unrelated donor) bone marrow transplants are also sometimes performed for patients with refractory/relapsed disease, particularly if few CD34⁺ cells are harvested from the patient in remission.

6.5 Plasma cell dyscrasias

Clonal proliferations of plasma cells usually result in secretion of the **monoclonal immunoglobulin into the plasma**, which is detectable on serum electrophoresis as a monoclonal band (also known as a paraprotein – see Chapter 19). Depending on the ability of the clonal cells to proliferate and to invade other tissues, the related clinical condition may be relatively benign for many years – benign paraproteinaemia – or frankly malignant with possible secondary deposits – multiple myeloma (Table 6.6).

6.5.1 Benign paraproteinaemia or monoclonal gammopathy of unknown significance

Monoclonal gammopathy of unknown significance (MGUS) is defined as the presence of a monoclonal protein in the serum of a person with no defining features of myeloma (see Case 6.5). About 25% of all patients with serum paraproteins have benign monoclonal gammopathy (Table 6.6). Benign paraproteinaemia is uncommon under 50 years of age, but occurs in 1% in those of 50 years, 3% of persons over 70 and 8% of people over 85 years. **Long-term follow-up** has shown that about a quarter of patients with a benign band will progress to a plasma cell malignancy, multiple myeloma, amyloidosis, macroglobulinaemia or other malignant lymphoproliferative disorder (Fig. 6.10). *All patients with a paraprotein should be investigated for multiple myeloma if they develop symptoms* of bone pains or pathological fractures, weight loss, night sweats, if the paraprotein level increases to ≥15 g/L or if the features described in Table 6.7 are present. It remains difficult to distinguish reliably at presentation those patients who will remain stable from those in whom a malignant condition will develop, although

Table 6.6 Comparison of monoclonal gammopathy of unknown significance (MGUS), smouldering myeloma and multiple myeloma

	MGUS	Asymptomatic myeloma	Multiple myeloma
Age at onset	Elderly	Elderly	Elderly
Symptoms	None	None	Defining feature
Concentration of paraprotein	<30 g/L	>30 g/L	>30 g/L
Bone marrow findings (plasma cells as % nucleated cells)	10%	>10%	>10%
Lytic bone lesions	None	None	May be present
Immunosuppression of other immunoglobulins in serum	Not typically	Not typically	Frequent
Haemoglobin, calcium, albumin	Normal	Usually normal	Often abnormal
Treatment	None	Wait for symptoms	Treat

Case 6.5 Benign paraproteinaemia

A 49-year-old woman presented with a six-month history of vague aches and pains in her chest. On examination, she was overweight but had no abnormal physical signs.

Her haemoglobin was 136 g/L with a white cell count of 6.7 × 10⁹/L and a normal differential. Her erythrocyte sedimentation rate (ESR) was 34 mm/h. Tests of thyroid function were normal. However, protein electrophoresis showed a small paraprotein band in the γ band; this band was an IgG of λ type. Her serum IgG was raised at 20.1 g/L (NR 7.2–19.0 g/L), with an IgA of 1.9 g/L (NR 0.8–5.0 g/L) and an IgM of 3.0 g/L (NR 0.5–2.0 g/L). Electrophoresis of concentrated urine showed no monoclonal light chains and the plasma ratio of free kappa : lambda light chains was normal. The serum paraprotein measured 10 g/L by densitometry (Chapter 19). A bone marrow examination showed only 2% plasma cells. Together with the absence of osteolytic lesions, the absence of monoclonal free light chains in the urine and normal serum IgA and IgM levels, these findings supported a diagnosis of benign monoclonal gammopathy, also known as a monoclonal gammopathy of unknown significance (MGUS). This woman has been followed at six-monthly intervals for 22 years with no increase in the paraprotein level. She will continue to be seen at yearly intervals.

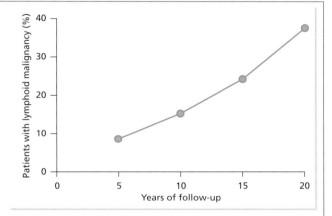

Fig. 6.10 Development of lymphoid malignancy after monoclonal gammopathy of unknown significance diagnosis. Source: Data from Kyle, 2002.

Box 6.4 Differential diagnosis in patients found to have a paraprotein

- Monoclonal gammopathy of unknown significance (MGUS)
- Myeloma
- Waldenström's macroglobulinaemia
- Lymphoproliferative disorders, including non-Hodgkin's lymphoma and chronic lymphocytic leukaemia
- Plasmacytoma
- Reactive or transient paraproteinaemias, e.g. due to infection in immunodeficient patients

All patients must have serial measurements of the serum paraprotein at least yearly (more frequently initially) and plasma checked for monoclonal light chains (Box 6.4).

The underlying causes of MGUS are not well understood.

6.5.2 Multiple myeloma

Multiple myeloma is the malignant proliferation of plasma cells (see Fig. 6.2), thought to be provoked by a translocation (probably during class switching in the germinal centre) resulting in activation of an oncogene in an immunoglobulin locus. In the bone marrow, interaction of the malignant plasma cells with stromal cells results in excess production of IL-6 and other cytokines that enables these malignant cells to survive. The malignant clones of plasma cells overproduce their specific heavy- and light-chain immunoglobulin molecules, which are easily detected in serum (whole immunoglobulin) or urine (free light chains) or both (Fig. 6.11 and Chapter 19, Fig. 19.4).

Multiple myeloma is a relatively common malignancy among elderly people (prevalence of 3 per 10⁵ population), but is very rare below the age of 40 years. Patients **commonly present** with recurrent infections (which may be due to immune paresis, or deficiencies in the other immunoglobulin classes), renal failure (due to hypercalcaemia or deposition of light

Table 6.7 Cytogenetic factors contributing to prognosis in multiple myeloma

Poor risk	Good risk
Del 13q14	T(11 : 14)
T(4 : 14)	T(6 : 14)
T(14 : 16)	Hyperdiploidy
T(14 : 20)	Normality
Del 17p13	
Hypodiploidy	

a non-IgG immunoglobulin, higher paraprotein concentrations, high beta-2 microglobulin level and an abnormal serum free light-chain ratio are suggestive of a higher risk of progression.

IgM paraproteins are associated with progression to Waldenström's macroglobulinaemia or lymphoma (see section 6.5.3). High IgM levels can cause hyperviscosity.

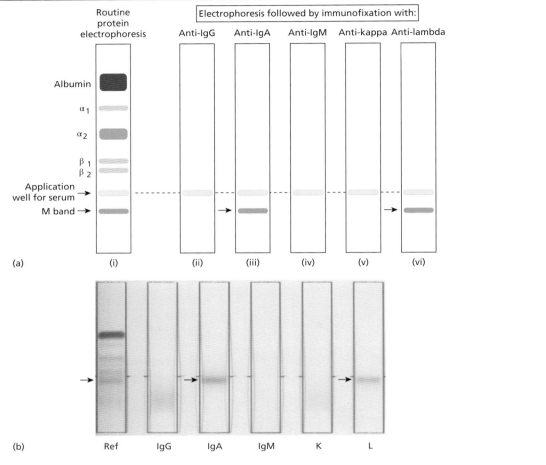

Fig. 6.11 Typing an M band by immunofixation. In this schematic example (a), the M band found on electrophoresis (i) is identified as an IgA (type λ), as shown on the actual fixation gel (b).

Case 6.6 Multiple myeloma

A 66-year-old man presented with sharp, constant low back pain, dating from a fall from a ladder six weeks earlier. On direct questioning, he did admit to vague malaise for over six months. On examination, he was in considerable pain but otherwise seemed fairly fit. He was mildly anaemic but had no lymphadenopathy and no fever. There were no signs of bruising, no finger clubbing, no hepatosplenomegaly and no abdominal masses. On investigation, his haemoglobin was low (102 g/L), but his white cell count was normal (6.2 × 10⁹/L). He had a normal differential white cell count and a normal platelet count, but his erythrocyte sedimentation rate (ESR) was 98 mm/h. Total serum proteins were raised at 98 g/L (NR 65–75 g/L) and his serum albumin was low; plasma creatinine and urea were normal. He had a raised serum calcium level (3.2 mmol/L) but a normal alkaline phosphatase. Serum protein electrophoresis revealed a monoclonal band in the γ region (see Chapter 19, Fig. 19.3), with considerable immunosuppression of the rest of this region (see Fig. 6.11). The band was typed by immunofixation (Fig. 6.11) and shown to be IgA of λ type. Quantification of serum immunoglobulins showed a low IgG of 6.0 g/L (NR 7.2–19.0 g/L), a high IgA of 15.3 g/L (NR 0.8–5.0 g/L) and a low IgM of 0.2 g/L (NR 0.5–2.0 g/L). Electrophoretic examination of concentrated urine showed a monoclonal band in the α region, which was composed of free λ light chains. X-rays of his back showed a small, punched-out lesion in the second lumbar vertebra, but a subsequent skeletal survey did not show any other bone lesions. Bone marrow examination showed an increased number of atypical plasma cells; these constituted 45% of the nucleated cells found on the film. This man showed the features required for a diagnosis of multiple myeloma (see Box 6.5).

chains in the kidney), pathological fractures or bone pain, as in Case 6.6 (due to osteolytic lesions or osteoporosis; see Fig. 6.12), or anaemia (due to marrow failure; see Fig. 6.13). Myeloma may also be a rare cause of peripheral neuropathy or the hyperviscosity syndrome.

It is believed that most cases of multiple myeloma are preceded by an MGUS. This premalignant condition can progress to myeloma at a rate of approximately 1% per year.

The **diagnostic criteria** (used in Case 6.6) are shown in Box 6.5. The finding of a paraprotein in the serum is not diagnostic of multiple myeloma. The paraproteins found in the sera of patients with myeloma are usually IgG, IgA or free monoclonal light chains; IgM myelomas are rare and large amounts of IgM monoclonal protein nearly always indicate the relatively more benign disease, Waldenström's macroglobulinaemia (see section 6.5.3). Rare cases of myeloma in which the clonal cells

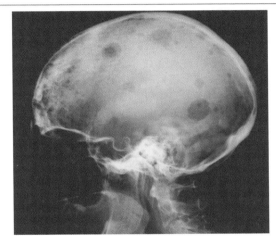

Fig. 6.12 Skull X-ray in myeloma showing lytic lesions. Source: Axford J & O'Callaghan C (Eds) *Medicine*, 2nd Ed (2004). Reproduced with permission of John Wiley & Sons Ltd.

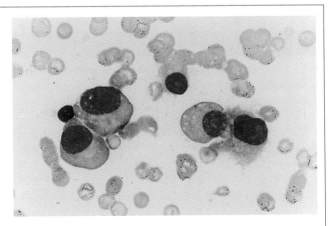

Fig. 6.13 Bone marrow in myeloma showing an excess of plasma cells. Source: Axford J & O'Callaghan C (Eds) *Medicine*, 2nd Ed (2004). Reproduced with permission of John Wiley & Sons Ltd.

Box 6.5 Criteria required for a diagnosis of multiple myeloma (all three required)

1 Serum /urine paraprotein
2 Clone of plasma cells in bone marrow or tissues (plasmacytoma)
3 End-organ damage related to plasma cell dyscrasia
  a Increased calcium levels
  b Lytic bone lesions/osteoporosis
  c Anaemia
  d Renal failure

are non-secretory are therefore very difficult to diagnose by routine methods.

Free monoclonal light chains can be detected in **serum or urine** in myeloma, where they are known as Bence Jones proteins. They may be associated with a serum paraprotein and, if so, then the urinary light chains are, of course, the same light-chain type: either kappa or lambda subtype. Only proteins of small molecular size are filtered by the normal renal glomerulus, so light chains (mol. wt. 22 kDa) can be excreted, but whole immunoglobulin molecules (mol. wt. of IgG 150 kDa; mol. wt. of IgM 800 kDa) are too large unless there is glomerular damage. When a normal plasma cell makes immunoglobulin, it always produces an excess of the particular light chains compared with heavy chains. This normal polyclonal excess is excreted in the urine and rapidly metabolized by the renal tubules. Since all plasma cells synthesize both heavy and light chains, the free light-chain excess in normal individuals is polyclonal, can be detected only in highly concentrated urine and is of no clinical consequence. The products of the monoclonal plasma cells in myeloma result in excess kappa or lambda light chains and therefore an abnormal κ : λ **serum free light-chain ratio**.

It is important to realize that *light chains are not detected by routine chemical/dipstick methods* for detecting protein in the urine. Free light chains are detected only by immunofixation, using specific antisera (see Chapter 19). In patients who have significant glomerular damage, leakage of all serum proteins into the urine may occur, including the serum paraprotein, and these may even obscure the band.

The bone marrow in myeloma shows abnormal **plasma cells in excess of 10%** (Fig. 6.13). This figure can be reached in some reactive conditions and is not, by itself, diagnostic, but if in doubt, immunohistology of the marrow trephine will confirm the monoclonal nature of the cells (Table 6.6).

Osteolytic bone lesions occur in many patients. These are best imaged by X-ray (rather than CT or magnetic resonance imaging [MRI]) and the typical **X-ray appearance** of a myeloma deposit in bone is a 'punched-out' lesion (Fig. 6.12), often found in the skull and axial skeleton, *although any part of the skeleton can be involved*. Osteoporosis also occurs, and myeloma may present with pathological (or osteoporotic) fractures. Multiple myeloma lytic bone lesions result from increased osteoclastic and osteoblastic dysfunction. This is thought to involve increased secretion of cytokines, including myeloma-derived macrophage-inflammatory protein (MIP1α) and IL-6, which activates osteoclasts and osteoblasts via nuclear factor kappa B (NFκB); some of these cytokines are released by benign stromal cells rather than the malignant plasma cells. About a third of patients have hypercalcaemia. Anaemia is ubiquitous.

The **suppression of** polyclonal immunoglobulin production to frank hypogammaglobulinaemia and failure to produce antibodies, demonstrated by a poor response to immunization, are associated with recurrent bacterial infections.

Light-chain myeloma is particularly associated with **renal tubular damage** (see Chapter 9, Case 9.11). The excessive production of free light chains causes the renal tubules to become dilated and plugged with eosinophilic, homogeneous casts. If this material is not removed by diuresis, the tubular cells eventually atrophy or even undergo frank necrosis. Forced diuresis of patients who present with a raised serum creatinine improves their early survival. A longer-term complication of myeloma is light-chain-associated amyloid (compare with Chapter 9, Case 9.9).

If untreated, myeloma can be rapidly progressive and patients die within a year. The overall prognosis depends on the presence of complications, such as anaemia, renal failure, hypercalcaemia or immunosuppression (see Table 6.6), which provide the staging; prognostic factors include serum albumin and serum beta-2 microglobulin levels, taken in conjunction with cytogenetic findings (Table 6.7). Of note is the finding that most translocations in multiple myeloma involved chromosome 14, which includes the genes for the immunoglobulin heavy chains.

Myeloma remains an incurable malignancy, though the outlook has improved somewhat in the last decade. Earlier therapy in Europe was based on melphalan and prednisone, and these are still used in those with significant co-morbidities or in very elderly patients. However, **intensive regimens** incorporating agents such as thalidomide, cyclophosphamide and steroids are more commonly used now. Bortezomib, a proteasome inhibitor that promotes normal apoptosis, and daratumumab (anti-CD38 monoclonal antibody) are also effective. Younger patients who respond well to chemotherapy may be eligible for autologous stem cell transplant. Initial responses are almost 90% successful, with about half of the patients also responding after first relapse. Overall survival extends from a median of 5 years for stage 1 to 2.5 years for stage 3.

Supportive measures are important, such as bisphosphonates to prevent osteoporosis and sometimes replacement immunoglobulin therapy for those with recurrent infections due to poor antibody production. G-CSF is used to increase the number of circulating CD34+ stem cells in the blood before harvesting to store for **subsequent autologous transplantation**; following high-dose chemotherapy, these stem cells then recolonize the marrow. However, multiple myeloma remains a fatal disease, possibly due to premalignant CD34+ stem cells themselves, though this remains controversial.

The search for curative therapies includes the possibility of CAR-T cell therapy targeted at B-cell maturation antigen (BCMA), a B-cell lineage-specific antigen whose strong expression on malignant plasma cells makes it an attractive therapeutic target.

6.5.3 Waldenström's macroglobulinaemia

Waldenström's macroglobulinaemia is a malignancy of IgM producing plasma cells that, unlike myeloma, do not metastasize to the bones or other tissues. The clinical **presentation** of Waldenström's macroglobulinaemia is variable. It tends to present after the age of 50 years and, in most patients, follows a relatively benign course.

Unlike myeloma, **symptoms** of Waldenström's macroglobulinaemia are usually directly attributable to the effects of the monoclonal IgM (see Case 6.7 and Table 6.8). IgM is a large molecule (mol. wt. 800 kDa) confined entirely to the intravascular pool. Increased IgM concentrations (particularly in excess of 40 g/L) cause a marked rise in serum viscosity. Although there is considerable variation in the level of viscosity that induces symptoms, these are

---

(🔍) Case 6.7 Waldenström's macroglobulinaemia

A 76-year-old woman presented with a six-month history of weakness, malaise, exertional dyspnoea and abdominal discomfort. In the previous month she had experienced epistaxes and headaches, but did not have visual disturbances, weight loss, bone pain or recurrent infections. On examination she was pale, with moderate axillary and cervical lymphadenopathy. Her liver and spleen were enlarged.

On investigation, she had an erythrocyte sedimentation rate (ESR) of 112 mm/h and a haemoglobin of 108 g/L. Her white cell count and differential were normal. The total serum protein was increased to 130 g/L. Protein electrophoresis (Chapter 19) and immunofixation (Chapter 19) showed a dense paraprotein in the γ region, which proved to be an IgM of κ type. Quantification of the serum immunoglobulins showed normal IgG (9.4 g/L) and IgA levels (1.1 g/L), but her IgM was markedly raised at 64.5 g/L (NR 0.5–2.0 g/L). By densitometry (Chapter 19), the paraprotein (see Chapter 19, Fig. 19.5) measured 63 g/L. Electrophoresis of concentrated urine showed no free monoclonal light chains and there were no bone lesions on X-rays of her chest and skull. Her serum viscosity, relative to water, was 4.7 (NR 1.4–1.8). A bone marrow examination showed a pleomorphic cellular infiltrate composed of a mixture of small lymphocytes, plasma cells and cells of an intermediate appearance, called lymphoplasmacytoid cells. These are features of Waldenström's macroglobulinaemia.

Table 6.8 Comparison of clinical features of multiple myeloma and Waldenström's macroglobulinaemia

	Multiple myeloma	Waldenström's macroglobulinaemia
Lytic bone lesions	+++	
Bone pain	+++	
Pathological fractures	++	
Anaemia	+++	++
Recurrent infection	++	
Hypercalcaemia	++	
Renal failure	++	
Thrombocytopenia	++	
Leucopenia	+	
Neuropathy	+	+
Lymphadenopathy	+	+++
Hepatosplenomegaly	+/–	+++
Hyperviscosity	+	+++

unusual if the relative serum viscosity (see Chapter 19) is below 4.0. The symptoms of **hyperviscosity** include headaches, confusion, dizziness and changes in visual acuity or, in some cases, sudden deafness. Nose bleeds and bruising may also occur. Examination of the optic fundi may reveal dilated vessels, haemorrhages, exudates, intravascular rouleaux formation or papilloedema.

Vigorous plasmapheresis can reduce the serum IgM level quite quickly and, once the viscosity has been lowered, maintenance **plasmapheresis** will keep the patient asymptomatic. However, plasmapheresis does not affect the disease itself; **chemotherapy (usually incorporating rituximab) or BTK inhibitors** are often used in symptomatic patients to control the monoclonal proliferation.

The mean survival of macroglobulinaemia is 4–5 years, but many patients live for 10 years or more following diagnosis. **Complications** are due to hyperviscosity or cryoglobulinaemia (see Chapter 11, section 11.5.3); infections are uncommon since serum immunoglobulin and neutrophil levels usually remain normal. A small proportion of patients have a rapidly progressive disease; symptoms resemble those of NHL, and are usually followed by the appearance of circulating lymphoplasmacytoid cells in peripheral blood.

6.5.4 Other plasma cell dyscrasias

Almost all malignant plasma cells produce an excess of monoclonal light chains, resulting in a high risk of **light chain–associated amyloid** (see Chapter 9, section 9.8.4). Amyloid may be associated with frank myeloma or can be 'idiopathic' if the malignant clone is not detected. These diseases are fully discussed in Chapter 9.

CHAPTER 7
Immune Manipulation

Key topics

Visit the companion website at **www.wiley.com/go/misbah/immunology** to download cases with additional figures on these topics.

Chapel and Haeney's Essentials of Clinical Immunology, Seventh Edition. Edited by Siraj A. Misbah, Gavin P. Spickett, and Virgil A.S.H. Dalm.
© 2022 John Wiley & Sons Ltd. Published 2022 by John Wiley & Sons Ltd.

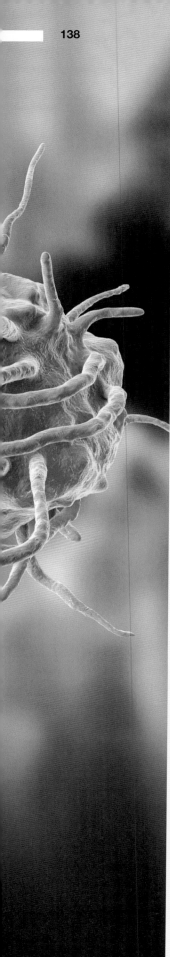
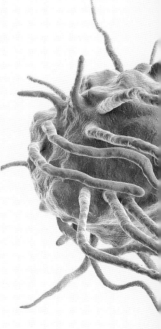

7.1 Introduction

Although the immune system usually responds appropriately to foreign antigens, there are patients whose disease is caused by immune responses that are excessive or defective. The aim of clinical immunology is to correct these abnormalities. Two major approaches are possible: immunosuppression or immunopotentiation. An overactive, self-damaging immune system requires some degree of **immunosuppression**; this is the mainstay of the management of organ transplantation and certain life-threatening autoimmune diseases. Until recently, with the major exceptions of immunization and human stem cell transplantation, **immunopotentiation** to improve a naive or defective immune system was still unproven. Recently however, immunopotentiation in the form of monoclonal antibody directed against immune checkpoints leading to enhanced T-cell function is now well established as a key component of cancer therapy for many malignancies. Gene therapy is now beginning to fulfil its potential as curative therapy for certain inherited immunodeficiencies (see section 7.4.2). Genetic manipulation of T cells involving the attachment of antigen-specific antibody fragments to certain T-cell receptor stimulatory domains, known as chimeric antigen receptor T (CAR-T) cells has been a recent revolutionary advance in the treatment of patients with certain B-cell malignancies.

Some methods of immune manipulation produce definite clinical benefit by mechanisms that are poorly understood, e.g. therapy with intravenous and subcutaneous immunoglobulin (IVIg, SCIg), though monoclonal antibodies can suppress, potentiate or modify immune responses depending on their action, specificity and the clinical circumstances.

7.2 Immunosuppression

7.2.1 Drugs

There are several groups of immunosuppressive drugs (Fig. 7.1). Their effects on the immune system are divided into *short-lived changes on cell traffic* and *more persistent effects on individual cell functions*. Their antiinflammatory properties are separate from those on the immune system. In general, azathioprine and cyclophosphamide act on the maturation of cells, while steroids and fungal derivatives inhibit the functions of mature cells.

Corticosteroids are primarily antiinflammatory, though they also affect cell trafficking. A single dose of corticosteroids causes changes in cell traffic within 2 hours of administration;

the result is a transient lymphopenia, which peaks at 4 hours but is no longer apparent after 24 hours. Lymphopenia occurs largely because Th cells are redistributed and Tc cells sequestered in the bone marrow; in addition, though, there is increased lymphocyte apoptosis (Table 7.1).

The **influence of steroids on cell function** varies according to species, dose and timing. *The major effect in humans is on 'resting' macrophages* (Table 7.1); *activated macrophages are not sensitive to corticosteroids*. Reduced antigen handling by macrophages probably accounts for the poor primary antibody

Table 7.1 Actions of corticosteroids on the human immune system

Inhibition of inflammation:
- Altered gene transcription, particularly via NFkB pathway
- Reduced production of prostaglandins, cytokines (IL-1, IL-6, TNF-α), histamine
- Reduced activity of neutrophils and maturation of macrophages
- Reduced proliferation of T cells

Inhibition of wound healing and repair:
- ↓ Endothelial cell function
- ↓ Natural killer cell function (↓ nitric oxide synthase activity)
- ↓ Antigen handling (↓ maturation of monocytes to macrophages)
- Reduced expression of adhesion molecules on neutrophils (to prevent export into tissues)

Changes in cell traffic;
- ↑ Neutrophils in blood (released from bone marrow as well as failed exit to tissues)
- ↓ Monocytes in blood
- ↓ Lymphocytes in blood (↑ apoptosis of CD4+ cells)
- T$_C$ sequestered in bone marrow

IFN-γ, interferon-γ; IL, interleukin; NFkB, nuclear factor kappa B; T$_C$, cytotoxic T cells; Th, helper T cells; TNF-α, tumour necrosis factor-α.

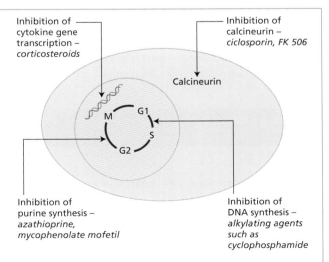

Fig. 7.1 Schematic depiction of the main intracellular sites of action of the major groups of immunosuppressive drugs.

response seen following corticosteroid administration. *The secondary antibody response is not affected, as memory cells are resistant to the effects of corticosteroids.*

In humans, corticosteroids are used for several purposes: the prevention or reversal of graft rejection and the treatment of autoimmune, allergic and malignant diseases. In transplantation (see Chapter 8) their antiinflammatory action and reduction of macrophage activity result in reduced cellular infiltration. *Steroids alone are ineffective in preventing rejection in the early phase*, although high doses (methyl prednisolone) do reverse acute rejection. Corticosteroids have a wide range of **side effects** (Fig. 7.2). They are known to increase the patient's susceptibility to infections of all kinds. Failure to export neutrophils into the tissues (Table 7.1) and reduced macrophage function are most relevant to this increased risk. Adverse effects are related to the duration of treatment as well as the dose; by giving larger doses for shorter periods, it is often possible to reduce infection risk while conserving immunosuppression. Alternate-day therapy or using steroid-sparing agents also reduces the unwanted effects.

The development of **thiopurines** in the 1950s provided another important immunosuppressive drug, namely **azathioprine**. It is inactive until metabolized by the liver and *takes a few weeks to be effective*. The metabolites can affect all dividing cells by inhibition of DNA synthesis (Fig. 7.1). Azathioprine is widely used in two main clinical situations:

(i) prevention of rejection after organ transplantation and (ii) treatment of systemic autoimmune disease. Azathioprine affects several aspects of immune function (Table 7.2), which accounts for its bone marrow toxicity. Most patients on long-term therapy eventually show granulocytopenia and thrombocytopenia. Homozygous deficiency of **thiopurine methyl transferase** (**TPMT**), a key enzyme responsible for metabolizing azathioprine, is associated with life-threatening marrow aplasia. This homozygous deficiency is present in approximately 1 in 300 individuals, whereas the heterozygous state is found in 10% of the population. Measurement of TPMT enzyme activity and/or TPMT genotypes prior to initiating therapy with azathioprine, or the related compound 6-mercaptopurine, can help prevent the toxicity associated with slow metabolism. Close monitoring of leukocyte and platelet counts is critical in all patients.

Mycophenolate mofetil is a purine inhibitor that inhibits inosine monophosphate dehydrogenase (IMP), a key enzyme in the *de novo* synthesis of purines in activated T and B lymphocytes. It is an excellent substitute for azathioprine if treatment fails or there is marrow toxicity, and is now a well-established component of maintenance immunosuppressive regimens following organ transplantation.

Alkylating agents, such as **cyclophosphamide**, interfere with DNA duplication at the premitotic phase and are most effective in rapidly dividing cells. Tissues vary in their ability to repair DNA after alkylation, which accounts for their differing sensitivities to this group of drugs. *They have little antiinflammatory activity* and so are often given with steroids. Cyclophosphamide also requires metabolism by the liver to form its active metabolites. When cyclophosphamide is given with, or immediately after, an antigen, there is **reduced antibody production** and **impaired delayed-type hypersensitivity**. At low doses, CD8$^+$ cells show a short-lived fall in number. As the dose is increased, numbers of CD4$^+$ cells fall progressively, increasing infection risk considerably. After stopping cyclophosphamide, recovery takes weeks or months, as in Case 7.1. Cyclophosphamide therapy is also associated with reactivation of latent viral infectious agents such as cytomegalovirus (CMV) and varicella zoster. Prolonged high doses are associated with bladder cancer, due to the carcinogenic metabolite acrolein. Clinically, cyclophosphamide is particularly

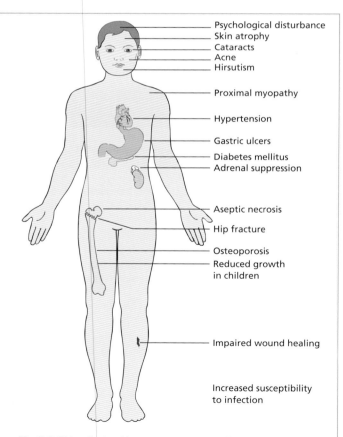

Psychological disturbance
Skin atrophy
Cataracts
Acne
Hirsutism

Proximal myopathy

Hypertension

Gastric ulcers

Diabetes mellitus
Adrenal suppression

Aseptic necrosis

Hip fracture

Osteoporosis
Reduced growth
in children

Impaired wound healing

Increased susceptibility
to infection

Fig. 7.2 Side effects of long-term treatment with corticosteroids.

Table 7.2 Actions of thiopurines on the human immune system
1 Cell traffic
Acute
• ↓ Lymphocytes, especially natural killer and T cells
• ↓ Monocytes
Chronic
• ↓ Granulocytes due to bone marrow suppression
• ↓ Platelets due to bone marrow suppression
2 Effects on inflammation
• ↓ Inflammatory infiltrate correlates with ↓ monocytes in blood

> ### (icon) Case 7.1 Pneumocystis pneumonia complicating immunosuppressive therapy
>
> A 35-year-old man with granulomatosis with polyangiitis (GPA; formerly Wegener's granulomatosis) was admitted to hospital with a two-week history of fever and shortness of breath. The diagnosis of GPA had been made 18 months earlier when he presented with haemoptysis and glomerulonephritis. Disease remission was achieved with aggressive immunosuppressive therapy using a combination of pulse methylprednisolone and cyclophosphamide, enabling him to be maintained on his current tapering dose of steroids and azathioprine. The results of investigations on his current hospital admission were as follows:
>
> - Chest X-ray: diffuse bilateral shadowing.
> - Serum C-reactive protein (CRP): 80 mg/L (NR <10).
> - Antineutrophil cytoplasmic antibody directed against proteinase 3: weakly positive at a titre of 1 : 40 (>1 : 640 at disease diagnosis).
> - Serum creatinine: 102 μmol/L (NR 50–140).
> - Urea: 4.5 mmol/L (NR 2.5–7.1).
> - Urine microscopy: clear.
>
> The differential diagnosis was between active GPA and infection complicating immunosuppressive therapy. It was crucial to distinguish between infection and active vasculitis in this situation, since an increase in immunosuppressive therapy in the face of sepsis could be potentially fatal. Further investigations, including bronchoalveolar lavage, revealed the presence of Pneumocystis carinii (Pneumocystis jiroveci), a recognized lung pathogen in patients on long-term immunosuppressive therapy. He made a full clinical and radiological recovery following two weeks of co-trimoxazole therapy and was discharged home on his usual dose of maintenance immunosuppression.

useful in aggressive autoimmune diseases (such as granulomatosis with polyangiitis or vasculitis associated with systemic lupus erythematosus) and in conditioning haematopoietic stem cell transplant (HSCT) recipients (see Chapter 8). It is also used with other antineoplastic treatments in many haematological and solid malignancies. Another alkylating agent, **chlorambucil**, is widely used for treating low-grade B-cell neoplasms, such as chronic lymphocytic leukaemia and non-Hodgkin's lymphoma. It appears to act on B cells directly. Chlorambucil is given either intermittently or in low dosage, because persistently high doses are associated with subsequent development of leukaemia.

Ciclosporin is a naturally occurring fungal metabolite. It has no effect on lymphocyte traffic, but suppresses both humoral and cell-mediated immunity by the effect on CD4⁺ T cells. Ciclosporin inhibits calcium-dependent signal transduction pathways downstream of the T-cell receptor, particularly the activation of several cytokine genes (Fig. 7.3). The major effect is **inhibition of IL-2 production** and thus CD4⁺ cell-dependent proliferative responses. Natural killer (NK) cell activity is also affected, because of its dependence on interleukin (IL)-2 production. A similar agent, **tacrolimus**, is derived from a soil fungus. Although its structure is quite different from that of ciclosporin and it binds to a different intracellular protein – immunophilin – it has a similar mode of action, but is 10–100 times more potent. Like ciclosporin, it inhibits IL-2, IL-3, IL-4 and interferon (IFN)-γ secretion, so preventing early activation of CD4⁺ T lymphocytes.

Both these agents cause a striking **prolongation of graft survival** and virtually all transplantation protocols now include a 'calcineurin inhibitor', usually in association with prednisolone

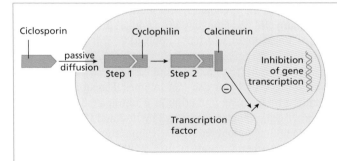

Fig. 7.3 Mechanism of immunosuppressive action of ciclosporin. In step 2 the Ciclo–Cyp complex binds to and inhibits calcineurin, a key enzyme responsible for translocation of transcription factors from the cytoplasm to the nucleus. Interruption of this event prevents gene transcription for interleukins IL-2, IL-3, IL-4, IL-5 and interferon (IFN)-γ.

and an antimetabolite such as azathioprine (see Chapter 8). Calcineurin inhibitors are partially successful in both preventing and reversing acute graft-versus-host disease following bone marrow transplant. Calcineurin inhibitors have also been used in a range of **autoimmune diseases mediated by helper T cells**. Efficacy has been established in controlled trials in conditions such as psoriasis (Chapter 11, Fig. 11.5), uveitis and severe rheumatoid arthritis. Several features are common to these reports (Box 7.1).

The timing and dose of calcineurin inhibitors must be balanced against the risk of toxicity, including **nephrotoxicity**, **hepatotoxicity** and **hypertension**. Other side effects include tremor, increased susceptibility to infections, and metabolic

---

Box 7.1 Features of calcineurin inhibitors

- These agents have a quick effect (within 2–12 weeks).
- Relapse occurs when the drug is stopped.
- The long-term course of the disease may be unaffected.
- High doses are nephrotoxic and cause hypertension.

---

disturbances such as hyperglycaemia. Both ciclosporin and tacrolimus are associated with an increased risk of squamous cell skin cancers and both benign and malignant lymphoproliferative diseases. This may reflect direct effects of calcineurin inhibitors or the result of altered immune surveillance of cells infected with oncogenic viruses such as human papilloma virus (HPV) or Epstein–Barr virus (EBV). This risk of malignancy is not a contraindication to its use in transplantation, as the risk of such proliferation is considerably less than that of rejection of the graft.

In contrast to immunocompetent individuals who are able to contain EBV as a chronic latent infection, patients with defective cellular immunity, either secondarily to drugs or as part of a primary immunodeficiency, are unable to do so and are at risk of developing B-cell lymphoma, as in Case 7.2. EBV-induced lymphoma in transplant patients often regresses on withdrawal or reduction of immunosuppressive medication, but this has to be balanced with the attendant risk of inducing graft rejection.

Rapamycin (sirolimus) is yet another immunosuppressive drug of fungal origin, which in combination with ciclosporin and steroids is successful in preventing renal transplant rejection. It is structurally similar to tacrolimus, but has a different immunosuppressive effect: sirolimus does not inhibit calcineurin and consequently cytokine gene transcription is unimpaired. However, it inhibits T-cell proliferation induced by IL-2 and IL-4.

Despite its undoubted efficacy, immunosuppressive drug therapy is inherently unsatisfactory, as illustrated in Cases 7.1 and 7.2. One method of maximizing local therapeutic immunosuppression without systemic adverse effects is the development of **topical immunosuppressive agents**. Tacrolimus and a related agent, pimecrolimus, are effective in ointment form in the treatment of moderate to severe eczema unresponsive to conventional therapy (see Chapter 4, section 4.8.2 and Case 4.11).

7.2.2 Polyclonal antibodies for prevention of responses

Antibodies can be used to prevent an immune response or to suppress ongoing immune responses.

Prevention of sensitization by removal of antigen is illustrated by the use of antibodies to the rhesus D blood group antigen. Haemolytic disease of the newborn due to rhesus incompatibility between the mother (rhesus D negative) and a rhesus D-positive fetus (see Chapter 18) is prevented by the administration of human anti-D antibodies to rhesus D-negative mothers immediately after delivery. These antibodies destroy any rhesus-positive fetal red cells, thus preventing an antibody response in the mother (Chapter 18, section 18.4.4).

Case 7.2 Epstein–Barr virus-induced lymphoma in a transplant recipient

A 65-year-old insulin-dependent diabetic man underwent cadaveric renal transplantation for end-stage renal failure. The immediate postoperative course was complicated by acute rejection, which was successfully reversed by steroids and then antithymocyte globulin. He was discharged from hospital two weeks later on insulin, prednisolone, azathioprine and ciclosporin (to prevent further transplant rejection), co-trimoxazole (to prevent Pneumocystis infection), erythropoietin and ranitidine. Five months later, he developed progressive dyspnoea, fever and fatigue. Clinical examination revealed bilateral lung crackles and hepatosplenomegaly. Bilateral diffuse interstitial shadowing was noted on chest X-ray. The differential diagnosis is summarized in Box 7.2. His haemoglobin was 84 g/L and he was severely leucopenic at 1.0×10^9/L. Blood cultures were sterile and a bone marrow biopsy showed normal myeloid and erythroid maturation, with no acid-fast bacilli or fungi evident on special stains. A transbronchial biopsy showed no histological abnormality; polymerase chain reaction (PCR) for acid-fast bacilli, Pneumocystis and cytomegalovirus was negative. Open lung biopsy showed fibrinous pneumonia with obstructive bronchiolitis associated with a dense cellular infiltrate of highly atypical lymphoid cells containing pleomorphic nuclei. The lymphoid cells expressed B-cell markers (CD20, CD79) and stained positively for a number of Epstein–Barr virus gene products (EBV nuclear antigens, EBV latent membrane proteins).

The lung biopsy results were diagnostic of a B-cell lymphoma secondary to EBV. Following the diagnosis, his immunosuppressive medication was stopped, but the patient died two weeks later from progressive respiratory failure.

Box 7.2 Differential diagnosis of fever and lung shadows in a renal transplant recipient

- Bacterial pneumonia (unlikely at five months post transplant).
- Reactivation of tuberculosis.
- Fungal infection (Aspergillus, Pneumocystis).
- Viral infection (cytomegalovirus).
- Epstein–Barr virus–induced lymphoproliferative disease (post-transplant lymphoproliferative disorder, PTLD).

7.2.3 Non-specific immunomodulation by therapeutic immunoglobulin

Immunoglobulin replacement is essential for patients with primary antibody deficiencies (see Chapter 3, section 3.2.5) and is of proven value in several forms of secondary hypogammaglobulinaemia (section 3.5.1). The serendipitous observation that IVIg raised the platelet count in two hypogammaglobulinaemic children with idiopathic thrombocytopenia inspired a new approach to the therapy of **autoimmune disease**. In these diseases, IVIg is given usually at a daily dose of 1 g/kg body weight for 1–2 days, with some patients requiring maintenance therapy at variable intervals (every 4–12 weeks) for chronic disease. The beneficial effect of IVIg has been established by controlled trials against placebo or conventional treatment in several disorders (Table 7.3), but benefit has also been claimed from open trials or anecdotal reports, though these provide inconclusive evidence for general use. Some trials have shown no benefit (Table 7.3).

In acute immune thrombocytopenia (ITP), the rise in platelet count occurs within 24–72 hours of infusion, but is often only transient; in other diseases, the effect of IVIg may be long-lasting. These differing patterns of response imply that **different mechanisms** operate. One mechanism of particular interest in autoimmune disease is the role of FcRn, the major histocompatibility complex (MHC) class I–related Fc receptor for IgG (also binds albumin) that protects IgG from lysosomal degradation. Blockade of FcRn by high-dose exogenous IgG is likely to result in accelerated catabolism of endogenous pathogenic IgG with consequent clinical improvement (Fig. 7.4). FcRn blockade by monoclonal antibodies results in dose-dependent reductions in serum IgG and pathogenic autoantibodies. A number of anti-FcRn antibodies are currently undergoing clinical trials in patients with systemic autoimmune diseases. Fc blockade of IgG receptors on macrophages in the spleen has been shown to be one of the mech-

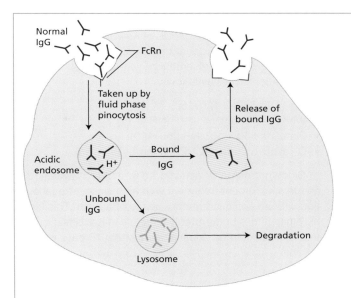

Fig. 7.4 Schematic representation of the role of the endothelial FcRn receptor in IgG homeostasis.

anisms involved in effectiveness in idiopathic thrombocytopenia. The mechanism of IVIg as the treatment of choice for Kawasaki's disease in children (Case 7.3) is unknown, though neutralization of an unknown infective trigger may play a role.

7.2.4 Monoclonal antibodies for specific immunomodulation

A major concern of using rodent monoclonal antibodies is the potential for triggering reactions after repeated usage, with loss of efficacy due to antibodies to the species part of the therapeutic antibody, particularly if effectiveness depends on multiple uses. Production of human monoclonal antibodies, by transforming B cells with EBV or fusing antibody-producing cells with human cell lines, has overcome this problem. An alternative approach has been to **humanize** mouse monoclonal antibodies genetically by transposing their antigen-binding sites (hypervariable regions) onto a human antibody framework (Fig. 7.6); this retains the full range of effector properties of human Fc regions while minimizing the immunogenicity of the mouse component (see Case 7.4).

A wide array of monoclonal antibodies have been developed with the aim of **interrupting interaction between antigen-presenting cells, T cells and B cells** (Fig. 7.7), though not all have been either safe or efficacious (Table 7.4). One volunteer trial in 2006 proved to be positively dangerous, since the anti-CD28 monoclonal antibody resulted in a cytokine storm (Box 7.3). These new therapies require extensive safety and efficacy testing in non-human primates as well as volunteers, which makes them expensive to develop unless the market is large and persistent. However, the advent of monoclonal antibody therapies has transformed several chronic immunological conditions as well as some surprises, e.g. paroxysmal nocturnal

---

Table 7.3 Intravenous immunoglobulin as an immunomodulatory therapeutic agent

Efficacy proven in randomized controlled trials (RCTs)

- Immune thrombocytopenia
- Guillain–Barré syndrome
- Chronic inflammatory demyelinating polyneuropathy
- Kawasaki's disease
- Dermatomyositis
- Lambert–Eaton myasthenic syndrome
- Multifocal motor neuropathy
- Myasthenia gravis in crisis

Ineffective in RCTs

- Post-viral fatigue (chronic fatigue syndrome)
- Rheumatoid arthritis
- Juvenile rheumatoid arthritis
- Multiple sclerosis

A 2-year-old boy was admitted to hospital with a seven-day history of high fever, lymphadenopathy, conjunctivitis and an erythematous exfoliative rash affecting his trunk and extremities (see Fig. 7.5). On the basis of the characteristic clinical picture, a clinical diagnosis of Kawasaki's disease (also known as acute mucocutaneous lymph node syndrome), an acute vasculitic disorder of infants affecting small and medium-sized blood vessels, was made. Other infective causes of a similar clinical presentation were excluded on the basis of negative blood and urine cultures. The results of initial investigations were as follows:

- Hb 110 g/L (NR 120–150).
- White cell count 14 × 10^9 (NR 4–11).
- Platelets 550 × 10^9 (NR 250–400).
- C-reactive protein (CRP) 80 mg/L (NR < 10).

Since untreated or delayed treatment of Kawasaki's disease is associated with the development of coronary artery aneurysms, urgent treatment with high-dose intravenous immunoglobulin (IVIg; total dose 2 g/kg) was given in conjunction with an antiinflammatory doses of aspirin. This led to rapid resolution of fever and normalization of CRP (within 48 h). While IVIg is undoubtedly effective in Kawasaki's disease, the mechanism of action is unclear. For maximum benefit, treatment should be administered within 10 days of onset of fever.

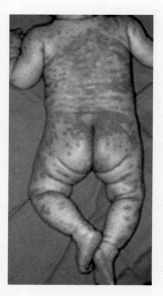

Fig. 7.5 Infant with Kawasaki's disease with an erythematous, predominantly truncal rash. Courtesy of Alexander F. Freeman and Stanford T. Shulman.

Fig. 7.6 Schematic depiction of humanized and chimeric antibodies.

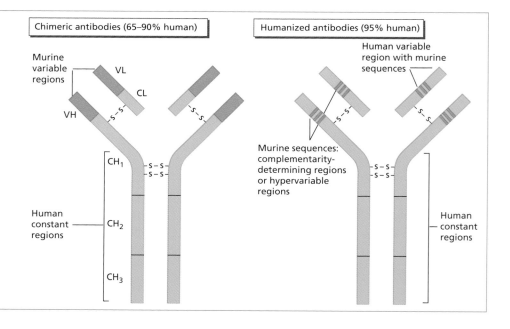

> ### 🔍 Case 7.4 Severe rheumatoid arthritis treated with anti-tumour necrosis factor-α monoclonal antibodies
>
> A 55-year-old woman with active rheumatoid arthritis, previously unresponsive to multiple disease-modifying agents, was treated with a humanized mouse monoclonal antibody to tumour necrosis factor-α (anti-TNF-α) as part of a clinical trial. Following her first uneventful infusion of anti-TNF-α, a significant reduction (60–70%) in clinical indices of inflammation (number of swollen and tender joints, duration of morning stiffness and pain score) and serum C-reactive protein was noted within three days. Clinical and laboratory improvement was sustained for six weeks following the first infusion.

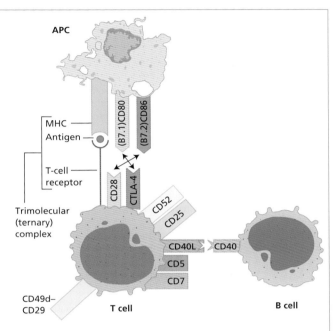

Fig. 7.7 Targets for monoclonal antibodies as immunosuppressive agents. APC, antigen-presenting cell; MHC, major histocompatibility complex.

haemoglobinuria (Chapter 16, section 16.2.4) and wet age-related macular degeneration (ARMD).

The use of **anti-tumour necrosis factor antibodies** (anti-TNF) as a therapeutic agent is an excellent example of targeted immunotherapy (Case 7.4). The success of TNF blockade in rheumatoid arthritis underlines the pivotal proinflammatory role of TNF in this disease (see Chapter 10, Fig. 10.4). TNF blockade can be achieved by the use of either a chimeric anti-TNF antibody (infliximab, adalimumab) or a soluble TNF receptor (etanercept). In clinical practice, therapeutic TNF inhibition is associated with a range of infective complications, in particular a significant risk of reactivation of Mycobacterium tuberculosis. In contrast to tuberculosis (TB) in the immuno-competent, characteristics of TB in the setting of anti-TNF therapy include a preponderance of extrapulmonary disease and poor granuloma formation on histology. The risk of latent TB (which might be activated by anti-TNF therapy) is assessed routinely in immunosuppressed patients by interferon release assays on whole blood (see Chapter 19), which were developed particularly for this indication. New immunological assays to monitor these potent therapies and their side effects are urgently needed.

7.2.5 Other uses of monoclonal antibodies

Monoclonal antibodies also have great potential in diagnosis and in combination treatment. Monoclonal antibodies have promise as **antitumour agents** (Box 7.4). Specific targeting and killing of tumour cells can be achieved by linking the monoclonal antibody to a cytotoxic drug (e.g. methotrexate or vincristine), a toxin (e.g. ricin) or a radioisotope (e.g. iodine-131 or yttrium-90), but cross-reactions of the antibody with normal tissues must be avoided. An example of a licensed antibody–drug conjugate (ADC) is Brentuximab vedotin, a chimeric monoclonal antibody linked to a chemotherapeutic agent (monomethyl auristatin) for the treatment of CD30-positive Hodgkin's lymphoma. Delivery of the ADC to tumour cells by virtue of binding to CD30 leads to internalization and intracellular release of the chemotherapeutic drug to induce cell-cycle arrest and apoptosis.

Radiolabelled antibodies have also been used for **immunolocalization** of tumour deposits, staging of malignant disease and determining the whole-body distribution of amyloid deposits (Chapter 9). Technetium (^{99m}Tc) sulesomab is a mouse monoclonal antibody labelled with technetium-99m, a radionuclide. It is approved for the imaging of infections and inflammations in patients with suspected osteomyelitis. The concern of using mouse monoclonal antibodies applies as much to diagnosis as it does to treatment (section 7.2.4).

Autologous stem cell grafting requires removal of bone marrow from the patient prior to supralethal therapy. Graft-versus-host disease is avoided, but, if tumour cells have already metastasized to bone marrow, they may be returned to the patient. Methods have been developed for **purging bone marrow** of tumour cells. Monoclonal antibodies can kill targeted cells by subsequent addition of complement; however, tumour cells of low antigen density may escape cytolysis, and some tumours are relatively resistant to complement-mediated lysis. An alternative approach has been to link the antibody to toxins such as ricin or abrin. Cells can also be physically trapped, using monoclonal antibodies attached to magnetic beads, and removed with cobalt magnets, before being returned to the patient.

7.2.6 Fusion proteins for blocking receptors

Blocking of specific lymphocyte/monocyte surface receptors has been shown to be useful in a number of conditions, particularly where a **short-term effect** is required as the blockade

Table 7.4 Monoclonal antibodies in current or potential therapeutic use

Antibody	Targets	Clinical use	Comments
Anti-thymocyte globulin (ATG)	T lymphocytes	Rabbit or equine antibodies used for treatment of steroid-resistant graft rejection in Europe and prevention of graft rejection in USA. ATG can induce cytokine release syndrome and increases the risk of post-transplant lymphoproliferative disorder (PTLD), though not when lower doses are used	
Alemtuzumab (CAMPATH-1H)	CD52 on lymphocytes and monocytes	T-cell depletion of bone marrow grafts to prevent graft-versus-host disease; multiple sclerosis, previously used in chronic lymphocytic leukaemia (CLL), rheumatoid arthritis (RA)	Marked prolonged CD4 lymphopenia; prevention of graft rejection in organ transplantation; useful in some patients with multiple sclerosis
Anti-CD3 (OKT-3) Otelixizumab Teplizumab Visilizumab	CD3	Treatment of renal and cardiac graft rejection Currently under investigation in Crohn's disease, ulcerative colitis and type 1 diabetes	Induces cytokine release from all mature T cells, leading to fever, rigors, meningism and hypotension, especially during first infusion Incidence of malignancy among recipients increased
Infliximab	Tumour necrosis factor (TNF)-α	RA, Crohn's disease resistant to conventional immunosuppression, severe ulcerative colitis, ankylosing spondylitis, psoriatic arthritis	Mouse–human chimeric antibody was licensed once benefit confirmed in double-blind placebo-controlled trials
Adalimumab (Humira®)		RA, psoriatic arthritis, ankylosing spondylitis, Crohn's disease, moderate to severe chronic psoriasis, juvenile idiopathic arthritis, and ulcerative colitis	Fully human monoclonal antibody also licensed following several double-blind placebo-controlled trials Both increased risk of developing infections – tuberculosis, histoplasmosis and pneumococcal sepsis
Ruplizumab anti-CD40 L	Activated T cells	Encouraging results in murine lupus But human trials abandoned due to thrombosis in recipients New formulations are being devised	Caution required in humans in view of immunodeficiency associated with lack of CD40L
Rituximab anti-CD20	CD20 on B cells	Refractory B-cell lymphoma/B-cell CLL Granulomatosis with polyangiitis RA and systemic lupus erythematosus (SLE)	Transient B-cell lymphopenia, but B cells in spleen and lymph nodes remain; modest fall in serum immunoglobulins usually recovers within a year Sustained hypogammaglobulinaemia in a minority of patients with B-cell malignancies
Ofatumumab	CD20 on B cells	Chronic lymphocytic leukaemia that is refractory to fludarabine and alemtuzumab; follicular non-Hodgkin's lymphoma, diffuse large B-cell lymphoma	Humanized monoclonal antibody to inhibit early-stage B lymphocyte
Natalizumab (anti-α4-integrins)	α4-integrins (CD49d– CD29)	Multiple sclerosis – severe	Inhibits leucocyte–endothelial interaction, preventing egress of lymphocytes into sites of inflammation, consequently associated with reduced immunosurveillance and high risk of progressive multifocal leucoencephalopathy (JC virus-related PML)
Ipilimumab	CD152	Either as mono- or combination therapy in advanced melanoma or advanced renal cell carcinoma	Anti- cytotoxic T-lymphocyte antigen 4 (CTLA-4) human monoclonal antibody that turns off inhibition of cytotoxic T lymphocytes

Table 7.4 (*Continued*)

Antibody	Targets	Clinical use	Comments
Tocilizumab	Interleukin (IL)-6R	RA, systemic juvenile idiopathic arthritis, giant cell arteritis, treatment of cytokine storm associated with chimeric antigen receptor T (CAR-T) cell therapy	Humanized monoclonal antibody against the interleukin-6 receptor (IL-6R). IL-6 is a cytokine that plays an important role in immune and inflammatory responses
Ustekinumab	IL-12 and IL-23	Moderate to severe plaque psoriasis, Crohn's disease unresponsive to conventional treatment/anti-TNF, ulcerative colitis	Human monoclonal antibody; clinical benefit for psoriasis patients who failed to respond to etanercept. Little long-term data as yet
Eculizumab	Complement protein C5, inhibits MAC formation to prevent uncontrolled intravascular haemolysis	Paroxysmal nocturnal haemoglobulinuria (PNH)	Only treatment available for PNH and atypical haemolytic uremic syndrome (aHUS). Little long-term data as yet
Basiliximab, daclizumab	α chain of the IL-2 receptor on T cells (CD25)	To prevent rejection in organ transplantation, especially in kidney transplants	Blocking chimeric antibody binding to the surface of the activated T lymphocytes Humanized blocking antibody
Mepolizumab	IL-5	Reduces asthma exacerbations in patients with severe eosinophilic asthma (<5% of all asthma); reduced the need for corticosteroids. Also in development for the management of hypereosinophilic syndrome and eosinophilic granulomatosis and polyangiitis	Humanized monoclonal antibody that recognizes IL-5 and eliminates eosinophils from blood, lungs and bone marrow
Omalizumab	IgE	Moderate to severe allergic asthma in patients >6 years old whose asthma is not controlled even with high doses of corticosteroids; severe chronic spontaneous urticaria	Recombinant DNA-derived humanized monoclonal antibody binding to free IgE in blood and interstitial fluid and to membrane-bound form of IgE on mIgE-expressing B lymphocytes; does not bind to IgE that is already bound by the high affinity IgE receptor (FcεRI) on the surface of mast cells, basophils and antigen-presenting dendritic cells. Long-term consequences are unknown
Palivizumab	Respiratory syncytial Virus (RSV)	Prevention (not treatment) in RSV season in high-risk babies because of prematurity or congenital heart disease	Monoclonal antibody produced by recombinant DNA technology directed against the fusion protein of RSV, inhibiting entry into epithelial cell and preventing infection
Bevacizumab (Avastin®) Ranibizumab (Lucentis®)	Vascular endothelial growth factor A (VEGF-A)	'Wet' type of age-related macular degeneration	Monoclonal antibody with anti-angiogenic properties. Clinical trials have shown both to be equally effective
Pembrolizumab	Enhances T-cell function by blocking programmed death (PD-1) on lymphocyte surface	Melanoma, metastatic non-small-cell lung carcinoma, relapsed/refractory Hodgkin's lymphoma, advanced urothelial carcinoma, metastatic head and neck squamous cell carcinoma, renal cell carcinoma	Its efficacy in a wide range of cancers has led pembrolizumab to be regarded as a tissue agnostic monoclonal antibody. Selection of some cancers for treatment depends on tumour expression of PD-L1, the ligand for PD-1
Rozanolixizumab	Anti-FcRn inhibitor; treatment rationale based on reduction in pathogenic autoantibodies	Currently undergoing phase 3 trials in myasthenia gravis	Lowers total serum IgG
Trastuzumab (Herceptin®)	HER receptors in cell membrane that respond to endothelial growth factors to stimulate cell proliferation	Breast cancers in which HER2 is overexpressed	Monoclonal antibody that interferes with the HER2/neu receptor. Controversial – especially in metastatic breast cancer. Also given to prevent recurrence of lesions if given in early stage

---

Box 7.3 Cytokine storm (TeGenero incident)

- A first-in-human volunteer trial with anti-CD28 humanized monoclonal antibody to activate T cells without involving the T-cell receptor; this antibody was termed a 'superagonist'.
- Intended as a treatment for rheumatoid arthritis and other autoimmune diseases (to stimulate regulatory T cells).
- Six individuals were admitted to the ITU at Northwick Park Hospital, UK.
- Life-threatening symptoms occurred <5 min after intravenous infusion.
- Symptoms included headache, fever, joint pains, burning skin, vomiting, abdominal pain, angioedema, hypovolaemia.
- Generalized T-cell activation via CD28 (Fig. 7.4) resulted in polyclonal T-cell expansion, activation and concentration-dependent interleukin (IL)-2 production.
- Eosinophils and neutrophils (CD28⁺) also activated, releasing neurotoxins and other cytokines.
- While the trial drug had been correctly formulated and had met regulatory requirements, subsequent investigations showed that testing in non-human primates appears not to 'predict' cytokine release, probably due to lack of CD28 expression on CD4+ effector memory T cells, thus engendering a false sense of security. In addition human volunteers had, in fact, received a near maximum immunostimulatory dose rather than a low starting dose.

Box 7.4 Criteria for therapeutic targeting of tumour antigens by monoclonal antibodies

- Antigenic target is stable – many tumours have mechanisms to avoid immune surveillance.
- Antigens are expressed homogeneously by tumour cells.
- Antigen is expressed negligibly/not at all in healthy tissues.
- Antigen has little or no soluble form of antigen (to avoid rapid antibody clearance).
- Antigen is easily accessible to plasma/monoclonal antibody given intravenously/subcutaneously.
- Antigen should not be internalized by cells

has a limited time span. Etanercept was the first such product, used to treat autoimmune diseases by acting as a TNF inhibitor over 10 years ago. Recombinant technology is used to fuse the TNF receptor to the Fc region of an IgG1 antibody. The protein binds to TNF-α and has been shown to decrease excess inflammation in patients with several inflammatory arthritides. Belatacept is an IgG Fc linked to the extracellular domain of CTLA-4 to selectively block T-cell activation and is intended to provide extended graft survival. Abatacept is similar and binds with higher avidity to CD80 (B7-1) than to CD86 (B7-2), so blocking co-stimulation of T cells selectively. It is licensed for treatment of rheumatoid arthritis patients who fail to respond to anti-TNF-α therapy (Fig. 7.8).

7.2.7 Small molecule inhibitors

A number of small molecule inhibitors targeting key enzymes involved in cell signalling have been developed as examples of targeted immune-mediated therapies for the treatment of certain cancers and autoimmune diseases. Licensed examples include ibrutinib, an inhibitor of Bruton tyrosine kinase (Btk) in the treatment of B-cell malignancies such as chronic lymphocytic leukaemia and Waldenström's macroglobulinaemia. While germ-line mutations in the Btk gene are associated with X-linked agammaglobulinaemia, in clinical practice the suppressive effects of Btk inhibitors on serum immunoglobulin levels have been modest.

Fig. 7.8 Impact of CTLA-4 fusion protein on T-cell activation.

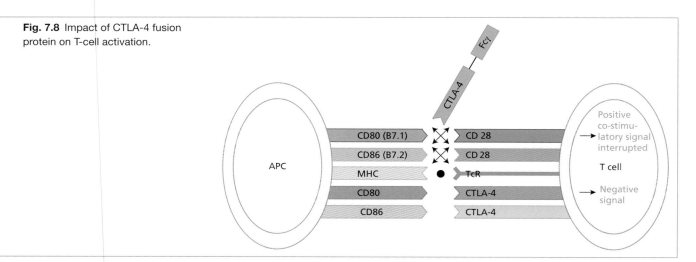

Small molecule inhibitors of the Janus associated kinases (JAK), which act as key intracellular signalling molecules of the JAK-STAT (signal transducer and activator of transcription) pathway, have been licensed for the treatment of refractory rheumatoid arthritis. Examples of licensed JAK inhibitors, also known as jakinibs, include tofacitinib and baricitinib.

7.2.8 Plasmapheresis and plasma exchange

Plasmapheresis involves taking blood, separating off the plasma and returning the red cell-enriched fraction to the patient. In contrast, **plasma exchange** involves the withdrawal of blood, removal of plasma and the return to the patient of the red cell-enriched fraction plus donor plasma. Both are done using mechanical separators, though the returning product varies. In plasmapheresis improvement may be due to the removal of mediators of tissue damage, whereas in plasma exchange it may be due to the replacement of deficient factors. Therapeutic plasmapheresis is used as an adjunct in many diseases in which autoantibodies or high levels of abnormal immunoglobulin are proven or suspected, but clear benefit has been shown in only a few of these diseases (Table 7.5). It is useful in the emergency treatment of hyperviscosity (see Chapter 6), but long-term treatment also requires correction of the underlying disorder.

7.2.9 Total lymphoid irradiation

Total lymphoid irradiation (TLI) produces long-term suppression of helper T-lymphocyte function and is currently used in many centres for human stem cell transplantation (HSCT) for haematological malignancies. Several studies have confirmed that when TLI is used in conjunction with antithymocyte globulin (see Table 7.4), the combination protects against graft-versus-host disease while maintaining the graft-versus-tumour effect (see Chapters 6 and 8). The resulting multilineage chimerism protects against rejection and it may even result in long-term tolerance, since some patients are able to stop immunosuppression completely with specific unresponsiveness to donor alloantigens.

7.2.10 Ultra-violet light

The known value of psoralen and ultra-violet A treatment in psoriasis has led investigators to assess the use of psoralens in other autoimmune diseases. **Extracorporeal photochemotherapy (photopheresis)** is a form of immunotherapy in which peripheral blood lymphocytes, pretreated with the photosensitizing compound 8-methoxypsoralen, are exposed to ultra-violet A irradiation and reinfused into the patient. Psoralens, once photoactivated, bind covalently to target molecules and interrupt function. Photopheresis is largely used for skin diseases: it is of palliative benefit for patients with advanced forms of cutaneous T-cell lymphoma and improves survival; it may be of benefit in the treatment of patients with pemphigus vulgaris and graft-versus-host disease.

7.3 Immunization against infection

Control of infectious diseases depends on eliminating the source of infection, breaking transmission and increasing the resistance of other individuals to new infections. Supply of clean water, better nutrition and improved personal hygiene were major factors in the reduction of infectious diseases in the last two centuries; immunization with vaccines against common diseases reduced this further in the last century; and now new approaches to generate safe, cheap and effective vaccines and greater political will to provide universal coverage will lead to even greater reductions worldwide.

7.3.1 Theoretical basis of immunization

There are two methods of achieving immunity: active and passive immunization. These may be naturally acquired or artificially induced (Fig. 7.9).

Table 7.5 Effects of plasmapheresis in various diseases

System	Examples of diseases	Benefit/indications
Renal	Goodpasture's syndrome Rapidly progressive glomerulonephritis	Treatment of choice in severe disease
	Systemic lupus erythematosus	Only if desperate
Neurological disease	Myasthenia gravis	Yes – in severe disease only
	Guillain–Barré syndrome	Yes – as efficacious as high-dose intravenous immunoglobulin therapy
Haematological disease	Isoimmunization in pregnancy	Yes – maybe several courses
	Thrombotic thrombocytopenic purpura	No – only if plasma replacement therapy is given
Lymphoproliferative disorders	Waldenström's macroglobulinaemia	Yes – for hyperviscosity
	Myeloma	Yes – for hyperviscosity
	Cold agglutinin disease	
	Cryoglobulinaemia	

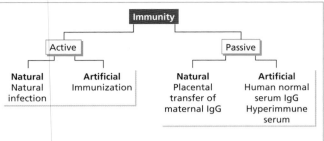

Fig. 7.9 Classification of immunity.

Active immunity is acquired when exposure to an immunogenic stimulus triggers an immune response by the host. The best type of active immunization follows **natural infection**, which may be clinical or subclinical; with many diseases, this gives lifelong protection at minimal cost to the individual (provided they recover without sequelae) or to the community. Artificial active immunization involves the deliberate administration of an immunogen in the form of a vaccine. **Vaccines** may be live organisms, killed organisms, part of the pathogen, modified toxins or coding genes incorporated into a vector such as an adenovirus. The latter rely on uptake of the vector into the recipient's cells, where the gene is transcribed into an immunogenic protein, for example to produce the immunogenic spike glycoprotein in Covid vaccines (see section 7.3.4). Another recent novel approach to Covid vaccines was the injection of the mRNA construct for the spike glycoprotein of SARS-CoV-2. An ideal vaccine should mimic the immunological stimulus associated with natural infection, have no side effects, be readily available, cheap, stable, easily administered and produce long-lasting immunity. This last property is dependent on its fulfilling certain immunological requirements. No current vaccine is ideal; each has its problems. Those encountered with live vaccines are generally related to their safety, while those of killed vaccines relate mainly to effectiveness (Table 7.6).

Live vaccines are selected so that they infect, replicate and immunize in a similar manner to natural infection without causing significant illness. Examples include Bacillus Calmette–Guérin (BCG) for TB, and measles, mumps and rubella (MMR) virus vaccines. Live vaccines must not contain fully virulent organisms and the organisms are therefore **attenuated**, so that their virulence is decreased without

reducing the immune response. The final vaccine represents a balance (see Table 7.6) between diminished pathogenicity and retained immunoreactivity. Even attenuated vaccines may induce disease in the immunocompromised host; an example is disseminated BCG in infants with severe combined immune deficiency (SCID). **Killed vaccines** consist either of suspensions of killed organisms (e.g. typhoid, cholera and whole pertussis) or of products or fractions of the microorganisms (acellular pertussis). They also include toxoids, modified toxins of diphtheria or tetanus, subunits of viruses (split vaccines) and recombinant vaccines. All killed vaccines are immunogenic but not infectious.

The high infection risk for encapsulated bacteria (see Chapter 17, Case 17.1) in infancy has led to the development of **protein–polysaccharide conjugate** vaccines. Unlike pure polysaccharides, conjugate vaccines elicit sustained antibody responses and induce B- and T-cell memory even before the age of 2 years. Examples of conjugate vaccines include those against Haemophilus influenzae type B (Hib), Neisseria meningitidis group C and certain serotypes of Streptococcus pneumoniae. The success of conjugate vaccines is seen by the dramatic reduction in invasive Hib disease following the inclusion of Hib conjugate vaccine in the routine immunization schedule for infants (Fig. 7.10). Similarly, the introduction of the 13-valent pneumococcal conjugate vaccine has led to an over 50% reduction in the incidence of invasive pneumococcal disease, albeit accompanied by a significant increase in disease due to non-vaccine serotypes.

In general, killed vaccines are less successful than live vaccines; when a live vaccine is used, the replicating agent provides an immunogenic stimulus over many days (Box 7.5). To produce the equivalent stimulus with killed vaccine would require a vast dose of antigen, with the risk of producing severe reactions. This problem is partly overcome by combining the vaccine with an adjuvant, a substance that enhances the immune response to the antigen (see section 7.3.2).

7.3.2 Adjuvants

Many purified or synthetic antigenic determinants show poor immunogenicity. *Adjuvants enhance the immune response to an antigen given simultaneously.* Thus, combinations of antigenic subunits and appropriate immunostimulatory compounds may provide a safe and effective vaccine. The best-known adjuvant is

	Live vaccines	Killed vaccines
Advantages	1 Single, small dose 2 Sometimes given by natural route 3 Invokes local and systemic immunity 4 Resembles natural infection	1 Safe 2 Stable, therefore the potential of single batch of vaccine is known (i.e. safety and efficacy)
Disadvantages	1 Contaminating virus? Oncogenic 2 Reversion to virulence by mutation 3 Inactivation by climatic changes 4 Disease in immunocompromised hosts	1 Multiple doses and boosters required 2 Given by injection – unnatural route 3 High antigen concentration needed 4 Variable efficiency

Table 7.6 Relative advantages and disadvantages of vaccines

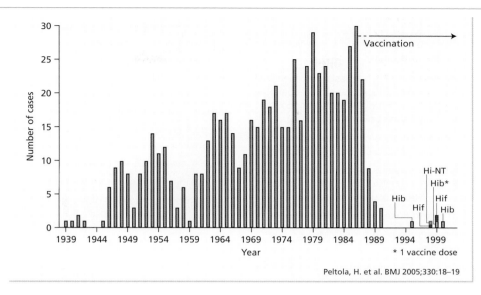

Peltola, H. et al. BMJ 2005;330:18–19

Fig. 7.10 Effect of introduction of Haemophilus influenzae type B (Hib) conjugate vaccine on the incidence of Hib meningitis in Helsinki. Hif, H. influenzae type f; Hi-NT, non-typeable H. influenzae. Source: Peltola et al. Incidence of Haemophilus influenzae type B meningitis during 18 years of vaccine use: observational study using routine hospital data. *BMJ* 2005; 330: 18–19. Reproduced with permission of BMJ Publishing.

Box 7.5 Immunological requirements of a vaccine

1 Activation of antigen-presenting cells to initiate antigen processing and production of cytokines.
2 Activation of both T and B cells to give a high yield of memory cells.
3 Generation of T cells to several epitopes to overcome:
   a Antigenic variation of pathogens.
   b Genetic variability in the host's immune response due to major histocompatibility complex polymorphism.
4 Persistence of antigen on follicular dendritic cells in lymphoid tissue where memory B cells are recruited.

Live attenuated vaccines fulfil these criteria *par excellence* and component vaccines may need adjuvants.

Freund's complete adjuvant, which has been used for many years to stimulate specific antibody production in animals. It contains mycobacteria, oil and a detergent. *Unfortunately, it cannot be used in humans because it induces granulomatous reactions in the spleen, liver and skin.* The active component of mycobacterial membranes is **muramyl dipeptide** (**MDP**), an adjuvant that seems free of toxic side effects and has now been synthesized. Its major action is dendritic cell and macrophage stimulation, with enhancement of T- and B-cell functions.

In humans, the most widely used adjuvants are **aluminium compounds** (**alums**). These form a precipitate with protein antigens and result in slow release of the antigen. Alums

are present in vaccines such as tetanus toxoid and diphtheria toxoid. **Biodegradable polymers** can be used as delayed-release agents, degenerating weeks after injection to release a booster dose of antigen. Numerous adjuvants are under development, many based on an increased understanding of the interplay between the innate and adaptive immune systems. Adjuvants can be designed to target specific innate pattern recognition receptors and thus direct adaptive responses (e.g. Th1, Th2 or Th17).

7.3.3 Routine immunization

Immunization of **children** is one of the most cost-effective activities in healthcare. Table 7.7 shows the schedule currently recommended in the UK, but recommendations for most other developed countries are similar.

Rubella vaccine is given to females to avoid the potentially disastrous effects of rubella on the fetus during early pregnancy. When maternal rubella occurs in the first three months of pregnancy, the risk of congenital infection is about 80%. At present, the vaccine is offered to all infants and to any seronegative women with an occupational risk of acquiring rubella (e.g. nurses). Immunized women must be warned against becoming pregnant for 8–12 weeks after vaccination, because the attenuated vaccine virus can also infect the fetus.

The risk of TB is now so low in the UK that **BCG is not given** unless there is a special indication (Table 7.7). This policy is not applicable in countries where the prevalence of human immunodeficiency virus (HIV) infection is high and there is an increase in tuberculosis (see Chapter 3).

Every vaccine can produce unwanted **side effects** in some people. *The risk of these reactions must be weighed against the*

Table 7.7 Current recommended immunization schedule for the UK

Age	Vaccine and timing
2 months	Diphtheria/tetanus/pertussis + polio vaccine + Haemophilus influenzae type b-conjugate vaccine (Hib) (first dose) + Pneumococcal conjugate vaccine (Pneu) (first dose)
3 months	Diphtheria/tetanus/pertussis + polio vaccine + Hib (second dose) + Men C (first dose)
4 months	Diphtheria/tetanus/pertussis + polio vaccine + Hib (third dose) + Pneu (second dose) + Men C (second dose)
12–13 months	Hib (fourth dose) + Men C (third dose)
	Measles/mumps/rubella (MMR) + Pneu (third dose)
3.4–5 years (school entry)	Diphtheria/tetanus/pertussis + polio Measles/mumps/rubella (MMR) (second dose)
12–13 years (girls only)	Human papillomavirus ×3
13–18 years (school-leaving)	Tetanus/diphtheria + polio vaccine booster

The BCG vaccine is no longer given as part of the UK routine childhood vaccination schedule unless a baby is thought to have an increased risk of coming into contact with TB (i.e. areas where TB rates are higher than in the rest of the country).

Table 7.8 General contraindications to immunization

Absolute contraindications
- Acute systemic febrile illness
- Any severe, local or generalized or neurological reaction to a previous dose of vaccine, particularly pertussis

Particular consideration needed, e.g. about timing
- A documented history of cerebral damage in the neonatal period, convulsions or idiopathic epilepsy
- Severe reaction to previous immunization
- Children with evolving neurological disease
- Immunosuppressed patients – primary or secondary
- Pregnancy

consequences of natural infection. A historical example is whooping cough. The acceptance rate of whooping cough immunization in the UK fell from 80% in 1974 to 31% in 1978 following widespread adverse publicity about unfounded risks of severe nervous system reactions. Whooping cough is a highly infectious and serious disease; over 110 000 cases of whooping cough were notified in the UK between 1977 and 1979, an incidence many times higher than that before the scare; in this time, 26 children died and a similar number suffered brain damage. In contrast, the risk of serious nervous system damage attributable to the full course of pertussis immunization is about 1 : 100 000 children. About 750 000 children die from pertussis in countries without immunization; it is a tragedy that **preventable deaths** on such a scale were to continue because lack of confidence in a vaccine led to failure to implement immunization programmes. Immunization uptake also falls if the public see scientific controversy. Fraudulent evidence relating to adverse effects of MMR vaccine led to reduced immunization rates and deaths from measles rose; the

promulgation of the 'controversy' was ultimately found to be scientific misconduct. The benefits of MMR immunization, both for a child and for society, clearly outweigh the risks, provided that there are no contraindications to immunization (Table 7.8).

Patients with hyposplenism and those who have undergone splenectomy are at risk from overwhelming pneumococcal infection (Case 7.5). This is because splenic B lymphocytes are important in the production of protective antibody (IgG_2) against pneumococcal cell wall and other carbohydrate antigens. **Polysaccharide pneumococcal vaccine** contains polysaccharide antigens of the 23 most common serotypes encountered in Europe, while the pneumococcal conjugate vaccine contains 13 serotypes. Immunization offers some protection (about 60% efficacy) in these patients and should therefore be performed before elective splenectomy and in all patients with known functional hyposplenism. In the UK, immunization is also offered to patients with lymphoma, chronic renal failure, HIV infection and to those undergoing transplantation; in the USA, the recommendations are more liberal.

Children under 2 years old respond poorly to this carbohydrate vaccine, but mount adequate antibody responses to pneumococcal conjugate vaccines.

Polypeptide vaccines from immunogenic subunits lack infectious viral activity, but individually are less immunogenic; the way in which the subunits are presented to the host greatly influences the response. The HPV vaccine is an example in which viral surface proteins are aggregated to form noninfectious virus-like particles.

Despite new methods for producing vaccines (section 7.3.6), there are many infections for which no vaccines are available at

Case 7.5 Fatal pneumococcal sepsis eight years following splenectomy

A 35-year-old man felt non-specifically unwell for 24 h before being found collapsed at home. Despite intensive attempts at resuscitation by ambulance staff, he was pronounced dead on arrival in hospital. Post-mortem examination revealed acute bacterial pneumonia and meningitis due to Streptococcus pneumoniae. His previous medical history was unremarkable except for a ruptured spleen following a road traffic accident, necessitating emergency splenectomy, eight years previously. It transpired that immunization with 'Pneumovax' (23 valent pneumococcal polysaccharide) had been overlooked at the time and the patient's compliance with subsequent antibiotic prophylaxis had been erratic.

present, for instance HIV, Epstein–Barr virus (EBV), leprosy and malaria.

7.3.4 Immunization against SARS-CoV-2

The Covid-19 pandemic caused by the SARS-CoV-2 virus resulted in a concerted scientific effort leading to the development of effective vaccines at breakneck speed. Unlike conventional vaccine development, which typically takes 10–15 years or longer from animal studies to human trials followed by regulatory approval, remarkably the first approved vaccines were administered to humans less than a year following publication of the viral genome (Fig. 7.11). The fact that this was achieved without compromising on safety is testament to the heroic efforts of scientists and clinicians in developing suitable vaccine platforms and undertaking robust international clinical trials to provide evidence of immunogenicity, efficacy and safety.

Vaccine development against SARS-CoV-2 uses the spike glycoprotein of SARS-CoV-2 as the target antigen and the key component of the virus responsible for entry into host cells. A range of approaches have been used. These include the use of inactivated or weakened virus, encapsulating the spike glycoprotein into a non-replicating adenoviral vector, mRNA-based technology to instruct host cells to produce spike protein and the use of protein subunit vaccines. Of these approaches, vaccines based on adenoviral vectors and mRNA technology are now in worldwide use. Vaccine efficacy is dependent on producing durable antibody and T-cell-based immune responses.

7.3.5 Immunization for travellers

Although no vaccine is 100% effective, vaccine-preventable diseases affect significant numbers of UK travellers each year. A very high proportion of typhoid and paratyphoid cases in the UK are acquired abroad, mainly in South Asia. **Typhoid vaccine** should be considered for any UK resident travelling to endemic areas, as should inactivated **hepatitis A** vaccine, which is safe and immunogenic in 86% of recipients. Other vaccines that may be offered include rabies (inactivated rabies virus particles) and hepatitis B (recombinant).

Many diseases acquired by travellers are not preventable by vaccination. Cases of malaria continue to increase, particularly among travellers to West Africa. Travellers should be advised of mosquito bite-prevention methods, such as nets and repellents,

and the use of chemoprophylaxis. All travellers should also be **informed and educated** on food and water consumption, personal hygiene and the high risks of sexually transmitted diseases, particularly HIV infection.

7.3.6 Passive immunization

At-risk patients exposed to certain infections can be given some degree of passive protection using human normal immunoglobulin or human-specific immunoglobulin. Passive immunity is short-lived because these IgG antibodies are slowly catabolized (half-life 3–4 weeks). **Human normal immunoglobulin**, in the form of intravenous or subcutaneous immunoglobulin, is essential treatment for patients with primary antibody deficiency (see Chapter 3, section 3.2.8). Units selected for high-titre specific antibodies, **human-specific immunoglobulins**, are used in particular exposure situations: these include short-term prophylaxis against measles in immunosuppressed children and immediate short-lived protection against hepatitis A in non-immunized individuals. High-titre anti-CMV antibody products are used for CMV prophylaxis, most often in kidney transplant patients, and varicella zoster hyperimmune immunoglobulin may be indicated in exposed children and adults with acute leukaemia or on chemotherapy, though with effective antiviral therapies to hand this becomes less necessary.

Monoclonal antibodies allow more specific protection against infection, but the results to date in humans have been largely disappointing, though the first rabies-specific monoclonal antibodies are undergoing clinical trials to replace polyclonal or equine products.

7.4 Immune potentiation other than vaccines

Immune potentiation as a form of treatment is evolving. The need to increase an immune response generally runs the risk of autoimmune diseases or cytokine storms (Box 7.3). The most specific forms of immune restoration involve replacement of a missing enzyme (adenosine deaminase – see Chapter 3), adjunct cytokine therapy or gene therapy. Potentiation by infusion of specific T cells, adoptive immunization, involves the transfer of mature circulating lymphocytes, but is rarely used in humans as it requires MHC histocompatible donors and carries severe risks of graft-versus-host disease. This technique has been used in humans to treat certain diseases, including some types of cancer and immunodeficiency.

7.4.1 Cytokine therapy

The most widely used cytokines in clinical practice are the **interferons**. These are antiviral glycoproteins produced in response to virus infections and they have wide-ranging immunomodulatory and antitumour effects (Table 7.9). There are

---

Covid-19 vaccines developed at breakneck speed

- Publication of Covid-19 genome 11.1.20
- Declaration of pandemic by WHO 30.1.20
- First trial participants in phase I trials vaccinated 16.3.20
- Approval by UK MHRA 2.12.20

Fig. 7.11 Timeline of Covid vaccine development.

Table 7.9 Antitumour and immunomodulatory properties of interferons

Antitumour effects	Immunomodulatory effects
1 Direct antiproliferative effect on certain tumour cells 2 Increased tumour cell antigenicity • Enhanced MHC expression • Enhanced expression of receptors for TNF • Stimulation of NK cell activity	1 Macrophage activation 2 Induction of MHC antigens 3 Stimulation of NK cell activity 4 Activation of cytotoxic T cells

MHC, major histocompatibility complex; NK cells, natural killer cells; TNF, tumour necrosis factor.

three families of human interferon: alpha (α), beta (β) (the type I interferons) and gamma (γ) (type II interferon). Interferons bind to cell-surface receptors and trigger secondary intracellular changes that inhibit viral replication. Genetically engineered, recombinant IFN-α, -β and -γ are available, but **IFN-α** is the best studied and since IFN-α is now conjugated to polyethylene glycol (PEG), the half-life is considerably extended, making PEG–IFN-α treatment regimens more acceptable. Response rates to IFN-α therapy vary in different malignancies. In hairy cell leukaemia, cutaneous T-cell lymphoma and metastatic renal cell carcinoma, IFN-α has a role in management of these otherwise poorly responsive malignancies.

PEG–IFN-α, in combination with antiviral medications, was previously included in treatment regimens for **hepatitis B and C**. Given systemically, IFN-α produces significant clearing of hepatitis B (HBV) in chronic carriers infected during adolescence or adult life, but has no effect on those infected at birth (see Chapter 14). PEG–IFN and ribavirin treatment leads to a sustained virological response (equivalent to cure of infection) in around 50–60% of patients with chronic hepatitis C (HCV). However, a revolution in HBV and HCV treatment has led to the development of effective interferon-free regimens using protease inhibitors. Quantification of viral genomes and analysis of their sequence to determine the genotype or subtype and identification of nucleotide or amino acid substitutions associated with resistance to antiviral drugs are already available. Although IFN-α has **toxic effects**, these are usually tolerable, such as flu-like symptoms, fever, malaise, anorexia and mental confusion. However, more serious problems include reversible bone marrow suppression, proteinuria, liver dysfunction and cardiotoxicity. Exacerbations of autoimmune disease, including thyroiditis, have also been reported. Some patients make low-titre antibodies to IFN-α while on treatment, but have not developed clinical problems as a result.

IFN-β (interferon β-1b, interferon β-1a) has been shown, in randomized trials, to reduce the frequency of attacks in 50% of patients with relapsing–remitting multiple sclerosis (see Chapter 17). IFN-β-1a also slowed progression of disability, and patients remained attack free for several years. Recent work

shows that the pathogenesis in those who do not respond involves a pathway involving Th17 cells and hence IFN-β is ineffective.

IFN-γ is a potent activator of macrophages and is most impressive in conditions in which defective macrophage function occurs, for instance lepromatous leprosy, leishmaniasis and chronic granulomatous disease (CGD). In CGD (Chapter 3), IFN-γ increases phagocyte bactericidal activity, but only some patients show enhanced superoxide production, implying that IFN-γ works by several mechanisms. IFN-γ is currently used in selected patients with CGD in whom prophylactic co-trimoxazole is inadequate to prevent infection; in these patients there is a 70% reduction of severe infections.

IL-2 is produced by stimulated CD4$^+$ T cells (see Chapter 1) and acts on recently synthesized IL-2 receptors (CD25 antigen) to induce clonal expansion of IL-2-positive T and B cells and stimulating activity of NK cells. IL-2 is used in malignant diseases or infections where weak immune responses are amplified by IL-2 (Fig. 7.12). Genetically engineered, recombinant IL-2 has been used in the treatment of metastatic renal cell carcinoma and malignant melanoma, but has recently been overshadowed by more effective immunotherapy targeted at immune check-point molecules. Treatment is limited by the **toxicity of IL-2**: common side effects are flu-like malaise, mild bone marrow suppression and abnormal liver function. The most serious side effect is the vascular leak syndrome: IL-2 infusion provokes massive release of IL-1, IFN-γ and TNF, all mediators of vascular permeability, with consequent marked hypotension, fluid retention, pulmonary oedema and neuropsychiatric symptoms.

Granulocyte colony-stimulating factor (G-CSF) and **granulocyte/macrophage colony-stimulating factor (GM-CSF)** are cytokines readily synthesized by recombinant DNA technology. They not only have a powerful stimulating effect on production of granulocytes (G-CSF) and monocytes/macrophages (GM-CSF), but also enhance the function of mature granulocytes and monocytes. When infused into patients, G-CSFs shorten the period of severe neutropenia caused by radiotherapy or cytotoxic drugs, in which infections are the major cause of morbidity and mortality. The myeloprotective effect of these factors has allowed oncologists to boost the doses of cytotoxics used, with a consequent improvement in the chance of cure, without apparently increasing the morbidity of treatment. Growth factors have **other uses** (Table 7.10).

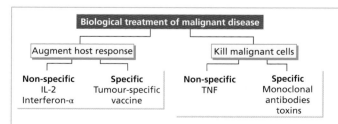

Fig. 7.12 Biological treatments in malignant disease. IL-2, interleukin-2; TNF, tumour necrosis factor.

Table 7.10 Potential clinical applications of recombinant haematopoietic colony-stimulating factors

Use	Examples
1 Reduce duration/degree of myelosuppression following chemotherapy	Small-cell lung cancer Carcinoma of bladder Carcinoma of breast Metastatic melanoma
2 Augment haematological reconstitution following haematopoietic stem cell transplantation (HSCT)	Non-Hodgkin's lymphoma Severe combined immune deficiency (SCID)
3 Facilitate harvesting of bone marrow stem cells	Prior to autologous HSCT
4 Treatment of leukaemia with cytotoxic drugs or toxins	Acute myeloid leukaemia
5 Treatment of other neutropenic states	Aplastic anaemia Cyclical/congenital neutropenias Myelodysplastic syndromes AIDS
6 Improve host defence against potential infection	Burns

7.4.2 Gene therapy

Since the demonstration that genes could be successfully transferred into humans in 1990, gene therapy has become established as an alternative strategy to HSCT in carefully selected individuals (Box 7.6).

Building on promising results in SCID due to adenosine deaminase deficiency, gene therapy has recently been extended to X-linked SCID associated with mutations in the common γ-chain cytokine receptor and CGD. Using a retroviral vector (Fig. 7.13), several children with this form of SCID are currently in remission, with durable restitution of T- and B-cell function. Delight at the apparent success of gene therapy was dampened by the development of T-cell leukaemia several years after engraftment due to **insertional mutagenesis** affecting the LMO2 oncogene, a possibility that had been feared. Instead, the use of a lentiviral vector has proved to be more successful, leading to sustained broad immune reconstitution without leukaemogenesis. Recovery of B-cell function was sufficiently robust to allow cessation of immunoglobulin replacement therapy in up to 50% of children.

The potential for somatic gene therapy is enormous, but this form of treatment must be shown to be ethically acceptable. Cloning of non-reproductive cells is permitted under strict regulatory approval in the UK purely for the purposes of therapeutic research. Recipients face the **risk** of vector-induced inflammation (as seen with some adenoviral vectors in cystic fibrosis), overwhelming viral infection by the vector (not seen yet) and the possibility, with retroviral vectors, of insertional mutagenesis, though inclusion of inactivation genes may prevent this. Encouraging results with an adenoviral vector given intravenously in haemophilia B indicate that progress is possible.

7.4.3 Cancer immunotherapy

Cancer immunotherapy offers a potentially exciting method of generating an effective antitumour immune response. It builds upon the widely recognized concept of immunosurveillance against cancer (Boxes 7.7 and 7.8), which has provided the impetus for immunotherapy.

Most cancers express tumour-associated antigens that are presented by antigen-presenting cells to T cells through either the MHC class II or I pathways. The principles of immunotherapy in cancer are summarized in Box 7.8. Since malignant melanoma fulfils the criteria for immunotherapy, there has been much interest in developing vaccines containing peptides derived from melanoma-specific antigens such as MAGE or melanocyte differentiation antigens. However, peptide-based immunotherapy has been overtaken by the dramatic tumour regression observed with monoclonal antibodies targeting T-cell inhibitory cell-surface molecules – cytotoxic T-lymphocyte associated protein 4 (CTLA-4), programmed cell death 1 receptor (PD-1) – and the ligand for PD-1 on cancer cells, known as PD-L1. Given that these agents enhance T-cell function, the emergence of severe iatrogenic systemic autoimmune disease (colitis, endocrinopathies, hypophysitis, myasthenia gravis, pneumonitis) has been a predictable but manageable adverse effect. For metastatic melanoma, the success of immunotherapy with anti-CTLA-4 and anti-PD1 agents is such that it has supplanted conventional chemotherapy as the treatment of choice.

Monoclonal antibody-based therapies that recognize particular target antigens on tumours are highly successful; more than 15 monoclonal antibodies have been approved for clinical use in the European Union and in the USA. Trastuzumab (Herceptin®) is probably the best known; this monoclonal antibody blocks HER receptors in the cell membrane of breast cancer cells that

---

Box 7.6 Requirements for successful gene therapy

- A single genetic abnormality being responsible for the defect.
- The normal gene being identified, cloned and inserted into a suitable vector (retroviruses, lentiviruses, adenoviruses, plasmid–liposomal complexes).
- Cells with the inserted gene proliferating normally when reintroduced into the host to replace the defective cell population.
- The gene product being detectable, to allow evaluation of the outcome.
- Consistent insertion of the vector, avoiding oncogenic sites.

Fig. 7.13 Gene therapy for severe combined immunodeficiency (SCID) associated with mutations in the common γ-chain gene. The use of a retroviral vector has now been supplanted by a lentivirus.

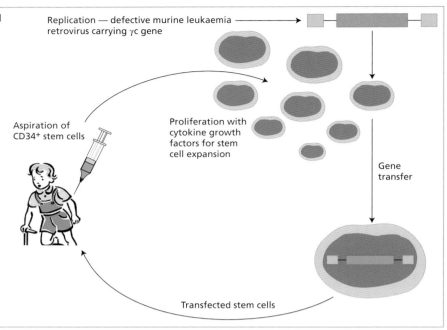

Replication — defective murine leukaemia retrovirus carrying γc gene

Aspiration of CD34+ stem cells

Proliferation with cytokine growth factors for stem cell expansion

Gene transfer

Transfected stem cells

Box 7.7 Evidence for immunosurveillance against cancer in humans

- Tumours arise frequently at periods of relative immune incompetence in the young and the old.
- Tumours arise frequently in primary immunodeficient patients.
- Kaposi sarcoma and lymphoid tumours in HIV patients.
- Skin and lymphoid tumours in those on long-term immunosuppressive therapy for transplantation.
- Presence of tumour-infiltrating lymphocytes correlates with longer survival and rare instances of spontaneous tumour regression.
- Immune responses to tumour-specific antigens can be demonstrated *in vivo* and *in vitro*.
- Clinical success of immune check-point inhibitors (anti-PD1, anti-PD-L1, anti-CTLA-4) in enhancing T-cell mediated therapeutic responses against various cancers.

Box 7.8 Requirements for effective immunotherapy in cancer

- For a particular tumour-associated antigen to be used as a target, it must be expressed exclusively in the tumour.
- A sufficient number of tumour-reactive lymphocytes must be capable of infiltrating the cancer.
- Intratumoural lymphocytes should have the appropriate effector mechanisms to destroy cancer cells.

7.4.4 Chimeric antigen receptor T-cell therapy

Genetically engineered host or allogeneic T cells containing immunoglobulin-derived heavy and light chains specific for a target antigen (single-chain variable fragment, scFv) grafted onto a T-cell-activating domain are known as CAR-T cells (Fig. 7.14).

CAR-T cells with this combination of antibody-directed specificity and T-cell-activating domains (CD28 or 4-1BB, also known as CD137) contained in a single molecule have proven to be remarkably successful in children with refractory B-cell acute lymphoblastic leukaemia (B-ALL) in whom conventional chemotherapy has failed, and in adults with B-cell lymphoma. In contrast to conventional T cells, recognition of target antigen by CAR-T cells is not HLA restricted. To date, two autologous anti-CD19 CAR-T cell products (tisagenlecleucel and axicabtagene ciloleucel) have been approved by the US Food and Drug Administration (FDA). Autologous CAR-T cells are a good example of personalized cellular therapy involving the removal of peripheral blood T cells from the patient by apheresis, followed by sequential steps in a specialist laboratory involving T-cell activation, incorporation of the virus encoding the relevant CAR,

would otherwise respond to epithelial growth factor stimulation and result in cell proliferation. Breast cancers in which HER2 is overexpressed are susceptible to long-term therapy with this monoclonal antibody and treatment may prevent recurrence of lesions if given in the early stages (Table 7.4). Rituximab, the anti-CD20 monoclonal, has transformed the treatment of lymphoid malignancies. Other monoclonal antibody-based therapies are in clinical trials, including bispecific monoclonal antibodies and multispecific fusion proteins and monoclonal antibodies conjugated with small molecule drugs. However, problems remain, including resistance to therapy, access to target cells and managing the iatrogenic adverse effects associated with suppressing physiological immune interactions.

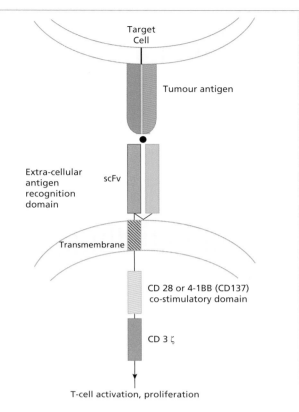

Fig. 7.14 Schematic representation of a CAR-T cell.

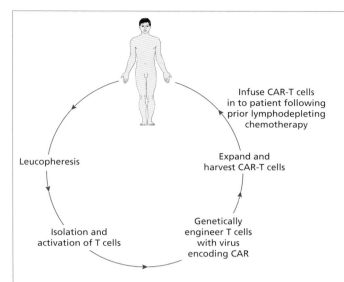

Fig. 7.15 Schematic representation of adoptive cell therapy with CAR-T cells.

expansion and harvest of CAR-T cells prior to reinfusion into the patient (Fig. 7.15).

The remarkable efficacy of CD19 CAR-T cells needs to be balanced with a range of significant adverse effects. B-cell aplasia is a recognized and predictable direct on-target pharmacodynamic consequence of therapy and is mitigated by immunoglobulin replacement therapy in most patients, until B-cell reconstitution occurs. Current evidence suggests that this is likely to take over a year in children, with a shorter time period in adults. Another on-target adverse effect of CAR-T cells is an acute cytokine release syndrome occurring within days of infusion. It is characterized by fever, hypotension, hypoxia and confusion and associated with widespread cytokine release, in particular IL-6. Consequently, tocilizumab (anti-IL-6 receptor) is used to dampen the inflammatory process and its efficacy in doing so has led to its being licensed by the FDA for this purpose.

CHAPTER 8
Transplantation

Key topics

 Visit the companion website at **www.wiley.com/go/misbah/immunology** to download cases with additional figures on these topics.

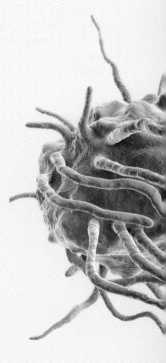

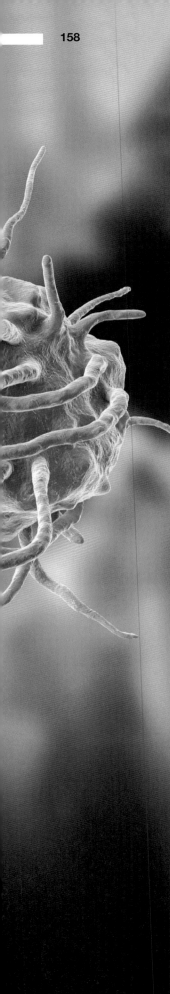

Chapel and Haeney's Essentials of Clinical Immunology, Seventh Edition. Edited by Siraj A. Misbah, Gavin P. Spickett, and Virgil A.S.H. Dalm.

8.1 Introduction

Transplantation of living cells, tissues or organs is well established as a routine practice. Cells (e.g. red blood cells, stem cells), tissues (e.g. skin grafting in extensively burned patients) or whole organs (such as kidney, heart, lung, pancreas or liver) may be successfully transferred between genetically dissimilar individuals (**allogeneic grafting**). The outcome depends on the degree of 'matching' of the relevant transplantation antigens of the two individuals and successful therapeutic immunosuppressive measures to prevent rejection. In contrast, grafting of an individual's tissue from one part of the body to another (**autologous grafting**) is always successful, provided there are no procedural setbacks.

8.2 Histocompatibility genetics in humans

The surfaces of all human cells express a series of molecules that are recognized by other individuals as foreign antigens. Some antigens, such as those of the rhesus blood group, are not relevant to the successful transplantation of human organs. In contrast, the **ABO blood group** system on red blood cells and the **human leucocyte antigens** (HLA) on lymphocytes and other tissues are extremely important in blood transfusion and organ transplantation. HLA antigens are also called 'histocompatibility antigens', since they play a crucial role in determining the survival of transplanted organs. They are encoded in humans by a segment of chromosome 6 known as the **major histocompatibility complex** (**MHC**; see Chapter 1). Additional antigenic systems (minor histocompatibility systems) play only a minor role in transplantation and are largely ignored in clinical practice.

At least six HLA loci are recognized (Fig. 8.1). The HLA-A and HLA-B loci were the first to be defined and these encode a large number of antigens (see Chapter 1). Together with the HLA-C locus, these **MHC class I genes** code for products of similar biochemical structure that serve similar functions (see Chapter 1). They are detectable on all nucleated cells in the body. The methods of **tissue typing**, i.e. the detection of HLA antigens, are described in Chapter 19.

In contrast to antigens of the HLA-A, -B and -C loci, HLA-DR, -DQ and -DP loci antigens are restricted to B lymphocytes, macrophages, epidermal cells and sperm. The antigens of the D loci differ from MHC class I antigens in their chemical structure and interactions with immune cell populations; they are called **MHC class II antigens** (see Chapter 1).

In renal transplantation, **matching** for the MHC class II antigens is more important than MHC class I antigen compatibility in determining graft survival. Matching for the ABO blood group system is also important; naturally occurring anti-A and anti-B antibodies can lead to hyperacute rejection of ABO-incompatible kidneys, since A and B antigens are expressed on endothelium.

In bone marrow transplantation, a complete HLA class I and II match gives the best survival; this is provided by an autologous graft, HLA-identical sibling or matched unrelated donor. Mismatched bone marrow invariably induces graft-versus-host disease (GVHD), with reduced survival of the graft (see section 8.5.3). The proximity of the HLA loci means that their antigenic products tend to be inherited together as an 'HLA haplotype'. Because one haplotype is inherited from each parent, there is a one in four chance that two siblings will possess identical pairs of haplotypes (Fig. 8.2).

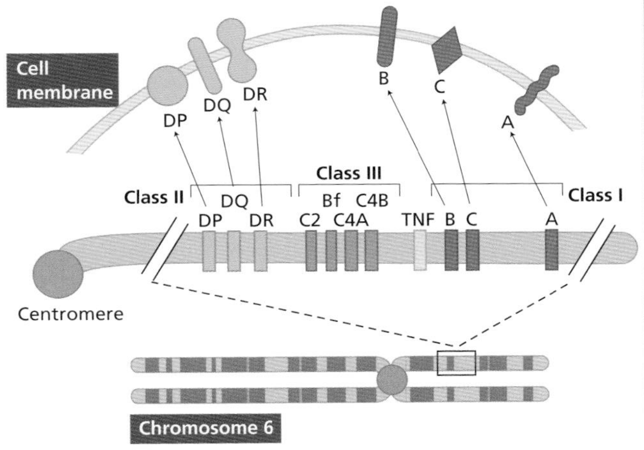

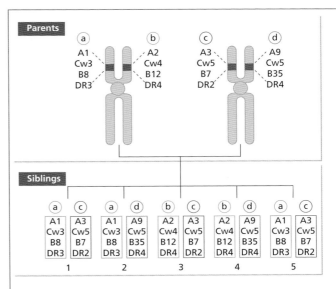

Fig. 8.2 Inheritance of human leucocyte antigen (HLA) haplotypes in a family. Siblings 1 and 5 are HLA identical. Haplotypes are denoted as a, b, c, d.

Fig. 8.1 Major histocompatibility complex on chromosome 6; class III antigens include complement components.

8.3 Renal transplantation

Kidney transplantation is now widely available for the treatment of end-stage chronic renal failure. Haemodialysis and continuous ambulatory peritoneal dialysis have enabled patients to come to transplantation in a state fit to withstand major surgery. The survival figures for transplanted kidneys have shown progressive improvement over the decades because of better immunosuppression, with consequent reduction in mortality of patients. A kidney transplant is the treatment of choice for most patients in end-stage renal failure.

8.3.1 Selection of recipient and donor

Criteria for **selection of patients** for renal transplantation vary between centres. Extreme old age, severe sepsis, a severe bleeding tendency or any other contraindications to high-dose steroids make a patient unacceptable as a potential recipient. Once selected, the patient has to wait for a suitably matched kidney to become available. Kidneys may be donated by living or deceased individuals.

The **selection of deceased donor (also known as cadaveric) kidneys** is rigorous (Fig. 8.3). A donor blood sample is taken as a source of DNA used to identify MHC class I and class II by molecular methods. In addition to the kidney, the spleen and some lymph nodes are also removed and may be disrupted, to extract lymphocytes for HLA typing (see Chapter 19). *Only patients with an ABO blood group compatible with the kidney donor* are considered suitable recipients; as in blood transfusion, a group O kidney can be transplanted to any recipient. Once the ABO blood group and HLA type of a deceased donor kidney are known, the national register of potential recipients is searched to find an ABO-compatible patient who matches the donor at as many loci as possible. Having selected the recipient, the **recipient's serum is then crossmatched against the donor's lymphocytes** (Fig. 8.4). The presence of any antibody against

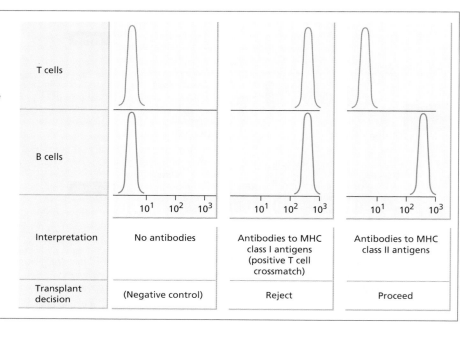

From living relative
• Donor has two functioning kidneys • No transmissible disease • No anomalous blood vessels • Psychologically stable • Excellent health

From cadaver
• Good renal fuction • No infection (clinical sepsis, HIV) • No malignancy or systemic disease (diabetes, hypertension) • Short warm ischaemia time

Recipient selection
• ABO compatible (not identical) • Negative serum cross match with donor's T lymphocytes • HLA match – as near as possible, especially at D loci

Fig. 8.3 Requirements for successful renal transplantation: selection of donor/recipient. HIV, human immunodeficiency virus; HLA, human leucocyte antigen.

donor HLA is a risk factor for rejection and if the patient has cytotoxic antibodies to donor class I antigens (positive T-cell crossmatch), then the kidney is unsuitable for that recipient.

Relatives who are anxious to donate a **live donor kidney** must be screened clinically and psychologically (see Fig. 8.3), and ABO and HLA typed so that the most suitable donor can be chosen. As discussed earlier, there is a one in four chance that a sibling will have the identical HLA haplotype (see Fig. 8.2). Where a compatible donor cannot be found, an

Fig. 8.4 Schematic representation of detection of cytotoxic antibodies in renal transplant recipients by flow cytometric crossmatching. Fluorescence intensity is depicted on the horizontal axis and the number of donor cells on the vertical axis (see Chapter 19 for discussion of flow cytometry). Major histocompatibility (MHC) class II antigens are expressed on B cells but not on T cells; MHC class I antigens are expressed on both.

T cells			
B cells			
Interpretation	No antibodies	Antibodies to MHC class I antigens (positive T cell crossmatch)	Antibodies to MHC class II antigens
Transplant decision	(Negative control)	Reject	Proceed

attempt is made to choose someone with the least disparity at the HLA-B and HLA-DR loci, as these are the most important loci governing rejection of the graft.

Once the kidneys have been removed from either donor type, they are perfused mechanically with physiological fluids. Provided that cooling is begun within 30 minutes of cessation of the renal blood supply (**warm ischaemia time**), these kidneys have an excellent chance of functioning in the selected recipient. The duration of the perfusion (**cold ischaemia time**) should be less than 48 hours. Damage to the graft during the ischaemic period leads to expression of tissue injury molecules (DAMPs: damage-associated molecular patterns), including heparan sulphate, heat-shock proteins and expression of Toll-like receptors, which activate the immune response and damage the graft when the vascular anastomosis is completed and circulation restored. The transplanted kidney is usually sited in the iliac fossa. Great care is taken with the vascular anastomoses and ureteric implantation. Once the vascular anastomoses are complete, the graft often starts to function immediately.

8.3.2 Post-transplantation period

In the post-transplantation period, the graft and the patient must both be monitored. There are several reasons why renal function may deteriorate immediately after surgery (Fig. 8.5). **Acute tubular necrosis** can occur due to low blood pressure in either the recipient or the donor. If this happens, the recipient can be dialysed until renal function recovers; this rarely takes longer than 3–4 weeks. Alternatively, poor renal function may indicate **hyperacute rejection**, **urinary obstruction**, which must be relieved surgically, or a **vascular event**; arterial perfusion and venous drainage can be assessed by duplex ultrasonography.

It is crucial to *distinguish rejection from infection*, since the treatment for a bacterial infection is an antibiotic, not an increase in immunosuppressive therapy. Regular core renal biopsies may be performed, but the procedure can damage the kidney and should not be done more than once every few

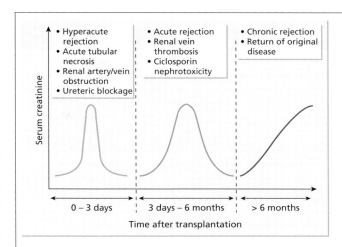

Fig. 8.5 Causes of graft failure.

weeks. Detection of rejection by **frequent percutaneous fine-needle aspiration** is much less traumatic, gives quick results and allows identification of infiltrating monocytes and increased expression of MHC class II molecules on renal tubular cells in the cortex – features of rejection (Case 8.1).

Immunosuppressive therapy (Table 8.1) is intended to prevent graft rejection and remains an essential component of management. Immunosuppressive drugs are fully discussed in Chapter 7.

The introduction of **calcineurin inhibitors** – ciclosporin and later tacrolimus – in the mid-1980s significantly improved short-term renal graft survival by lowering acute rejection rates, but chronic nephrotoxicity was a cause of declining transplant function. Hence, *various combinations are used to avoid such nephrotoxicity*, including monoclonal antibodies, mycophenolate mofetil or rapamycin (sirolimus) or everolimus. Most protocols reserve lymphocyte-depleting monoclonal antibodies for rejection therapy, and use steroids and ciclosporin or tacrolimus for prophylaxis. Conversion from a calcineurin inhibitor-based

---

🔍 Case 8.1 Acute rejection

An 18-year-old student with end-stage renal failure due to chronic glomerulonephritis was given a deceased donor kidney transplant. He had been on maintenance haemodialysis for 2 months, and on antihypertensive therapy for several years. His major blood group was A and his tissue type was HLA-A1, -A9, -B8, -B40, -Cw1, -Cw3, -DR3, -DR7. The donor kidney was also blood group A and was matched for one HLA-DR antigen and four of six HLA-ABC antigens. The patient was given triple immunosuppressive therapy with ciclosporin, azathioprine and prednisolone.

He passed 5 L of urine on the second post-operative day and his urea and creatinine fell appreciably. However, on the seventh post-operative day, his graft became slightly tender, his serum creatinine increased and he had a mild pyrexia (37.8 °C). A clinical diagnosis of acute rejection was confirmed by a finding of lymphocytic infiltration of the renal cortex on fine-needle aspiration. A 3-day course of intravenous methylprednisolone was started; 24 hours later his creatinine had fallen and urine volume increased.

Subsequently, the patient had similar rejection episodes 5 and 7 weeks post-operatively. Both were treated with intravenous corticosteroids, and he has since remained well for over 3 years. Ciclosporin A was discontinued after 9 months, but he still takes a daily maintenance dose of immunosuppressive drugs, namely 5 mg prednisolone and 50 mg azathioprine.

Table 8.1 Drugs used as antirejection therapy in renal transplantation

Prevention of graft rejection	Treatment of acute rejection
Prednisolone	Methylprednisolone
Ciclosporin	Antithymocyte globulin
Tacrolimus (FK506)	Rituximab
Mycophenolate mofetil	Intravenous immunoglobulin
Sirolimus/everolimus	Eculizumab
Monoclonal antibodies against the α chain of the interleukin (IL)-2 receptor (CD25) on T cells or CD52 (CAMPATH-1)	
Belatacept (CTLA-4-IgG1 Fc fusion molecule)	
OKT3, anti-CD3 monoclonal antibody.	

regimen to another long-term agent such as rapamycin (sirolimus) or everolimus (mTOR inhibitors) is undertaken between 3 and 6 months post transplant. Immunosuppression in **children** undergoing kidney transplantation is more difficult and mycophenolate mofetil-based regimens with low-dose calcineurin inhibitor therapy and corticosteroids are preferable. In patients with chronic allograft dysfunction and over-immunosuppression leading to recurrent infections, **mycophenolate mofetil and corticosteroids** are more appropriate. Results show that for regimens consisting of a calcineurin inhibitor combined with mycophenolate mofetil and corticosteroids, > 90% of all renal grafts are functioning after 1 year, with 77% and 56% at 5 and 10 years, respectively. Additionally, in some centres monoclonal antibody therapy is included in the induction stage to reduce the risk of acute rejection. The most commonly used are basiliximab or daclizumab (against the α-chain of the interleukin [IL]-2 receptor on T cells [CD25]) and alemtuzumab (CAMPATH-1H, anti-CD52) (see Chapter 7).

8.3.3 Clinical rejection

Rejection may occur at any time following transplantation. The classification of rejection into early, short term and long term reflects the differing underlying mechanisms (see Fig. 8.5).

Hyperacute rejection may occur a few minutes to hours following revascularization of the graft. It is due to preformed circulating cytotoxic antibodies in the recipient that react with MHC class I antigens in the donor kidney. A similar picture is seen if an ABO-incompatible kidney is inadvertently used. Activation of complement results in an influx of polymorphonuclear leucocytes, platelet aggregation, obstruction of the blood vessels and ischaemia. The patient may be pyrexial with a blood leucocytosis. Histologically, the microvasculature becomes plugged with leucocytes and platelets, resulting in infarction. The kidney swells dramatically and is tender. Red cells and desquamated tubular cells are often found in the urine. Renal function, which normally starts within minutes of revascularization of the graft, declines; oliguria or anuria follows. Eculizumab, which blocks the activation of the terminal complement cascade, and purified C1-esterase inhibitor can be used to block complement-mediated damage and may salvage the kidney. With improved crossmatch techniques (see Fig. 8.4), hyperacute rejection has become very uncommon.

Accelerated rejection occurs within the first 3–5 days after transplantation. **Acute rejection** occurs within 6–90 days following transplantation. This can be acute antibody-mediated rejection or cell-mediated rejection; cell-mediated rejection can be enhanced by antibody (antibody-dependent cell-mediated cytotoxicity). Early diagnosis is important, because prompt treatment with intravenous methyl prednisolone and/or anti-CD3/ATG reverses renal damage. Rituximab can be used to suppress antibody production. Clinical features may be masked by ciclosporin; a rising serum creatinine and a mild fever may be the only signs. It is important to exclude urinary obstruction or perirenal collections of urine, blood or pus. Histologically, there is a mononuclear infiltrate in cellular rejection with necrosis of arterial walls; after successful treatment, the inflammatory infiltrate clears (Fig. 8.6). Acute rejection is associated with increased expression of MHC class I and class II antigens in inflamed grafts, and with early infiltration of CD8+ T lymphocytes. Biopsy helps to distinguish rejection from ciclosporin toxicity and acute humoral rejection with granulocytes and complement deposition or cell-mediated rejection.

Chronic allograft nephropathy occurs after 90 days, resulting from a number of causes, including rejection, and is seen after months or years of good renal function. There is slowly progressive renal failure and hypertension. Dominant histological findings are double contouring of the glomerular

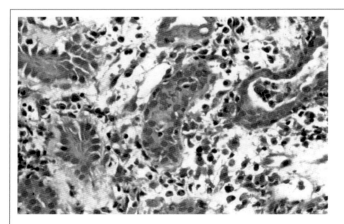

Fig. 8.6 Acute renal transplant rejection (cellular) showing interstitial oedema and a lymphoid infiltrate with tubulitis, typical of steroid-responsive acute rejection.

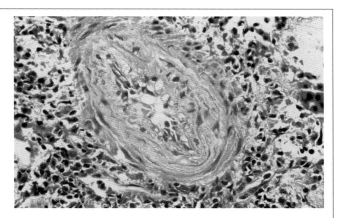

Fig. 8.7 Chronic renal transplant rejection showing intimal proliferation with narrowing of arteriolar lumen.

basement membrane, hyalinization of the glomeruli, interstitial fibrosis and proliferation of endothelial cells. Many of these findings are non-specific, except for concentric endothelial proliferation in arteries, which is characteristically associated with chronic rejection (Fig. 8.7). The Banff criteria identify the key features of different forms of chronic rejection. Occasionally, a short course of steroids may be effective if a renal biopsy shows a predominantly cellular infiltrate, but fibrosis is not reversible. Chronic rejection must be distinguished from recurrence of the original glomerular disease (see section 8.3.6).

8.3.4 Immunopathology of rejection (the allograft response)

CD4+ T cells play a central role in rejection of allogeneic grafts; such grafts persist without requiring immunosuppression in 'nude' mice and rats, which congenitally lack CD4+ T cells. Furthermore, ciclosporin, which blocks IL-2 production by CD4+ T cells, and the monoclonal antibodies daclizumab and basiliximab, which affect IL-2 receptor signalling, prevent rejection.

The rejection process has two parts: an **afferent** (initiation or sensitizing component) and an **efferent** phase (effector component). In the afferent phase, donor MHC molecules found on 'passenger leucocytes' (dendritic cells) are recognized by the recipient's CD4+ T cells, a process called allorecognition. CD4+ T cells are responsible for orchestrating rejection by recruiting a range of effector cells responsible for the damage seen in rejection – macrophages, CD8+ T cells, natural killer cells and B cells, as well as antibodies and complement. Co-stimulation of T cells is crucial to activation or tolerance. **Belatacept**, a fusion molecule of CTLA-4 with immunoglobulin (Ig)G1 Fc, inhibits the co-stimulation and blocks the activation of T cells and increases T-cell tolerance. It is being trialled as an agent to increase T-cell tolerance in transplantation, and long-term data suggest that graft function is better and vascular complications reduced in the treated group. The main risk appears to be an increase in B-lymphoproliferative disease.

Recognition of foreign antigens (**allorecognition**) can occur in either the graft itself or in the lymphoid tissue of the recipient. Allorecognition occurs in one of two ways (Fig. 8.8): either donor MHC may be recognized as an intact molecule on

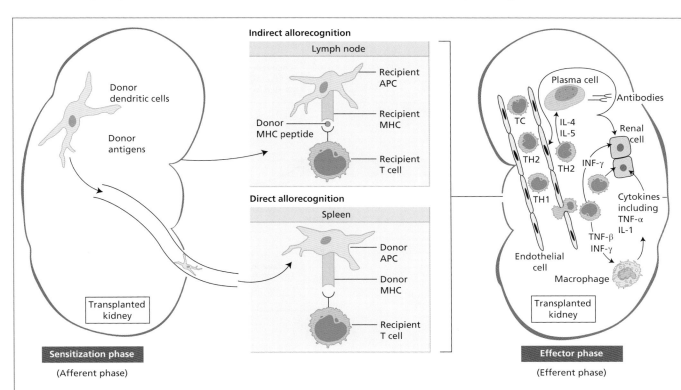

Fig. 8.8 Immunopathology of rejection (the allograft response). APC, antigen-presenting cell; IL, interleukin; INF, interferon; MHC, major histocompatibility complex; TNF, tumour necrosis factor.

the surface of donor antigen-presenting cells (APC) by the recipient's T cells (direct allorecognition), or a peptide fragment derived from donor MHC may be presented by the recipient's APC (indirect allorecognition).

The direct alloresponse is important for initiating acute rejection, with a highly significant proportion (approximately 2%) of recipient peripheral blood lymphocytes responding to any particular alloantigen. The strength of the indirect alloresponse is much weaker, with only about 0.2% of lymphocytes being capable of responding to a particular alloantigen.

8.3.5 Graft survival

Long-term graft survival is closely correlated with the **degree of HLA matching** (Fig. 8.9), particularly at the class II locus in deceased donor transplantation. Extrapolation from the graph (data displayed in months) shows that 50% of fully matched deceased donor grafts will survive approximately 17 years, in contrast to mismatched grafts that survive for only 8 years. While the advent of modern immunosuppression has minimized the need for a close match at the entire class II locus, it

is still important to obtain a good match at the HLA-DR locus (but less important at HLA-DP and HLA-DQ).

Patients who have previously rejected one graft or have been pregnant may have **cytotoxic antibodies** that are associated with hyperacute rejection. Efforts to remove or neutralize cytotoxic antibodies with the use of intravenous immunoglobulin, in combination with rituximab, have met with some success. **Retransplantation** is only possible provided there is a completely negative MHC class I antigen crossmatch (see Fig. 8.4), i.e. no relevant cytotoxic antibodies; there may be a need to wait a considerable time before a second suitable donor kidney is found. Sensitized patients who have a potential living donor with whom they are incompatible may be transplanted through a kidney donor exchange scheme.

8.3.6 Complications

An important aspect of the management of post-transplant patients is an awareness of their **increased susceptibility to infection** (see Chapter 3). *Death of the patient following transplantation is usually due to infection or malignancy*, and rarely

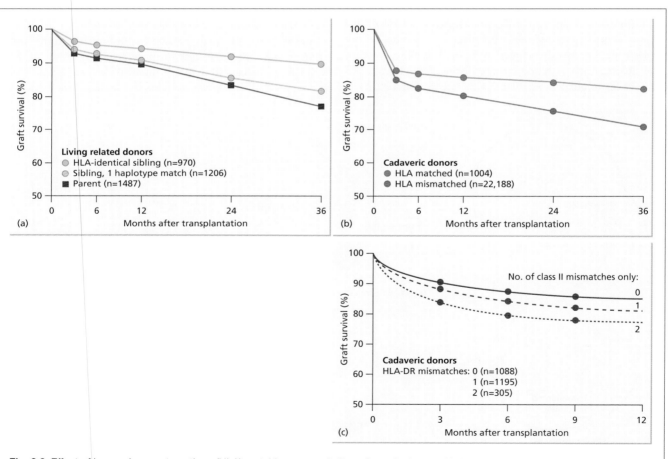

Fig. 8.9 Effect of human leucocyte antigen (HLA) matching on renal allograft survival rates. (a) Effect of matching on grafts obtained from living related donors. (b) Effect of matching on grafts obtained from cadaveric donors. (c) Effect of different degrees of HLA-DR mismatches on survival of cadaveric grafts. Figures have improved overall in the last two decades – see text. Data from Suthanthiran M, Strom TB. N Engl J Med 1994;331:370.

to graft failure, since, if the kidney fails, the patient can be maintained on haemodialysis. Mortality due to infection has fallen dramatically in the past two decades. Infections may be bacterial, fungal, viral, protozoal or mixed, and tend to occur at predictable time intervals following transplantation (Fig. 8.10). Infection with cytomegalovirus (CMV) is often associated with rejection of the graft, so CMV-negative recipients must receive CMV-negative blood products (Case 8.2). Excessive immunosuppression has recently led to the emergence of BK polyoma virus in nephropathy; this may account for 1–10% of allograft failures. Epstein–Barr virus (EBV)

can lead to post-transplant B-lymphoproliferative disorder (BLPD; see Chapter 7, Case 7.2). Infections in immunosuppressed patients are discussed in Chapter 3.

A late complication of renal transplantation is **recurrence of the original disease** (see Chapter 9). This should always be considered in patients in whom there is functional deterioration following long periods of stable graft function. Although glomerulonephritis recurs histologically in about one in four transplants, the *clinical recurrence rate is much less*. For example, in type II membranoproliferative glomerulonephritis (dense deposit disease), recurrent disease is histologically demonstrable

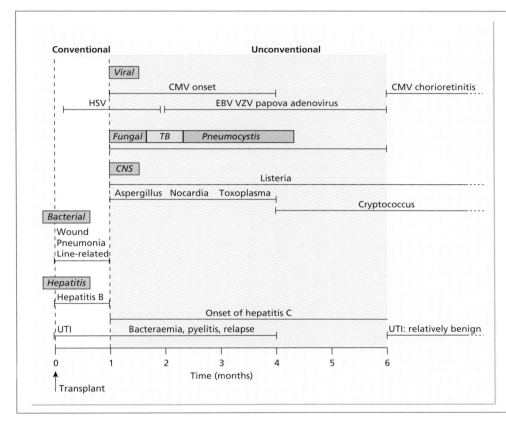

Fig. 8.10 Timetable for the occurrence of infection in renal transplant recipients (Rubin's table). CMV, cytomegalovirus; CNS, central nervous system; EBV, Epstein–Barr virus; HSV, herpes simplex virus; UTI, urinary tract infection; VZV, varicella zoster virus. Source: Rubin RH. Kidney Int 1993;44:221–236. Reproduced with permission of Nature Publishing.

Case 8.2 Primary cytomegalovirus infection in a renal transplant recipient

A 22-year-old welder was given a deceased donor renal graft after a month of haemodialysis for end-stage renal failure. His immediate post-operative course was uneventful and he was discharged home on maintenance immunosuppressive therapy (ciclosporin A 5 mg/kg, prednisolone 30 mg and tacrolimus 0.20 mg/kg body weight daily).

He was readmitted on the 37th day with general malaise, muscle aches and fever, but able to maintain a reasonable urine output (1700 mL/24 h). On examination, he had tender muscles and hepatomegaly; the transplanted kidney was not tender. Investigation showed a leucopenia but a normal serum creatinine.

In view of the leucopenia, tacrolimus was withheld for 8 days, and intravenous corticosteroids were substituted. However, his serum creatinine began to rise and urine output fell, necessitating haemodialysis. Stored pre-transplant serum samples showed no evidence of anti-cytomegalovirus (CMV) antibodies or CMV antigen by polymerase chain reaction (PCR) analysis. However immunoglobulin (Ig)M anti-CMV antibodies were detected in a current serum sample accompanied by a positive PCR signal for CMV antigen. These findings indicated primary CMV infection in the recipient due to transplantation of a CMV-positive kidney into a CMV-negative recipient. The patient made a complete recovery following prompt treatment with a combination of ganciclovir (a CMV-specific drug) and CMV-specific immune globulin.

in three-quarters of renal grafts, but less than 10% of graft failure in this group of patients is due to recurrence. Anti-glomerular basement membrane (GBM) disease may recur in transplanted kidneys.

Another late complication is the development of some types of **malignancy** in the recipient (see section 6.4) and malignancy is the third most common cause of death post transplant. There is a 20-fold increase in the incidence of non-melanoma skin cancers, non-Hodgkin's lymphoma and Kaposi's sarcoma, also seen in the acquired immune deficiency syndrome (AIDS; see Chapter 3, Case 3.7). These malignancies are more common because immunosuppression reduces 'tumour immune surveillance', but also because viral infections are implicated in their pathogenesis. Human papilloma virus is important in the carcinogenesis of non-melanoma skin cancer, EBV activation plays a role in non-Hodgkin's lymphoma (see Chapter 7, Case 7.2) and Kaposi's sarcoma is due to the human herpes virus 8.

Transplanted patients also have an increased risk of **acute myocardial infarction**. This may be linked to hypertension, hypertriglyceridaemia or insulin-resistant diabetes, since these conditions are often present before transplantation and are aggravated by steroids. Newer treatment regimens may reduce vascular damage.

8.4 Other types of transplantation

8.4.1 Liver transplantation

Liver transplantation has become the treatment of choice in patients with end-stage liver diseases. Great improvements in graft preservation, surgical skills, anaesthetic techniques and perioperative management have increased 5-year survival rates to almost 80% (Table 8.2). However, severe bleeding is still a major cause of morbidity and mortality, due to haemostatic abnormalities. The liver surgeon faces unique problems, including the bleeding tendency of a recipient with liver failure and the technically difficult surgery required to revascularize a grafted liver. However, compared with transplants of other organs, rejection episodes may be milder and require **less immunosuppression**. HLA matching and crossmatching are not routinely performed, although retrospective studies show a correlation between patient survival and DR compatibility. ABO compatibility is important, but livers have been

successfully transplanted across the ABO barrier in emergency situations. Recipients with life-threatening disease but some residual liver function are selected since they are best able to withstand major surgery. Indications for liver transplantation now include biliary atresia, primary biliary cirrhosis, end-stage hepatitis B and C and alcoholic cirrhosis. Even salvage liver transplantation can be effectively performed for patients with recurrence or deterioration of liver function after removal of liver for hepatocellular carcinoma, and the survival rates are no worse than those for primary liver transplantation.

8.4.2 Heart transplantation

Increased experience and the use of ciclosporin have resulted in rapid improvement in the survival of heart grafts (Fig. 8.11). Hearts are allocated according to ABO compatibility. HLA matching is not required, although retrospective studies have shown a correlation between graft survival and MHC class II compatibility. The immunosuppressive regimens are the same as those used for kidney transplantation. However, unlike with renal patients, there is no satisfactory life-support facility (comparable to dialysis) if the donated heart is rejected, so **early diagnosis of rejection** is crucial. To this end, changes in the

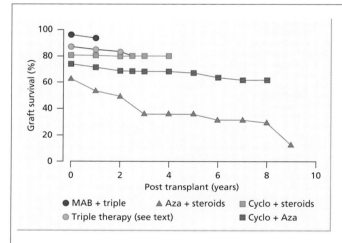

Fig. 8.11 Heart graft survival. Aza, azathioprine; Cyclo, cyclophosphamide; MAB, monoclonal antibodies.

Table 8.2 Patient survival in various forms of transplantation

Organ	Actuarial survival at				
	1 year	2 years	3 years	4 years	5 years
Liver*	93%	–	–	–	78%
Single lung+	90%	–	72%	–	63%
Heart and lungs+	87%	–		–	76%
Pancreas+	90–95%		84%	–	77%

* Figures from Pittsburgh, USA.
+ Columbia University, New York City, USA.

electrocardiograph are closely monitored; serial endomyocardial biopsies (with increasing use of fine-needle aspirates) show grossly increased MHC class I expression by myocardial cells in early rejection.

A major post-operative problem is accelerated atherosclerosis in the graft coronary arteries – cardiac allograft vasculopathy (CAV). This is a major cause of death in patients who survive more than 1 year; it is estimated that 50% of patients have angiographic evidence of coronary artery disease in the graft after 5 years. Recipients are therefore treated with antithrombotic and statin therapy. Sirolimus, in addition to its role as an immunosuppressive agent, has antiproliferative effects on allograft vasculature and is used in the prevention and treatment of CAV. As the transplanted heart is denervated when transplanted, and reinervation is generally incomplete, transplant patients are less likely to present with typical symptoms of ischaemia.

Acute allograft rejection and CMV infection of the donor heart are other major causes of morbidity and mortality in the first year. However, the survival data are good and survivors report good, stable quality of life 5–10 years after heart transplantation.

8.4.3 Lung transplantation

Lung transplantation is now a well-established treatment for irreversible and potentially fatal lung disease. The most common indications are cryptogenic fibrosing alveolitis, cystic fibrosis, primary pulmonary hypertension and severe chronic airways disease. Single, bilateral and heart–lung transplantation may be performed, with the last being particularly used when there is severe right-sided heart disease. Current immunosuppressive regimens and refinement of surgical technique give a 5-year survival of more than 75% in some centres. After the immediate post-operative period, the major causes of death are infection, acute rejection and obliterative bronchiolitis, a fibroblast proliferation process that may have a similar pathogenesis to chronic rejection of the kidney and heart and chronic GVHD. More than 20% of lung transplant recipients developed bronchiolitis obliterans by 2 years after transplantation and 50% by 6 years. The risk of this complication seems to be less among tacrolimus-treated patients than among those receiving ciclosporin. New-onset diabetes is a particularly serious complication after transplantation and is associated with the use of tacrolimus.

8.4.4 Pancreatic transplantation

Clinical islet transplantation is being offered currently to a subset of approximately 15% of patients with type 1 diabetes (IDDM) with refractory hypoglycaemia or marked glycaemic lability, which cannot be corrected by other means. Improvements in surgical technique and better immunosuppression have resulted in 90–95% survival at 1 year of transplanted vascularized pancreatic grafts. In diabetics with labile glycaemic control, serial transplantation of several pancreases results in excellent glycaemic control and improved quality of life. Pancreatic transplants have

been combined with kidney transplants in diabetics with poor renal function and graft survival for both organs correlates with HLA compatibility. Recently, the use of T-depletional immunosuppression with sirolimus has been shown to substantially improve long-term islet graft survival and 50% insulin independence beyond 5 years after transplantation has now been achieved routinely for islets alone. In stable non-uraemic diabetics, medical management is preferred to pancreatic transplantation.

8.4.5 Skin grafting

Allogeneic skin grafting in humans is useful in providing skin cover in **severely burned patients**. Although HLA-matched skin survives longer than mismatched skin, HLA typing is not done in practice because the endogenous immunosuppressive effect of severe burns allows prolonged survival of unmatched skin. Although the graft is finally rejected, the short-term protective barrier afforded by covering burns during this time is of enormous benefit to the patient in resisting infection. If there is sufficient normal skin, cells from the patient are taken for culture and the resulting sheets are used for grafting, as autografts do survive *in vivo*. For those patients that need large amounts of grafting, skin taken from cadavers soon after death and stored in liquid nitrogen until required is excellent, and more recently, to minimize postburn deformity, an acellular human dermis (also from cadavers) has been used as a dermal replacement for treating massive burns.

8.4.6 Corneal grafting

Corneal transplantation has been routine for over 50 years. Corneas are obtained from cadaveric donors. There is no need to HLA type or systemically immunosuppress the recipient, because corneal rejection does not occur unless the graft becomes vascularized. In grafts that do become vascularized, particularly those that follow chemical burns or chronic viral infections, HLA matching significantly improves survival (Chapter 12).

8.5 Haematopoietic stem cell transplantation

The transplantation of haematopoietic stem cells (HSCT) from bone marrow, peripheral blood or cord blood offers the only chance of cure for many patients with a wide range of disorders (Table 8.3). As in other transplant systems graft rejection is common, but allogeneic HSCT has the *unique, and often fatal, complication of GVHD*, in which the grafted immunocompetent cells recognize the host as foreign and mount an immunological attack.

8.5.1 Indications and selection of patients

Theoretically, any abnormality of bone marrow stem cells is correctable by the transplantation of healthy stem cells; such abnormalities include absence of cells (aplastic anaemia), malignancy and functional defects (Table 8.3). The **risks of allogeneic transplantation** are high and success depends on

Table 8.3 Indications for haemopoietic stem cell transplantation

1 Severe aplastic anaemia
   Idiopathic (Diamond–Blackfan anaemia; Fanconi anaemia; thalassaemia major) Iatrogenic
2 Acute/chronic myeloid leukaemia – in first remission
3 Acute lymphoblastic leukaemia
4 Non-Hodgkin's lymphoma for young patients in remission
5 Immunodeficiency
   Severe combined immunodeficiency
   Chronic granulomatous disease and other severe neutrophil defects
   Wiskott–Aldrich syndrome
   CD40 ligand deficiency
   Other genetically defined combined immunodeficiencies (adults/children)
6 Inborn errors of metabolism (osteopetrosis, Gaucher's disease, mucopolysaccharidoses)
7 Juvenile chronic arthritis

balancing the severity of the disease against the risks of the procedure.

Ideally, the donor and recipient should be ABO compatible and MHC identical, but there is only a one in four chance that two siblings will have identical pairs of haplotypes (see Fig. 8.2). Advances in pharmacological immunosuppressive agents have enabled bone marrow or peripheral blood stem cells to be used from HLA-matched but unrelated donors, as well as donors with one haplotype mismatch, such as parents.

8.5.2 Management of patients

Preparation for transplantation usually begins 10 days before grafting. Measures to **reduce infection risk** include reverse-barrier nursing, decontamination of the skin and gut, the use of appropriate antibiotics and antimycotics. Intravenous feeding and immunoglobulin replacement are required for those with failure to thrive associated with immune deficiencies.

The grafting procedure is straightforward; small amounts of marrow are taken from multiple sites under general anaesthetic. Commonly CD34+ are purified from peripheral blood after the donor has taken granulocyte colony-stimulating factor (G-CSF) to increase the stem cell count peripherally, or cord blood is used

as a source enriched in CD34+ cells. Stem cells can then be given either without fractionation (only in leukaemia; Case 8.3) or after removal of immunocompetent T lymphocytes responsible for GVHD (in immunodeficiency; Case 8.4). Cells are then transplanted by intravenous infusion. The optimal size of the graft is probably between 10^8 and 10^9 nucleated cells per kg body weight, although fewer cells are needed in immune-deficient infants.

For malignant disease, stem cell transplantation may be autologous (i.e. from the patient): stem cells harvested and purified while the patient is given intensive chemoradiotherapy followed by reinfusion of purified stem cells. This has the advantage of minimal risk of graft failure or rejection, and more rapid engraftment. Post-transplant immunosuppression is not usually required. The risk is contamination of the graft with malignant cells. The procedure cannot be undertaken where normal stem cells cannot be harvested, for example in myelodysplasia or chronic myeloid leukaemia. Allogeneic stem cell transplantation (from a healthy donor) has a slower engraftment, with a higher risk of GVHD, but also a higher change of beneficial graft-versus-tumour or -leukaemia activity (GVT or GVL).

Three major problems dominate the post-transplant period: failure of the graft to 'take', infection and GVHD. **Failure of engraftment** can be due to using insufficient bone marrow cells or rejection of the grafted cells by the host. Patients with some functional immunity (e.g. as in leukaemia in remission or those with partial immune deficiencies) require immune suppression prior to grafting ('conditioning') to ensure that rejection does not occur. Leukaemia or high-risk lymphoma patients are pretreated with bone marrow obliterative-conditioning regimes (e.g. bulsulphan, cyclophosphamide), with or without total body irradiation, immediately prior to transplantation. Those patients with no immune function (e.g. severe combined immune deficiency [SCID]; Case 8.4) do not, in theory, require conditioning since they are unable to reject the graft, but some pretreatment is beneficial.

Recombinant growth factors, such as G-CSF or granulocyte/macrophage colony-stimulating factor (GM-CSF), are used to shorten the duration of neutropenia post transplantation and so reduce **infection risk**.

A successful graft is indicated by a rise in the peripheral white cell count and the appearance of haematopoietic precursors in the marrow 10–20 days post transplantation. The **rate of recovery**

Case 8.3 Haematopoietic stem cell transplantation for acute myeloid leukaemia

A 22-year-old man was treated for acute myeloid leukaemia (AML) with cyclical combination chemotherapy, and complete clinical remission was obtained after three courses. However, remission in AML is generally short; half the patients relapse within a year and second remissions are difficult to achieve. Stem cell transplantation after high-dose chemoradiotherapy is therefore considered in young patients with suitable family members. The brother of this patient was HLA identical and willing to act as a marrow donor. The patient was given cyclophosphamide (120 mg/kg) followed by a dose of total body irradiation that is ordinarily lethal. Immediately after irradiation, he was given an intravenous transfusion of 10^9 unfractionated bone marrow cells per kg obtained from his brother. He was supported with granulocyte colony-stimulating factor and platelet transfusions during the days of aplasia before engraftment occurred. Methotrexate was administered intermittently to try to prevent graft-versus-host disease. The patient was discharged home, well, 7 weeks after transplantation, and remains free of leukaemia 7 years later.

is influenced by many factors, including prior chemotherapy, conditioning regimen, presence of GVHD and infection. Post-transplant immune reconstitution is a lengthy process (Fig. 8.12). Significant impairment of T- and B-cell function is common during the first few months and underlies the increase in susceptibility to both viral and bacterial infections during this period.

The pace of immunological recovery is slower in recipients of T cell–depleted, HLA-incompatible marrow than in recipients of HLA-identical marrow. While T-cell function usually returns to normal within 6–12 months, B-cell function may take longer,

up to 2 years; in some cases B-cell reconstitution fails and replacement immunoglobulin therapy is needed for life.

8.5.3 Complications of allogeneic haematopoietic stem cell transplantation and their prevention: graft-versus-host disease and infection

GVHD occurs in most patients who receive allogeneic transplants and even in transplants between HLA-identical siblings, differences in minor histocompatibility antigens (small peptides derived from cytoplasmic proteins and presented by the MHC) provoke mild GVHD in 20–50% of cases. As in Case 8.4, the cause may be blood products containing viable T cells. Consequently, the *use of unirradiated blood products in immunosuppressed hosts* (whether due to SCID or drugs) is *fraught with danger* and must be avoided. If blood-derived cells are required, it is essential to ensure that they are irradiated to inactivate all immunocompetent T cells.

GVHD manifests **clinically** as a rash, fever, hepatosplenomegaly, bloody diarrhoea and breathlessness 7–14 days after transplantation. In severe cases, the rash may progress from a maculopapular eruption to generalized erythroderma and exfoliative dermatitis. A skin biopsy (as in Case 8.4) shows basal cell degeneration and lymphocytic infiltration with vascular cuffing. The **mortality** of GVHD is considerable; over 70% of those with severe GVHD and about one-third with mild GVHD will die. Treatment requires an increase in immunosuppression but, once established, GVHD is very difficult to eradicate. Since not all patients have suitable HLA-matched

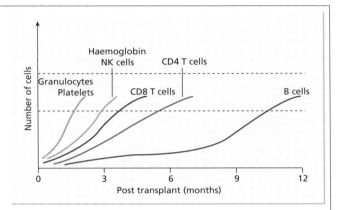

Fig. 8.12 Haematological and immune reconstitution following bone marrow transplantation. Dotted lines represent upper and lower reference ranges. NK, natural killer.

Case 8.4 Graft-versus-host disease in an infant with severe combined immune deficiency

A 3-month-old boy was admitted to hospital with failure to thrive and a persistent cough. On examination his height and weight were below the third centile. Initial investigations revealed marked anaemia: haemoglobin 50 g/L, white cell count 8.9×10^9/L, platelet count 260×10^9/L. A chest X-ray was reported to be compatible with right lower lobe pneumonia, but no organism was identified on blood culture. The patient was treated empirically with broad-spectrum antibiotics but failed to improve.

In view of the anaemia he was transfused with two units of packed red cells (before the advent of irradiation policies for all blood/cellular blood products being irradiated before transfusion). Six days following transfusion he developed a widespread erythematous maculopapular rash and abnormal liver function tests. A skin biopsy showed diffuse vacuolar degeneration of basal epidermal cells with a mononuclear inflammatory cell infiltrate and aberrant expression of human leucocyte antigen (HLA)-DR on epidermal keratinocytes. These findings were indicative of graft-versus-host disease (GVHD) and raised the possibility of underlying immunodeficiency in the baby. Subsequent immunological investigations were diagnostic of severe combined immune deficiency (SCID): i.e. marked T- and B-cell lymphopenia and hypogammaglobulinaemia.

In the light of this diagnosis, the baby was bronchoscoped and analysis of bronchial secretions revealed *Pneumocystis carinii*, a common pathogen in babies with defective cellular immunity. The baby was treated aggressively with co-trimoxazole, intravenous immunoglobulin and prophylactic antifungal therapy. Despite his poor outlook, it was decided to perform a single haplotype-matched stem cell transplant from his father. Sadly, this was unsuccessful and the baby died 3 days later from overwhelming sepsis. This was not unexpected, since transplantation in the face of established GVHD and sepsis often proves difficult. GVHD as a result of the use of non-irradiated blood should not occur now that there is greater awareness of SCID, but is included here to demonstrate the obvious similarity of findings between GVHD due to blood T lymphocytes and stem cells.

While the general principles of bone marrow transplantation for leukaemia and SCID are similar, comparison of this case with Case 8.3 highlights some important differences (Table 8.4).

siblings (especially children with congenital immune deficiencies), ways have been sought to prevent GVHD.

Elimination or reduction of the numbers of immunocompetent T cells involves the use of T cell–specific monoclonal antibodies and complement to lyse mature T cells *in vitro* before transplantation. **T-cell depletion** of bone marrow can prevent GVHD. However, it is associated with an increased failure of engraftment and/or relapse of leukaemia (Table 8.4). This suggests that donor T cells have a role in eliminating leukaemic cells (GVL). New protocols, using incomplete depletion and mild immunosuppression, are under investigation to find a balance between GVHD, rejection of the graft and leukaemia relapse. Attempts to separate beneficial effects of GVL from GVHD remain experimental, but results are encouraging. GVHD is usually not a problem in autologous HSCT.

Even in autologous HSCT serious bacterial, fungal and viral **infections** occur despite measures aimed at reducing their incidence and severity. CMV infection is a common cause of death; evidence of CMV reactivation is seen in 75% of patients who are CMV positive pre transplant, due to the time taken for the graft to function (see Figure 8.12). Wherever possible both donor and recipient are matched for CMV status. Patients are divided into two groups in terms of risk of CMV infection (Fig. 8.13).

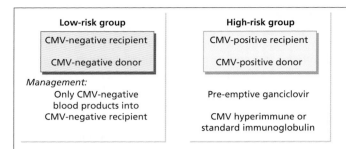

Fig. 8.13 Strategies for cytomegalovirus (CMV) prophylaxis.

Recombinant growth factors (G-CSF/GM-CSF) are used to shorten the post-transplant risk period by stimulating rapid maturation of neutrophils; intravenous immunoglobulin will be used for the period of inadequate B-lymphocyte function together with antibiotic, antiviral and antifungal agents.

Patients receiving HSCT should be monitored for the return of cells as engraftment takes place: this should include T and B lymphocytes and subsets of CD4+ T cells and the appearance of class-switch memory B cells. In HSCT for chronic granulomatous disease, the return of functioning neutrophils can easily be followed by flow cytometry, and will give an easy measure of chimerism (i.e. the percentage of normal donor neutrophils versus the non-functioning recovering recipient neutrophils). For allogeneic HSCT for other types of immunodeficiency, monitoring cellular chimerism using genetic markers is usually undertaken and repeated at intervals to check for graft failure.

8.5.4 Results

The results of HSCT vary according to the indications for performing the procedure.

Infants with **SCID** die before they are 2 years old unless marrow or stem cells can be grafted. As the siblings of infants with SCID are often too young to be donors, grafting with incompatible tissue was originally attempted, but nearly always failed due to GVHD. The best results are still obtained when completely matched marrow is used, but T-cell depletion has dramatically improved the outcome if partially matched marrow is used. A **good prognosis** is associated with transplantation within the first 6 months of life, absence of infection and ablative therapy to the recipient's marrow before transplantation to ensure engraftment. Many SCID babies are now diagnosed at birth (or even antenatally) due to a positive family history; these infants have > 98% survival when compared, regardless of matching, with those who are a first presenting member in the family (overall survival 40%), with one-third of children dying before HSCT. With good matching, survival post transplant can reach > 90% in experienced centres.

In **aplastic anaemia**, long-term survival following transplantation of selected cases is about 80%, compared with only 5% without transplantation. Survival is better in younger patients who are relatively fit at the time of transplantation.

The results of chemotherapy for **acute lymphoblastic leukaemia** (ALL) are now good, with most patients achieving

Table 8.4 Comparison of haemopoietic stem cell transplantation (HSCT) for primary immune deficiency with HSCT for myeloid leukaemia

	Primary immune deficiency	Leukaemia
Age	Infants and young children	Adults/ children
Need for pre-transplant conditioning	On theoretical grounds not required, but in practice some conditioning is beneficial	Yes
T-cell depletion of graft	Yes	Yes (but certain degree of GVHD is beneficial in view of its antileukaemia effect)
Complications (infections, GVHD)	Similar	Similar
Pace of immunological and haematological reconstitution	Similar	Similar

GVHD, graft-versus-host disease.

remission, although not all are permanently cured (see Chapter 6). Patients now undergo ablative therapy followed by bone marrow transplantation. Survival for this group of patients, who otherwise have a poor prognosis, is now 90% at 10 years, with most patients disease free. Cord blood from an unrelated donor is an alternative source of haematopoietic stem cells for adults with acute leukaemia who lack an HLA-matched bone marrow donor. A recent meta-analysis showed that sibling donor allogeneic HSCT is more effective than chemotherapy in adult acute myeloid leukaemia (AML; except in good-risk patients) in first remission, with similar results for childhood AML and adult ALL. The technique of **autologous bone marrow transplantation** in leukaemia is established in many centres, although leukaemia relapse remains a problem. This involves cryopreservation of bone marrow taken from the patient during remission. The marrow is then 'transplanted' after total body irradiation has eradicated residual leukaemic cells. The technique has the advantage of eliminating the problem of GVHD, but depends on the removal of leukaemic cells from the preserved marrow; however, autologous HSCT is equal to or less effective than chemotherapy.

CHAPTER 9
Kidney Diseases

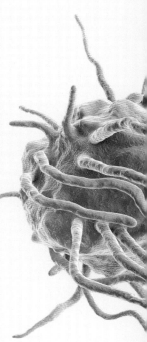

Key topics

 Visit the companion website at **www.wiley.com/go/misbah/immunology** to download cases with additional figures on these topics.

Chapel and Haeney's Essentials of Clinical Immunology, Seventh Edition. Edited by Siraj A. Misbah, Gavin P. Spickett, and Virgil A.S.H. Dalm.
© 2022 John Wiley & Sons Ltd. Published 2022 by John Wiley & Sons Ltd.

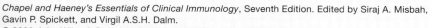

9.1 Introduction

Renal disease includes damage to the glomeruli, the tubules or the interstitial tissue. Immunological components are involved in most cases of glomerular damage (glomerulonephritis) and for some forms of injury to the renal tubules and interstitium (tubulointerstitial nephritis), although the precise mechanisms are not always clear. Humoral and cell-mediated immune mechanisms (Box 9.1a, b) play a part in the pathogenesis of nephritis, but some common types of glomerulonephritis (e.g. minimal-change disease) and tubulointerstitial disease do not have a clear-cut immune basis.

The terminology of glomerulonephritis is confusing because three descriptive classifications have been in simultaneous use for many years, but none is entirely satisfactory in isolation. There is a clinical classification, describing the commoner modes of presentation; a morphological classification, based on light and electron microscope findings; and an immunological classification, based on the proposed immune mechanism of renal damage.

Box 9.1a Ways in which antibodies can induce damage

- Antibody may react directly with the glomerular or tubular basement membrane
- Antibody may form immune complexes with antigens that subsequently lodge in the kidney
- Antigen may bind with, or be trapped in, the glomerular basement membrane and react with antibody subsequently
- Antibody may induce a vasculitic process that damages the capillary plexus of the glomerulus

---

Box 9.1b Evidence that T-cell-mediated mechanisms are involved in pathogenesis of glomerulonephritis

- Adoptive transfer of sensitized T cells to rats treated with sub-nephritogenic doses of antibody causes glomerular hypercellularity due to proliferation of resident glomerular cells and an influx of mononuclear leucocytes
- Severe proliferative nephritis can develop after immunization with glomerular basement membrane in bursectomized chickens unable to mount antibody responses
- In humans, T lymphocytes have been found in proliferative and non-proliferative glomerulopathies
- Treatment with ciclosporin is effective in some glomerular disorders

---

9.2 Clinical syndromes

Several clinical syndromes are recognized, but with considerable overlap.

Recurrent haematuria may be the first manifestation of renal or extrarenal disease. It can be macroscopic or microscopic. Haematuria of unknown origin requires urological investigation to exclude a site of bleeding in the upper and lower urinary tracts, particularly since tumours of the bladder are the second most common cause after infections.

Persistent proteinuria. A small amount of albumin (up to 30 mg/day) is normally present in urine of healthy adults. Amounts in excess of this are pathological. Excretion of >300 mg albumin per 24 h is termed 'overt albuminuria', while excretion of amounts between 30 and 300 mg/day is called 'microalbuminuria'. **Overt proteinuria** is a cardinal sign of established glomerular damage and a risk factor for declining renal function. The higher the level of proteinuria, the faster the development of tubulointerstitial lesions and renal fibrosis progressing to chronic renal failure. Proteinuria is often discovered by chance when urine is tested for some other reason. **Microalbuminuria** is used as a marker of early diabetic nephropathy and therapeutic interventions are increasingly targeted at the early microalbuminuric stage in the belief that pathological damage may be modifiable or even reversible at this point.

Nephrotic syndrome is defined as low plasma levels of albumin (hypoalbuminaemia) accompanied by dependent oedema resulting from severe proteinuria, usually in excess of 3.5 g/day. In children, this is a common presentation of glomerulonephritis.

Acute nephritis is characterized by sudden onset of haematuria, proteinuria, hypertension and oliguria.

Renal failure may be acute or chronic. Acute renal failure is a period of sudden, severe impairment of renal function, usually triggered by some vascular or inflammatory insult. Chronic renal failure may be the end result of any disorder that destroys normal renal architecture; although there are many causes, about half of cases are caused by some type of glomerulonephritis.

There is a poor correlation between the clinical picture and the underlying morphology. A specific form of glomerulonephritis can show different clinical features in different patients or even in the same patient at different times (Fig. 9.1). A definite diagnosis, allowing for more accurate assessment of prognosis, is best made by **renal biopsy**, the results of which tie up with patient outcome in terms of disease progression.

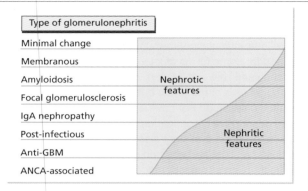

Type of glomerulonephritis		
Minimal change		
Membranous		
Amyloidosis	Nephrotic features	
Focal glomerulosclerosis		
IgA nephropathy		
Post-infectious		Nephritic features
Anti-GBM		
ANCA-associated		

Fig. 9.1 Overlap of nephritic and nephrotic features of various forms of glomerular disease. ANCA, antineutrophil cytoplasmic antibody; GBM, glomerular basement membrane.

9.3 Classifications of glomerulonephritis

An understanding of glomerulonephritis requires a grasp of normal **glomerular structure** (Fig. 9.2). The glomerulus is a unique capillary plexus, fed by an afferent arteriole and drained by an efferent arteriole, supported by a stalk called the mesangium. As the afferent arteriole enters the glomerulus, it divides into numerous capillary loops. The wall of the capillary loop (Fig. 9.3) acts as the glomerular filter and is composed of three layers: an inner layer of glomerular endothelial cells, an outer (i.e. urinary side) layer of glomerular epithelial cells, and the glomerular basement membrane between them. Each layer has specialized features distinguishing it from capillary walls elsewhere in the body.

Endothelial cells offer no anatomical barrier to the passage of molecules. The cytoplasm of the endothelial cells forms a thin layer perforated by fenestrations much larger in diameter than macromolecules in the plasma. These openings allow capillary blood to come into direct contact with the glomerular basement membrane.

Glomerular basement membrane (GBM) has unique constituents with restricted isoforms of laminin, type IV collagen and proteoglycans, highly negatively charged molecules that account for the charge-dependent filtration that normally conserves plasma proteins.

Epithelial cells or podocytes are arranged around the capillaries (Fig. 9.3). Epithelial cells are phagocytic. Each cell has multiple foot processes that interdigitate and are partly embedded in the outer layer of the GBM. A thin membrane – called the slit diaphragm – bridges the spaces between the foot processes of the podocytes and is vital for maintaining the barrier to plasma proteins. Several interacting slit diaphragm proteins have been identified and mutations in the genes coding for some of them are associated with inherited forms of nephrotic syndrome, strongly implying that podocytes are vital in preventing proteinuria in healthy people. Disruption of structural slit diaphragm proteins by proteinuria may predispose to apoptosis (death) of podocytes.

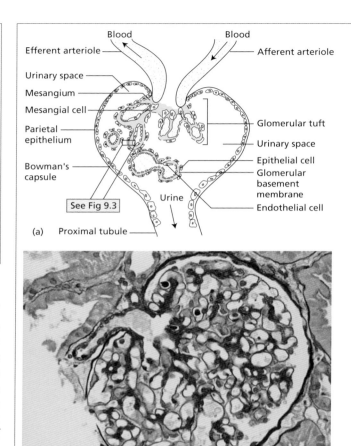

Fig. 9.2 (a) Normal glomerular structure. (b) Normal glomerular histology (periodic acid–Schiff stain).

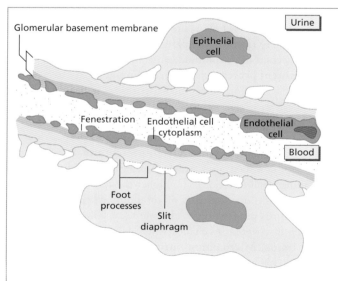

Fig. 9.3 A section across a normal capillary loop (see text for explanation).

The **mesangium**, the central core of tissue in the glomerulus, is made up of mesangial cells separated by an extensive matrix. The mesangial region can take up and dispose of large molecules, particularly immune complexes. The mesangial matrix ultimately drains into renal lymphatics and so, via paraaortic lymph nodes, to the venous blood supply.

9.3.1 Histological classification

Glomeruli are composed of three main cell types – mesangial, endothelial and epithelial – and any or all of these cells may increase in number in response to injury. The term glomerulonephritis must therefore be qualified (Table 9.1) by defining **the types of cells affected** and whether part or all of the **glomerulus is damaged**. Classification is based on light microscopy, electron microscopy and immunohistochemistry.

9.3.2 Mechanisms of glomerulonephritis

The evidence that human glomerulonephritides are immunological disorders relies heavily on animal experiments. At least two mechanisms are known to induce glomerulonephritis in animals:

- Deposition of circulating antigen–antibody complexes within glomeruli – 'immune-complex nephritis', an example of type III hypersensitivity (see Chapter 1).

- Reaction of circulating antibodies with antigens that are either part of the GBM (for instance, 'anti-GBM' nephritis), antigens that have been trapped there or antigenic components of renal vascular endothelium (Fig. 9.4), examples of type II hypersensitivity.

After the initiation of glomerular injury, a number of pro-inflammatory mediator pathways (Fig. 9.4) are activated both in infiltrating cells and in resident glomerular cells and participate in the destructive and restorative processes. Remodelling of extracellular matrix after injury generates signals that differ from those transmitted by normal glomerular matrix and induces activation and proliferation of resident and infiltrating cells in the glomerulus. Haemodynamic changes cause hyperfiltration, intraglomerular hypertension and abnormal intravascular shear forces that can worsen glomerular injury. Depending on the cells affected, apoptosis may have a crucial role either in resolution of damage or in causing glomerular scarring.

9.4 Asymptomatic haematuria

Some forms of glomerulonephritis often follow infections of the respiratory tract and usually involve mesangial deposits of IgA.

9.4.1 IgA nephropathy

IgA nephropathy ('mesangial IgA deposition' or 'Berger's disease') is the most common form of primary glomerulonephritis in the world. It accounts for about 10% of all cases of primary glomerular disease in the USA, 20% of cases in Europe and 30–40% in Asia. It affects mainly older children or young adults, is often asymptomatic (a chance finding of microscopic haematuria), but may **present** as recurrent episodes of macroscopic haematuria occurring after an upper respiratory tract infection (Case 9.1) or, less frequently, a gastrointestinal or urinary tract infection, or strenuous exercise; presentation with acute nephritis, hypertension or nephrotic syndrome is less frequent. In contrast to post-streptococcal glomerulonephritis (see later Case 9.3), the period between infection and haematuria is short, ranging from hours to a few days.

The clinical features are variable and yet the **biopsy findings** are constant and probably persist indefinitely. On light microscopy, the glomeruli show focal and segmental mesangial proliferation and, as the name of the condition implies, prominent deposits of IgA are found in the mesangium of every glomerulus (Fig. 9.5), together with complement components of the alternate pathway.

In terms of **pathogenesis**, IgA nephropathy can be considered a type of renal limited vasculitis caused by an innate defect in IgA mucosal immunity in the gut or lung: repeated exposure to a variety of environmental antigens results in an abnormal IgA response, namely the generation of nephritogenic polymeric IgA antibodies with defective galactosylation of the IgA hinge region, resulting in deposition in the

Table 9.1 Some descriptive terms used in the morphological classification of nephritis	
Extent of damage	
• Diffuse	Involving all glomeruli
• Focal	Involving some glomeruli only
• Segmental	Involving part of a glomerulus while the rest of that glomerulus appears normal
Cellular changes	
• Proliferative	An increase in the numbers of cells within the glomerular tuft. Subgroups exist in which proliferation is predominantly confined to a particular cell type
• Membranous	Thickening of the glomerular capillary wall by abnormal deposits on the epithelial aspect of the basement membrane
• Membranoproliferative	Proliferation of cells **plus** thickening of the glomerular capillary wall
• Crescents	Proliferation of parietal epithelial cells (extracapillary proliferation)

Fig. 9.4 Immunopathological mechanisms involved in the clinical syndromes of nephritis. ANCA, antineutrophil cytoplasmic antibody; GBM, glomerular basement membrane.

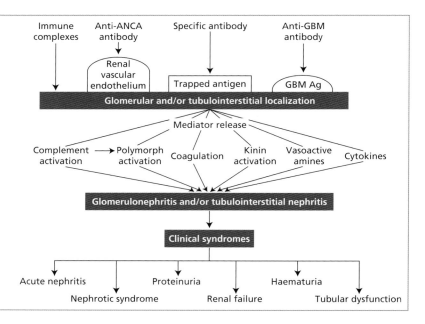

Case 9.1 IgA nephropathy

A 14-year-old boy presented with an 18-month history of intermittent, painless haematuria, usually occurring after strenuous exercise, but without dysuria or increased frequency of micturition. He also had frequent colds and sore throats and believed that the haematuria also happened at these times. On examination, he appeared fit and healthy; his blood pressure was 120/75. Urine analysis showed microscopic haematuria (3+) and a trace of protein. Intravenous urography, a micturating cystogram and cystoscopy were normal. His haemoglobin, white cell count, blood urea and creatinine clearance were normal; the urinary protein excretion was 0.95 g/day. Immunoglobulin, CH_{50}, C4 and C3 levels were within normal limits. In view of the duration of haematuria, a renal biopsy was performed. Twelve glomeruli were present: all showed a diffuse increase in mesangial cells with thickening of the matrix. Immunofluorescent examination of the biopsy showed mesangial deposits of IgA and C3 (Fig. 9.5a). The appearances were characteristic of IgA nephropathy.

mesangium and the induction of inflammation in genetically susceptible individuals. Genome-wide association studies (GWAS) have shown a number of genetic polymorphisms relating to susceptibility such as those involved in the response to pathogens (Toll-like receptor [TLR]-9 polymorphisms), the response to IgA immune deposits (FcγR 2a, 3a and 3b polymorphisms) or the activity of the renin–angiotensin pathway (angiotensin-converting enzyme [ACE] polymorphisms). Clinical evidence includes an association between IgA nephropathy and chronic liver disease, coeliac disease and dermatitis herpetiformis, other disorders that are also linked with immune complexes containing IgA.

Predictors for **prognosis** are being sought actively, but currently depend on the biopsy and clinical findings. Patients presenting with nephrotic-range proteinuria, hypertension or crescents on biopsy are more likely to progress to renal failure. Spontaneous clinical remission occurs in about 10% of patients. Of the remainder, renal survival of 80–90% at 10 years and 50–70% at 20 years implies that IgA nephropathy

can be a relatively benign disease with a good prognosis but, because IgA nephropathy is so common, it contributes significantly to the population with end-stage renal failure (ESRF) (30% of cases). The risk of developing renal failure increases by about 1% per year.

Renal transplantation has provided the strongest support for IgA nephropathy as a systemic disease. Recurrence in the donor kidney can be demonstrated in around one-third of patients who receive a transplant for ESRF due to IgA nephropathy. Further, when a kidney is inadvertently sourced from a patient with asymptomatic IgA nephropathy and transplanted to a recipient, histological evidence of IgA nephropathy quickly disappears.

There is no specific **treatment** and trials of immunosuppression and plasma exchange have been controversial. Treatment is limited to those with a poor long-term prognosis. Angiotensin II receptor blockers, ACE inhibitors and fish oil supplements have been used for their protective and antiproteinuria effects, with some benefit.

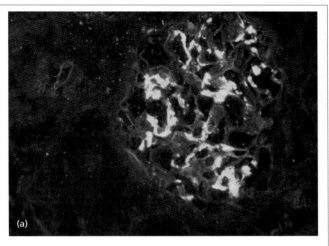

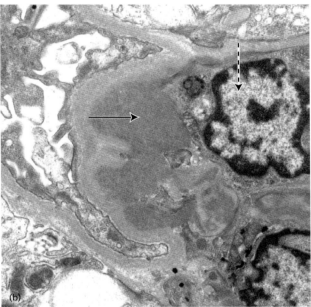

Fig. 9.5 (a) IgA nephropathy showing IgA deposits in the mesangium on immunofluorescence. (b) Electron micrograph of IgA nephropathy showing an IgA deposit (arrowed) and an adjacent mesangial cell (interrupted arrow).

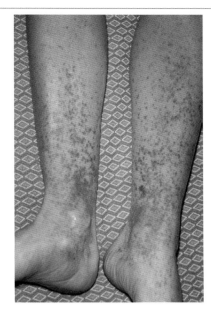

Fig. 9.6 Henoch–Schönlein purpura in an adult.

9.4.2 Henoch–Schönlein nephritis

Henoch–Schönlein nephritis (HSN; Henoch–Schönlein purpura or anaphylactoid purpura) is a common form of systemic vasculitis in which small blood vessels in a number of organs are involved. It is usually a disease of children, with a peak age of onset between 4 and 10 years. The syndrome is characterized by non-thrombocytopenic purpura of the skin (particularly around joints; Fig. 9.6), arthralgia, gastrointestinal pain and glomerulonephritis, as in Case 9.2. *Kidney disease is the most important manifestation of HSN as renal failure is the main cause of death.* The overall **prevalence of renal disease** varies from 40% to 100%, but in most patients this is mild; *progression to renal failure occurs in fewer than 10%.* Those with the most severe clinical presentation have the worst outcome: about 40% of those with nephritic or nephrotic syndromes at onset show long-term impairment of renal function. Treatment is largely empirical, controversial and, at best, only partially effective. Steroids seem to control the joint and abdominal pain, but have no effect on the skin or renal involvement at routinely used doses. Despite the uncertainty regarding therapy, the short-term prognosis is favourable. However, recurrence of HSN is common.

Immunohistology of the renal biopsy shows irregular, granular deposits of IgA, C3 and fibrin in the glomeruli. Deposits of IgA and C3 are also found in the skin, even in non-affected areas, and are diagnostic of the condition. As in IgA nephropathy, the available evidence suggests an IgA-dominant immune-complex pathogenesis with complement activation occurring via the alternate pathway. A variety of bacterial or viral antigens could be involved, as there is an association with preceding upper respiratory tract infection. In addition, HSN is a seasonal disease: most patients present during the winter. The clinical and immunological similarity between HSN and IgA nephropathy suggests that IgA nephropathy is a renal limited form of HSN.

9.5 Acute glomerulonephritis

9.5.1 Acute immune-complex nephritis

A single intravenous injection of a foreign protein into a rabbit causes vasculitis, arthritis and glomerulonephritis about 10 days later ('**one-shot' serum sickness**; Fig. 9.7). This occurs when the amount of circulating antigen is still in excess of specific IgG antibody produced in response to the stimulus (see Chapter 1); the small immune complexes so formed are soluble but become trapped in capillary membranes, particularly in the kidney. Immunofluorescent examination of the kidney shows deposition of the injected antigen,

Case 9.2 Henoch–Schönlein nephritis

A 12-year-old boy presented with a 1-week history of pain in the left loin. This was diagnosed as a urinary tract infection and treated with amoxicillin. One week later, he developed a purpuric rash around the ankles, accompanied by some blistering and superficial necrosis. Shortly afterwards, he developed pain in the left elbow joint. On admission to hospital, he was noted to have haematuria and proteinuria and a blood pressure of 130/90. Over the next month, he suffered further episodes of abdominal colic and purpura. His haemoglobin was 95 g/l with a normal white cell count. Antinuclear antibodies were negative and total haemolytic complement, C4 and C3 levels were normal. Although his blood urea was normal, his creatinine clearance was low at 31 ml/min per m² with proteinuria of 4.5 g/day.

A skin biopsy of a purpuric lesion showed vasculitic changes in the dermis, with IgA and C3 deposition in the blood-vessel walls. A renal biopsy, containing 21 glomeruli per section, showed epithelial crescents and diffuse mesangial hypercellularity in seven glomeruli. On immunofluorescence, granular deposits of IgA and C3 and, to a lesser extent, IgG and properdin were present in the mesangium. The clinical and histological features were those of Henoch–Schönlein nephritis. Because of the heavy proteinuria and diminished creatinine clearance, he was treated with a limited course of corticosteroids. Over a 9-month follow-up period, the purpura and episodes of abdominal colic subsided, his creatinine clearance increased to 47 ml/min, but he continued to have moderately heavy proteinuria (3.2 g/day). The prognosis is uncertain.

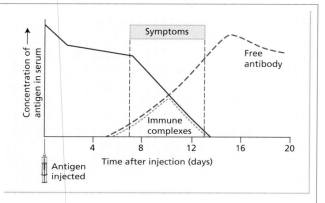

Fig. 9.7 Immune-complex formation in acute serum sickness.

specific antibodies and complement components in an irregular, granular ('lumpy-bumpy') distribution along the GBM. Renal injury is due to the resultant attraction and accumulation of polymorphs in the glomeruli and release of inflammatory mediators.

The symptomatic phase is usually transient and subsides, with complete healing, as the complexes, both soluble and fixed, are cleared in around 2–4 weeks.

9.5.2 Acute post-infectious glomerulonephritis

Post-infectious glomerulonephritis is seen increasingly in immunocompromised adults and in elderly people. It is frequently linked to staphylococcal and Gram-negative bacterial infections, often at multiple sites. The clinical presentation can be insidious and the diagnosis made only after renal biopsy suggests an infectious cause. In contrast to post-streptococcal disease, the destructive glomerular proliferation often persists and the prognosis is poor. Post-infectious glomerulonephritis may also follow parasitic (malaria, filariasis) and viral (hepatitis B or C) infections (Case 9.3).

Acute post-streptococcal glomerulonephritis (PSGN) is mainly seen in countries in which antibiotics for streptococcal infections are not widely available and accounts for about a third of cases of acute glomerulonephritis. It is a disease of children aged 2–10 years, but adolescents and adults may be affected. Over 90% of cases are preceded by streptococcal infection of the throat or skin. Patients **typically present** with acute nephritis 7–12 days after a throat infection or about 3 weeks after a skin infection. The diagnosis of PSGN rests on prior microbiological culture, increasing titres of streptococcal antibodies and a low serum C3 level. Laboratories can often test for a range of antistreptococcal antibodies including antistreptolysin (ASO), antihyaluronidase (AHase), antistreptokinase (ASKase), antinicotinamide-adenine dinucleotidase (anti-NAD) and anti-DNAse B antibodies. These antibodies are useful in approximately 95% of cases following pharyngitis and 80% in those following pyoderma.

The **histological features** depend on the timing of biopsy. Acute post-streptococcal glomerulonephritis is characterized by the presence of electron-dense deposits ('humps') on the epithelial side of the GBM (Fig. 9.8): these represent the discrete 'lumpy-bumpy' deposits of IgG and C3 found by immunofluorescence along the capillary loop in sites corresponding to the 'humps' (Fig. 9.9). There is also diffuse proliferation of endothelial and mesangial cells and polymorph infiltration of the glomerulus. Antigenic fragments from nephritogenic strains of streptococci bind to the GBM, so localizing specific antibody to this site.

The **clinical and immunological** features of this condition are similar to acute ('one-shot') immune-complex nephritis in rabbits. Serum complement C3 is markedly reduced during the early phase, with a gradual return to normal over 6–10 weeks in uncomplicated cases. *A low C3 persisting beyond 12 weeks suggests a different diagnosis* (see section 9.6.2 and Case 9.4).

The **prognosis** of acute post-streptococcal glomerulonephritis is good in children, worse in adults. Almost all preschool children will recover, with less than 1% developing crescentic glomerulonephritis.

Case 9.3 Post-streptococcal glomerulonephritis

A 9-year-old boy was admitted as an emergency with puffiness of the face, eyes and trunk. A week previously he had complained of a sore throat. On examination, he was mildly pyrexial (temperature 37.5 °C) and hypertensive (BP 170/110). There was periorbital and scrotal oedema. His urine showed proteinuria, haematuria and red cell casts. He was anaemic (Hb 107 g/l) with a normal white cell count and differential. A throat swab grew normal flora, but antibodies to strepto-coccal antigens were present in high titre: antistreptolysin O titre 1600 IU/ml (normal <300 IU/ml). Serum complement studies done 3 days after admission showed a very low C3 (0.10 g/l; NR 0.8–1.40) and a normal C4 (0.23 g/l; NR 0.2–0.4). His creatinine clearance was 46 ml/min, serum albumin 29 g/l and urinary protein excretion 1.5 g/day.

These findings were typical of post-streptococcal glomerulonephritis and so renal biopsy was not performed. As anticipated, the serum complement returned to normal in 4 weeks, accompanied by disappearance of the proteinuria and hypertension, although a small amount of microscopic haematuria persisted. The prognosis is good. An unusual feature of this case was the degree of hypertension.

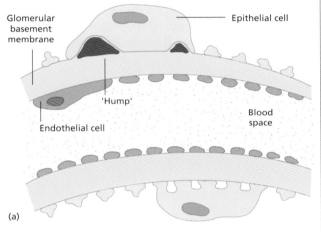

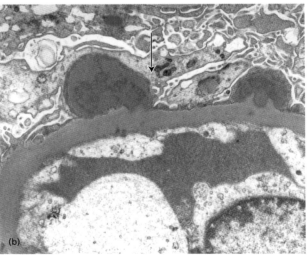

Fig. 9.8 (a) Characteristic 'humps' seen in post-streptococcal glomerulonephritis. These are localized, epimembranous, electron-dense deposits found in several forms of acute post-infectious glomerulonephritis. (b) Electron micrograph of acute proliferative post-streptococcal glomerulonephritis showing subepithelial 'humps' (arrow) (see also Fig. 9.13).

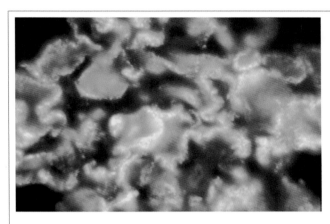

Fig. 9.9 Post-streptococcal glomerulonephritis showing 'lumpy-bumpy' deposits on immunofluorescence. Compare this with antiglomerular basement membrane nephritis (Fig. 9.15b).

9.6 Chronic glomerulonephritis

9.6.1 Chronic immune-complex glomerulonephritis

Immune-complex nephritis is believed to account for the majority of cases of human glomerulonephritis, but certain criteria should be fulfilled for complexes to be considered relevant to the pathogenesis of renal disease (Box 9.2). In practice, however, the diagnosis of immune-complex nephritis usually rests solely on immunofluorescent findings similar to those of experimental models of immune-complex disease.

The **pathogenesis** of experimental immune-complex nephritis is well defined. When rabbits are given repeated intravenous injections of a foreign protein, some develop a chronic progressive glomerulonephritis. Damage depends on producing a state of antigen excess after every injection, which saturates free antibody and generates loads of immune complexes. If animals fail to produce any antibody or, instead, mount a strong humoral response that rapidly eliminates the antigen, they do not develop glomerulonephritis. Affected animals produce non-precipitating, low-affinity antibody that is poor at antigen elimination. Even good antibody producers develop nephritis if the repeated antigen dose is increased to maintain antigen excess.

Reasons for chronic immune-complex disease in humans are not fully understood, but comparisons with this experimental model suggest some specific situations in which this is likely to occur (Box 9.3 and Fig. 9.10). Examples of **persistent antigen exposure** that give rise to immune-complex nephritis are shown in Table 9.2. Chronic infection is the best-recognized source of prolonged antigen exposure.

Variations in host responses are often due to genetic differences. Associations exist between various forms of glomerulonephritis and certain human leukocyte antigen (HLA) types may, at least in part, reflect linked, partial deficiencies of complement components C4 and C2. Patients with inherited complement defects (see Chapter 3) are unduly prone to immune-complex disease (including nephritis), since high levels of circulating immune complexes are not cleared from the blood. Classical complement pathway activity is important in

preventing the formation of large insoluble immune complexes, while the alternate pathway is concerned with disruption of large insoluble complexes. Failure of any of these functions, particularly dysregulation of the alternate pathway of complement, can result in deposition of immune complexes (see Chapter 10, Fig. 10.10). Paradoxically, complement both protects against immune-complex disease and yet is a mediator of immune-complex-mediated tissue damage.

The reticuloendothelial system (mononuclear-phagocyte system) is a major mechanism for clearance of complexes (Fig. 9.10, see also Chapter 1, Fig. 1.21) and this also applies to the mesangium of the kidney. Clinically troublesome complexes seem to be of intermediate size (Fig. 9.11). Larger complexes, formed in excess of either antibody or antigen, are deposited mainly in the mesangium or, to a lesser extent, between the endothelium and the basement membrane.

Host factors may also be involved in renal damage. Certain genetic polymorphisms in factors H and B, membrane cofactor protein and C3 are also associated with membranoproliferative glomerulonephritis (MPGN) and may act as susceptibility genes, though these are not the whole story as family members with similar genetic changes are healthy and

---

Box 9.2 Criteria in support of an immune-complex-mediated aetiology of glomerulonephritis

- Immune complexes are present at the site of tissue damage
- The antigen component of the immune complex is identifiable
- Removal of immune complexes produces clinical improvement

Box 9.3 Experimental situations that tend to immune-complex disease

- Antigen exposure persists (Table 9.2)
- The host makes an abnormal response
- Local factors, such as C3 receptors or changes in permeability that promote deposition of circulating complexes
- Complexes are made less soluble by defects in complement factors

---

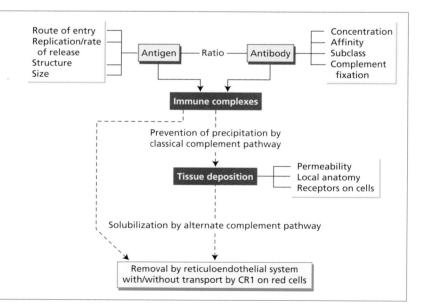

Fig. 9.10 Factors influencing the development of immune-complex disease. CR1, complement receptor 1.

Table 9.2 Examples of immune-complex nephritis in humans

	Antigen*	Associated disease†
Exogenous antigens		
Virus	Hepatitis B virus	Hepatitis B
		Polyarteritis nodosa
	Hepatitis C virus	Mixed essential cryoglobulinaemia
	Cytomegalovirus	Glomerulonephritis
Bacteria	Streptococcus	Post-streptococcal glomerulonephritis
	Streptococcus viridans	Bacterial endocarditis
	Staphylococcus	Shunt nephritis
	Mycobacterium leprae	Lepromatous leprosy
Parasites	Plasmodium malariae	Quartan malarial nephropathy
	Schistosoma mansoni	Schistosoma nephritis
	Toxoplasma gondii	Toxoplasma nephritis
Drugs	Penicillamine	
	Gold	Drug-induced nephropathy
	Foreign serum	Serum sickness
Endogenous antigens		
Autoantigens	Nuclear antigens	Systemic lupus erythematosus
	Renal tubular antigen	Membranous nephropathy
	IgG	Cryoglobulinaemia
	Tumour antigens	Neoplasia

*In many disorders with features suggestive of immune-complex deposition, no specific antigen has been incriminated.
†While immune complexes have been detected in these conditions, other mechanisms may also contribute to tissue damage.

glomerulonephritis usually develops later in life, suggesting environmental factors are important too.

While some glomerular damage is due to deposition of circulating complexes, other forms of glomerulonephritis are due to formation of **complexes *in situ***. Charged antigens, such as lectins or certain bacterial products, can be trapped electrostatically in the GBM or mesangium and then attract antibody and immune reactants. For instance, DNA binds to the capillary wall and may localize anti-DNA antibodies to this site in systemic lupus erythematosus (SLE).

The **diagnosis** of immune-complex nephritis is nearly always made by direct immunofluorescence or immunoperoxidase

staining of kidney biopsies. Immunoglobulins and complement may be deposited in tubular basement membrane, interstitial tissue and blood vessels, as well as in the glomeruli. An irregular, interrupted granular or 'lumpy-bumpy' pattern of deposition is characteristic of immune complexes (Fig. 9.9). Deposition may be mainly in the GBM or confined to the mesangium (Fig. 9.12).

9.6.2 Membranoproliferative glomerulonephritis (mesangiocapillary glomerulonephritis)

MPGN is one of the most severe glomerular diseases of late childhood and adolescence. At least two distinct types of MPGN exist (Fig. 9.13 and Table 9.3), although the differences are only detectable by electron or immunofluorescent microscopy.

Two-thirds of patients have electron-dense deposits in the mesangium and in the subendothelial space – **type I MPGN**. Immunohistology shows that these contain IgG, IgM, C4, C3 and C1q. Serum C3 levels do not show a consistent pattern and, when complement activation is demonstrated, the classical or alternate pathways or both may be involved. These immune deposits are not specific and can occur in any of the chronic immune-complex disorders shown in Table 9.3, but particularly hepatitis B or C, or SLE.

In the remaining one-third, deposits are present within the GBM, as in Case 9.4, giving a 'ribbon-like' appearance – **type II MPGN** ('dense-deposit disease') (Fig. 9.13). In type II MPGN there is almost exclusive fixation of C3 along the margin of the dense-deposit material in the mesangium and in the GBM. Serum levels of C3 are extremely low, with normal levels of C1q and C4, implying that complement activation is occurring via the alternate pathway. Nearly all patients with type II MPGN have circulating C3 nephritic factor (C3 NeF) and absent Factor H (which inhibits C3b – see Chapter 1) due to genetic factors or autoantibodies, suggesting dysregulation of the alternate complement pathway. This is consistent with animal data implicating deletion of this gene in the development of a dense-deposit renal phenotype. C3 NeF is an autoantibody of IgG class that binds to the alternate pathway C3 convertase to create a stable enzyme complex that is resistant to breakdown. As a result, more C3 is cleaved to C3b and this positive feedback loop continues until most of the serum C3 is consumed. The overproduction of C3b by C3Nef, along with failure of Factor H, the C3b inhibitor, results in deposition of C3b in the GBM and subsequent activation of C5 and the membrane attack complex (see Chapter 1).

C3 NeF alone is not sufficient to cause MPGN: its presence is not related to the clinical state of the patient or to the prognosis, as some patients with C3 NeF do not develop MPGN. As an IgG antibody, C3 NeF may be transported across the placenta and cause transient hypocomplementaemia in the newborn. However, renal function is not altered in these children, suggesting that C3 NeF is a marker of MPGN rather than the cause of the renal damage. There is a strong association between type II MPGN and partial lipodystrophy,

Fig. 9.11 Sites of immune-complex deposition in humans. The size of the complexes and their rates of deposition influence the clinical presentation and eventual renal morphology. GBM, glomerular basement membrane.

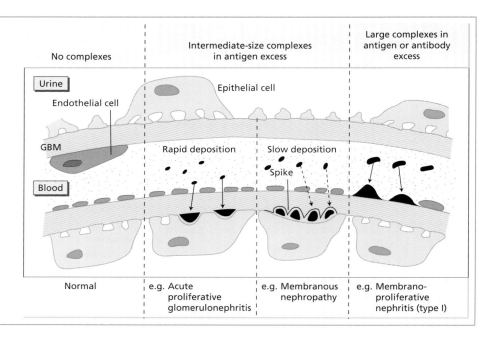

Fig. 9.12 Schematic representation of direct immunohistological staining of renal biopsies. Immune complexes may be present as granular deposits or aggregates in the glomerular capillary loops (1a), mesangium (2), tubular basement membrane (3a) or the interstitium (4). Linear staining is typical of antibodies reacting with antigens present in the glomerular (1b) or tubular (3b) basement membranes.

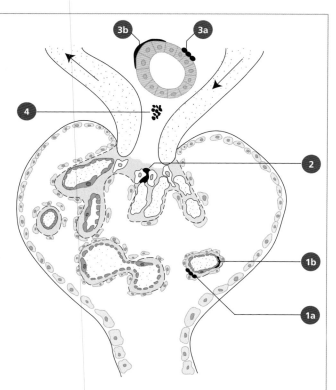

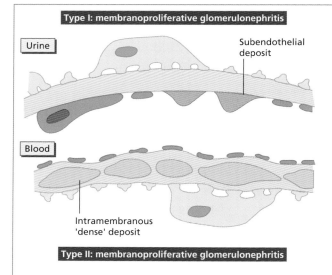

Fig. 9.13 Membranoproliferative glomerulonephritis. Two major types can be recognized, depending on whether the deposits are subendothelial (type I) or intramembranous (type II).

a condition characterized by loss of subcutaneous fat from the upper half of the body.

These two types of glomerulonephritis show significant clinical differences (Table 9.3) and **differences in therapy**. Various types of treatment have been tried in type I MPGN, with little evidence of any benefit. In type II MPGN patients with mutations in the Factor H gene (CFH), infusion of fresh frozen plasma to provide functionally intact Factor H or plasmapheresis (to remove C3Nef), or both, are reported to be helpful (Case 9.4).

Atypical haemolytic–uraemic syndrome (aHUS) is a severe illness, characterized by haemolytic anaemia, thrombocytopenia and acute renal failure. Diarrhoea, peripheral ischaemia, vasculopathy and myocardial infarction are also described. Some 90% of cases are due to shiga-toxin-producing E. coli (STEC). The remaining 10% are due to congenital or acquired defects in the complement system. This can include deficiency of Factor H and Factor I, and acquired autoantibodies to these two proteins. The acquired form may be seen in the context of connective tissue diseases such as SLE, during pregnancy and associated with malignancy. Eculizumab, an antibody that blocks the activation of C5, has been used successfully in patients with atypical haemolytic–uraemic syndrome due to complement abnormalities in the alternate complement pathway. This may be used in type II MPGN patients, since the safety and efficacy of eculizumab were established in patients with paroxysmal nocturnal haemoglobinuria (PNH). Avacopan is an oral anti-C5a, which is being trialled in aHUS and to prevent renal damage in antineutrophil cytoplasmic antibody (ANCA)-associated vasculitis.

Without specific therapy, the overall 10-year survival rate for both forms of MPGN is about 50%. Prognosis is worse in patients who have a persisting nephrotic syndrome, hypertension, crescents on the renal biopsy or decrease in the glomerular

Table 9.3 A comparison of type I and type II membranoproliferative glomerulonephritis

Feature	Type I	Type II
Acute nephritic episode	Uncommon	Common
Nephrotic syndrome	Common	Common
Serum C3 level	Normal or low	Very low
Genetic association	Not with Factor H deficiency	Factor H deficiency
Clinical associations	Hepatitis C malignancy	Partial lipodystrophy
Recurrence following renal transplantation	Frequent	Invariable

---

(icon) Case 9.4 Membranoproliferative glomerulonephritis – type II

A 13-year-old boy had been well until 4 weeks before admission, when he developed a cough, periorbital oedema, ankle swelling, headaches and upper abdominal discomfort. On admission, he was febrile with facial and ankle oedema; there was generalized, superficial lymphadenopathy, numerous adventitial sounds in the lungs and hypertension (BP 140/110). His haemoglobin was 72 g/l with a normal white cell count and an erythrocyte sedimentation rate (ESR) of 137 mm/h. His blood urea was high (27.5 mmol/l) with a low serum bicarbonate (13.6 mmol/l) and serum albumin (19 g/l). His creatinine clearance was 45 ml/min per m^2 with urinary protein loss of 6.7 g/day. His serum CH_{50} was low (14 U/ml; NR 25–45), as was his C3 level (0.20 g/l; NR 0.8–1.4); his C4 level was normal (0.30 g/l; NR 0.2–0.4). A chest X-ray showed several rounded opacities in both lungs. These were presumed to be infective and treated with amoxicillin and flucloxacillin with resolution of the radiological findings.

The association of a low C3 with acute glomerulonephritis suggested acute post-streptococcal disease as the most likely diagnosis (see Case 9.1), although no streptococci were isolated and streptococcal antibodies were not raised. Over the following 3 weeks, his blood urea fell but the proteinuria and hypertension persisted.

Three months later, he felt better but still had heavy proteinuria with a low serum albumin (22 g/l; NR 35–50). Surprisingly, the serum CH_{50} and C3 levels were still low at 18 U/ml and 0.4 g/l, respectively. This pattern was not consistent with the working diagnosis. It suggested continued complement activation via the alternate pathway, due either to some circulating activating factor or a regulatory defect caused by absence of the inhibitors I or H (see Chapter 1). However, serum levels of I and H were normal. Electrophoresis of fresh serum and plasma showed the presence of C3 breakdown products and his serum was able to break down C3 in normal serum due to the presence of C3 nephritic factor.

C3 nephritic factor shows a strong association with membranoproliferative glomerulonephritis (MPGN), but not with acute post-streptococcal glomerulonephritis. Since these conditions have different prognoses, a renal biopsy was performed at this late stage. This showed 11 glomeruli, all of which were swollen with proliferation of mesangial, endothelial and epithelial cells. On electron microscopy, the capillary loops showed basement membrane thickening with electron-dense deposits within the glomerular basement membrane (GBM; Fig. 9.13). On immunofluorescence, intense C3 deposition was present in the GBM without immunoglobulin staining. These appearances, together with the finding of circulating C3 nephritic factor, are characteristic of MPGN with dense intramembranous deposits (type II MPGN). Alternate-day prednisolone therapy was started; as this condition nearly always shows a slow progression to chronic renal failure, plasmapheresis was attempted with additional immunosuppression in the hope that progression could be avoided, since there were no crescents seen on histology.

filtration rate. Transplantation is successful in 60% of patients with type I MPGN, but type II MPGN recurs histologically in almost all grafts (see later Table 9.8) in line with the systemic causes of the renal depositions.

9.6.3 Lupus nephritis

Although only 25% of patients with SLE present with renal disease as the first manifestation of lupus (see Chapter 10), clinical glomerulonephritis occurs in about 50% of cases of SLE at some time, and evidence of renal involvement can be detected in most patients, even in the absence of proteinuria. The development of nephritis is closely linked to morbidity and survival in lupus. The **histological appearances** have been classified by the World Health Organization (WHO) according to the pattern and extent of immune deposition and inflammation (Table 9.4). The clinical features of lupus nephritis do not predict the severity of the glomerular lesion on biopsy.

The **prognosis** in SLE is not as dismal as was once believed, but the development of renal disease is a strong predictor of ESRF and early mortality. The 10-year survival in patients with all forms of the disease is over 80%. Patients with ESRF are excellent candidates for renal transplantation. Disease activity post transplantation is sporadic and infrequent; recurrence of lupus nephritis is rare.

The major cause of early **deaths** is active systemic disease – particularly central nervous system, cardiac, thrombotic and renal disease. Late deaths are often caused by disease progression (e.g. ESRF). Infection is an important cause of mortality at all stages of the condition. Overwhelming infection occurs typically in patients treated with high-dose steroids and other immunosuppressive drugs. While aggressive induction treatment reduces renal disease, it may increase susceptibility to infection (Chapter 3).

Most **treatment** data suggest that WHO class II nephritis has a benign course, and treatment, in the absence of other indications, is not usually needed. The outcome and treatment of class V nephritis are hotly debated. The decision to treat active WHO class III and IV lupus nephritis is less controversial. Systematic review of available trials supports treatment with corticosteroids and an immunosuppressive agent, usually cyclophosphamide or azathioprine. Mycophenolate mofetil can be used in place of azathioprine. A Cochrane review showed that cyclophosphamide plus steroids slowed progression to ESRF, but had no impact on mortality and with a significant risk of ovarian failure. Azathioprine plus steroids reduced the risk of mortality, but did not alter renal outcomes. Ciclosporin is an alternative agent, particularly used in children to reduce corticosteroid complications. Monoclonal antibodies to CD20 are being used (rituximab, ocrelizumab) with benefit in selected subgroups. Belimumab, which targets BAFF/BLyS, has been approved as an adjunctive therapy for active lupus nephritis, and abatacept, which binds to T-cell activation antigens CD80/CD86, and Janus kinase (JAK) inhibitors are undergoing trials.

Table 9.4 Modified World Health Organization classification of lupus nephritis

Class 0	Normal
Class I	Light microscopy normal, immune deposits on immunofluorescence involving part of a glomerulus while the rest of that glomerulus appears normal
Class II	A. Mesangial deposits
	B. Mesangial hypercellularity
Class III	Focal segmental proliferative glomerulonephritis (<50% glomeruli)
	Immune deposits in mesangium
Class IV	As class III but 'diffuse' (>50% glomeruli)
	Includes membranoproliferative type
Class V	Membranous nephropathy with subepithelial immune-complex deposition
	A. Membranous nephropathy (MN) alone
	B. MN plus class II
	C. MN plus class III
	D. MN plus class IV
Class VI	Glomerulosclerosis

9.7 Rapidly progressive glomerulonephritis

Rapidly progressive glomerulonephritis (RPGN) describes a group of diseases with aggressive glomerular injury that can lead to ESRF within days or weeks if not diagnosed and treated early. The usual pathological lesion is **crescentic glomerulonephritis**. RPGN constitutes 3–5% of all cases of glomerulonephritis. It is not a single entity but has multiple aetiologies involving several pathogenic mechanisms. Based on the immunological findings, patients fall into three broad groups, as shown in Fig. 9.14. The prognosis is especially grave when over 70% of glomeruli are involved, there are diffuse circumferential crescents and there is prolonged oliguria.

9.7.1 Antiglomerular basement membrane disease

Acute glomerulonephritis mediated by anti-GBM antibody accounts for about 1–2% of all cases of glomerulonephritis, but about 20% of cases presenting as acute renal failure due to RPGN. Anti-GBM nephritis is more common in those who possess HLA-DR15 or DR4, and less common in those with DR1 or DR7. Patients present with nephritis alone (Case 9.5) or commonly with glomerulonephritis and lung haemorrhage, a combination termed **Goodpasture's syndrome**. However, rapidly progressive nephritis and pulmonary haemorrhage can occur in other multisystem disorders such as SLE or granulomatosis with polyangiitis (GPA), so *the combination of renal and lung involvement is not synonymous with anti-GBM disease.*

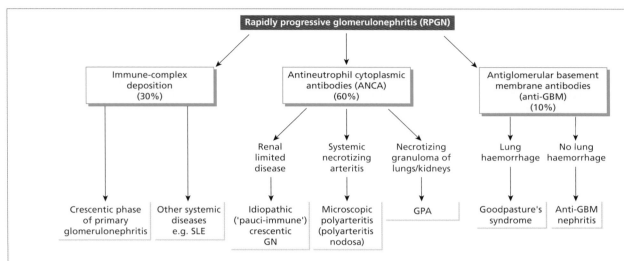

Fig. 9.14 Clinical and immunological classification of rapidly progressive glomerulonephritis. GN, glomerulonephritis; GPA, granulomatosis with polyangiitis; SLE, systemic lupus erythematosus

Case 9.5 Antiglomerular basement membrane glomerulonephritis

A 55-year-old man presented with a 3-week history of malaise, nausea, fever and shivering. Although there were no urinary symptoms, analysis of a mid-stream urine specimen showed microscopic haematuria and proteinuria (2+). There was no cough or haemoptysis and no family history of renal disease or hypertension. On examination, he was mildly pyrexial but there were no vasculitic lesions, oedema or hypertension. Cystoscopy and renal ultrasound showed no cause for his haematuria. Over the next week, his blood urea rose steadily from 10 to 23 mmol/l (NR 2.5–7.5) and the serum creatinine from 164 to 515 μmol/l (NR 60–120). His haemoglobin was 89 g/l with a white cell count of 10.4 × 10^9/l and a normal differential. His urine contained red cell casts and he rapidly became oliguric. Antinuclear antibodies, including anti-DNA antibodies, were not detected and serum C3 and C4 levels were normal.

A renal biopsy specimen contained seven glomeruli: four showed focal necrotizing glomerulonephritis with epithelial crescents, but the remaining three were normal. On immunofluorescence, linear staining with IgG was present along the glomerular capillary basement membrane (Fig. 9.15b). The patient's serum contained antibodies to glomerular basement membrane (GBM; see Chapter 19). The diagnosis was therefore rapidly progressive glomerulonephritis due to antibodies to GBM. Although oliguric, he was treated with high doses of prednisolone and cyclophosphamide, and underwent daily plasma exchanges for 2 weeks, until anti-GBM antibodies were no longer detectable. However, renal function failed to recover; cytotoxic therapy was stopped and regular haemodialysis started.

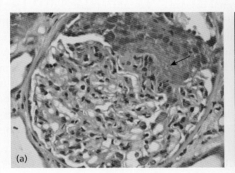
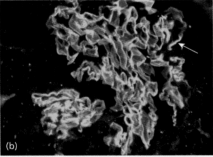

Fig. 9.15 Antiglomerular basement membrane nephritis showing (a) a crescent with fibrin necrosis (arrowed) and (b) linear fluorescent staining along the basement membrane (arrowed).

The target antigen is the α3 chain of type IV collagen, a major constituent of the GBM. **Lung damage** results from antibodies to antigens common to both alveolar and glomerular basement membranes. In Goodpasture's syndrome, respiratory symptoms often precede renal disease by 1 year or longer. Haemoptysis, sometimes severe enough to cause anaemia, is a prominent feature and the sputum typically contains haemosiderin-laden macrophages. Lung biopsies show

> ### Box 9.4 Evidence that anti-glomerular basement membrane (GBM) antibodies are pathogenic
>
> - Linear deposition of IgG reflects binding to regularly spaced antigenic determinants rather than deposition as immune complexes
> - IgG eluted from the kidneys of patients with anti-GBM nephritis causes identical glomerular damage when injected into monkeys
> - Removal of anti-GBM antibodies from the circulation can prevent irreversible organ damage if done early
> - Anti-GBM nephritis can recur rapidly in a renal allograft if transplantation is performed while circulating anti-GBM antibodies are still present

> ### Box 9.5 Evidence that anti-neutrophil cytoplasmic antibodies (ANCA) may be pathogenic
>
> - *in vitro*, ANCA activate primed neutrophils and react with endothelial cells that express PR3
> - *in vitro*, ANCA promote recruitment and adhesion between neutrophils and endothelial cells
> - ANCA accelerate apoptosis of tumour necrosis factor (TNF)-primed neutrophils
> - Spleen cells from MPO-knockout mice immunized with MPO cause necrotizing, crescentic glomerulonephritis and systemic vasculitis when injected into the immunodeficient Rag 2–/– mouse. Anti-MPO IgG was also able to induce crescentic nephritis

intraalveolar haemorrhage and necrotizing alveolitis. There is convincing evidence that anti-GBM antibodies are responsible for the nephritis (Box 9.4). Renal biopsy reveals crescenteric glomerulonephritis with linear deposition of IgG along the glomerular capillaries.

Although the **trigger** is unknown, anti-GBM disease follows upper respiratory tract infections in 20–60% of patients, or exposure to certain hydrocarbons as in smoking. These agents may damage alveolar basement membrane, generating new, previously hidden ('cryptic') and potent antigens that are highly susceptible in antigen processing by endosomal proteases and so able to stimulate autoantibody production. Pulmonary haemorrhage in anti-GBM disease is strongly associated with cigarette smoking. Experimental data implicate both autoantibodies and cell-mediated immunity in pathogenesis, and there are reports that regulatory T cells are increased in the convalescent phase. Unlike other systemic autoimmune diseases, patients rarely suffer a relapse once the autoantibodies are eliminated.

The **prognosis** of anti-GBM disease is extremely poor: without appropriate treatment the likelihood of requiring dialysis or dying from the disease is over 90%. **Aggressive immunosuppressive therapy**, usually a high-dose steroid combined with cyclophosphamide, coupled with intensive plasmapheresis, is the treatment of choice. *Prompt treatment can lead to long-term recovery*, but no improvement in renal function can be expected in patients with established anuria or where crescents involve over 85% of glomeruli. The main risk to life in these circumstances is massive lung haemorrhage. While renal transplantation is successful, nephritis can recur if antibodies are still present, so transplantation should be deferred until anti-GBM antibodies are no longer detectable.

9.7.2 Antineutrophil cytoplasmic antibody-associated glomerulonephritis

Serum IgG antibodies reacting with cytoplasmic components of neutrophils and monocytes are a diagnostic marker for active granulomatosis with polyangiitis (formerly Wegener's granulomatosis; Chapter 11) and reflect disease activity. *Two patterns of antineutrophil cytoplasmic antibody (ANCA) reactivity are important clinically*: generalized cytoplasmic staining (**C-ANCA**) and a perinuclear pattern (**P-ANCA**). Most C-ANCA sera react with a serine proteinase called proteinase 3 (PR3), while most pANCA sera react with myeloperoxidase (MPO). A further pattern is associated with inflammatory bowel disease, particularly ulcerative colitis. Some C-ANCA/P-ANCA-positive sera react with neutrophil antigens other than PR3/MPO, particularly after infections.

Raised ANCA titres are generally detectable during active granulomatosis with polyangiitis, and rising titres may herald a relapse. There has been debate whether ANCAs are pathogenic in vasculitis or simply a marker, but there is mounting evidence that they are pathogenic (Box 9.5). The exact pathogenesis of granulomatosis with polyangiitis is not completely understood, but T cells, B cells, neutrophils and endothelial cells have all been implicated in the process.

Patients with ANCA-associated glomerulonephritis are usually aged from 40 to 70 years and most have had a flu-like illness with arthralgia and myalgia a few days or weeks prior to the onset of renal disease or vasculitis (Case 9.6). A **spectrum of vasculitis** is seen, ranging from disease limited to the kidneys in about 25% of cases to a systemic vasculitic process with pulmonary involvement in 50%. ANCA-associated glomerulonephritis is now the commonest form of crescentic or RPGN. As in Case 9.6, the renal lesion is characterized by few or no deposits of immunoglobulin or complement in the kidney (so-called pauci-immune glomerulonephritis) and by necrosis and crescent formation (Fig. 9.16).

Over 75% of patients with ANCA-associated glomerulonephritis go into remission following aggressive immunosuppression, although 30–50% relapse within 2 years and require further therapy. Cyclophosphamide and glucocorticoids are first-line therapy, giving a survival rate of 80% at a mean follow-up of 8 years. Rituximab can be used if cyclophosphamide is contraindicated, and plasmapheresis has shown benefit in some cases of severe disease.

Case 9.6 Antineutrophil cytoplasmic antibody-associated necrotizing crescentic glomerulonephritis

A 64-year-old man presented with a 1-month history of nausea and malaise and a 1-week history of flu-like symptoms, rigors and vomiting. Eight weeks earlier, while on holiday, he had developed infected insect bites around his left ankle and was treated with erythromycin. He had no urinary or joint symptoms and no family history of renal disease. On examination, he was pale, with mild pitting oedema of both ankles and a blood pressure of 170/90. Analysis of a mid-stream urine specimen showed proteinuria (3+) with microscopic haematuria and granular casts. His haemoglobin was 92 g/l with a white cell count of 17.7×10^9/l and an erythrocyte sedimentation rate (ESR) of 122 mm/h. His blood urea was 42.6 mmol/l (NR 2.5–7.5) and serum creatinine 1094 μmol/l (NR 60–120). Malarial parasites and hepatitis B surface antigen were not detected in his blood. Over the next 72 h, his urine output fell to 30 ml/day with further increases in his blood urea and serum creatinine.

Ultrasound examination showed bilaterally enlarged kidneys but no evidence of obstruction. Serum immunoglobulin levels were normal, but C3 (1.56 g/l; NR 0.8–1.40) and C4 (0.46 g/l; NR 0.2–0.4) were raised. There was no paraproteinaemia and no free monoclonal light chains in his urine. Antinuclear, anti-dsDNA, and antiglomerular basement membrane antibodies were negative. However, the patient's serum contained IgG antibodies that reacted strongly with cytoplasmic antigens of alcohol-fixed neutrophils, producing a granular pattern characteristic of classical antineutrophil cytoplasmic antibodies (C-ANCA). Further analysis showed antibodies to a neutrophil enzyme called serine proteinase 3 (PR3) by enzyme-linked immunosorbent assay (ELISA; see Chapter 19).

A renal biopsy was performed to confirm the cause of his rapidly progressive glomerulonephritis. The biopsy specimen contained 30 glomeruli: one-third of these were totally sclerosed and all but one of the remainder showed necrotizing, crescentic glomerulonephritis. Cellular crescents, with extensive tuft necrosis (Fig. 9.16b), were seen in most glomeruli. Immunofluorescence showed no immune deposits in the glomeruli, so-called 'pauci-immune' disease. The diagnosis was that of ANCA-associated, necrotizing crescentic glomerulonephritis.

He was treated with pulse cyclophosphamide (500 mg/m^2) and pulse methylprednisolone (1 g daily for 3 days), followed by 60 mg of prednisolone daily. For the next 12 days he required peritoneal dialysis until his renal function improved. He was discharged on maintenance therapy of prednisolone 40 mg/day with pulse intravenous cyclophosphamide at monthly intervals. He continued on this regimen until his C-ANCA became negative; his treatment was then changed to oral prednisolone and azathioprine.

9.8 Nephrotic syndrome

The three essential features of the nephrotic syndrome are:

- Marked proteinuria.
- Hypoalbuminaemia.
- Oedema.

In adults, the proteinuria generally exceeds 3.5 g/day with a serum albumin concentration below 25 g/l. In children, the proteinuria is usually more than 50 mg/kg per day. Although hypercholesterolaemia and hypertriglyceridaemia often accompany the nephrotic syndrome, they are not essential for diagnosis.

Diagnosis of the nephrotic syndrome does not imply any particular renal histology or any specific disease: it reflects an underlying glomerular disease that increases the permeability of the glomerular basement membrane to protein; there are many causes (Fig. 9.17). There are three distinct histological variants of primary nephrotic syndrome: minimal-change nephropathy, focal glomerulosclerosis and membranous nephropathy.

9.8.1 Minimal-change nephropathy

The major features of minimal-change nephropathy (MCN) are exemplified by Case 9.7. It accounts for over 90% of cases of nephrotic syndrome in children and 20% of adult cases (Fig. 9.17). No age is exempt.

The **cause and pathogenesis** of MCN are unknown. There is no realistic animal model. Cell-mediated immune reactions leading to podocyte dysfunction may play an important role (Box 9.6). Mutations in several genes coding for split diaphragm proteins – nephrin and podocin – are known to cause MCN, severe congenital forms of nephrotic syndrome and some cases of steroid-resistant nephrotic syndrome, the suggestion being that disruption of slit diaphragm proteins is thought to lead to podocyte apoptosis (see Figure 9.3). Renal pathology of MCN shows normal glomeruli on light microscopy but fusion of podocytes on electron microscopy. Current theory suggests that MCN is a result of abnormal T-cell function and that T cells secrete some sort of 'permeable factor' affecting susceptible podocytes in the GBM. However, evidence of the involvement of T cells is sketchy and even B cells may play a role since rituximab has shown some efficacy.

MCN responds predictably and consistently to **corticosteroids**; 95% of patients have a complete remission within 8 weeks. Failure to respond to steroids or the presence of unselective proteinuria would negate a diagnosis of minimal-change disease (see Case 9.7) and a renal biopsy be necessary. Once symptoms improve, alternate-day steroid **therapy** can be used to reduce the likelihood of Cushing's syndrome. The aim is to

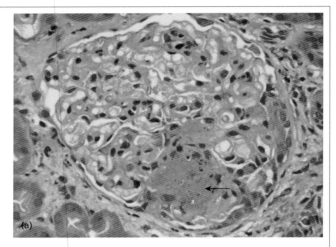

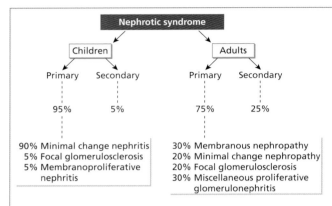

Fig. 9.17 Renal morphology in patients with the nephrotic syndrome. Primary glomerulonephritis is more common than secondary renal disease (see section 9.8.5).

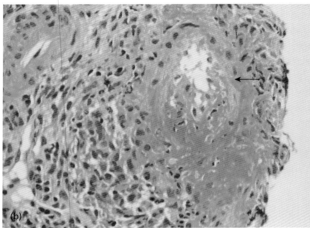

Fig. 9.16 Antineutrophil cytoplasmic antibody (ANCA)-associated glomerulonephritis showing (a) a segmental area of tuft necrosis (arrowed) and (b) vasculitis of a renal arteriole (arrowed).

keep patients on steroids for 3–4 months: this is associated with a lower relapse rate at 2 years than if steroids are given for a shorter period. About 25% of children have one attack only; the remainder relapse, 50% on more than four occasions, usually as steroids are stopped or the dose reduced. Relapses usually respond to further steroid therapy, but in some frequent relapsers treatment with ciclosporin, cyclophosphamide, tacrolimus or levamisole may produce prolonged remissions.

MCN has a very good **prognosis**, even when therapy is required for years. The earlier the age at onset of symptoms, the longer the illness persists, but death occurs in about 3% of cases only, usually from avoidable complications such as septicaemia, hypovolaemia, thromboembolism or acute renal failure.

9.8.2 Focal glomerulosclerosis

In some cases of the nephrotic syndrome, the clinical picture resembles MCN except that proteinuria is only moderately or poorly selective, hypertension is relatively common and the

---

Case 9.7 Minimal-change nephropathy

An 8-year-old girl presented with a 3-day history of swelling of the legs and puffiness around the eyes following a cold 1 week earlier. She had some mild abdominal discomfort and a headache for 2 days. Examination revealed a generally oedematous girl with ascites and a blood pressure of 120/70. Her height was on the 50th centile but her weight was above the 90th centile. Urinalysis showed marked proteinuria without haematuria. Her haemoglobin, white cell count and urea and electrolytes were normal, but there was marked hypoalbuminaemia (11 g/l) and proteinuria (26 g/day). The urinary clearance of IgG relative to that of transferrin was less than 0.1, indicating highly selective proteinuria. Creatinine clearance, CH_{50}, C4 and C3 levels were all normal. A throat swab grew commensal flora only and the antibody titre to streptococcal antigens was normal.

Highly selective proteinuria in a child with nephrotic syndrome is virtually diagnostic of minimal-change nephropathy. For this reason, renal biopsy was not performed but a trial of steroid therapy (prednisolone 60 mg/day) was started, with dramatic effect. Over the next week, her serum albumin rose to 26 g/l and the proteinuria subsided. At discharge, only a trace of proteinuria was detectable but she continued to take 40 mg prednisolone on alternate days for a further 3 months. The nephrotic syndrome did not relapse when steroids were withdrawn.

Box 9.6 Evidence that T-cell-mediated reactions are involved in minimal-change nephropathy (MCN)

- The condition responds dramatically to corticosteroid therapy
- Hodgkin's disease, lymphoma, leukaemia and thymoma are associated with MCN
- Spontaneous clinical improvement has been seen following infections that depress cellular immunity, such as measles
- Changes are demonstrated in lymphocyte cytotoxicity to human kidney tissue in some patients with MCN
- Cultured T cells from MCN patients synthesize a factor causing transient proteinuria when injected into rats

---

patient responds poorly to steroids. Subsequent renal biopsies may show focal segmental glomerulosclerosis. *Because this disorder involves juxtamedullary glomeruli initially, superficial biopsies of the cortex can be normal.* As the disease progresses, more glomeruli become sclerosed until the outer cortex is also involved. Focal glomerulosclerosis is a **histological** diagnosis that can either arise without a clear cause ('primary' or 'idiopathic') or due to glomerular injury – commonly due to hypertension.

The **pathogenesis** of primary focal glomerulosclerosis, like that of minimal-change disease, is not well characterized, but several genetic mutations in split diaphragm proteins have been described and give rise to an autosomal dominant form of the condition.

The **incidence** of focal glomerulosclerosis seems to be increasing in adults and children and the *prognosis is quite different from minimal-change disease.* Progressive renal impairment occurs in 50% of patients. A small number of patients follow a rapidly downhill course and the lesion may recur after renal transplantation. An especially malignant variant of focal glomerulosclerosis occurs in patients with human immunodeficiency virus (HIV) infection. This HIV-associated nephropathy has a strong predilection for African-Americans and runs a fulminant downhill course.

Treatment remains controversial, although up to 20% of patients respond to immunosuppressive therapy with complete remission and long-term renal survival. Unfortunately, there is little in the way of good evidence to identify those who will respond.

9.8.3 Membranous glomerulonephritis

About 80% of patients with membranous glomerulonephritis present with a florid nephrotic syndrome; the remainder present with hypertension, poorly selective proteinuria or microscopic haematuria discovered on routine examination of the urine. Membranous glomerulonephritis can occur at any age, with the peak incidence in adults aged between 40 and 70 years (Case 9.8). The **characteristic lesion** is uniform thickening of the GBM without proliferation of cells. The lesions uniformly affect every glomerulus, but the degree of membranous thickening is not related to the severity of proteinuria.

The membranous thickening is produced mainly by **subepithelial deposits of immune complexes, followed by secondary formation of projections ('spikes')** of basement membrane material between the deposits (see Fig. 9.11). The deposits are characteristically granular and may contain C3, IgA and IgM as well as IgG. About 80% of cases of membranous glomerulonephritis are primary, i.e. no known cause has been found. Some cases are now associated with antibodies to the phospholipase A2 receptor (PLA2R) or to the thrombospondin type 1 domain containing 7A (THSD7A). Unusually, the autoantibody may be of IgG_4 subclass. The remaining 20% of cases are secondary to another disease or to drugs. The most important causes are drugs (gold, penicillamine, non-steroidal antiinflammatory drugs [NSAIDs], captopril, heroin), infections (hepatitis B or C, malaria, syphilis), SLE or tumours (carcinoma of the

---

 Case 9.8 Membranous glomerulonephritis

A 48-year-old man presented with a 3-month history of intermittent swelling of his ankles and puffiness of his face. There were no urinary symptoms and no family history of renal disease. He was taking no medication. On examination, he was pale and thin, with ankle oedema and a blood pressure of 130/80. Investigations showed a normal haemoglobin and white cell count and an erythrocyte sedimentation rate (ESR) of 32 mm/h. His blood urea was 9.1 mmol/l (NR 2.5–7.5), serum albumin 26 g/l, with a urinary protein loss of 7.8 g/day and a creatinine clearance of 106 ml/min. His serum immunoglobulin IgM and IgA, C3 and C4 levels were normal, but his IgG was low at 5.1 g/l (NR 7.2–19.0). Antinuclear antibodies, hepatitis B surface antigen and antibody, and hepatitis C antibody were not detected. There were no free light chains in his urine.

A renal biopsy was done to find the cause of his nephrotic syndrome; this showed no obvious increase in cellularity. However, the basement membrane of all glomeruli showed marked but uniform thickening with numerous subepithelial 'spikes'. Immunofluorescent examination showed granular deposits of IgG and C3 along all the glomerular capillary walls. The biopsy appearances were typical of membranous glomerulonephritis (Fig. 9.9). No specific treatment was given at this stage. One year later, he is asymptomatic but still has severe, non-selective proteinuria of 14 g/day.

Table 9.5 Protein component of amyloid fibrils

Type of amyloid	Major protein of fibril	Chemically related protein (? precursor) in serum
Light-chain-associated amyloidosis		
Idiopathic	AL	Light chain
Myeloma	AL	Light chain
Other monoclonal gammopathies	AL	Light chain
Acute-phase-associated amyloidosis		
Chronic inflammation/ suppuration	AA	SAA
Senile systemic amyloid	ATTR (senile) amyloid	Transthyretin
Haemodialysis-associated amyloidosis	β_2M	β_2M
Transmissible spongiform encephalopathies	Prion protein	?

AA, amyloid A protein; AL, light-chain amyloid protein; ATTR, amyloid transthyretin; β_2M, β_2-microglobulin; SAA, serum amyloid A protein.

bronchus, breast or colon). Some 10% of patients with membranous nephropathy have an underlying malignancy. It is presumed that nephropathy is the result of either antigenic cross-reactivity between the tumour and an unknown renal antigen, or the deposition of tumour antigens in the glomerulus followed by immune-complex formation.

There is considerable evidence that the **pathogenesis** of membranous nephropathy is immunologically mediated (Box 9.7). There is increasing evidence that complexes are formed *in situ* in the subepithelial space. Recently, the identification of several target antigens in human podocytes has led to the finding of specific autoantibodies, though their pathogenic role is as yet uncertain. A GWAS has provided further evidence for a highly significant association between a gene for one such antigen (PLA2R1) and HLA-DQA1 in some patients.

Membranous glomerulonephritis accounts for 30% of nephrotic syndrome in adults. The prognosis of idiopathic disease is variable: one-third of patients undergo spontaneous remission of proteinuria with excellent long-term survival; another third have persistent proteinuria; and the final third progress to renal failure, usually within 10 years of diagnosis.

Treatment of idiopathic membranous nephropathy is controversial and usually reserved for those patients showing definite evidence of renal deterioration. Urinary excretion of β_2-microglobulin is a marker of disease activity and may identify those patients likely to deteriorate relentlessly. In these patients, controlled trials have shown that prednisolone alone is of little benefit, but the addition of cyclophosphamide can induce remission.

9.8.4 Amyloid disease

Amyloidosis is a disorder of protein folding that results in fibrils. There have been many attempts to classify amyloidosis. Amyloidosis can be hereditary or acquired and the deposits can be focal, localized or systemic. Hereditary types are very rare though important models for studying pathogenesis. The main clinical problems are the systemic, acquired types. Classifications of these into 'primary' or 'secondary' types and those based on histological grounds or on the pattern of organ involvement have proved unreliable. *The best classification is one based on the nature of the amyloid protein found on biopsy.*

The fibrillary structure confers on amyloid the characteristic staining appearance with dyes such as Congo red or Sirius red or thioflavine T, and its birefringence under polarized light. Many different proteins make up these amyloid fibrils (Table 9.5). **Light-chain-associated amyloidosis** (or **AL amyloidosis**) is almost always associated with an abnormality of lymphoid cells and excessive production of monoclonal free light chains. About 20% of patients have frank multiple myeloma (see Chapter 6), but in 70% the immunocyte dyscrasia is subtler and clonal disease is undetectable in the remaining 10%. Most patients are over 50 years and almost any organ, except the brain, can be involved.

The amyloid protein found in **acute phase-associated amyloidosis** (or **AA amyloidosis**) is not derived from light chains. This protein is called amyloid A protein (AA). Its circulating serum precursor, serum amyloid A protein (SAA), is an acute-phase reactant with similarities to C-reactive protein. AA amyloidosis occurs in three main types of chronic disease: inflammatory disorders, local or systemic bacterial infections, and malignant disease. Previously amyloid was inevitable in autoinflammatory diseases, including familial Mediterranean fever (see Chapter 10), but a dramatic change in treatment has resulted in reducing amyloid in the past 10 years, following the discovery that most are driven by abnormal IL-1β secretion and can be controlled with anti-IL-1 agents. In the UK, rheumatic diseases are the commonest underlying disorders, with about 1% of patients with rheumatoid arthritis or juvenile chronic arthritis developing amyloidosis.

All forms of amyloid also contain **P-component**, which is identical to a plasma glycoprotein called serum amyloid P-component (SAP). SAP does not behave as an acute-phase reactant in humans, although SAP and C-reactive protein belong to the same protein 'superfamily' called pentraxins. SAP binds specifically to all amyloid fibrils as well as to DNA and chromatin, and protects fibrils from proteolysis and digestion by macrophages. Amyloid deposits mostly exert their pathological effects through physical disruption of normal tissue structure and function, although they may also have a cytotoxic effect by inducing apoptosis.

Case 9.9 shows that the clinical and biochemical picture produced by amyloid deposition in the kidneys has no unique features. Where the **diagnosis** is considered, *it is essential that the pathologist is made aware of this possibility so that the appropriate stains are used.* However, biopsies do not provide information on the extent of amyloid deposition. This can be achieved by scintigraphy using radiolabelled SAP. The tracer does not accumulate in normal subjects, but binds rapidly and specifically to all amyloid fibrils, allowing measurement of the whole-body amyloid load and the tissue distribution of the deposits. Repeat scans are used to monitor the progression of amyloid.

Renal and cardiac failure are the major causes of death in systemic amyloidosis and this poor prognosis has led to many trials. Treatment of AL amyloid now involves intensive chemotherapy, often including **bortezomib** (a proteasome inhibitor) followed by stem-cell transplantation. Thalidomide derivatives are also in the primary treatment (lenalidomide, pomalidomide). **Tafamidis** is a novel drug that binds to transthyretin (TTR) and is proving useful in amyloid due to TTR (ATTR). Measures that reduce the supply of the respective amyloid fibril precursor proteins (Table 9.6) can preserve organ function and improve survival, such as anti-tumour

Table 9.6 Principles of treatment of amyloidosis

Fibril type	Aim of treatment	Example
AL amyloidosis	Suppress monoclonal light-chain production	Chemotherapy for myeloma or immunocyte dyscrasia; thalidomide derivatives; bortezomib; stem-cell transplantation
AA amyloidosis	Suppress acute-phase response	Immunosuppression for underlying disease, e.g. RA, autoinflammatory disease; anti-Il-1, anti-Il-6 Surgery to remove chronic infection, e.g. osteomyelitis
ATTR amyloidosis	Prevent formation of abnormal fibrils	Tafamidis (binds to altered TTR)

AA, Amyloid A protein; AL, light-chain amyloid protein; ATTR, amyloid transthyretin; RA, rheumatoid arthritis; TTR, transthyretin.

 Case 9.9 Idiopathic light-chain-associated (AL) amyloid

A 52-year-old woman presented with increasing swelling of both legs over a period of 3 months. Fourteen years earlier she had been treated for tuberculosis. On examination, she was pale, with gross bilateral leg oedema extending to the umbilicus and a large infected ulcer on the medial aspect of the right leg. Chest X-ray and electrocardiogram were normal, but she had a microcytic anaemia (Hb 75 g/l) with an erythrocyte sedimentation rate (ESR) of 140 mm/h. Her initial biochemical results showed a low serum albumin (14 g/l) and marked proteinuria (12 g/day), but a normal blood urea, serum creatinine and creatinine clearance. Serum electrophoresis showed no monoclonal band. Serum immunoglobulin levels were: IgG 2.2 g/l (NR 7.2–19.0); IgA 1.2 g/l (NR 0.8–5.0); and IgM 1.2 g/l (NR 0.5–2.0). Electrophoresis of a concentrated (×20) urine sample showed considerable amounts of albumin and gammaglobulin and an M band in the β region. Immunofixation of the serum and urine showed the presence of monoclonal free λ light chains in the urine only.

The presence of urinary monoclonal light chains suggested a possible diagnosis of light-chain myeloma or renal amyloid. A rectal biopsy was performed to look for amyloid deposits: this showed deposition of small amounts of amorphous material around blood vessels. This material stained strongly with Congo red and showed green birefringence when viewed under polarized light, an appearance that is characteristic of amyloid. A renal biopsy was also performed: striking deposits of amyloid were found in the glomerular basement membrane, in the tubular basement membrane and in the walls of several arterioles.

In view of her past medical history, the amyloid could have been associated with the previous tuberculosis or with the chronic infection of her leg ulcer – acute-phase-associated (AA) amyloid (see Table 9.5). However, antisera to λ light chains stained the material in both biopsies, showing that the amyloid was light-chain-associated (Table 9.5) and thus idiopathic or due to multiple myeloma. The absence of suppression of IgA and IgM levels, the lack of plasma cell infiltration of the bone marrow and the absence of osteolytic lesions on X-ray excluded the diagnosis of multiple myeloma. Therefore, this was idiopathic AL amyloid. In view of her reasonable renal function, only supportive treatment was given; this consisted of a low-salt, high-protein diet and diuretics. To date, her proteinuria has persisted but has not worsened.

necrosis factor (TNF) agents in rheumatoid arthritis. Many patients with underlying B-cell dyscrasias die from established amyloidosis of the kidneys or heart before cytotoxic drugs can produce benefit.

9.8.5 Other causes of nephrotic syndrome

In adults, the nephrotic syndrome may be secondary to a number of conditions (see Fig. 9.17 and Table 9.2). In the UK, the commonest causes are amyloid disease, SLE and diabetes mellitus, but elsewhere in the world chronic parasitic infestation dominates the list of causes.

9.9 Tubulointerstitial nephropathy

Tubulointerstitial nephropathy (TIN) or 'interstitial nephritis' describes a group of diverse renal disorders with predominant involvement of the renal tubules and interstitial tissue. Immunological mechanisms similar to those causing glomerulonephritis can also cause tubulointerstitial injury. Thus, antibodies to tubular basement membrane, immune complexes and cell-mediated reactions can produce TIN in experimental animals and in humans.

In general, there are three types of **functional defect** caused by TIN (Box 9.8).

Clinically, TIN can is divided into acute and chronic forms. Acute TIN is most commonly due to acute bacterial pyelonephritis or to drugs, although Epstein–Barr virus infection has been implicated in some cases. Chronic TIN may be idiopathic or secondary to a wide range of infective, toxic,

neo-plastic, hereditary or immunological conditions as well as eating disorders. Those conditions in which immunological mechanisms are thought to be involved are discussed in the cases.

9.9.1 Acute drug-induced tubulointerstitial nephritis

Acute TIN is a rare but well-recognized complication of an increasing list of drugs; these include the β-lactam antibiotics (both penicillins and cephalosporins), sulphonamides, rifampicin, anticonvulsants, cimetidine, diuretics, allopurinol and various NSAIDs. Antibiotics and NSAIDs are the most important triggers. Whatever the drug, TIN occurs about 10–15 days after the start of treatment and is not dose dependent. It is characterized by fever, haematuria, proteinuria, arthralgia and a maculopapular skin rash. The majority of patients recover completely, usually within a few days of stopping the drug.

The **mechanism of damage** is unclear, but blood and tissue eosinophilia, a rash, lack of correlation with the dose of the drug and the latent period between treatment and symptoms suggest an idiosyncratic or hypersensitivity reaction, possibly mediated by Th2 cells, since the interstitial infiltrate consists predominantly of CD4+ T cells, and *in vitro* lymphocyte transformation responses to the drug have been demonstrated in some patients. Circulating antibodies to tubular basement membrane, with characteristic linear IgG staining on immunofluorescent examination of the biopsy, suggest that the drug, or its hapten, may also bind to components of the tubular basement membrane, forming new antigens (Case 9.10).

9.9.2 Multiple myeloma and myeloma kidney

Multiple myeloma (see Chapter 6) is associated with many renal problems (Box 9.9). The most characteristic renal lesion is irreversible chronic renal failure due to **tubular atrophy (myeloma kidney)** with associated acidification and concentration defects (Case 9.11). Poor renal function correlates with the presence of light-chain proteinuria. Because of their size, light chains are readily filtered at the glomerulus and

---

> ### Box 9.8 Functional defects in tubulointerstitial nephropathy
>
> - Proximal tubular lesion, causing proximal renal tubular acidosis with or without the Fanconi syndrome (phosphaturia, glycosuria and aminoaciduria)
> - Distal tubular dysfunction, resulting in distal renal tubular acidosis, hyperkalaemia and salt-wasting
> - Medullary dysfunction, causing impaired urine-concentrating ability

---

Case 9.10 Acute tubulointerstitial nephritis (TIN)

A 37-year-old woman was admitted to hospital with a diagnosis of bacterial endocarditis. Blood cultures grew Streptococcus faecalis. She was treated with intravenous gentamicin and ampicillin with considerable improvement. However, on the 12th day of treatment, she developed a further fever and a macular rash on her trunk and limbs. Her white cell count was normal with an absolute eosinophil count of $0.32 \times 10^9/l$. Further blood cultures were negative, but her serum creatinine rose from 140 μmol/l (NR 60–120) to 475 μmol/l over the next 3 days, with a rise in the eosinophil count to $0.92 \times 10^9/l$. Serum complement levels were normal. A renal biopsy showed marked interstitial oedema and infiltration of tubules by mononuclear cells, neutrophils and eosinophils. A diagnosis of acute TIN, probably drug induced, was made; antibiotics were discontinued and prednisolone started instead. Her serum creatinine rose to a peak of 640 μmol/l, but she never became oliguric and did not require dialysis. After 3 days of steroids, her renal function began to improve and the eosinophil count fell.

Box 9.9 Renal complications of multiple myeloma

These include:

- Manifestations of the paraprotein itself, such as proteinuria, myeloma kidney or renal amyloidosis
- Secondary metabolic disturbances, including hypercalcaemia, hyperuricaemia and proximal renal tubular defects
- Adverse effects resulting from treatment (drug nephrotoxicity or pyelonephritis)

catabolized in the proximal tubular cells. When the amount of filtered free light chains exceeds the metabolic capacity of the tubules, two kinds of toxicity occur: first, tubular cells are damaged by intracellular deposits of crystals; and, second, protein precipitates out in the distal tubules and collects in ducts, forming casts. This is accelerated by dehydration. Other patients with excessive monoclonal light-chain excretion develop renal tubular acidosis and the Fanconi syndrome (phosphaturia, glycosuria and aminoaciduria) or amyloidosis (similar to Case 9.9).

The key principles in the prevention and **management** of the renal complications of myeloma are:

- Maintenance of adequate hydration and institution of a diuresis if urinary casts are seen.
- Avoidance of dehydration before diagnostic procedures.
- Vigorous treatment of any hypercalcaemia or hyperuricaemia.
- Careful monitoring of all potentially nephrotoxic drugs.
- Reduction of free lights in plasma by use of thalidomide, lenalidomide and bortezomib (see Chapter 6) in combination with dexamethasone, to reduce rapidly the monoclonal plasma cells that are producing light chains.
- Monitoring of serum free light chains.
- Patients whose myeloma responds to chemotherapy are considered for places on maintenance dialysis programmes.

9.9.3 Other immunologically mediated tubulointerstitial nephritides

Immune complexes formed in the circulation may be deposited in the tubulointerstitial tissue of the kidney. In humans, the best example is SLE. Over 50% of renal biopsies from patients with **SLE** show evidence of tubulointerstitial immune complexes; these are seen as granular deposits of immunoglobulins and complement along the tubular basement membrane or in the interstitium. The deposits contain nuclear antigens analogous to those seen in glomerular deposits. *The TIN may sometimes be severe enough to cause acute renal failure with minimal glomerular involvement.*

Evidence that TIN is also induced by antitubular basement membrane (TBM) antibodies includes linear deposits of immunoglobulin and complement along the TBM (see Fig. 9.12). In humans, **anti-TBM antibodies** have been detected in over 70% of patients with anti-GBM nephritis (see section 9.7.1) and in about 20% of patients after renal transplantation, although the importance of anti-TBM antibodies in graft rejection is unknown.

Renal tubular acidosis is often found in association with hypergammaglobulinaemic conditions such as SLE, Sjögren's syndrome, chronic active hepatitis, primary biliary cirrhosis and fibrosing alveolitis. The most common functional defect is an **inability to concentrate and acidify the urine**. The immunological mechanism responsible for renal tubular acidosis in hypergammaglobulinaemia is not known, but an excess of polyclonal free light chains, normally metabolized in the tubules, may be the cause.

9.10 Chronic renal failure

Glomerulonephritis is a common cause of chronic renal failure (Table 9.7), although there are major differences in causation in different ethnic groups. Because renal biopsies are not always performed in patients with ESRF, it is difficult to reconstruct a complete picture of the evolution of these disorders. Treatment to halt or reverse the progress of the renal damage remains empirical; management consists mainly of the preservation of

 Case 9.11 Myeloma kidney

A 76-year-old man was admitted with a history of progressive weakness over a period of several months. On examination, he was unkempt, thin, pale and acidotic. His blood pressure was 110/60. He was markedly anaemic (Hb 64 g/l) with an erythrocyte sedimentation rate (ESR) of 116 mm/h. His initial biochemical results showed a raised blood urea of 48 mmol/l (NR 2.5–7.5) and a grossly raised serum creatinine of 1910 µmol/l (NR 60–120), but a normal serum calcium. Urinary protein excretion was 2.8 g/day. A diagnosis of chronic renal failure of unknown cause was made. Peritoneal dialysis was started while other investigations were performed.

Serum electrophoresis showed a decreased γ fraction with a monoclonal band in the β region. Serum immunoglobulin levels were IgG 1.4 g/l (NR 7.2–19.0); IgA 24.5 g/l (NR 0.8–5.0); and IgM 0.3 g/l (NR 0.5–2.0). Immunofixation of the serum and urine showed an IgA (λ type) paraprotein in the serum, with monoclonal free λ light chains in the urine. A bone marrow aspirate showed marked infiltration of atypical plasma cells. Radiology of the skeleton revealed osteolytic lesions in the pelvis and skull. A diagnosis of myeloma kidney was therefore made. Despite symptomatic treatment of his renal failure and therapy for myelomatosis, he died from renal failure 5 weeks after admission.

Table 9.7 Causes of end-stage renal failure

Cause	Proportion (%)
Chronic glomerulonephritis	20
Diabetes mellitus	30
Hypertension	20
Pyelonephritis/reflux nephropathy	5
Polycystic kidneys	10
Interstitial nephritis	5
Other	15

Table 9.8 Recurrence of original disease in kidney grafts

Original renal disease	Proportion showing histological recurrence (%)
Focal glomerulosclerosis	30
Henoch–Schönlein nephritis	35
IgA nephropathy	50
Membranoproliferative glomerulonephritis	
Type I	20–30
Type II	50–100
Antiglomerular basement membrane disease	<1

surviving nephrons by conservative measures. Renal dialysis followed by transplantation is the only therapeutic option.

9.11 Recurrent glomerulonephritis in transplanted kidneys

Glomerulonephritis can recur in the allografted kidney. On average, this happens in about one in four transplants, although the prevalence and severity depend on the original disease: it is very likely in MPGN and rare in SLE (Table 9.8). The graft shows the same lesions that existed in the patient's own kidneys. However, the presence of a form of glomerulonephritis that may recur is not a contraindication to transplantation, since symptomatic recurrence is less frequent.

CHAPTER 10
Joints and Muscles

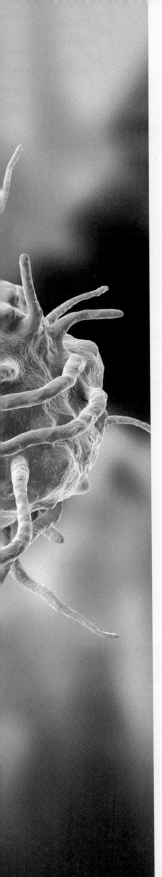

Key topics

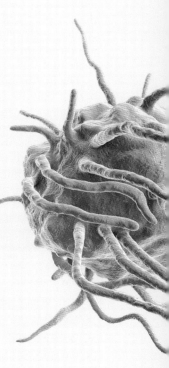

 Visit the companion website at **www.wiley.com/go/misbah/immunology** to download cases with additional figures on these topics.

Chapel and Haeney's Essentials of Clinical Immunology, Seventh Edition. Edited by Siraj A. Misbah, Gavin P. Spickett, and Virgil A.S.H. Dalm.
© 2022 John Wiley & Sons Ltd. Published 2022 by John Wiley & Sons Ltd.

10.1 Introduction

Immunological mechanisms are responsible for many rheumatological diseases. Although these disorders often present with joint or muscle inflammation, many have multisystem involvement with a particular tendency to involve skin, lungs and kidney. These disorders are often autoimmune and include rheumatoid arthritis (RA), systemic lupus erythematosus (SLE), dermatomyositis, scleroderma and some forms of vasculitis. They used to be referred to as the 'connective tissue diseases'; *this woolly phrase was meaningless in pathophysiological terms*, and the phrase largely dropped from usage. Discussion of these disorders can also be found in other organ-based chapters in relation to the particular organ involved. These systemic autoimmune diseases are characteristically associated with non-organ-specific autoantibody production, particularly against components of cell nuclei. *These autoantibodies are not necessarily responsible for joint or tissue damage*, but can be helpful markers in diagnosis or prognosis (see Chapter 19).

10.2 Patterns of joint disease

Joint diseases fall into two broad categories: degenerative conditions of cartilage (osteoarthritis) or disorders characterized by inflammation of the joint lining or synovium (**inflammatory arthritis or synovitis**). The diagnosis of a particular form of inflammatory arthritis is rarely made using a single diagnostic test, notable exceptions being the presence in synovial fluid of uric acid crystals in gout or of bacteria in septic arthritis. Instead, the *diagnostic process relies heavily upon clinical assessment*, with a smaller role being played by various immunological tests (Table 10.1). Most forms of chronic inflammatory joint diseases can be defined using clinical criteria alone, and this, in part, reflects our ignorance of the underlying aetiopathogenesis. The major common patterns of joint inflammation and the common underlying causes are summarized in Table 10.2.

The healthy synovial lining (Fig. 10.1) consists of a single layer of cells overlying loose, well-vascularized stromal tissue. The lining cells are of two kinds: one fibroblastic, which synthesizes the proteoglycans that act as a lubricant within the joint, and one derived from macrophages, which probably have a scavenging function. Unlike most body surfaces, free passage of intercellular fluid can occur across the synovial membrane, a factor that may explain why antigens tend to be deposited within the joint. The synovial response to injury is relatively limited, and the *pathology of most forms of inflammatory arthritis consists of hyperplasia of the lining layer and cellular infiltration of the vascular tissues beneath the lining*. Cytokine production in chronic synovial inflammation may also be limited in its variety: most synovial diseases show some response to treatments that block the action of tumour necrosis factor (TNF)-α.

10.3 Arthritis and infection

There are two principal mechanisms whereby microorganisms can cause inflammatory arthritis: direct invasion of the synovium (infective or septic arthritis) or a hypersensitivity response (mediated by T-cell or immune complexes) against microbial antigen deposited within the joint.

Table 10.1 Major factors in the assessment of the patient with joint disease

Age/sex

Acute or chronic

Pattern of joint disease
- Monoarticular
- Oligoarticular
- Polyarticular

Extraarticular disease

Rheumatoid factor positive

Antinuclear antibody positive

Table 10.2 Common patterns of inflammatory joint disease

Pattern of joint inflammation	Common causes
Monoarthritis	Bacterial infection
	Gout/pseudogout
	Spondyloarthropathy (especially reactive arthritis)
Oligoarthritis	Spondyloarthritis (especially reactive and psoriatic)
	Gout/pseudogout
Polyarthritis	
Symmetrical	Rheumatoid arthritis
	Systemic lupus erythematosus
	Viral arthritis
Asymmetrical	Psoriatic arthritis

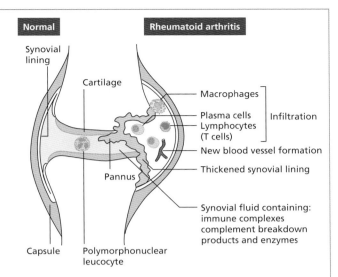

Fig. 10.1 Diagrammatic representation of a joint. One side is normal, the other shows characteristic pathological features of rheumatoid arthritis.

10.3.1 Septic arthritis

Pyogenic arthritis can occur in previously healthy joints in immunocompetent subjects, but the risk is increased by previous joint damage, recent joint surgery or injection, or defective immunity, particularly abnormalities of antibody production or neutrophils (the latter being most often a consequence of chemotherapy). Joint damage probably increases the risk of sepsis by allowing increased entry of organisms into the joint. Patients with RA have a particular propensity to joint sepsis, this being partly due to corticosteroid therapy and joint damage, but also related to subtle defects in immunity associated with the disease itself (Case 10.1). The organisms most frequently associated with septic arthritis are summarized in Table 10.3.

Septic arthritis is a medical emergency. Delay in treatment is associated with an increasing risk of severe joint damage and with high mortality, especially in immunocompromised subjects.

Gonococcal and meningococcal infection can be associated with arthritis. This is most often associated with a subacute septicaemic illness, and organisms can be isolated from the blood and synovial fluid. However, in gonococcal (and less commonly meningococcal) infection, an **immune complex-mediated arthropathy** can also occur, which usually presents 7–10 days after the onset of infection and is associated with falling levels of antigen in serum, rising levels of antibody and evidence of complement consumption, all features suggesting an immune complex-mediated disease.

Lyme disease, which is caused by the tick-borne spirochaete Borrelia burgdorferi, is associated with a chronic large-joint arthritis. Borrelia are invasive, non-toxigenic, persistent pathogens, and little is known about the pathogenesis of Lyme disease. The arthritis first appears some months after the initial tick bite, and usually has a relapsing and remitting course, but can be persistent and associated with joint destruction. Organisms are difficult to isolate from the joint, but an antibody response can be detected. The arthritis may be partly mediated by hypersensitivity mechanisms but improves after antibiotic treatment, suggesting that live organisms also play a role in pathogenesis.

Case 10.1 Septic arthritis

A 37-year-old woman developed a symmetrical polyarthritis. A test for cyclic citrullinated peptide (CCP) antibodies was positive and erosive changes were seen on X-ray, confirming a clinical diagnosis of rheumatoid arthritis (RA). The arthritis followed an aggressive course with poor response to a variety of disease-modifying antirheumatic drugs and she became increasingly disabled due to severe destructive changes in the knees, wrists and shoulders. A moderate dose of prednisolone was introduced at the age of 42, with some symptomatic improvement in her joints, and she was referred to an orthopaedic surgeon with a view to knee replacements. However, 1 month before her orthopaedic appointment, she presented to the emergency department with a painful swollen right knee. On examination she was unwell, febrile (38 °C) and had a hot, red right knee with a sizeable effusion. Then 80 ml of purulent synovial fluid was aspirated from the joint and microscopy of the fluid revealed numerous Gram-positive cocci. A diagnosis of septic arthritis was made on a background of severe RA and steroid therapy. She was treated with high-dose intravenous antibiotics and the joint was washed out via an arthroscope. Culture of blood and synovial fluid grew Staphylococcus aureus. She received 6 weeks' antibiotic treatment in total together with vigorous physiotherapy. Her knee, however, was significantly worsened by the infection and she could no longer straighten the leg or walk more than a few yards. Joint replacement was deferred for 6 months to reduce the risk of infection in the prosthesis.

Table 10.3 Relative frequency of bacterial causes of septic arthritis in the UK

Staphylococcus aureus	40%
Pneumococcus	10%
Other streptococci	18%
Haemophilus influenzae	7%
Gram-negative bacilli	12%
Gonococcus*	<1%

*Gonococcal joint infection is much more common in North America and Australia.

Viral arthritis

Joint and muscle pain is very common in acute viral infections, but inflammatory arthritis is much less common. Infections such as rubella, mumps and hepatitis B can cause a **transient arthritis** that is probably due to a combination of direct infection and hypersensitivity, since immunization with attenuated rubella virus can also cause a transient arthritis. The most common viral cause of arthritis in adults is parvovirus B19 (which in children usually only produces a mild febrile illness with a characteristic 'slapped cheek' rash). This produces an acute, symmetrical, peripheral polyarthritis (clinically similar to early RA), which usually remits within 3 weeks but which can occasionally persist for several months.

Immune-mediated arthritides

The distinction between active infection and immune-mediated arthritis is not always clear-cut, as the earlier account makes clear. There are other forms of arthritis that appear to be triggered by infection and follow a subacute, relapsing or chronic course. The most common of these, **reactive arthritis**, is discussed further in section 10.5. It will also be apparent from the sections on RA, other spondyloarthritides and juvenile chronic arthritis that attempts have been made to explain most forms of chronic inflammatory joint disease in terms of inappropriate response to an unidentified organism. This model has perhaps been most successfully applied to the spondyloarthritides (see section 10.5). Other disorders in which arthritis is immune mediated include rheumatic fever, which is discussed in Chapter 2, and Henoch–Schönlein purpura, discussed in Chapter 9.

10.4 Rheumatoid arthritis

10.4.1 Diagnosis

RA is a common disease affecting 1–2% of the adult population and is twice as common in women as men. It is most common between the ages of 25 and 55 years, and the most frequent presentation is an insidious, symmetrical polyarthritis, although the disease can begin abruptly. Although systemic manifestations (Table 10.4) may be present at the outset, they develop more usually as the disease progresses (see later Case 10.3). *The diagnosis of RA is made on clinical grounds*, as illustrated in Case 10.2.

10.4.2 Serology

A test measuring levels of **antibodies that bind citrulline modified proteins** (anti-CCP) is used in the diagnostic work-up for RA. It is specific for rheumatoid disease, as it is elevated in patients with RA or in those about to develop RA and not in other forms of arthritis (see later in the text).

Patients with RA fall into two groups: those with usually less severe disease who lack circulating **rheumatoid factor**

Table 10.4 Extraarticular features of rheumatoid arthritis (RA): the commonest features are marked in bold

Intrinsic or essential systemic features of rheumatoid disease
Rheumatoid nodules
Serositis (pleurisy, pericarditis)
Vasculitis
Neuropathy (often caused by vasculitic damage to nerves)
Felty's syndrome (neutropenia and splenomegaly)
Consequences of chronic inflammation and immune stimulation
Anaemia
Weight loss and fever
Lymphadenopathy
Complications of rheumatoid disease
Entrapment neuropathy, e.g. carpal tunnel syndrome
Accelerated atherosclerosis
Infection
Amyloidosis
Cervical myelopathy
Complications of treatment
Osteoporosis (corticosteroids)
Accelerated atherosclerosis
Infection
Drug-specific side effects
Associated syndromes (also occur without RA)
Keratoconjunctivitis sicca
Interstitial lung diseases
Episcleritis and scleritis

(RF) (seronegative RA); and a larger group (70%) with more aggressive disease who have, or develop, a RF in the serum (seropositive RA). Extraarticular disease occurs predominantly in this seropositive group. *RF is of value in diagnosis and prognosis, but is not of sufficient specificity alone to establish the diagnosis of RA.* RF, in this context, refers only to the IgM antibody that binds aggregated IgG as its antigen; rheumatoid factors of the IgG or IgA class are not clinically helpful, although they may play a role in joint inflammation. The presence of anti-CCP antibodies can also be used to predict which patients will get more severe RA. Other serological tests are of little value in RA. Antinuclear antibody (ANA) is present in 40%, but is usually of low titre and often of IgM class; such ANAs are found in many other conditions. Serum complement C3 and C4 levels may be normal or raised due to an 'acute-phase' reaction (see Chapter 1).

C-reactive protein (CRP) (another 'acute-phase' reactant) is an important test in any inflammatory arthritis, being raised particularly in active RA; this helps to distinguish active RA from active SLE, in which there is not an acute-phase response (see later Fig. 10.8). Also **erythrocyte sedimentation rate** (ESR) values can be measured, which tend to correlate with disease activity and severity in RA. Radiological damage is more likely to progress when CRP and ESR are elevated.

🔍 Case 10.2 Rheumatoid arthritis – classical course

A 37-year-old woman gradually developed painful wrists over 3 months; she consulted her doctor only when the pain and early-morning stiffness stopped her from gardening. On examination, both wrists and the metacarpophalangeal joints of both hands were swollen and tender but not deformed (Fig. 10.2). There were no nodules or vasculitic lesions. On investigation, she was found to have a raised C-reactive protein (CRP) level (27 mg/l; NR <10), but a normal haemoglobin and white cell count. A latex test for rheumatoid factor was negative, but autoantibodies to cyclic citrullinated peptides (CCP) were detected.

The clinical diagnosis was early rheumatoid arthritis and she was treated with ibuprofen. Despite some initial symptomatic improvement, the pain, stiffness and swelling of the hands persisted and 1 month later both knees became similarly affected. She was referred to a rheumatologist.

She was seen 3 months after the initial presentation. By this time she was struggling to work, drive and carry heavy objects. A test for rheumatoid factor was now positive (titre 1/256) and anti-CCP antibodies were strongly positive. X-rays of the feet showed small but definite erosions in two metatarsal heads. She still had a raised CRP (43 mg/l), but normal serum complement (C3 and C4) levels.

This woman had rheumatoid arthritis, with some features suggesting a poor prognosis. Her treatment was changed to weekly low-dose methotrexate. This controlled the arthritis and no further erosions developed for several years. When the disease flared, she received anti-tumour necrosis factor (TNF) therapy. In view of the poor prognosis, she would nowadays be started on anti-TNF therapy by her rheumatologist when first seen in clinic.

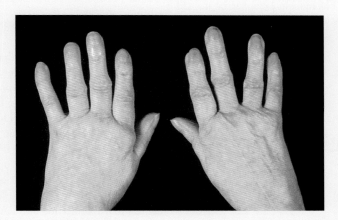

Fig. 10.2 Symmetrical synovitis in early rheumatoid arthritis. Source: From *Medical Masterclass. Rheumatology and Clinical Immunology*. Copyright © 2001 Royal College of Physicians. Reproduced with permission.

10.4.3 Pathology

The earliest pathological change in RA appears to be an **infiltrate of neutrophils and mononuclear cells around small blood vessels** in the loose connective tissue beneath the synovium. As the disease progresses, large numbers of T cells, macrophages, B cells and plasma cells accumulate in this tissue, and the synovium becomes markedly thickened due to **fibroblast proliferation** and macrophage migration. The surface area increases and becomes folded into villi. New vessel formation (**angiogenesis**) occurs and some blood vessels develop into structures specialized for lymphocyte migration: so-called high endothelial venules (see Chapter 1, section 1.7). **Secondary lymphoid follicles** also develop. In consequence, the histological structure comes to resemble that of an activated lymph node, emphasizing the high degree of immunological activity in RA. Increased amounts of synovial fluid can

form (especially in large joints), and this contains large numbers of neutrophil polymorphs, which have migrated from the blood.

This chronic inflammatory tissue has several destructive effects upon the joint. First, the hypertrophied lining layer at the margins of the joint (known as **pannus**) **erodes cartilage** and underlying bone. Second, cytokines induce chondrocytes and fibroblasts to produce enzymes that break down the extracellular matrix. Third, degranulation of neutrophils in the synovial fluid can directly damage the surface of cartilage (Fig. 10.1).

10.4.4 Immunopathogenesis

The immunohistology of rheumatoid synovium suggests that the disease results from an immunological response to an

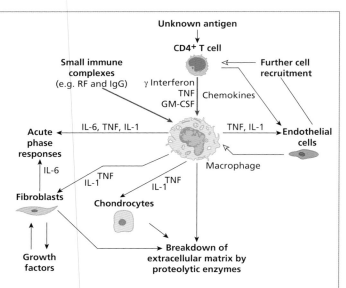

Fig. 10.3 How CD4⁺ T cells and immune complexes may control the events leading to joint damage in rheumatoid arthritis. GM-CSF, granulocyte macrophage colony-stimulating factor; IL, interleukin; TNF, tumour necrosis factor.

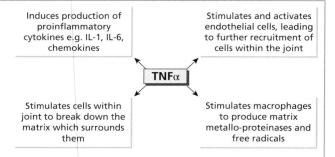

Fig. 10.4 The central role of tumour necrosis factor (TNF)-α in rheumatoid synovial inflammation. IL, interleukin.

Table 10.5 Evidence that T and B cells play a central role in the pathogenesis of rheumatoid arthritis (RA)

T cells

- Rheumatoid synovium densely infiltrated with activated mature T cells (mainly CD4⁺)
- Disease closely associated with particular MHC class II polymorphism, i.e. DR4
- Therapy directed against T cells (e.g. ciclosporin and anti-TNF agents) effective in treatment
- RA improves with progression of HIV infection
- Most animal models critically dependent upon T cells

B cells

- Rheumatoid synovium contains large numbers of plasma cells
- Disease closely associated with autoantibodies: anticitrullinated peptide antibodies (and rheumatoid factor in some patients)
- Efficacy of therapy specifically directed against B cells (rituximab)
- B cells also important in animal models

HIV, human immunodeficiency virus; MHC, major histocompatibility complex; TNF, tumour necrosis factor.

There is probably more than one immunological mechanism leading to macrophage activation in rheumatoid synovium. *The most widely accepted model is a process driven by CD4⁺ Th1 cells.* The evidence for T-cell involvement in RA is summarized in Table 10.5. However, the model of RA as a T-cell-driven disease has been criticized, as T-cell cytokines such as IL-2 and interferon (IFN)-γ are hard to detect in RA synovium, in contrast to macrophage-derived cytokines such as TNF-α, IL-1 and IL-6, IL-21 and IL-23, which are present in abundance. Following the descriptions of **Th17 cells** being central to inflammation and RA being an inflammatory disease *par excellence*, the role of these cells makes sense given the pathology. Th17 cells form a subset that produces IL-17A, IL-17F, IL-21 and IL-22 as well as TNF-α. Th17 differentiation is promoted by macrophage- and dendritic cell-derived transforming growth factor (TGF)-β as well as the cytokines mentioned, IL-1β, IL-6, IL-21 and IL-23. At the same time regulatory T cells (Tregs) are suppressed, shifting T-cell homeostasis toward inflammation. Th17 cells primarily produce IL-17A, which together with TNF-α activates fibroblasts and chondrocytes. Foxp3+ Tregs, although detected in tissues from patients with RA, have limited function.

Inflammation driven by antibodies may also be important. The synovium is infiltrated by B cells and may even form ectopic lymphoid follicles. **Plasmablasts and plasma cells are widely distributed in the synovium** and in juxtaarticular bone marrow. Clinical demonstration that depletion of B cells (with an anti-CD20 monoclonal antibody, rituximab – see Chapter 7) dramatically improves the clinical features of RA in a subset of patients shows that antibody-mediated inflammation does play a crucial role in the disease (Table 10.5), though the elimination of activated B cells that can present

unknown antigen within the joint. It is, however, clear that joint destruction in RA is driven by activated macrophages (Fig. 10.3), which secrete TNF-α and other cytokines to cause tissue breakdown directly as well as activating other cells in the joint. A large number of **inflammatory mediators** are produced in RA synovium (Fig. 10.3), and early descriptions of cytokine production in RA talked of a 'cytokine soup', suggesting no simple way of inhibiting this process. However **TNF-α plays a central role** (Fig. 10.4), since inhibition with neutralizing antibodies reduces the production of other inflammatory mediators in cell culture. Furthermore, when these antibodies are administered to patients, a dramatic improvement in joint inflammation occurs. The members of the interleukin (IL)-1 family, IL-1α and IL-1β, also play an important role, although a less crucial one than TNF.

autoantigen to more T cells and produce inflammatory cytokines such as IL-6 is important too. The role of innate immunity is uncertain as yet, but the ability of macrophages and neutrophils to be activated directly by triggering factors, through Toll-like receptors (TLRs) or intracellular receptors, to produce inflammatory cytokines is likely as the monoclonal antibody tocilizumab, an IL-6 receptor inhibitor, has been shown to have excellent clinical effects.

Since RA is an immunologically mediated disease, then it should be possible to define the main antigens driving the T- and B-cell responses in the joint. These autoantigens could be self-molecules expressed in the joint or could be foreign (e.g. bacterial or viral) antigens sequestered in joint tissue. T- and B-cell responses to a number of **autoantigens** have been described in RA (Table 10.6), but most are not specific for RA and the role of responses against these antigens in the disease is unclear. One of the most plausible autoimmune models of RA would be for the disease to be driven by an immune response against an antigen whose expression is confined to joints, such as type II collagen, the main protein of articular cartilage. However, although immune responses against cartilage and synovial proteins can be found in some patients with RA, these are not found in all patients and are also found in other diseases. Antibodies against a number of peptides containing the unusual amino acid citrulline (known as **anticyclic citrullinated peptide antibodies, CCP antibodies**) have recently been found to be highly specific to RA and to predict aggressive and persistent disease. It seems likely that RA is not caused by a single antigen, but rather by a response against a range of 'citrullinated' joint-specific proteins in genetically susceptible patients. In patients with the 'shared epitope' (see section 10.4.5), smoking produces detectable citrullinated proteins in the lungs, mechanistically linking genetic and environmental risk factors.

There is also evidence that macrophage-induced inflammation can become **self-sustaining** and independent of any triggering immune response: cytokines such as TNF-α produced by macrophages induce further macrophage activation. It is plausible that different mechanisms may predominate at different stages of this chronic disease.

10.4.5 Aetiology

In Europeans there is an association between possession of HLA-DR4 and -DR1 and RF-positive RA. This association becomes stronger with increasing severity of disease, and the presence of extraarticular manifestations (Table 10.4). Once the detailed structure of DR molecules was known at the amino acid level, comparison of different DR alleles associated with RA showed that almost all alleles associated with RA (HLA-DRB1*0101, 0401 and 0404) have a distinctive five amino acid sequence near the peptide-binding region of the DRβ chain; this sequence is known as the '**shared epitope**'. Possession of two copies of the 'shared epitope' (one inherited from each parent) is not only associated with a high risk of severe disease (Table 10.7), but also with presence of anti-CCP antibodies. Genome-wide association studies have shown that other genes involved in T-cell activation and the NFκB inflammation pathways are important. Female sex is an important genetic risk factor, and it seems plausible that this risk is mediated hormonally, as there is an increased risk of onset of RA in the post-partum period.

Environmental factors predisposing to RA remain poorly understood. Smoking is a relatively weak risk factor, but can increase the risk of RA 20- to 40-fold in genetically susceptible individuals. Many attempts have been made to link RA to infectious agents such as parvovirus, Epstein–Barr virus, mycoplasma and mycobacteria. However, while the idea of RA as a disease either initiated or perpetuated by an immune response against an infection has many attractions, no convincing evidence exists to implicate any known agent (see Chapter 5 for discussion of how infections may trigger autoimmunity).

Table 10.6 Autoimmune responses identified in patients with rheumatoid arthritis (RA)

Autoantigen	Antibodies in RA	T-cell response in RA	Specificity for RA
IgG	Yes: rheumatoid factor		No
Type II collagen and other cartilage antigens	Yes: in 10–20%	Yes: in 10–20%	No
Citrullinated proteins (CCP)	Yes	Yes	Yes

Table 10.7 How possession of an HLA-DRB1 allele containing the 'shared epitope' influences absolute risk of developing rheumatoid arthritis (RA) in a Caucasian population

	Approximate risk of developing RA
Total population	1 in 100
Subjects with no copies of shared epitope	1 in 580
DRB1*0401	1 in 35
DRB1*0404	1 in 20
DRB1*0101	1 in 80
DRB1*0401 *and* 0404	1 in 7

The risk is highest in those who inherit a copy of a different DRB1 gene from each of their parents.

Many animal models of RA have been developed, centred on both infection and autoimmunity, all with some similarity to the human disease. If nothing else, these models emphasize that the synovial response to injury is limited in scope and most of the aetiological factors are plausible and not mutually exclusive.

10.4.6 Outcome

Although the outcome of RA is variable and a few patients have mild or remitting disease, *for most it is a severe and disabling illness*. Most (70%) of RA patients have many periods of remission and relapse over decades (polycyclic disease as in Case 10.2) though sustained remission is rarely achieved. Joint damage begins in the early stages of the disease and once established is effectively irreversible. Early studies suggested that 5 years after diagnosis, one-third of patients are unable to work at all and only one-third are still in full-time work. Subsequent surveys have shown that treatment with biologics was associated with a 35% increase in employment rate. Factors predicting a poor prognosis are detailed in Table 10.8.

RA is associated with increased mortality as well as disability. *Life expectancy in RA is reduced by approximately 7 years compared with age- and sex-matched controls.* In severe, disabling RA, the 5-year mortality is around 50%. The causes of these premature deaths are multiple and in general not directly attributable to the arthritis, although some patients die of extraarticular disease such as pulmonary fibrosis (Case 10.3), vasculitis, amyloid (see Chapter 9) or lymphoma and others from the side effects of drug treatment. Patients with RA also show an increased susceptibility to severe or recurrent infection. The largest single contributor to increased mortality in RA is, however, an increased risk of **ischaemic heart disease (IHD)**. Mortality from IHD in RA is increased by approximately two- to threefold, a comparable increase in risk to that seen in diabetes mellitus. Similar increased mortality from IHD has also been described in other chronic inflammatory diseases, particularly SLE. The mechanisms underlying this increased risk are unclear, but conventional risk factors alone (such as smoking, hyperlipidaemia and hypertension) cannot explain the increased risk, and immunosuppressive treatment and disease-specific factors make substantial contributions.

10.4.7 Management

Although **management of RA** is a multidisciplinary process, aiming to control the disease and minimize pain and disability, the paramount aim of treatment is the pharmacological

Table 10.8 Predictors of a poor prognosis in early rheumatoid arthritis

High-titre serum rheumatoid factor
Female sex
High levels of acute-phase proteins (ESR, CRP)
High levels of disability
Extraarticular disease
Radiological evidence of joint damage
High-titre anticitrullated peptide (anti-CCP) antibodies
Possession of the shared epitope: two copies are worse than one

CRP, C-reactive protein; ESR, erythrocyte sedimentation rate.

Case 10.3 Pulmonary fibrosis in rheumatoid arthritis (RA)

A 61-year-old man, with a 15-year history of seropositive RA, was admitted with increasing shortness of breath, myalgia and weight loss. He had previously smoked 40 cigarettes a day, but had never been exposed to coal or silica dust. On examination, he was pale and thin, with generalized muscle tenderness. Widespread crepitations were heard over both lung fields. His joints were tender and he had subluxation of the metacarpophalangeal joints of both hands. There was bilateral cervical and axillary lymph node enlargement but no splenomegaly. Neurological and cardiac examinations were normal.

Investigations showed a raised C-reactive protein (CRP; 81 mg/l) and a normochromic anaemia (Hb 95 g/l) but a normal white cell count. His serum IgG was raised at 44 g/l (NR 7.2–19.0), although IgA and IgM levels were normal. He had a strongly positive rheumatoid factor and anticyclic citrullinated peptide (CCP) antibody titres. There were no detectable antibodies to DNA or to extractable nuclear antigens (ENA; see Chapter 19) and the serum levels of muscle enzymes were normal. A chest X-ray suggested pulmonary fibrosis. High-resolution computed tomographic scanning of the chest confirmed severe pulmonary fibrosis, with no evidence of any ground-glass shadowing (a feature that would suggest a good response to immunosuppression). Pulmonary function tests showed a severe restrictive defect, with an forced expiratory volume in 1 sec/forced expiratory vital capacity of 1.1/1.3. He was too unwell to undergo a lung biopsy.

This man's dyspnoea was rapidly progressive and he continued to deteriorate despite intravenous corticosteroids and cyclophosphamide. At autopsy, both lungs showed severe fibrosis, with the pattern of interstitial pneumonia (see Chapter 13, section 13.4.3), which is a rare complication of RA with a poor prognosis. The onset of serious complications of RA so long after the initial diagnosis is not unusual.

limitation of joint inflammation and damage, using drugs that modify the natural history of the disease (**disease-modifying antirheumatic drugs, DMARDs**). Joint damage in RA begins early, is effectively irreversible and has a poor outcome: *these are compelling reasons to introduce effective, aggressive treatment early in the disease.*

Recognition of these factors has led to early use of disease-modifying drugs, particularly in subjects felt to have a poor prognosis; in addition to anti-TNF agents, methotrexate, leflunomide and sulfasalazine (Chapter 7) are commonly used drugs. There is an increasing tendency to use drugs in combination in severe or aggressive disease; these combinations are more effective and often no more toxic than single drug regimens. The goal is to achieve low disease activity (determined by affected joints) within 3–6 months to prevent irreversible damage. If this fails, another conventional DMARD is added or the patient is switched to another DMARD plus a glucocorticoid.

Patients who have failed treatment with methotrexate and similar drugs within 6 months, or those that have a poor prognosis (Table 10.8), are now usually treated with **anti-TNF agents**, such as etanercept and infliximab, which can control RA in >70% of patients. Dramatic responses in patients with refractory disease have also been reported following treatment with the anti-B-cell monoclonal antibody, rituximab. Recombinant IL-1 receptor antagonist has also been used to block the action of IL-1α and IL-1β, but the response is not as striking as that seen with anti-TNF agents. Other biological agents approved for RA therapy include tocilizumab (anti-IL-6), and the co-stimulation blocking agent abatacept (CTLA4-Ig). Janus kinase (JAK) inhibitors have been recently introduced in RA, either alone or in combination with methotrexate, and may be appropriate for patients who prefer to avoid medications requiring intravenous or subcutaneous administration. Small numbers of patients have been treated with highly aggressive chemotherapy and autologous stem cell transplantation with some success (see section 8.5), but the long-term utility of this approach is not yet clear.

10.5 Seronegative spondyloarthritis

This group of disorders includes ankylosing spondylitis, reactive arthritis, psoriatic arthropathy and enteropathic arthritis.

These syndromes are characterized by absence of RF (seronegative), spinal (spondylo-) involvement and often asymmetrical peripheral arthritis, tending to involve large joints. Inflammation at the insertion of muscles, ligaments or tendons into bone (enthesitis) is a core feature in these disorders. It has been recognized for many years that enthesitis underlies the spinal involvement. Magnetic resonance imaging (MRI) or ultrasounds have demonstrated that synovial inflammation begins with enthesitis at the joint margins. Ossification can occur at the site of enthesitis, and in the spine this can lead to fusion (ankylosis) of adjacent vertebrae. All of these disorders are strongly associated with **HLA-B27**, the association being strongest in subjects with predominantly spinal disease. Most

of these disorders show a therapeutic response to anti-TNF agents (see Case 7.4).

The use of the label *reactive arthritis* requires comment: while any arthritic process triggered by infection could be reasonably called reactive, the diagnostic label is usually reserved for one of the forms of spondyloarthritis described in more detail later in the chapter.

10.5.1 Ankylosing spondylitis

Ankylosing spondylitis is a chronic inflammatory condition of the spine and sacroiliac joints. It is a progressive disease in which restriction of movement of the lower spine and the sacroiliac joints is associated with **ossification of the intervertebral ligaments**. As in Case 10.4, this disease mainly affects men aged between 15 and 30 years. Four men in 1000 are affected and 5% have a positive family history. Complications are common: 25% develop iritis and 20% have a peripheral arthritis, although either condition may be the sole presenting symptom. Rarer complications include pulmonary fibrosis, aortic incompetence, cardiac conduction defects and amyloidosis.

The association between HLA-B27 and ankylosing spondylitis is very strong; over 95% of affected individuals are positive for this antigen. The frequency (3–10%) of HLA-B27 in an unaffected, healthy population makes a positive test useless, but the absence of HLA-B27 in a patient with suspected disease makes ankylosing spondylitis very unlikely.

The precise aetiology is unknown. The association of ankylosing spondylitis with HLA-B27 is shared with other arthritides that follow infection, such as reactive arthritis following mucosal infections (see section 10.5.2) in which the specific antigens of the infecting organisms have been demonstrated in joint tissues. This suggests that ankylosing spondylitis may also be triggered by infection (possibly in the gastrointestinal [GI] tract) in susceptible HLA-B27-positive individuals. The finding that two-thirds of patients with ankylosing spondylitis have asymptomatic inflammatory gut lesions supports this, although these may be caused by antiinflammatory drugs used for therapy.

The relationship of arthritides and HLA-B27 remains uncertain, but has been clarified by studies using transgenic rats. The introduction of the gene for human HLA-B27 into otherwise normal rats results in a multisystem disease resembling ankylosing spondylitis. The development of this disease is dependent upon exposure to gut commensal organisms, particularly bacteroides. This model confirmed that the gene is an important predisposing factor.

The most important aspect of treatment is exercise to maintain full mobility, with antiinflammatory drugs to reduce the pain. Joint replacement and occasionally spinal surgery may be required. Anti-TNF agents have been shown to have a significant effect on the spinal inflammation and use of non-steroidal antiinflammatory drugs (NSAIDs) results in symptom relief, including back pain and stiffness. IL-17 inhibitors are reasonable alternatives in patients with an inadequate response to a TNF inhibitor.

Case 10.4 Ankylosing spondylitis

A 21-year-old man presented to his local emergency department with acute pain and swelling of one knee. On examination, the joint was tender and restricted in movement. X-ray
of the knee showed periarticular osteoporosis. On investigation, he had a raised erythrocyte sedimentation rate (ESR) of
102 mm/h, a mild anaemia (Hb 106 g/l), but no detectable
serum rheumatoid factor. The knee effusion was aspirated;
the fluid contained a polymorphonuclear leucocytosis but no
organisms or rheumatoid factor. No diagnosis was made at
this stage, but he was treated empirically with diclofenac; his
arthritis improved.

Fifteen months later he developed an iritis in his left eye.
At this point, a history was also elicited of low back pain and
prolonged early-morning stiffness dating back to his late
teenage years. His peripheral joints were normal, but his
lumbar spine was rigid and he had some pain and restriction
of the neck. X-rays of his lumbar spine and pelvis showed
the classical changes of ankylosing spondylitis and tissue
typing revealed that he was HLA-B27 positive (Fig. 10.5). He
continues to have widespread spinal discomfort, although
daily exercises have reduced the stiffness in his neck. At his
last clinic visit he asked whether he should receive an anti-
TNF drug as he does fit the criteria.

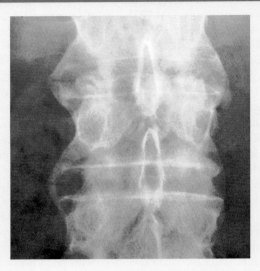

Fig. 10.5 Bamboo lumbar spine in ankylosing spondylitis.
Source: From *Medical Masterclass. Rheumatology and
Clinical Immunology*, 1st Ed. Copyright © 2001 Royal College
of Physicians. Reproduced with permission.

Case 10.5 Reactive arthritis following infection (previously Reiter's disease)

A 19-year-old man presented with acute swelling of his right knee and left ankle and extremely painful heels. On questioning, he admitted to a penile discharge and dysuria for 4 days. On examination, he had bilateral Achilles tendonitis
and his right knee and left ankle were red, hot and tender. He had aphthous-like mouth ulcers and ulcers around the
glans penis. There were no skin lesions and, in particular, no evidence of keratoderma blenorrhagica or subungual
pustules.

On investigation, he was found to have a raised erythrocyte sedimentation rate (ESR; 60 mm/h) but a normal haemoglobin and white cell count. A latex test for rheumatoid factor was negative. X-rays of the joints were normal. Joint fluid
aspirated from the right knee showed a polymorphonuclear leucocytosis but no organisms. Gonococci were not cultured from the urethral pus or from the joint fluid, but chlamydial DNA was detected by the polymerase chain reaction.
Tissue typing showed him to be HLA-B27 positive. A diagnosis of Reiter's disease was made. He was given diclofenac
for symptomatic relief of the arthritis and tendonitis. The chlamydial urethritis was treated with doxycycline and his partner was screened for sexually transmitted infection. Four days later, he developed bilateral conjunctivitis and some
photophobia. However, 6 weeks later he had fully recovered and did not relapse.

10.5.2 Other seronegative spondyloarthritides

Reactive arthritis

Reactive arthritis (previously known as Reiter's syndrome;
Case 10.5) can be regarded as a spectrum of disease, ranging
from a multisystem disorder characterized by an inflammatory
arthritis, urethritis, conjunctivitis, uveitis or skin changes to
disease that is confined to the joints. Of all the spondyloarthritides, the link to infection is clearest in reactive arthritis: the
majority of cases appear to be triggered by either Chlamydia
trachomatis infection or by certain bacterial infections of the

gut (in particular, Shigella, Salmonella, Campylobacter or
Yersinia infection). The overall risk of this syndrome following
a triggering infection is around 1%, and HLA-B27 is an
important risk factor (80% of patients are B27 positive). The
syndrome is more common in men than women (by about 3 to 1),
and tends to affect those under 40 years old.

Bacterial/chlamydial proteins and DNA can be detected in
affected joints, but viable organisms have not been found. The
arthropathy results mainly from a T-cell response to the sequestered
bacterial antigens. Treatment is with intraarticular corticosteroid
injections, antiinflammatory drugs and physiotherapy; antibiotic

treatment of the triggering infection has no effect on the arthritis. Most cases remit within a few months, but up to 20% (largely B27-positive patients) develop chronic peripheral joint and spinal disease. Severe reactive arthritis can also occur in patients with human immunodeficiency virus (HIV) infection.

Enteropathic arthritis

Of patients with ulcerative colitis, 20% develop a mild seronegative inflammatory arthritis, enteropathic arthritis, which affects peripheral joints. Conversely, 5% of patients with ankylosing spondylitis have either clinical ulcerative colitis or Crohn's disease. **Inflammatory bowel disease** should be considered as an underlying cause in patients with features of a seronegative spondyloarthropathy.

The overlapping clinical features of HLA-B27-related arthropathies suggest that similar immunopathogenic mechanisms are involved.

Psoriatic arthritis

Psoriasis is a common skin disease (see Chapter 11). Of patients with psoriasis, 2% develop psoriatic arthropathy; this may affect the peripheral joints or the spine. The psoriasis generally precedes the arthritis by many years; in rare cases where the arthritis comes first, diagnosis may be difficult. A family history of psoriasis is a helpful diagnostic clue and the characteristic nail changes of psoriasis are present in 80% of patients with psoriatic arthritis. Dactylitis – inflammation of an entire digit to look like a sausage – is a distinctive feature. Treatment is similar to that for RA, including the use of anti-TNF drugs. The prognosis is usually good, although severe joint destruction can occur.

10.5.3 Other seronegative arthritides

The disorders discussed later do not share clinical and aetiological features with the spondyloarthritides, but are sometimes classified with them under the loose (and largely meaningless) banner of seronegative arthritis.

Relapsing polychondritis is a rare, non-hereditary condition characterized by inflammation of cartilage and is often associated with arthritis. Most patients have an episodic, migratory, asymmetrical polyarthritis. A provisional diagnosis of seronegative RA is often made until the characteristic attacks of cartilage inflammation occur, usually in the ears, nose and trachea. The aetiology of this condition is not well understood. Cartilage antibodies are found in some patients, and T lymphocytes sensitized to cartilage antigen have been reported in others; however, it is likely that these changes are secondary to cartilage damage rather than its cause. An immune-mediated pathogenesis in relapsing polychondritis is supported by its association with other immune-mediated diseases, an HLA-DR4 genetic predisposition, and by animal models where immunization with components of cartilage (e.g. type II collagen, matrillin-1) successfully reproduces many aspects of the disease.

Behçet's disease (Case 10.6) is a chronic, multisystem disorder affecting slightly more men than women. Oral and genital ulceration is most frequently reported, Other clinical features include recurrent, potentially blinding uveitis and arthritis, which develops in 45% of patients and is the presenting symptom in 15%. Vasculitis with thrombophlebitis and neurological involvement occurs in 25–30% of cases. There is no diagnostic test and the diagnosis is entirely clinical.

Behçet's disease shares class I major histocompatibility complex (MHC) associations in common with autoimmune diseases, but has clinical features that seem to be mostly autoinflammatory. Unknown triggering infections may cause disease in genetically predisposed patients. Genome-wide association studies reported associations with polymorphisms in IL-10 and IL-23R/IL-12RB2 genes, similar to other inflammatory diseases including Crohn's disease. Th17 responses and the suppression of Tregs by IL-21 correlate with disease activity. The finding of neutrophils, Th1, Th17, cytotoxic CD8$^+$ and $\gamma\delta$ T cells in inflammatory lesions paves the way for new therapies. In the meantime, no specific treatment is available, although corticosteroids may control symptoms and azathioprine and adalimumab (a humanized antibody to TNF-α) have been shown to reduce progression of visual loss. In severe cases, ciclosporin and tacrolimus may be effective. Thalidomide may be useful in refractory orogenital ulceration. There is an association between Behçet's disease and HLA-B51.

🔍 Case 10.6 Behçet's syndrome

A 32-year-old man from a Turkish family presented with deteriorating vision and painful swollen knees. Further questioning revealed a 10-year history of relapsing and remitting mouth ulcers and a less severe history of genital ulceration. On examination he had reduced visual acuity associated with a florid retinal vasculitis. Two 1-cm mouth ulcers were found, but no active genital ulceration. He had synovitis in both knees. Investigation revealed a raised erythrocyte sedimentation rate (ESR) at 94 mm/h, but a normal blood count and negative tests for rheumatoid factor, antinuclear antibodies, cytomegalovirus and human immunodeficiency virus (HIV) infection. A clinical diagnosis of Behçet's syndrome was made. He was treated with high-dose corticosteroids and azathioprine with good response, although his visual acuity remains permanently impaired. He might have benefited from therapy with adalimumab (a humanized antibody to tumour necrosis factor [TNF]-α), but this was not available at the time.

10.6 Chronic arthritis in children

Juvenile idiopathic arthritis (JIA) is the generic term for a group of diseases in which an inflammatory arthritis begins before the age of 16 years; there are several distinct syndromes. It is important first to exclude diseases that do not form part of the spectrum of JIA; these include juvenile dermatomyositis, acute rheumatic fever, SLE, post-infective arthropathies and joint disease associated with antibody deficiency or haemophilia.

Chronic arthritis in childhood is divided into six subgroups (Fig. 10.6). There is a juvenile version of seropositive RA in 10% of cases. This behaves like the adult disease, and the presence of CCP antibodies confirms the diagnosis. The condition tends to progress to severe joint destruction with extraarticular complications of RA, such as nodules and vasculitis. A further 15% have enthesitis-related arthritis (ERA), which is closely related to ankylosing spondylitis and the spondyloarthropathies (Fig. 10.5).

The majority (75%) of children with a chronic inflammatory arthritis have seronegative diseases that have no obvious counterpart in adult arthritic disorders, although rarely adults can develop a disorder that is very similar to systemic JIA: this is adult-onset Still's disease.

The aetiologies of the childhood-specific forms of JIA are poorly understood; no environmental triggers have been identified, but a number of genetic associations have been delineated, mainly within the HLA region. These genetic associations will further differentiate these disorders from adult forms of arthritis.

Potentially blinding chronic uveitis is a major complication of JIA, as in Case 10.7. This type of uveitis is usually clinically silent until vision is impaired (in contrast to acute uveitis, a common feature of spondyloarthropathies, which is painful). Chronic uveitis occurs predominantly, but not exclusively, in children with oligoarticular JIA. Therefore all children with JIA require screening for this silently progressive condition.

Useful investigations in children with chronic arthritis include the ESR, and acute-phase reactants such as CRP; both increase with disease activity. Anti-CCP antibodies can be detected in those with polyarticular IgM-RF; RF and antinuclear antibodies are helpful in classification. Antinuclear antibodies, directed against histones and other nuclear antigens, but not DNA, are found in a high proportion of cases.

The **mechanisms** of joint inflammation in the various forms of JIA seem to be similar to those in RA, with similar immunohistology. A major advance in the management of JIA has been the advent of biological agents including anti-TNF-α agents, especially etanercept and adalimumab, the fully humanized

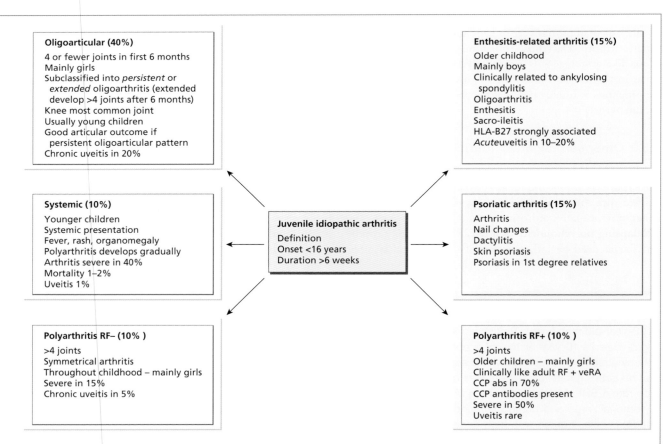

Fig. 10.6 Classification of juvenile idiopathic arthritis. Disorders on the left only occur in childhood, whereas those on the right are childhood equivalents of adult diseases. CCP, cyclic citrullinated peptide; RF, rheumatoid factor.

> ### Case 10.7 Juvenile idiopathic arthritis (JIA)
>
> A 2-year-old girl was taken to her GP because she was unwilling to walk. Her GP found her right knee to be swollen and tender and referred her to an orthopaedic surgeon, who was concerned that she may have septic arthritis, although she was systemically well. An X-ray was normal. Synovial fluid was aspirated under general anaesthetic, but was sterile on culture. The pain settled somewhat, although the knee was still swollen on examination. Two months later her left ankle also became swollen and painful. Blood tests showed a raised erythrocyte sedimentation rate (ESR) at 40 mm/h, a negative test for rheumatoid factor and a low-titre (1/40) homogeneous antinuclear antibodies (ANA). DNA antibodies were not detected. Serum immunoglobulins were normal. A diagnosis of early-onset pauciarticular JIA was made and she was treated with ibuprofen with a good response. However, 1 month later the knee was still swollen and she was given an intraarticular steroid injection, with complete resolution of the synovitis. Her vision seemed normal, but ophthalmological screening revealed a severe chronic uveitis, which was treated with topical steroids. At the age of 4 her joint disease was in complete remission, but her uveitis remained intermittently active, and she has developed a cataract in the right eye. She remains under long-term ophthalmological follow-up; *this emphasizes the need for rapid ophthalmological screening as soon as a diagnosis of JIA is made.*

monoclonal antibody that binds soluble and membrane-bound TNF-α. **Treatment** with anakinra, the recombinant form of the human IL-1 receptor antagonist that competitively binds the IL-1 receptor and thus blocks endogenous IL-1 signalling, led to rapid (within days) remission in some patients, but not all responded to this treatment and the response was not always sustained. Tocilizumab, the humanized monoclonal antibody that binds to the IL-6 receptor and blocks downstream signalling of IL-6, is promising.

10.7 Systemic lupus erythematosus

10.7.1 Clinical features

SLE is a **multisystem disorder** that typically affects young women, with a prevalence of around 1 in 2000. It is characterized by the presence of autoantibodies to nuclear antigens. The most common presenting feature is arthritis or arthralgia (Table 10.9). Nearly all patients eventually experience joint problems and skin lesions, as in Case 10.8, while about one-half to two-thirds also have pulmonary, renal, neurological or haematological involvement at some time (Table 10.10).

Atypical and non-specific **presentations** of SLE often cause difficulty in diagnosis. Pleuropericardial inflammation is common, but usually mild and transient; a few patients (10%) have clinical and radiological evidence of diffuse, progressive interstitial lung disease. The renal complications of SLE are described in Chapter 9. Neurological features of SLE (see Chapter 17, section 17.6) span the spectrum of neurological and psychiatric disease from headaches to psychosis. Common manifestations include dementia, depression, convulsions, chorea and migraine (see Chapter 17).

Recurrent venous or cerebral arterial thrombosis, thrombocytopenia and recurrent abortions are associated with the presence of the 'lupus anticoagulant' and/or antiphospholipid antibodies. The lupus anticoagulant causes a prolonged clotting time *in vitro* but thrombosis *in vivo*. It is often found in association with other autoantibodies to phospholipids, such as anticardiolipin antibodies and false-positive tests for syphilis.

Table 10.9 Presenting features of systemic lupus erythematosus

Features	%
Constitutional symptoms	50
Joints/muscles	62
Skin	50
Blood	8
Brain	15
Kidney	25

Table 10.10 Cumulative organ involvement in patients with systemic lupus erythematosus

Organ/tissue	Patients (%) who eventually develop organ involvement
Skin	80
Joints/muscles	80
Lung/pleura	30
Blood	60
Brain	30
Kidney	40
Heart	15

The distinction between SLE with antiphospholipid antibodies and the primary antiphospholipid antibody syndrome is discussed in Chapter 16.

In such a varied disease as SLE, it is important to have agreed criteria if comparisons are to be made. The American College of Rheumatology criteria are internationally accepted and were revised in 1982 and slightly modified in 1997 (Table 10.11). *These criteria are designed primarily for use in research rather than everyday clinical work.*

Table 10.11 American College of Rheumatology criteria for diagnosis of systemic lupus erythematosus (SLE)

Entry criterion

Antinuclear antibodies (ANA) at a titre of ≥1: 80 on HEp-2 cells or an equivalent positive test (ever)

↓

If absent, do not classify as SLE

If present, apply additive criteria

↓

Additive criteria

Do not count a criterion if there is a more likely explanation than SLE

Occurrence of a criterion on at least one occasion is sufficient

SLE classification requires at least one clinical criterion and ≥10 points

Criteria need not occur simultaneously

Within each domain, only the highest weighted criterion is counted towards the total score

Clinical domains and criteria	Weight	Immunology domains and criteria	Weight
Constitutional		*Antiphospholipid antibodies*	
Fever	2	Anti-cardiolipin antibodies OR	
Haematological		Anti-β2GP1 antibodies OR	
Leukopenia	3	Lupus anticoagulant	2
Thrombocytopenia	4	*Complement proteins*	
Autoimmune hemolysis	4	Low C3 OR low C4	3
Neuropsychiatry		Low C3 AND low C4	4
Delirium	2	*SLE-specific antibodies*	
Psychosis	3	• Anti-dsDNA antibody OR	
Seizure	5	• Anti-Smith antibody	6
Mucocutaneous			
Non-scarring alopecia	2		
Oral ulcers	2		
Subacute cutaneous OR discoid lupus	4		
Acute cutaneous lupus	6		
Serosal			
Pleural or pericardial effusion	5		
Acute pericarditis	6		
Musculoskeletal			
Joint involvement	6		
Renal			
Proteinuria >0.5 g/24 h	4		
Renal biopsy Class II or V lupus nephritis	8		
Renal biopsy Class III or IV lupus nephritis	10		

Total score:

↓

Classify as systemic lupus erythematosus with a score of 10 or more if entry criterion fulfilled

Case 10.8 Systemic lupus erythematosus (SLE)

A 26-year-old woman presented with fatigue and painful, stiff knees of 4 weeks' duration. She had a 6-year history of Raynaud's phenomenon, frequent mouth ulcers and had had a blotchy rash and ill-health after a recent holiday in Spain. On examination, she had bilateral effusions in both knee joints, but all other joints were normal. She had no skin lesions, muscle tenderness, proteinuria or fever. A full blood count showed mild thrombocytopenia with a platelet count of 95 (normal 150–400 × 10^{12}/l) and lymphopenia (0.7 × 10^9/l, normal 1.5–4.0). The results of relevant immunological investigations are shown in Table 10.12. On the basis of these findings, a diagnosis of SLE was made and the patient treated with aspirin for her painful knees. She improved over 4 weeks and then remained symptom free for 5 years. During this time, her antinuclear antibody remained positive at 1/1000, her anti-double-stranded (ds) DNA antibody level varied from 40 to 100 (normal <25) and her C3 and C4 levels were occasionally low. Later, she developed a bilateral, blotchy rash on her hands and thighs, consistent with active vasculitis. Her Raynaud's phenomenon concurrently became much worse. Following treatment with hydroxychloroquine, the skin manifestations gradually disappeared and the steroids were tailed off.

This patient presented with arthritis and Raynaud's phenomenon. She is unusual in that the arthritis of SLE usually involves small joints. It is important to note that she remained perfectly well without treatment for 5 years, despite persistently abnormal serology.

Table 10.12 Investigations in Case 10.8 (also see Chapter 19, Table 19.6)

C-reactive protein	8 mg/l (normal)
Rheumatoid factor	Negative
Antinuclear antibody	Positive (titre 1/1000; IgG class, homogeneous pattern)
Anti-dsDNA antibodies	80 (<25)
Antibodies to extractable nuclear antigens	Negative
Serum complement levels	
C3	0.35 g/l (NR 0.65–1.30)
C4	0.05 g/l (NR 0.20–0.50)
Serum immunoglobulins	
IgG	22.0 g/l (NR 7.2–19.0)
IgA	3.8 g/l (NR 2.0–5.0)
IgM	1.2 g/l (NR 0.5–2.0)
Biopsy of normal, sun-exposed skin (lupus band test)	Granular deposits of IgG and complement at dermo–epidermal junction

10.7.2 Laboratory findings

Almost all patients with SLE have ANAs, particularly antibodies to double-stranded DNA (dsDNA) (Table 10.13). A negative ANA does not completely exclude a suspected diagnosis of SLE, while positive dsDNA antibodies strongly support it. Antibodies to other, extractable nuclear antigens (ENAs) detected by non-fluorescent methods (see Chapter 19) are often present also (Table 10.13; Fig. 10.7). Other laboratory findings are positive in a varying proportion of patients (Table 10.13). In view of the wide range of presenting symptoms and the difficulties of making a definite diagnosis, all patients in whom SLE is suspected should be tested for **antinuclear antibodies, including those to dsDNA and ENA, including anti-Sm antibodies**, and for **antiphospholipid antibodies**, as well as having their serum levels of **IgG** and complement components, **C3 and C4**, measured.

10.7.3 Differential diagnosis

It is obviously important to distinguish between SLE and RA, since their management differs. The main differentiating features are shown in Fig. 10.8.

10.7.4 Drug-induced systemic lupus erythematosus

Some drug reactions can induce a lupus-like disease, especially the cutaneous manifestations; any of the clinical features of SLE may be present in drug-induced lupus, although renal and central nervous system involvement is rare. The most important diagnostic feature is resolution of the syndrome on withdrawal of the suspected offending drug, even though this may take several months. Most patients with drug-induced lupus have positive ANAs but negative dsDNA binding, negative lupus band tests and normal serum complement levels. Though in the past hydralazine, procainamide, certain anticonvulsants (phenytoin, hydantoins), isoniazid, chlorpromazine, penicillamine and minocycline (Chapter 5, Case 5.6) were likely suspects for inducing lupus, currently anti-TNF therapy with infliximab or etanercept, interferon-α and oncology drugs (doxorubicin and cyclophosphamide for breast cancer) are more common. Ticlopidine, an antiplatelet drug, has also been implicated.

Subjects with genetic defects in metabolism of these drugs (particularly those with reduced ability to acetylate these drugs, so-called slow acetylators) are at greatly increased risk of drug-induced SLE.

Table 10.13 Laboratory findings in untreated systemic lupus erythematosus (SLE)*

Immunological test	%	Haematological	%	Others	%
Anti-dsDNA	70–85	Raised ESR	60	C-reactive protein –often normal unless infection	
Antinuclear bodies (high titre; IgG class)**	>95%	Leucopenia	45	Proteinuria	30
Raised serum IgG level	65	Direct Coombs' test positive	40		
Low serum complement C3/ C4 levels	60	Lupus anticoagulant	10–20		
		Thrombocytopenia	8		
Antibodies to ENA:					
Sm	30				
RNP	35				
Ro	30				
La	15				
Antibodies to phospholipids	30–40				
Skin biopsy IgG, C3 and C4 deposits in normal skin	75				

* Figures show percentage of patients with positive tests.
** provided tested on human cell line (Hep2) cells.
ENA, extractable nuclear antigens; ESR, erythrocyte sedimentation rate; RNP, ribonucleoprotein.

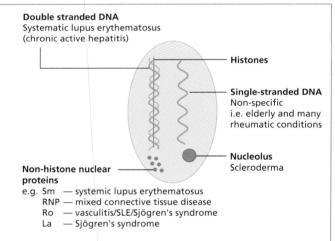

Fig. 10.7 Nuclear antigens: their role in diagnosis in rheumatic conditions. DNA + histones = nucleosome. RNP, ribonucleoprotein; SLE, systemic lupus erythematosus.

10.7.5 Management of systemic lupus erythematosus

SLE can be a mild disease, although even when mild, quality of life is often reduced. Patients may require no treatment or only small doses of NSAIDs. The major aims in management are:

- To avoid stimuli that may trigger an exacerbation.
- To control autoantibody production by immunosuppression.
- To limit damage.

Flare-up of activity often follows exposure to sunlight or infection; CRP is helpful to detect underlying infection, since disease activity alone rarely stimulates significant CRP synthesis.

SLE is a **relapsing and remitting disease**, and any immunosuppression required is therefore variable. Corticosteroids in moderate doses form the basis of treatment. Skin and joint symptoms respond well to antimalarials such as hydroxychloroquine, which also help prevent relapse. In persistent disease, mycophenolate is usually added as a steroid-sparing agent. Most patients can be controlled on a combination of mycophenolate, steroids and antimalarials. Cyclophosphamide, usually given as intravenous pulses, is widely used in vasculitis, severe cerebral SLE and severe lupus nephritis.

New therapies include several to limit the damaging effects of autoantibodies. The role of the anti-B-cell monoclonal antibody **rituximab** in treatment of patients with SLE remains controversial. Efficacy was reported in various observational studies on articular, cutaneous, renal and haematological manifestations, although severe infections occurred in 10% of patients (including multifocal leukoencephalopathy, PML); on the other hand, other studies reported no benefit of rituximab on disease activity. More studies are needed to determine the place of rituximab in treatment of SLE. **Belimumab** is a human monoclonal antibody that inhibits the biological activity of the soluble form of a B-cell survival factor BLyS. Belimumab has been shown effectives in patients with active cutaneous and musculoskeletal disease, and it is now licensed for use alongside standard care. **Epratazumab** is a humanized monoclonal antibody

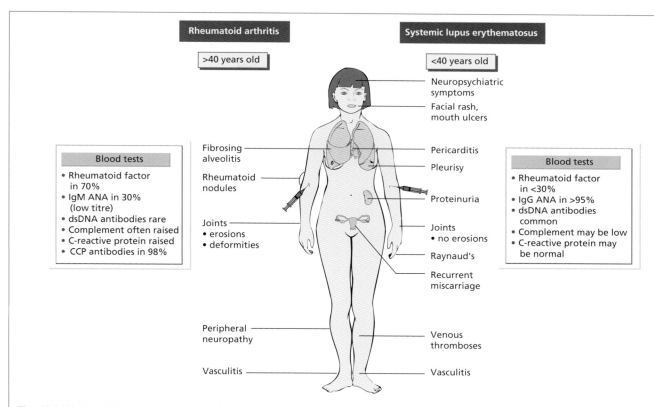

Fig. 10.8 Distinguishing clinical features of rheumatoid arthritis and systemic lupus erythematosus. ANA, antinuclear antibodies; CCP, cyclic citrullinated peptide.

against CD22 on B cells and showed success in early trials. Monoclonal antibodies to prevent or modulate T-cell activation seem to have no effective role in therapy. Current ongoing clinical trials using anti-interferon-α receptor monoclonal antibodies seem promising, but require further studies. The most exciting, though as yet unproven, therapies involve **small molecules incorporating dsDNA** that mop up a subset of anti-dsDNA antibodies that are pathogenic in the brain and kidney. If these can protect these vital organs from antibody-mediated damage, it may be possible to treat this autoimmune disease without inducing major immunosuppression and risking mortality due to severe infections as well as flares resulting from infections.

It is important to monitor the activity of SLE. This can be done by measuring serially the DNA antibody level and serum C3, C4 and CRP levels (Table 10.14). Anti-DNA antibody levels may rise before a major exacerbation and there is a strong association between the level of anti-dsDNA antibodies and glomerulonephritis. However, the level of anti-DNA antibodies does not reflect disease activity in all patients, so using this marker is not useful for all patients with SLE. In patients with renal damage, a fall in C4, followed by C3, may be the first indicator of renal damage and may occur 6 months before other features of renal involvement. Routine checks must also be made for proteinuria and renal dysfunction.

Table 10.14 Interpretation of serial serological changes in systemic lupus erythematosus

Result			
dsDNA antibodies	**C3**	**C4**	**Interpretation**
↑	Stable	Stable	Activity – watch for change in clinical state
Stable	↓	↓↓	Renal involvement should be suspected
Increased/stable	↑	–	Look for infection – measure C-reactive protein

10.7.6 Prognosis

The prognosis in SLE has improved considerably over the last 30 years. For all forms of SLE, the 5-year survival figure exceeds 90%, compared with 70–80% in the 1970s. Organ involvement correlates with severity; patients with skin and musculoskeletal disease have a good prognosis, whereas those with renal and central nervous system disease have a poorer prognosis. However, even in patients with proven nephritis, the 5-year survival is now over 80%. This reflects improvements in treatment of severe disease such as nephritis. *There is still, however, a considerable late mortality:* survival falls to 80% at 10 years and less than 70% at 20 years. The causes of death differ in early and late disease; in the first 5 years after diagnosis, **active SLE** accounts for about one-third of deaths and **infection** for most of the remainder. In later disease, infection is still a significant cause of death, but deaths from active lupus are much less common. The increased risk of death from infection in SLE is partly secondary to immunosuppressive treatment, but partly to the disease itself. **Secondary complement deficiency** (due to consumption of complement in active disease) and **functional hyposplenism** (due to overload of splenic mechanisms to clear immune complexes) both increase the risk of bacterial infection.

An increased prevalence of **atherosclerosis**, particularly IHD, accounts for much of the increased mortality in late disease. As in RA, some of this increased risk can be attributed to conventional risk factors and corticosteroid treatment, but there also appears to be a disease-specific risk that is greater in patients with severe or poorly controlled SLE. The risk of atherosclerosis seems much higher in SLE than in RA: *the risk of myocardial infarction in women with SLE is around 50 times higher than that in age- and sex-matched controls.* There is also an increased risk of certain **malignancies** in patients with SLE. Increased incidences of Hodgkin's lymphoma, non-Hodgkin's lymphoma, lung cancer and breast cancer have been noted. This predisposition seems to be the result of the SLE disease process itself, rather than the immunodeficiency associated with the disease and/or its treatment.

In addition to the continuing late mortality in SLE, there is also a considerable **late morbidity**, due to organ damage, vascular disease and other factors, such as osteoporosis (caused by corticosteroids). As in other severe, life-threatening diseases such as HIV infections and haematological cancers that have seen major improvements in treatment of the underlying disease, these late problems form a new challenge.

10.7.7 Aetiology and pathogenesis

The aetiology of SLE is complex, and many observations suggest a role for genetic, immunological, hormonal and environmental factors. SLE is largely an antibody-mediated disease, with both type II and type III hypersensitivity (see Chapter 1, section 1.8 and Chapter 5) playing major roles in **pathogenesis**. There is evidence that tissue damage in many patients is due to deposition of complexes of dsDNA with anti-DNA antibody, although complexes composed of other nuclear and cytoplasmic antigens are also thought to be important. Whether circulating complexes are deposited or whether dsDNA is first deposited in susceptible sites is still controversial. *Immunohistological studies of affected tissues show deposition of immunoglobulins and complement* and there is usually serological evidence for complement turnover and consumption. Antibodies have been eluted from affected tissues (particularly kidney) and are enriched for antinuclear antibodies compared with serum. **Maintenance** of the disease involves the process

centred around blood vessels, with overt vasculitis (i.e. damage to the vessel wall) in some cases, with ischaemic damage by plugging of small blood vessels with large numbers of inflammatory cells. In addition to immune-complex-mediated inflammation, antibodies to red blood cells, platelets and clotting factors can play a direct (type II) pathogenic role. The role of T cells is controversial; as yet there is no evidence of malfunction of Tregs, though there appears to be an expansion of Th17 cells in the blood and kidneys of those patients with renal disease. Increased levels of IL-17 correlate with disease activity in renal involvement, suggesting how inflammation in this site is maintained.

Since innate cells are activated by dsDNA via TLRs, this may account in part for **triggering** of SLE. IgG autoantibodies to dsDNA are produced when TLR9 is activated. In addition, plasmacytoid dendritic cells (pDC) produce large amounts of type I IFNs (IFN-α and IFN-β) in response to nucleic-acid–containing immune complexes. The evidence for a pathogenic role of type I IFNs in SLE includes a signature of mRNA for IFN-induced genes in the peripheral blood of patients, the identification of risk alleles involved in TLR and IFN pathways by genome-wide association studies (see later in the text) and disease acceleration by exogenous IFN-α in several lupus models.

The possible causes of the changes in DNA that enable an immune response to be triggered are legion, though failure of removal (apoptosis) or recycling (autophagy) nucleic acids may play a role (see later). A number of known factors contribute (Fig. 10.9) to this complex disease in susceptible individuals.

Genome-wide association studies have further highlighted the multifactorial pathogenesis of SLE. Approximately 40 polymorphisms associated with an increased risk of the disease have been identified. The majority of these polymorphisms were in genes either involved in the innate immune response

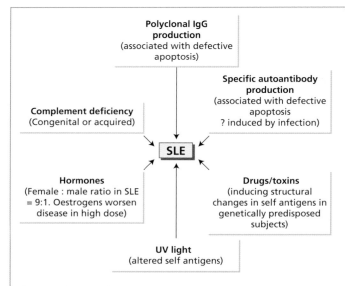

Fig. 10.9 Multiple factors combine in the aetiology of systemic lupus erythematosus (SLE).

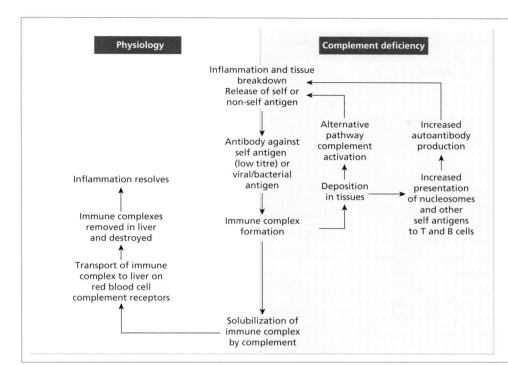

Fig. 10.10 Immune complex metabolism in normal subjects (left) and those with complement deficiency (right).

(e.g. STAT-4, IRF-5) or adaptive immunity (e.g. HLA loci, OX40L).

Inherited deficiency of components of the classical pathway of complement (C1, C4 or C2) is associated with a greatly increased risk of developing SLE. This is seen most strikingly in C1q deficiency, in which the risk of severe anti-dsDNA-positive SLE is almost 100%. A similar syndrome is also seen in C1q knockout mice. Metabolism of immune complexes is grossly abnormal in subjects with any complement deficiency, with a tendency for deposition in the tissues (Fig. 10.10). However, inherited severe complement deficiencies are rare, and make up only a handful of cases with SLE. Partial complement defects are common in SLE: non-coding or null alleles for C4 are important genetic risk factors for SLE, and the complement deficiency by consumption may, in turn, perpetuate the disease. Autoantibodies directed against complement components, especially C1q, have also been described, which may cause further complement deficiency.

Defective apoptosis was implicated in SLE when two animal models of spontaneous SLE were found to be due to deficiency of Fas and Fas ligand – two cell-surface counter-receptors with a key role in triggering apoptosis (see Chapters 1 and 5). Apoptosis, triggered through Fas, has an important role in deleting autoreactive lymphocytes and *Fas deficiency in humans causes a characteristic syndrome comprising red cell and platelet autoimmunity, lymphadenopathy and polyclonal increases in serum immunoglobulin levels: the autoimmune lymphoproliferative syndrome (ALPS),* though not classical SLE. Nevertheless, several genes involved in alternative apoptopic pathways were found in genome-wide association studies in human SLE. C1q

binds to apoptotic cells and plays a key role in clearance of these cells. C1q deficiency (whether genetic or acquired) may therefore predispose to lupus by both allowing access of nuclear material to the immune system, and allowing tissue deposition of immune complexes (Fig. 10.10). Acute-phase proteins called pentraxins, which include CRP and serum amyloid P (SAP), can bind to DNA and other nucleosomal particles, which are then cleared by the complement system. SAP gene knockout mice develop a lupus-like illness, and there is some evidence that CRP and SAP production are reduced in some humans with SLE. This suggests a further link between cell death, complement and lupus.

Sunlight is a well-recognized trigger for both skin and systemic manifestations of SLE. **Ultraviolet (UV) light** has a number of immunological actions on the skin, but perhaps most significant is induction of apoptosis of keratinocytes. This causes expression of lupus autoantigens (such as Ro and La) on the cell surface, where they can gain access to the immune system. Subjects with common genetic polymorphisms reducing their ability to handle UV-induced damage may be particularly liable to develop photosensitivity.

SLE is around 10 times more common in women than in men, and tends to present between the menarche and the menopause. This is due, in part, to the influence of sex steroid hormones: **oestrogens** can accelerate the disease in animal models of SLE, and reduction in oestrogen levels improves the disease. Similar observations have been made in humans, although sex-specific factors other than oestrogens may also play a role. Surprisingly little is known of the exact mechanisms underlying these hormonal influences upon immune function.

10.8 Other 'connective tissue' diseases

Generally, it is accepted that there are five major systemic auto-immune disorders: RA, SLE, scleroderma (Chapter 11), polymyositis (PM) and dermatomyositis (DM). Another disorder, Sjögren's syndrome, is commonly associated with each of these diseases and is called primary Sjögren's syndrome when it occurs alone.

10.8.1 Mixed connective tissue disease

The 'mixed connective tissue disease' (MCTD) was an additional syndrome first described in 1972 as an apparently distinct rheumatic disease with a specific diagnostic antibody. The clinical features in the original description included arthritis, polymyositis, pulmonary fibrosis and scleroderma-like changes in the skin. It is now apparent that patients with MCTD also develop features more commonly associated with SLE, as in Case 10.9 (Table 10.15) or other systemic autoimmune diseases. The length of this list makes some clinicians believe that it is not a separate disease; nevertheless, the most important distinguishing feature between MCTD and classic SLE is the relative scarcity of renal and cerebral involvement in MCTD.

The major serological finding is a high titre of antibody against the extractable nuclear antigen **RNP** (see Chapter 19). The presence of this antibody without other 'lupus' autoantibodies (such as anti-Sm) correlates with a good clinical outcome. There is usually a positive ANA, which typically shows a speckled pattern, but antibodies to dsDNA are absent and C3 and C4 levels are normal.

MCTD was once thought to have a better prognosis than SLE because of the relative lack of renal and cerebral involvement. However, longitudinal studies have shown that some patients do develop severe disease with attendant mortality, with pulmonary arterial hypertension being the main cause of death among patients with MCTD. Studies report a wide range of survival rates, with 10-year mortality approaching 20%. Pregnancy is uneventful. The response to treatment with corticosteroids is usually reasonable, although steroid-sparing drugs such as azathioprine or methotrexate are often required.

Table 10.15 Features of mixed connective tissue diseases

1. SLE or RA-like features

Arthritis (usually mild but can be erosive)

Constitutional symptoms: fever, malaise

Lymphadenopathy

Peripheral neuropathy (particularly trigeminal)

Erythematous rashes

Serositis

2. Polymyositis

3. Scleroderma-like features

Raynaud's phenomenon – may be severe

Puffy hands – fingers often sausage-like at presentation

Abnormal oesophageal motility

Interstitial lung disease

4. Antibodies to RNP at high titre

RA, rheumatoid arthritis; RNP, Ribonucleoprotein; SLE, systemic lupus erythematosus.

🔍 Case 10.9 Mixed connective tissue disease

A 19-year-old typist presented with acute, bilateral arthralgia of her wrists and knees. The pain prevented her from sleeping or typing. On examination, there were no effusions or tenderness of any joints. No diagnosis was made, but she was treated symptomatically. Two months later, she developed severe Raynaud's phenomenon, with arthralgia and pronounced sausage-like swelling of her fingers and some proximal muscle weakness. On investigation, she had a low haemoglobin (108 g/l) but a normal white cell count and differential. Her erythrocyte sedimentation rate (ESR) was raised (63 mm/h), and her serum contained antinuclear antibody (ANA; titre 1/160; speckled pattern; see Chapter 19). dsDNA binding was normal, but antibodies to extractable nuclear antigens (ENA) were detected and found to be largely directed against nuclear ribonucleoprotein (RNP); there were no antibodies to the Sm antigen (see Chapter 19). A latex test for rheumatoid factor was negative. Complement levels (C3 and C4) were normal, but she had a raised serum IgG of 21.8 g/l (NR 7.2–19.0). X-rays of the hands and knees were normal. There was no proteinuria and her serum creatinine and blood urea were normal. Her creatine kinase was elevated at 2100 IU/ml (normal <100) and a muscle biopsy showed features of a low-grade myositis.

A diagnosis of mixed connective tissue disease (MCTD) was made and the patient started on prednisolone 40 mg daily. The muscle weakness and joint pain improved dramatically, but attempts to reduce and discontinue the steroids were unsuccessful; muscle weakness returned each time the drug was discontinued. Azathioprine was introduced as a steroid-sparing immunosuppressive. Her Raynaud's phenomenon has slowly worsened and is now associated with progressive sclerodactyly.

10.8.2 Sjögren's syndrome

Dry eyes and a dry mouth can occur in otherwise healthy elderly people (around 1–2% of those over 70 years) and do not appear to be associated with any autoimmune process. However, these features should always raise a suspicion of Sjögren's syndrome, *particularly in the younger patient* (Case 10.10). The principal feature of Sjögren's syndrome is autoimmune destruction of **exocrine glands, most prominently the lacrimal and salivary glands**, but also glands at other sites including the respiratory mucosa and vagina. Sjögren's syndrome can occur as a syndrome in itself, associated with distinctive non-exocrine clinical features and antibodies against Ro and La (primary Sjögren's syndrome, Fig. 10.11) or can occur in association with another connective tissue disease such as RA, SLE or scleroderma (secondary Sjögren's syndrome). Sjögren's has a strong female predominance. The prevalence of Sjögren's is unclear, as the symptoms are often mild and hence unrecognized, but it appears to be at least as common as SLE. It is not clear whether the high prevalence of sicca features in elderly patients reflects mild Sjögren's or some other pathology. Lymphoma is a recognized complication of Sjögren's syndrome.

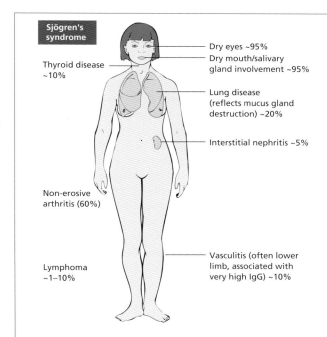

Fig. 10.11 Clinical features of primary Sjögren's syndrome.

Case 10.10 Sjögren's syndrome

A 38-year-old woman was referred to an oral surgeon for investigation of a dry mouth. She had a sister with arthritis. Examination and investigations were unremarkable except for a raised erythrocyte sedimentation rate (ESR; 42 mm/h). Six months later, she developed a mild conjunctivitis and complained of sore eyes. On testing, rheumatoid factor was now positive (Rose–Waaler titre 1/64); total serum proteins were raised (98 g/l); and immunoglobulin levels showed a raised IgG of 28 g/l (NR 7.2–19.0), with a slightly raised IgM of 2.8 g/l (NR 0.5–2.0) and a normal IgA. Schirmer's test was performed (see section 10.8.2). The test was markedly abnormal, as only 3.5 mm of the filter strip in the right eye and 1.5 mm of that in the left eye became wet (Fig. 10.12).

She was treated with methylcellulose eye drops to prevent corneal ulceration. Over a period of many years, her rheumatoid factor titre steadily increased and antinuclear antibodies (ANA) and antibodies to the extractable nuclear antigens Ro and La became detectable. Seven years after the development of the dry mouth and dry eyes (together known as the sicca complex), she developed a mild, bilateral non-erosive polyarthritis of her hands, wrists and knees. A diagnosis of secondary Sjögren's syndrome was made. The disease has remained mild. Non-steroidal antiinflammatory drugs (NSAIDs) have been given for the arthritis, but have had no effect on the sicca complex.

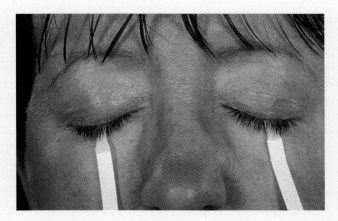

Fig. 10.12 Dry eyes in Sjögren's syndrome demonstrated by Schirmer's test. Source: From *Medical Masterclass. Rheumatology and Clinical Immunology*, 2nd Ed. Copyright © 2008 Royal College of Physicians. Reproduced with permission.

The simplest **diagnostic test** for suspected Sjögren's is the Schirmer test: a slip of sterile filter paper is placed over the lower eyelid. Failure to produce sufficient tears in 5 min to wet 10 mm of the paper suggests defective tear production and in the context of other features of connective tissue disease strongly suggests Sjögren's. Biopsy of glandular tissue involved by Sjögren's (minor salivary glands in the lip being the most accessible) shows a dense lymphocytic infiltrate of largely activated, cytokine-producing CD4⁺ T cells, with marked class II MHC expression on the remaining glandular structures. Autoantibodies to salivary gland tissue can be helpful.

Primary Sjögren's is strongly associated with the HLA A1 B8 DR3 haplotype, as well as polymorphisms in **genes** associated with innate immunity and mRNA expression of interferon genes in salivary gland tissues. Environmental triggers are unclear, but activation of type I interferon (IFN-α and IFN-β pathways) as well as production of B-cell survival factor, BAFF, have been demonstrated. In mice, stimulation of dendritic cells can result in dryness and lymphocytic infiltrates in salivary glands. Oestrogen deficiency, with or without Epstein–Barr virus (EBV) infection, can lead to autoimmune inflammation of the epithelium. Taken together, these findings suggest that the interaction of IFNs and BAFF with B cells is involved in the pathogenesis and rituximab is therefore in clinical trials.

Therapy of Sjögren's is usually supportive, with artificial tears and attention to oral hygiene, since the affected glands are usually irreversibly destroyed at presentation. The prognosis of primary Sjögren's is usually good, but some patients may have problems (Fig. 10.11) and there is also an increased risk of B-cell lymphoma.

10.8.3 Scleroderma

Scleroderma (progressive systemic sclerosis) is characterized by diffuse fibrosis affecting skin, lungs, GI tract, heart and muscle. It is described in detail in Chapter 11; a seronegative polyarthritis develops in 25% of patients, often early in the disease.

10.9 Systemic vasculitis

10.9.1 Polyarteritis nodosa

Polyarteritis nodosa (PAN) is antineutrophil cytoplasmic antibody (ANCA)-negative systemic necrotizing vasculitis characterized by swelling of muscle fibres within the media of medium-sized arteries. This is followed by fibrinoid change and intense infiltration of polymorphonuclear leucocytes. The process results in **multiple aneurysm** formation (which gives rise to the name 'nodosa'), often with total occlusion of the vessel (Fig. 10.13). The extent of involvement of a particular artery is variable and 'skip' lesions are often present.

The **aetiology** of the vasculitis is unknown. A small proportion of patients are positive for hepatitis B antigen or hepatitis C, regardless of overt clinical hepatitis in the past, while a drug reaction or infection may precede PAN. These observations support the view that PAN is triggered by a foreign agent(s), with deposition of the circulating immune complexes in the vessel wall.

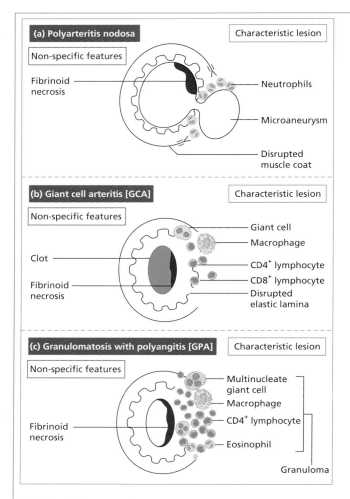

Fig. 10.13 Histology of three types of vasculitis in patients who may present with arthritides/arthralgia or myalgia.

The **clinical features** of PAN are extremely varied (Fig. 10.14) and investigations often unrewarding. Selective renal angiography may show arterial aneurysms, but in only 50% of cases. **Muscle biopsy** is positive in 40% of cases, provided that an affected, tender area of muscle is chosen, as in Case 10.11. It is mandatory to test hepatitis B and C serology. Non-specific findings include a raised ESR and CRP, low haemoglobin and a leucocytosis with an occasional eosinophilia. Renal function may be compromised with hypertension, but glomerulonephritis is not a feature. Immunological investigations are unhelpful.

It is important to distinguish PAN from microscopic polyarteritis (MPA) (see Chapters 9 and 11), in which lung involvement may lead to fatal pulmonary haemorrhage. The development of rapidly progressive crescentic glomerulonephritis (typical of granulomatosis with polyangiitis, GPA) and positive ANCA (see Chapters 9 and 19) has led to the view that MPA is related to GPA rather than PAN. This is important, not only for treatment (cyclophosphamide as well as steroids) but also for prognosis.

Without **treatment**, the prognosis of PAN is poor, with 1-year and 5-year survival rates of approximately 50% and 13%, respectively. The overall prognosis of PAN depends on

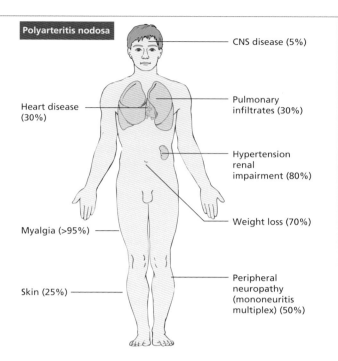

Fig. 10.14 Clinical features of polyarteritis nodosa. CNS, central nervous system.

the organs involved. Renal failure and cerebral or cardiac infarction are the major causes of death. Other severe complications include GI involvement and malignant hypertension. Treatment with high-dose corticosteroids in the acute stage has improved the prognosis. In patients with mild disease who are resistant to or intolerant of the dose of glucocorticoids required, methotrexate or azathioprine can be considered. Patients with moderate to severe disease manifestations, such as those with renal insufficiency or mononeuropathy multiplex, are treated with a combination of corticosteroids and cyclophosphamide.

10.9.2 Polymyalgia rheumatica and giant cell (temporal) arteritis

Polymyalgia rheumatica (PMR) and giant cell arteritis (GCA) are closely related conditions, best considered as part of a spectrum of disease, which are *relatively common in elderly people, particularly women*. About 1% of over 70-year-olds are affected. PMR alone is most common, but 20% of patients with PMR also have features of GCA. GCA may also occur without PMR. The disease is rare before the age of 55. The major presenting **symptoms** of PMR are acute onset of pain and morning stiffness in the muscles of the shoulders and pelvic girdle. Systemic symptoms include malaise, weight loss, depression and anorexia. Severe headaches, pain in the scalp, jaw and tongue and visual loss suggest a diagnosis of GCA (sometimes know as temporal or cranial arteritis). Vascular inflammation in GCA is usually confined to the branches of the external carotid artery. Sudden **blindness** can occur due to occlusion of the posterior ciliary artery, which supplies the optic disc.

Laboratory investigations in this disease are usually nonspecific. The ESR is considerably raised in 95% of patients and the **CRP** in 90%; temporal artery biopsy is abnormal in only 25–40% of cases, but may be helpful when there is diagnostic uncertainty. The response of polymyalgia rheumatica and temporal arteritis to corticosteroids is dramatic, as in Case 10.12. Because of the risk of blindness, suspected GCA requires immediate treatment with **high-dose prednisolone** 40–60 mg daily, but pure polymyalgia responds to lower doses, often as little as 10–15 mg prednisolone daily. Treatment can usually be reduced and gradually withdrawn over 1–2 years. Anti-TNF treatment is of no added value in either PMR or GCA. Tocilizumab (anti-IL6) was successfully used as a corticosteroid-sparing agent in (relapses of) GCA.

The **pathological changes** in GCA are distinctive: there is an arteritis of large and medium-sized arteries with large multinucleate giant cells in the media and around a swollen and

---

🔍 Case 10.11 Polyarteritis nodosa

A 64-year-old man developed diplopia due to a right sixth nerve palsy, lethargy, weight loss and skin lesions on the right leg, which were thought to be erythema nodosum. Six weeks later, he presented with aches and pains in his shoulders, which his doctor thought were due to polymyalgia rheumatica. He improved dramatically on steroids, but unfortunately they had to be withdrawn because of hypertension. On investigation, he had an erythrocyte sedimentation rate (ESR) of 104 mm/h, a polymorphonuclear leucocytosis and some proteinuria (1.5 g/24 h) with occasional granular casts. Biopsy of a skin lesion showed non-specific changes. A renal biopsy was normal. No diagnosis was possible.

Four weeks later, he developed profound malaise with fever, marked muscle weakness and anaemia. His haemoglobin was 77 g/l with a C-reactive protein (CRP) of 70 mg/l, a negative direct Coombs' test and a reticulocyte count of 5.4%. Blood urea, serum creatinine and creatinine clearance were normal, as was serum creatine kinase level. Antinuclear antibodies (ANA), dsDNA binding and antineutrophil cytoplasmic antibodies (ANCA) were negative, with normal C3 and C4 complement levels. Biopsy of an affected calf muscle showed a florid arteritis. All the medium-sized arteries showed reduction of their lumens or complete occlusion. On the basis of this muscle biopsy, a firm diagnosis of polyarteritis nodosa was made. The patient was started on 60 mg of prednisolone per day. Over the next few days his temperature fell and his symptoms improved.

🔍 Case 10.12 Polymyalgia rheumatica

A 73-year-old woman presented with sudden pain and stiffness of her shoulder muscles. She had become increasingly depressed over the preceding 3 months, with anorexia and loss of weight. On examination, there was limitation of movement of both shoulders with muscle tenderness; neurological examination was normal. The temporal arteries were extremely tender on palpation. On investigation, her haemoglobin was 101 g/l with a raised C-reactive protein (CRP) of 68 mg/l. A diagnosis of polymyalgia rheumatica and temporal arteritis was made and a temporal artery biopsy taken. Treatment was started immediately with 60 mg of prednisolone daily and within 24 h the patient was markedly improved; she became more alert and her muscle stiffness lessened. The temporal artery biopsy showed a vasculitis with infiltration by lymphocytes, macrophages and giant cells (Fig. 10.15). Improvement continued over the next few days. Steroids were gradually withdrawn over 2 months, but her polymyalgia relapsed a year later and she again improved on steroids.

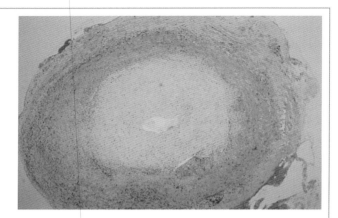

Fig. 10.15 Occluded, temporal artery in giant cell arteritis. The vessel wall is thickened and infiltrated with lymphocytes and macrophages. Source: From *Medical Masterclass. Rheumatology and Clinical Immunology*, 2nd Ed. Copyright © 2008 Royal College of Physicians. Reproduced with permission.

fragmented internal elastic lamina (Figs 10.13 and 10.15). The distribution of the arteritis corresponds to the amount of elastic tissue within the vessel; thus, arteries of the head and neck are especially affected, whereas pulmonary and renal vessels are usually spared.

The pathogenesis of temporal arteritis involves infiltration of the vessel wall by CD8+, and to a lesser extent CD4+, T cells and macrophages. There is evidence of both T-cell and macrophage cytokine production and of cytotoxic T-cell responses against cells within the vessel wall. The pathology of polymyalgia rheumatica remains obscure.

There are no real clues as to environmental triggers to temporal arteritis, although some have speculated that UV light may alter the antigenic structure of elastin and other components of the vessel wall.

10.9.3 Other vasculitides

Other vasculitides may involve the joints, resulting in arthralgia or arthropathy. In particular, patients with granulomatosis with polyangiitis (GPA; formerly Wegener's granulomatosis)

commonly present with vague joint pains before developing the more specific clinical features in the respiratory tract, nose or kidneys. The histological features of GPA are different from those of GCA and polyarteritis nodosa (Fig. 10.13). Vasculitis is fully discussed in Chapter 11 (see Table 11.3) and the treatment of GPA is also included in Chapters 9 and 13.

10.10 Inflammatory muscle disease or myositis

The spectrum of autoimmune myositis (Table 10.16) includes muscle inflammation in isolation (primary polymyositis; Case 10.13), in association with skin changes and vasculitis (dermatomyositis) or in association with other clinical features of MCTD. Childhood dermatomyositis appears to be a different disease from the adult form, with a greater tendency to vasculitis and soft tissue calcification.

Myositis usually **presents** with muscle weakness, principally involving the proximal muscles. Some pain and tenderness may be present, but this is usually mild. Respiratory muscle weakness and swallowing difficulty suggest a poor prognosis (see Case 10.3). **Investigations** show a raised level of skeletal muscle enzymes (such as creatine kinase), a non-specific finding in many kinds of muscle damage, and electromyography and magnetic resonance scanning provide supportive evidence. A definitive diagnosis is usually made by **muscle biopsy** that shows damaged fibres and infiltration by lymphocytes. As usual antinuclear antibodies are present in over 50% of patients, useful **specific autoantibodies are those to Jo 1**, which are associated with myositis, pulmonary fibrosis and sclerodermatous changes.

The **pathogenesis** of polymyositis and dermatomyositis seems to be different: polymyositis is associated with muscle damage caused by T cells, whereas antibody and complement appear to be more important in dermatomyositis as well as Type I interferons for autoantibody production.

The **aetiology** of myositis is unknown in most cases. There has been much interest in a viral cause, but no convincing evidence, although transient myositis is well documented after Coxsackie virus. Drugs, particularly statins, may trigger a syndrome resembling myositis, although it is hard to distinguish

---

🔍 Case 10.13 Polymyositis

A 32-year-old woman with a past history of ulcerative colitis (quiescent for the last 7 years) presented with a dry cough. The cough became productive of clear sputum and she was admitted 2 months later with increasing dyspnoea, myalgia and arthralgia. A clinical diagnosis of fibrosing alveolitis was made and confirmed by transbronchial biopsy. She was treated with prednisolone, which improved her arthralgia, and it became clear that she had a severe proximal myopathy. Serum creatine kinase was found to be very high and a muscle biopsy showed necrosis and a cellular infiltrate compatible with polymyositis. She had a circulating autoantibody to Jo 1 antigen (see Chapter 19).

She recovered eventually, after a stormy course that included treatment with pulsed methylprednisolone, oral azathioprine and three plasma exchanges of 2.5 l. She has persistent myalgia and some arthralgia and remains on 20 mg prednisolone daily; the prognosis is poor.

Table 10.16 Classification of autoimmune myositis

1 Primary idiopathic polymyositis

2 Primary idiopathic dermatomyositis

3 Myositis with malignancy

4 Juvenile dermatomyositis

5 Myositis as a feature of other autoimmune disease – myositis with systemic lupus erythematosus, scleroderma, and that associated with Jo 1 antibodies

toxic myopathies from immunologically mediated disease. *Around 10% of cases of adult dermatomyositis are associated with underlying carcinomas*, suggesting that the tumour is inducing the autoimmune muscle disease. Cancers of the ovary, lung, GI tract and lymphoma are most common in this context.

Treatment is with high-dose corticosteroids, often combined with azathioprine or another immunosuppressive drug. High-dose intravenous immunoglobulin is effective in adult dermatomyositis, but this relapses if treatment is withdrawn. The role of plasmapheresis remains controversial, but could be considered in specific patients. The 5-year mortality from myositis is 10–15%, but long-term morbidity from muscle weakness is much more common and is often severe.

10.11 Hereditary periodic fevers

The hereditary periodic fevers (also known as the **autoinflammatory syndromes**) are a group of genetic disorders of inflammation. All are characterized by episodic fever, often with inflammation involving joints, skin and serosal surfaces. The clinical phenotype and the pattern of inheritance of these disorders have been described for many years, but in the last few years the genetic basis of these disorders has been unravelled. The proteins encoded by the affected genes have mainly been found to play a regulatory role in inflammation. The proteins, pyrin and cryopyrin, are **regulators of cytokine production and apoptosis** and the **TNF receptor** that modulates the action of TNF is involved. Globally, the most common and serious of these disorders is familial Mediterranean fever (FMF), due to mutations in gene MEFV, which encodes pyrin; this has a prevalence of 1–5 per 1000 among Sephardic Jews, Armenians and

Table 10.17 Epidemiological, genetic and clinical features of the hereditary periodic fevers

	Familial Mediterranean fever	TNF receptor–associated periodic syndrome (TRAPS)	Hyper IgD syndrome	Muckle Wells syndrome	Familial cold autoinflammatory syndrome
Inheritance	Autosomal recessive	Autosomal dominant	Autosomal recessive	Autosomal dominant	Autosomal dominant
Ethnic distribution	Jewish, Arab, Turkish, Armenian	Irish, Scots plus sporadic families elsewhere	North European	North European	North European
Gene affected	MEFV	TNFRSF1A	MVK	CIAS1	CIAS1
Protein encoded by affected gene	Pyrin	55-kDa TNF-α receptor	Mevalonate kinase (involved in cholesterol synthesis – link with inflammation unclear)	Cryopyrin	Cryopyrin
Duration of febrile episode	1–3 days	>7 days	3–7 days	1–2 days	

TNF, tumour necrosis factor.

some Arabs. If untreated, patients with FMF have a high risk of developing systemic AA amyloidosis. Mutations in the gene for the p55 TNF receptor led to the renaming of familial Hibernian fever as TNF receptor–associated periodic syndrome (TRAPS). Both diseases lack the clinical and laboratory markers that indicate adaptive immune dysregulation, such as autoantibodies and antigen-specific T cells. There is no evidence of infection or classical immunodeficiency; disease triggers are not obvious, though stress and minor infections often induce flares.

Treatment of FMF with low-dose colchicine decreases the frequency of acute attacks of fever and pain and greatly reduces the risk of amyloid deposition. Following the discovery that most are driven by abnormal IL-1β secretion, most of the others can be controlled with anti-IL-1 agents, such as anakinra (an IL-1 receptor antagonist) or canakinumab (a monoclonal antibody to IL-1).

The genetics, clinical features and treatment of the main five hereditary periodic fevers are summarized in Table 10.17.

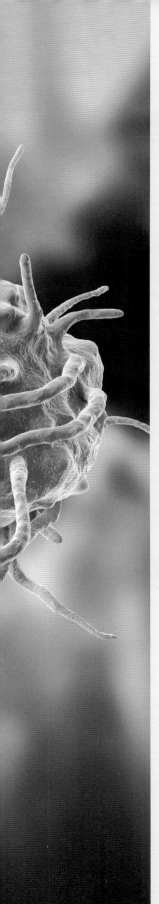

CHAPTER 11
Skin Diseases

Key topics

 Visit the companion website at **www.wiley.com/go/misbah/immunology** to download cases with additional figures on these topics.

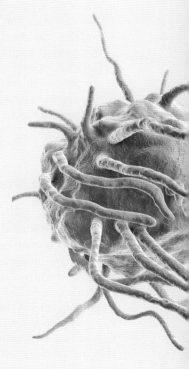

Chapel and Haeney's Essentials of Clinical Immunology, Seventh Edition. Edited by Siraj A. Misbah, Gavin P. Spickett, and Virgil A.S.H. Dalm.
© 2022 John Wiley & Sons Ltd. Published 2022 by John Wiley & Sons Ltd.

11.1 Introduction

The skin consists of an impervious horny layer of stratified squamous epithelial cells called keratinocytes (**epidermis**) overlying vascular connective tissue (**dermis**). The epidermis has an important mechanical function as a barrier from the outside world, but also plays a more active role in the skin's response to injury. The **keratinocyte** can synthesize a large number of cytokines and other inflammatory mediators in response to injury or ultraviolet radiation (UVR) (Fig. 11.1). These non-specific mediators increase vascular permeability, attract and activate immune cells and induce the expression of adhesion molecules on nearby endothelial cells to allow these cells access to the damaged tissue.

Intertwined with this innate response to injury is a system for adaptive immunity against antigens gaining access via the skin. Around 10% of the cells in the epidermis are a specialized antigen-presenting population known as **Langerhans cells**. These cells have a high capacity for the uptake and processing of antigen. Following any insult to the epidermis (such as invasion by microorganisms), they migrate along afferent lymphatics to the paracortex of the draining lymph nodes; during migration they differentiate into classical dendritic cells with high expression of major histocompatibility complex (MHC) class II and co-stimulatory molecules (see Chapter 1, section 1.3.4). They then activate specific naive T cells, via T-cell receptors (TCRs) for those peptides derived from antigens taken up in the skin, inducing proliferation and differentiation of T cells into effector cells. Most of these leave the lymph node, enter the blood and then migrate into inflamed skin. In order to return to the particular site of inflammation, T cells express receptors (integrins) that are specific for intercellular addressin cell adhesion molecules (ICAMs) found on endothelial cells in inflamed skin (the expression of which is induced by cytokine signals from keratinocytes). The best-characterized T-cell adhesion molecule for homing to skin is known as cutaneous lymphocyte-associated antigen (CLA), which binds to E-selectin on endothelial cells. Skin-homing T cells also express the chemokine receptors CCR4 and CCR10, which selectively bind a distinctive chemokine produced by cutaneous endothelial cells and keratinocytes. This leads to migration and retention of these T cells in the skin. Langerhans cells, keratinocytes, CLA-positive T cells and local lymph nodes have been regarded collectively as skin-associated lymphoid tissue (SALT). Although this tissue limits infection, it is also responsible for some types of skin disease (see section 11.3).

Unlike the rest of the body, the skin is exposed to UVR, which has important local and systemic immunological effects (Table 11.1). Chronic UVR exposure leads to skin cancer due to oncogenic human papilloma viruses (HPV). The risk of skin malignancy is increased in immunosuppressed patients, especially in skin exposed to high levels of UVR. This suggests that immune mechanisms normally control HPV infection. Particular strains of HPV produce E6 and E7 proteins that affect cell cycle components and can lead to reduced apoptosis and eventually uncontrolled growth, i.e. malignancy, if not checked by immune responses. UVR exposure depresses Langerhans cell function, reduces in vitro lymphocyte responses and impairs cell-mediated immunity (Table 11.1 and Fig. 11.1). Infection, autoimmunity or hypersensitivity can cause skin diseases. Skin damage may be triggered by autoantibodies to skin antigens (in the bullous diseases) or by deposition of immune complexes (in systemic lupus erythematosus, SLE). T cells are involved in some forms of dermatitis.

11.2 Infections and the skin

Bacterial, viral and fungal infections can occur when the physical barrier of the skin is breached following trauma (especially burns) or widespread eczema, or if immune defences are impaired by systemic or topical immunosuppressive treatment due to exposure to corticosteroids and cytotoxic drugs (Chapter 7) or due to primary or secondary immunodeficiency (see Chapter 3). Septicaemic infections, e.g. gonococcal or meningococcal septicaemia, may seed foci of infection into the skin. Certain viruses invade the skin to produce infected lesions (chickenpox, varicella-zoster virus; or warts, HPV), although a reactive, non-infective rash is a more common response to systemic viral infections (e.g. exanthemata of rubella or measles). Recurrent herpes labialis is caused by reactivation of persistent herpes simplex infection; attacks are often provoked by exposure to UV light, probably due to suppression of the skin immune system (Case 11.1). Atopic individuals have an increased tendency to herpes labialis, perhaps related to a less effective T-cell response against this virus. Skin granulomas, although rare in developed countries, are most commonly caused worldwide by invading microorganisms such as Mycobacterium tuberculosis, M. leprae or Treponema pallidum.

One of the best examples of the multiple skin manifestations associated with immunodeficiency is human immunodeficiency virus (HIV) (see Chapters 2 and 3). A wide spectrum of skin problems occurs in HIV-infected individuals (Fig. 11.2). Sometimes these are exacerbations of preexisting skin disease, such as psoriasis, but more often they are new conditions.

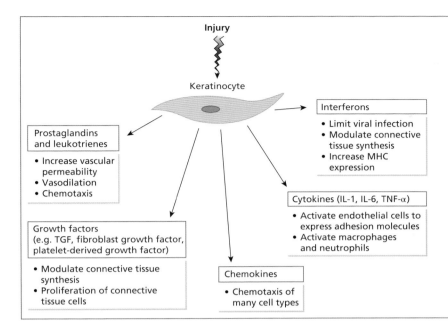

Injury

Keratinocyte

Prostaglandins and leukotrienes
- Increase vascular permeability
- Vasodilation
- Chemotaxis

Growth factors
(e.g. TGF, fibroblast growth factor, platelet-derived growth factor)
- Modulate connective tissue synthesis
- Proliferation of connective tissue cells

Chemokines
- Chemotaxis of many cell types

Interferons
- Limit viral infection
- Modulate connective tissue synthesis
- Increase MHC expression

Cytokines (IL-1, IL-6, TNF-α)
- Activate endothelial cells to express adhesion molecules
- Activate macrophages and neutrophils

Fig. 11.1 Multiple proinflammatory factors produced by keratinocytes in response to injury. IL, interleukin; MHC, major histocompatibility complex; TGF, transforming growth factor; TNF, tumour necrosis factor.

Table 11.1 Effects of ultraviolet radiation on the skin

Induces skin cancer formation

Effect on Langerhans cells
- Alters morphology
- Reduces expression of cell-surface receptors
- Reduces ability to present antigen

Effect on lymphocytes
- Alters cell trafficking
- Changes cell populations in peripheral blood (CD4+ lymphocytes ↓ CD8+ lymphocytes ↑)
- Suppresses contact hypersensitivity responses
- Impairs lymphocyte transformation responses to mitogens and antigens
- Alters cytokine production

Upregulates Ro52 antigen (E3 ubiquitin ligase) expression in epidermis
- Increases risk of skin disease in patients with anti-Ro52 autoantibodies

11.3 T cell–mediated skin disease

T cells play a central role in some of the most common skin diseases: the best understood are contact dermatitis, mediated by Th1 cells, and atopic eczema, mediated largely by Th2 cells. The chronic skin disease psoriasis also appears to be mediated largely by T cells, although the triggering antigen and the mechanism by which T cells induce the characteristic epidermal changes of psoriasis are not fully understood.

 Case 11.1 Recurrent cold sores

A 38-year-old woman had been troubled since the age of 8 by recurrent cold sores. Several times each year she would develop a distinctive tingling sensation around her nose or lips, followed several hours later by localized formation of small blisters that crusted, became more painful and gradually cleared over several days. The attacks were often provoked by exposure to strong sunlight. She had a history of troublesome hay fever but was otherwise well. She was able to prevent attacks by use of a high-factor sun block and treat any breakthrough episodes with prompt use of aciclovir tablets at the onset of symptoms.

11.3.1 Contact dermatitis

Contact dermatitis is an inflammatory skin disease caused by **Th1 cell–mediated (type IV) hypersensitivity to external agents** that come into contact with the skin. It is an important cause of occupational skin disease. The range of potential sensitizing antigens is enormous but, fortunately, a relatively small number of substances account for most cases (Table 11.2). These agents are usually of relatively low molecular weight (<1 kDa) and are not immunogenic in their own right; as small molecules they easily penetrate the epidermis and bind covalently to skin or tissue proteins to act as haptens combined with the host cells as carriers (see Chapter 1).

The **diagnosis** of contact dermatitis depends on a careful medical history, the distribution of the lesions and patch testing. In the patch test, the suspected contact sensitizer is applied to normal skin (usually on the upper back) and covered for 48 h. The reaction is read after 2 and 4 days. In a positive response,

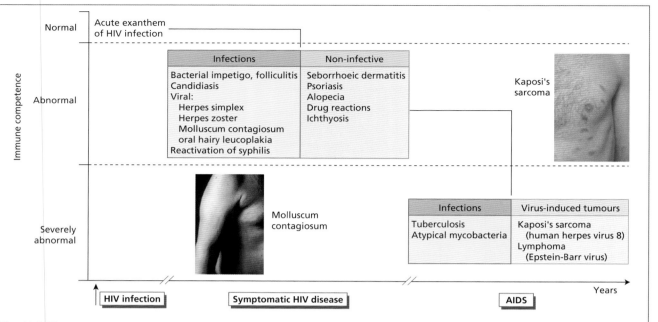

Fig. 11.2 The spectrum of skin disease in human immunodeficiency virus (HIV)-positive individuals. The disorder on the left is molluscum contagiosum and that on the right is early Kaposi's sarcoma.

Table 11.2 Some agents responsible for allergic contact dermatitis

	Agent	Examples of exposure
Metals	Nickel	Coins, clasps, necklaces, watch straps
	Chromate	Cement (building site workers)
	Cobalt	Metal-plated objects, jewellery, metal prostheses, cements, porcelain pigments, hair dyes, some types of vitamin B_{12}
Medications	'Para' group chemicals	Benzocaine-type anaesthetics, sulphonamide antibiotics, para-aminobenzoic acid (PABA)-containing substances (e.g. sunscreens), some diuretics and oral hypoglycaemic agents (sulfonylureas)
	Phenothiazines	Phenothiazine-based antihistamines
	Neomycin	Topical antibiotics
Plastics	Epoxy resins, acrylates; formaldehyde	Construction industry, glues
Rubber	Accelerators, antioxidants (mercapto mix; thiuram mix; carba mix)	Tyre industry, rubber gloves, shoes, clothing, household 'grips', etc.
Plants*	Poison ivy (USA only)	
	Primula	
	Daisy family (*Compositae*)	
	Geranium	
Cosmetics	PPD (4-phenylenediamine)	Hair dye (reactions may be severe and extensive)
	Fragrances (cinnamic alcohol, cinnamic aldehyde, hydroxycitronellal, amylcinnamaldehyde, geraniol, eugenol, isoeugenol, oakmoss absolute); balsam of Peru	Any perfumed products
	Lanolin	Wool fat; used as moisturizer
Plasters	Colphony	Adhesives on plasters
Disinfectants	Glutaraldehyde	Sterilizing instruments, leather tanning, embalming

Further information is available at **https://www.dermnetnz.org/topics/baseline-series-of-patch-test-allergens**
* Some plants are photosensitizers, i.e. the skin reaction requires both plant and sun exposure.

there is **inflammation and induration** at the test site. Although there are pitfalls in interpretation, patch testing is indispensable in the investigation of allergic contact dermatitis (Case 11.2).

Contact dermatitis is a prototype of T cell–mediated hypersensitivity (see Box 11.1). **Two phases of pathogenesis** are recognized: an **induction phase**, from the time of initial antigen contact to sensitization of T lymphocytes, and an elicitation phase, from antigen reexposure to the appearance of dermatitis. In the induction phase, Langerhans cells bind the hapten–carrier protein complex and present it, in association with MHC class II antigens, to T lymphocytes (Fig. 11.3). Induction of cellular immunity to a contact skin sensitizer can occur within 7–10 days of first contact, but it usually happens after many months or years of exposure to small amounts of antigen

(Case 11.2). Individual sensitivity varies according to the nature of the chemical, its concentration and the genetic susceptibility of the person exposed. Recently the contribution of innate immunity to inflammation during the induction phase, following recognition of the sensitizer by Toll-like receptors (TLRs) on dendritic cells, has been reported in mice. This has to be confirmed in humans, as does the role of natural killer (NK) cells that are found in significant numbers in biopsies from patients with contact dermatitis.

Reexposure to the relevant antigen triggers the **elicitation phase** that produces characteristic features of dermatitis. In this phase, effector T lymphocytes, previously carried via the circulation to the skin, meet the hapten–carrier complex. CD8 T cells have been identified as the crucial effector population. Th1 CD4⁺ T cells provide activation signals through the release

---

Case 11.2 Nickel dermatitis

A 47-year-old woman presented with a 3-week history of an acute rash that started beneath her watch. Two weeks later, a further patch appeared at the umbilicus. She had previously noted that she could not wear cheap earrings without triggering a rash on her ear lobes. There was no past medical history of note and no personal or family history of atopy. On examination, two patches of dermatitis were seen over the presenting areas. The appearances were suggestive of nickel-induced contact dermatitis corresponding to nickel in the watch and on a jeans stud. She was patch tested to a battery of commonly implicated agents (Table 11.2): strongly positive results were induced by nickel sulphate and cobalt chloride only. The final diagnosis was nickel dermatitis, which cleared spontaneously following avoidance of nickel-containing articles.

Box 11.1 Evidence supporting the hypothesis that psoriasis is a T cell–mediated disease

- Association between psoriasis and HLA-C6 and -DR7
- Relationship with streptococcal infection, which is known to cause other immunologically mediated hypersensitivity disorders
- Worsening of psoriasis in human immunodeficiency virus infection
- Response of psoriasis to therapeutic interventions directed against T cells (such as ultraviolet radiation, monoclonal antibodies and ciclosporin/tacrolimus, although the latter drugs also have direct effects on keratinocytes)
- Excellent responses to antitumour necrosis factor therapies

---

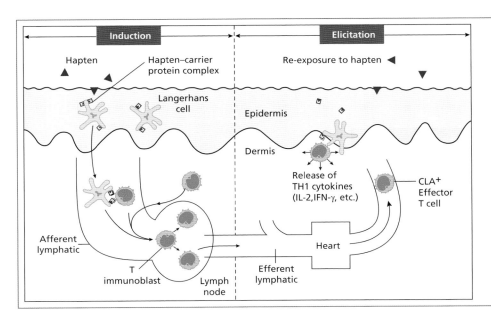

Fig. 11.3 The pathogenesis of allergic contact dermatitis. Langerhans cells bind and present the hapten–carrier protein complex to T lymphocytes (T). Subsequent reexposure to the hapten triggers a T cell–mediated (type IV) hypersensitivity reaction in the skin. CLA, cutaneous lymphocyte-associated antigen; IFN, interferon; IL, interleukin.

of cytokines such as interferon-γ and tumour necrosis factor; CD8⁺ and Th17 cells are activated to induce skin inflammation (Fig. 11.3), recruitment of more T cells and monocytes, keratinocyte proliferation, hyperplasia of the epidermis and consequent thickening.

The **management** of contact dermatitis involves two approaches: prevention and treatment. Identification and elimination of the responsible antigen form the most important goal.

Unfortunately, many common antigens are ubiquitous and antigen avoidance may be difficult to achieve. Preventative measures in industrial dermatitis depend on the use of protective gloves and clothing, improved ventilation or the substitution of non-antigenic chemicals. Some medicines used to treat skin disease are among the commonest culprits of contact dermatitis (see Table 11.2); they include topical antibiotics and antihistamines. As in atopic eczema, topical corticosteroids are useful therapeutic agents, together with antibacterial measures where indicated.

11.3.2 Atopic eczema

Atopic eczema is a common disorder, occurring predominantly in childhood, which appears to be caused by barrier dysfunction with subsequent altered exposure to microbes and allergens that results in a Th2 hypersensitivity reaction in the skin. Although it is usually a mild disorder (as in Case 11.3), patients with severe atopic eczema (especially children) are really disabled and on occasions there can be life-threatening complications. The disorder and its pathogenesis are discussed in more detail in Chapter 4. It is strongly associated with other atopic diseases (allergic rhinoconjunctivitis, asthma). **Dupilumab** is an anti-IL4 receptor-α antagonist that has shown great promise in the treatment of severe atopic eczema.

11.3.3 Psoriasis

Psoriasis is a common skin disease, affecting about 2–4.7% of the world's population. It is less common in sunny climates and in those with pigmented skins. Important risk factors include smoking and a high body mass index. It can present at any age, but most commonly appears between the ages of 15 and 30 years or 50 and 60 years.

Although very varied, the **usual clinical form** consists of chronic, raised, red, scaly, round or oval plaques, with sharply marginated edges, mainly occurring on the knees, elbows and scalp. Chronic plaques may remain static for years, resolve spontaneously or progress to the rest of the skin (Fig. 11.4), so-called erythrodermic psoriasis. The diagnosis (as for much of dermatology) is a clinical one; there are no helpful tests. The quality of life of a psoriatic patient is markedly reduced, not only due to the disfigurement but also to **co-morbidities** including cardiovascular disease, depression and diabetes. In addition, 2–19% of patients develop a seronegative arthropathy (see Chapter 8).

Numerous inflammatory **triggers** for psoriasis have been proposed, including trauma, bacterial infections, cellular stress and various medications. However, these are not consistently observed across patients. Guttate (drop-shaped) psoriasis may begin with several small lesions 1–2 weeks after a Group A streptococcal throat infection, but these usually resolve spontaneously after a few months (Fig. 11.4).

The **pathology** involves markedly increased proliferation and shedding of keratinocytes is disordered, as part of the chronic inflammation. An unknown trigger results in DNA being released from keratinocytes, forming a complex with the secreted keratinocyte cathelicidin antimicrobial protein LL-37. This acts on TLR9 on plasmacytoid dendritic cells to release type I interferons (α and β), which in turn activate myeloid dendritic cells; these cells then release interleukin (IL)-20 to stimulate keratinocyte proliferation. Some myeloid dendritic cells migrate to local lymph nodes, where they release IL-23 and activate naive T cells to differentiate into Th1 and Th17 cells that are recruited back to the skin and cause inflammation via interferon-γ, IL-17 and IL-22. This results in further keratinocyte proliferation and a vicious circle of keratinocytes activating dendritic cells, dendritic cells activating T cells, and T cells activating keratinocytes.

Genetic studies showed a familial trait and genome-wide association studies have confirmed at least 10 psoriasis susceptibility genes that are involved in immunity, including HLA-C6 and -DR7 (Box 11.1). Polymorphisms in the IL-12/IL-13 receptor, the p40 subunit of IL-12 and IL-23, and the p19 subunit of IL-23 are strongly associated with psoriasis, supporting their critical role in the disease process and providing targets for medical therapy.

Case 11.3 Atopic eczema

A 5-year-old boy had developed an itchy rash on his trunk and feet at the age of 18 months. This waxed and waned over the next 3 years and gradually came to involve predominantly his flanks, popliteal and antecubital fossae. He had mild asthma requiring occasional bronchodilators only. His mild atopic eczema was treated with bland emollient creams and occasionally 1% hydrocortisone. His prognosis was good and his skin problems resolved over the next few years.

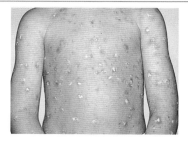

Fig. 11.4 Guttate psoriasis. Source: Miall L, Rudolf M & Smith D (2012) *Paediatrics at a Glance*, 3rd Ed. Reproduced with permission from Wiley.

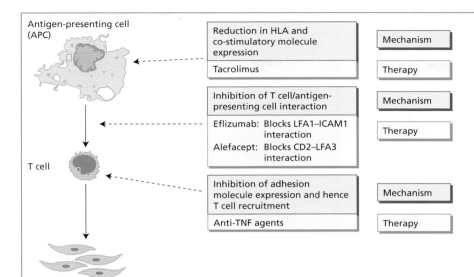

Fig. 11.5 Immunological mechanisms in psoriasis, and how targeted biological therapies may inhibit key steps in pathogenesis. HLA, human leucocyte antigen; TNF, tumour necrosis factor.

Antigen-presenting cell (APC)

Reduction in HLA and co-stimulatory molecule expression — Mechanism

Tacrolimus — Therapy

Inhibition of T cell/antigen-presenting cell interaction — Mechanism

Eflizumab: Blocks LFA1–ICAM1 interaction
Alefacept: Blocks CD2–LFA3 interaction — Therapy

T cell

Inhibition of adhesion molecule expression and hence T cell recruitment — Mechanism

Anti-TNF agents — Therapy

Proliferation of keratinocytes

Therapy of psoriasis is targeted at breaking this cycle. Many older treatments aimed to limit keratinocyte proliferation, often using coal tar–based drugs. Recent understanding of the role of inflammation and T cells has resulted in the use of immunosuppressant and antiinflammatory agents. Immunosuppressant therapy may be delivered topically, for example corticosteroids or T-cell-suppressant drugs such as tacrolimus, or physically in the form of UVR. Severe disease has been transformed by the use of targeted biological therapies (Fig. 11.5), providing confirmation of the role of both T cells and tumour necrosis factor (TNF)-α in psoriasis. This has largely replaced high doses of methotrexate or ciclosporin, the serious side effects (pulmonary fibrosis and renal disease, respectively) of which are considerable. The currently approved biological therapies include the TNF-α inhibitors and ustekinumab. The TNF inhibitors, infliximab, etanercept and adalimumab (Chapter 7), are highly effective, though contraindicated in infection or in patients with demyelinating disease. As with other indications for these drugs, patients are screened for active infection, including tuberculosis and hepatitis B, to avoid reactivation. Up to 80% of patients achieve clearance of psoriasis after three doses of infliximab, but efficacy is lost in the longer term due to neutralizing antibodies to the drug if given continuously; simultaneous treatment with methotrexate reduces the production of these antibodies. **Ustekinumab** is a monoclonal antibody directed against the common p40 subunit of IL-12 and IL-23, which has been shown to be at increased levels in psoriatic lesions. Up to 80% of patients achieve clearance of their disease, but long-term toxicities (serious infections, malignancies and a case of reversible posterior leukoencephalopathy) have been reported, so this should be reserved for patients with severe psoriasis in whom other treatments have failed.

11.4 Autoimmune skin disease

The autoimmune skin diseases offer a striking demonstration of the remarkable specificity of autoimmune responses. Many different antigens within the skin can be targeted, including several adhesion molecules, melanocytes and hair follicles. The disease phenotype varies accordingly, from life-threatening disruption of the integrity of the skin to patchy loss of pigmentation. *In contrast to the cell-mediated diseases described in section 11.3, autoantibodies can be detected in many of these disorders.* However, both B and T cells probably mediate tissue damage in these disorders.

11.4.1 Bullous skin diseases

The bullous skin diseases (which include pemphigus vulgaris, bullous pemphigoid, pemphigoid gestationis and dermatitis herpetiformis) are not common, but they are serious and, so far as pemphigus vulgaris is concerned, may occasionally prove fatal. Immunology has made important contributions to the understanding of these conditions (Box 11.2), which have characteristic appearances on **direct immunohistological examination** (Fig. 11.6) and/or serum antibodies detectable by indirect immunofluorescence of human skin. The autoantigens recognized by these antibodies are summarized in Fig. 11.7.

Pemphigus vulgaris

This is the **most serious** of the bullous skin disorders and was often fatal before systemic corticosteroids became available. The usual age of onset is between 40 and 60 years, but no age group is exempt. It often begins with ulceration of the oral mucosa, followed by widespread flaccid, weepy bullae (Case 11.4).

Box 11.2 Evidence that pemphigus is an autoimmune disease

- Over 90% of patients have circulating antibodies to desmosomal adhesion molecules, particularly desmoglein 3
- The titre of antibody sometimes correlates with disease activity
- Plasmapheresis reduces antibody titres and disease activity
- Some women with active disease have given birth to children with lesions typical of pemphigus vulgaris
- Pemphigus-like lesions can be produced in mouse and monkey skin by intradermal injections of sera from patients with pemphigus
- IgG fractions from pemphigus sera induce epithelial cell detachment in human skin cultures

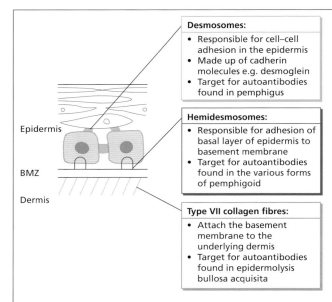

Desmosomes:
- Responsible for cell–cell adhesion in the epidermis
- Made up of cadherin molecules e.g. desmoglein
- Target for autoantibodies found in pemphigus

Hemidesmosomes:
- Responsible for adhesion of basal layer of epidermis to basement membrane
- Target for autoantibodies found in the various forms of pemphigoid

Type VII collagen fibres:
- Attach the basement membrane to the underlying dermis
- Target for autoantibodies found in epidermolysis bullosa acquisita

Fig. 11.7 Autoantigens in bullous skin disease. BMZ, basement membrane zone.

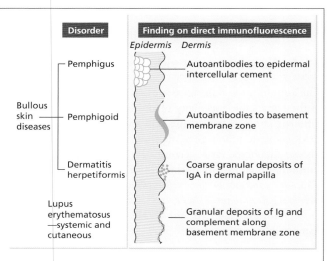

Disorder	Finding on direct immunofluorescence
	Epidermis *Dermis*
Pemphigus	Autoantibodies to epidermal intercellular cement
Pemphigoid	Autoantibodies to basement membrane zone
Dermatitis herpetiformis	Coarse granular deposits of IgA in dermal papilla
Lupus erythematosus —systemic and cutaneous	Granular deposits of Ig and complement along basement membrane zone

Bullous skin diseases

Fig. 11.6 Characteristic findings on direct immunofluorescent examination of skin biopsies.

Blisters occur **within the epidermis**; thus, epidermal cells line both the roof and floor of the blister. Spontaneous remissions are unusual, although the condition does fluctuate in severity over the years.

In virtually all cases, direct immunofluorescence of perilesional skin is diagnostic (Fig. 11.6): antibodies (IgG class) and complement (C3) react with the cell surfaces of keratinocytes in the epidermis, i.e. at the site of the pathological changes. The main antigenic target is the adhesion molecule, desmoglein 3. Primary **autoantibodies to desmoglein 3** synergize with serine proteases to activate cell death in keratinocytes. Keratinocyte shrinkage and detachment and death via apoptosis are called apoptolysis, since this involves the same signals and cell death enzymes as apoptosis. This understanding has enabled combination of immunosuppressive therapies with drugs with direct antiacantholytic effects (such as pilocarpine) to improve therapies substantially. The mainstay of **treatment**

Case 11.4 Pemphigus vulgaris

A 46-year-old woman presented with a generalized, blistering rash of 4 weeks' duration. Her trunk was mainly affected. On examination, there was extensive blistering and large areas of denuded skin. Ulcers were also present in her mouth. The provisional diagnosis was pemphigus vulgaris.

Laboratory investigations showed a normal haemoglobin, full blood count and biochemical profile. Her serum contained antibodies reacting strongly with the cell surfaces of keratinocytes in the epidermis. Direct immunofluorescent examination of a biopsy of normal skin taken from a site adjacent to one bulla showed deposition of IgG around the keratinocytes, giving a 'chicken-wire' appearance (see Fig. 11.6). These findings are characteristic of pemphigus vulgaris. She was treated with methyl prednisolone initially, reducing to prednisolone 40 mg/day when new blister formation ceased. She has been regularly followed for 2 years, during which therapy has been gradually reduced to maintenance levels and no new bullae have appeared.

is systemic corticosteroids. The initial dose should be high enough to suppress new blister formation and severe cases need pulsed methyl prednisolone that has an antiacantholytic effect as well as being immunosuppressive, but has little effect on antibody production. In milder cases oral prednisolone may start at 40–60 mg/day and be reduced gradually. Antibody titres may help to gauge the eventual maintenance dose. Azathioprine, cyclophosphamide and mycophenolate have been used for their 'steroid-sparing' effects, allowing lower maintenance doses of steroids to be given. Plasmapheresis has also proved successful in removing circulating antibodies, especially in steroid-resistant cases. Other options in recalcitrant cases include rituximab and intravenous immunoglobulin (IVIg).

A milder and rarer form of pemphigus, known as **pemphigus foliaceus,** which tends to spare mucous membranes, is associated with autoantibodies to a different desmosomal protein, desmoglein 1.

Paraneoplastic pemphigus is a rare, severe and usually fatal condition seen in association with lymphoma, chronic lymphocytic leukaemia and thymoma. Multiple autoantigens are thought to be involved, including desmoglein 1 and 3, desmoplakin I and II. There is necrosis of keratinocytes. Gastrointestinal and pulmonary involvement occurs and is the usual cause of death, along with infection. Treatment is with steroids and immunosuppressive drugs. Rituximab, alemtuzumab (anti-CD52) and daclizumab (anti-IL2 receptor-α) have shown some promise in small numbers of cases. Mortality is 90%.

Bullous pemphigoid

This condition shows close clinical similarity to pemphigus (hence its name), but the blisters are **subepidermal**, not intraepidermal. It is most common in people over the age of 60 years and is characterized by the presence of large, tense bullae, usually on the thighs, arms and abdomen (Fig. 11.8). Direct immunofluorescent staining of perilesional skin is diagnostic; it shows deposition of IgG and C3 as a continuous ('linear') band along the basement membrane zone (see Fig. 11.6). Almost all patients have **circulating antibodies to basement membrane zone (BMZ)** that bind to 180-kDa hemidesmosomal proteins localized in the lamina lucida, and these are also detectable by indirect immunofluorescence in 75–90% of patients with active disease. There are antibodies to 230-kDa hemidesmosomal proteins as well in 60% of patients. The autoantibodies directed against the 180-kDa antigen have been convincingly demonstrated to cause a similar disease in animal models and levels in patients correlate with disease activity, suggesting these are primary pathogenic antibodies.

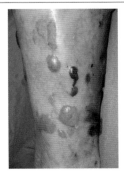

Fig. 11.8 Bullous pemphigoid. Source: Chowdhury M, Katugampola R, Finlay A (2013) *Dermatology at a Glance.* Reproduced with permission from Wiley.

The **treatment** of bullous pemphigoid is similar to that of pemphigus vulgaris, except that lower doses of prednisolone and azathioprine are usually sufficient to suppress blistering, and spontaneous fluctuations may sometimes occur.

Pemphigoid gestationis

Pemphigoid gestationis (herpes gestationis) is a rare, blistering skin disease of pregnancy. It resembles bullous pemphigoid in its macroscopic appearance, but the most common finding on direct immunofluorescence is a 'linear' band of C3 at the BMZ. Sera from women with herpes gestationis contain antibodies to the same 180-kDa hemidesmosomal proteins that act as one of the autoantigens in bullous pemphigoid. These IgG4 antibodies are present at low concentrations and are difficult to detect by conventional indirect immunofluorescence. However, nearly every patient can be shown to have circulating IgG antibodies that 'fix' C3 to normal basement membrane, so that the C3 can then be detected.

Epidermolysis bullosa acquisita

Epidermolysis bullosa acquisita (EBA) is a rare autoimmune blistering disorder with some similarities to the group of inherited blistering disorders known generically as dystrophic epidermolysis bullosa. The bullae in EBA tend to occur in the extremities and to be provoked by trauma. Direct immunofluorescence in EBA shows IgG deposited along the BMZ, but the antigenic target is different from that in the various forms of pemphigoid: the autoantigen appears to be type VII collagen, fibres of which anchor the BMZ to the underlying dermis. Mild cases may respond to dapsone. More severe cases require immunosuppression with corticosteroids, azathioprine, cyclophosphamide or ciclosporin. Rituximab and high-dose IVIg have been used with benefit.

Dermatitis herpetiformis

Dermatitis herpetiformis (DH) is characterized by groups of extremely itchy, small vesicles on extensor surfaces such as the elbows, knees, buttocks, neck and shoulders. Although most patients are aged 20–40 years at diagnosis, any age group can be affected. Like pemphigoid, the bullae are subepidermal, but the immunofluorescent findings are quite different.

Direct immunofluorescence of skin in DH shows deposition of IgA in a granular fashion in the tips of dermal papillae (Fig. 11.7). However, indirect immunofluorescence shows no autoantibodies to skin tissues in patients' blood. Some patients with large bullae show linear deposition of IgA instead, but this is now considered to be a different entity (linear IgA bullous dermatosis) because the lesion, the course of the disease, the genetic background and the treatment differ.

Most patients with DH also have an enteropathy indistinguishable from coeliac disease (see Chapter 14); this is usually mild, asymptomatic and demonstrable only by jejunal biopsy. About 70% of patients with DH will have antibodies to endomysium in their serum. In DH, as in coeliac disease, there is an increased risk of lymphoma and a markedly increased inheritance of the HLA-B8, -DR3, -DQ2 haplotype. Dietary wheat protein (gluten) is the cause of the enteropathy in DH and the intestinal abnormality improves on gluten withdrawal. The skin disease responds to a strict and prolonged gluten-free diet, with disappearance of the granular IgA deposits from the skin, although >2 years is often needed to control the rash. Reintroduction of dietary gluten causes recurrence of the rash within 3 months, proving that DH is gluten dependent. The pathogenesis of DH has been shown to involve the same antibodies to tissue transglutaminase, though the antigen in DH is the enzyme in the epidermis. Other treatments are available: dapsone produces prompt improvement in the skin but has no effect on the enteropathy. The mechanism of action of dapsone in DH is unknown.

11.4.2 Vitiligo

Vitiligo consists of patches of skin depigmentation anywhere on the body. These changes result from loss of melanocytes from the epidermis via a process that is thought to be autoimmune. IgG antibodies to melanocytes and, in particular, to tyrosinase, a key enzyme in melanin synthesis, have been found in about 80% of patients with vitiligo and there are strong clinical associations with organ-specific autoimmune diseases, such as thyroid disease, diabetes mellitus, pernicious anaemia and idiopathic Addison's disease. Immunological treatment is not used.

11.4.3 Alopecia areata

Alopecia is characterized by limited patchy loss of hair (alopecia areata) or loss of all scalp hair (alopecia totalis) or all body hair (alopecia universalis). Alopecia affects children and adults of all ages and races. Association with other organ-specific autoimmune diseases suggest that an autoimmune process may be responsible (Box 11.3). Recent evidence suggests that alopecia areata can be considered a T-cell–mediated autoimmune disease in which the gradual loss of protection provided by immune privilege of the normal hair follicle plays an important role. Recently, genome-wide association studies have identified susceptibility loci common to alopecia areata in some immune genes, namely in the MHC and IL-2R.

11.4.4 Lichen planus

Lichen planus is believed to be a T-cell–mediated inflammatory disease that affects the oral mucosa and skin (causing Whickham's striae). The cause is unknown. It may occur in association with other autoimmune conditions, such as alopecia, vitiligo and ulcerative colitis. It is also associated with infective hepatitis and drugs (gold, pencillamine, thiazides, beta-blockers and anti-TNFs). In the mouth it can predispose to oral cancer. Treatment is usually with topical steroids and tacrolimus/pimecrolimus. Curcumins (derived from turmeric)

> ### Box 11.3 Evidence for immunological involvement in alopecia areata
>
> *Association with autoimmune diseases*
>
> - Autoimmune polyendocrine disease
> - Hashimoto's thyroiditis
> - Myasthenia gravis
>
> *Immunopathological evidence of immune involvement*
>
> - Lymphocytic infiltration around the hair bulb, predominantly CD4+ T lymphocytes
> - Increased expression of major histocompatibility complex (MHC) class I and class II antigens by epithelial cells of the hair bulb
> - Increased infiltration by Langerhans cells adjacent to the hair bulb
>
> *Clinical response to immunosuppression in some patients*

are being investigated as a potential treatment. Patch testing is sometimes carried out to metals and trials of low-nickel and cinnamon diets help a few patients. Cure is rarely achieved.

11.5 Systemic diseases with skin involvement

11.5.1 C̄ī inhibitor deficiency

Hereditary angioedema is caused by deficiency of the inhibitor of the first component of complement (C inhibitor or C̄ī INH; see Chapter 1). It is the commonest known deficiency of a complement component. Patients suffer from recurrent attacks of **skin, laryngeal or intestinal oedema**. *In contrast to urticaria, localized oedema of the face, limbs and trunk is neither painful nor itchy.* Sometimes, however, oedema occurs in the intestinal tract, causing severe abdominal pain and vomiting when the jejunum is involved, or watery diarrhoea if the colon is affected. Laryngeal oedema may be fatal because of airways obstruction. The attacks develop over a few hours and subside spontaneously over 1–2 days (Case 11.5). Although often unheralded, episodes may occur after trauma, surgery, menstruation, stress or intercurrent infection. Attacks of angiooedema are infrequent in early childhood, but exacerbations occur during adolescence and continue throughout adult life.

C1-INH **inhibits activated proteins of several systems**, including plasmin and kallikrein as well as activated C1. Deficiency due to a disease causing mutation in the C1-INH gene results in an autosomal dominant condition in heterozygotes. A critical plasma level of C1-INH, about 30% of normal, is needed to maintain normal inhibitor function. Since C1-INH is consumed by its interactions with these other enzyme systems, the output of one normal gene cannot maintain plasma levels at 50% of normal in the face of normal utilization in the heterozygotes. Plasma C1-INH levels then fall below the critical threshold, allowing C̄ī to act on C4 and C2,

Case 11.5 Hereditary angioedema

Daniel, a 14-year-old boy, presented with a 6-month history of recurrent episodes of swelling of his lips, eyes and tongue (Fig. 11.9). The swellings came on suddenly, grew over a period of 15–20 min, and lasted from 12 to 48 h. They were not itchy but tended to give a prickly sensation. There was no obstruction of airways or abdominal pain during the attacks, which were often associated with intercurrent infection. Urticaria was absent. His sister, aged 21 years, had suffered from an identical problem for 4 years. Physical examination was normal.

The clinical story was typical of angioedema and the family history suggested that this might be hereditary angioedema (HAE). Blood samples taken for complement analysis during remission showed a normal C3 (0.85 g/l), but a rather low C4 of 0.12 g/l (NR 0.2–0.4) and a C1 inhibitor (C1̄-INH) level of 0.06 g/l (NR 0.18–0.26); these findings were consistent with the diagnosis of HAE. When the tests were repeated during a subsequent attack of angioedema, the C3 concentration was unchanged but the C4 level was extremely low at 0.04 g/l. Daniel was started on treatment with danazol. Although his C1̄- INH level only rose to 0.14 g/l, he had no further attacks of HAE. He was also issued with syringes of icatibant for emergency treatment of severe attacks. What is not clear is why neither parent has a history of HAE, since the condition is inherited in an autosomal dominant fashion. A new mutation is therefore likely.

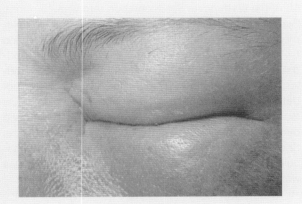

Fig. 11.9 Severe periorbital angioedema.

generating C2 kinin-like peptides (see Chapter 1), which produce angioedema. The diagnosis rests on finding low levels of C1-INH functionally or antigenically. In active disease, uninhibited C1̄ cleaves C4 and C2, causing increased turnover and low levels of these components. A low serum C4 and normal C3 thus provide a useful screening test for this condition. **Three major forms** of the disease exist: in the commoner form (85%) a low level of C1-INH is found, and in a rarer type

(10%) a functionally defective protein is synthesized with apparently 'normal' serum levels of a non-functioning inhibitor. In a patient with angioedema, a low C4 level with a normal immunochemical C1-INH concentration indicates the need for a functional assay. A normal C4 level *during an attack of angioedema* excludes the diagnosis of hereditary angioedema. The third type of HAE (predominantly in women) has similar clinical manifestations, but there are no abnormalities in C1-INH level or function and a gain-of-function mutation in coagulation factor XII protease (Hageman factor) has been documented.

Therapy for HAE consists of treatment of acute attacks, as well as short-term and long-term prophylaxis. All patients should carry a medical card stating the diagnosis and a contact doctor. **An acute attack** should be treated by infusion of pure C1-INH (manufactured either from plasma or a recombinant product) to increase serum levels of the inhibitor (Fig. 11.10). New treatment options for acute attacks work as kinin pathway modulators: one inhibits plasma kallikrein and the other is a **competitive antagonist of bradykinin B2 receptor (icatibant).** Symptoms do not respond to antihistamines or steroids.

Prophylaxis with modified androgens, danazol or oxandrolone, has been effective in stimulating synthesis of functional C1-INH in the liver. The long-term use of this drug may be limited by troublesome side effects, including acne, cholestatic jaundice, virilization of females and suppression of endogenous testosterone production in males. The protease inhibitor tranexamic acid is a fairly effective prophylactic agent; it probably functions by restricting activation of the various other enzymes with which C1-INH reacts, so minimizing its consumption. **Lanadelumab,** a monoclonal plasma kallikrein inhibitor, has recently been licenced for prophylaxis in the USA and the UK.

Deficiency of C1̄ inhibitor can also occur **secondary to underlying disorders**: the most frequent association is lymphoproliferative disease (splenic villous lymphoma), although cases have also been described in association with autoimmune haemolytic anaemia and chronic infection. An autoantibody to C1-INH has been described that blocks its function. In some

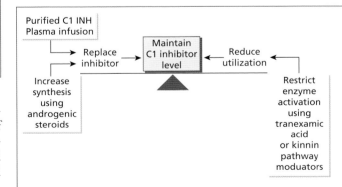

Fig. 11.10 Principles underlying the treatment of C1 inhibitor (INH) deficiency.

cases, circulating paraproteins may activate C1, with consumption of the inhibitor, resulting in very low levels of C1, C2 and C4. As in the hereditary form, danazol has proved successful in some cases. Treatment of the underlying disease, where feasible, may also stop the attacks.

11.5.2 Vasculitis

Vasculitis is a diagnosis that rests on histological evidence of **inflammation of blood vessels**. The diversity of clinical lesions seen in vasculitis is extensive, and the vasculitides are best considered as a diverse group of conditions with different pathogenic mechanisms (Box 11.4).

Many agents can **induce vasculitis** (Table 11.3), although the incriminating evidence is often circumstantial. Removal of the drug or treatment of the infection may clear the vasculitis, but this is not proof of causation. In most cases, no cause is found. A search must be made for systemic involvement in patients who present with cutaneous vasculitis. However, the disorder is confined to the skin in many cases (Case 11.6).

Box 11.4 Factors affecting clinical lesions of vasculitis

- The severity and type of vessel wall damage
- The size of the vessels affected
- The organ(s) supplied by these damaged vessels

Table 11.3 Some causes of vasculitis

1 Drugs	
2 Infections	
• Bacterial	Streptococci
	Mycobacterium tuberculosis
	Gonococci
	Bacterial endocarditis
• Viral	Hepatitis B
	Infectious mononucleosis
3 Injection of foreign protein	'Serum sickness'
4 Autoimmune diseases	Systemic lupus erythematosus
	Rheumatoid arthritis
	Chronic active hepatitis
	Ulcerative colitis
	Granulomatosis with polyangiitis
	Kawasaki's syndrome
5 Cryoglobulinaemia	Lymphoproliferative disease
	Hepatitis C

Immunopathogenesis is variable. Some forms of vasculitis are caused by **deposition of circulating antigen–antibody complexes** in blood vessel walls. A vasculitic skin rash is a common feature of acute ('one-shot') experimental serum sickness. Acute serum sickness is a self-limiting process: resolution occurs spontaneously as the injected antigen is cleared. However, when an endogenous source of antigen (i.e. an autoantigen) is available, or the antigen is replicating (e.g. a microorganism), circulating antigen is produced on an intermittent or continuous basis; the result may be chronic immune complex–induced injury (see Chapter 9). The best examples of this are nuclear antigens in SLE and hepatitis B antigen in some cases of polyarteritis nodosa or hepatitis C antigens in mixed cryoglobulinaemia. In most other cases of vasculitis, positive direct immunofluorescence on fresh lesions is the only evidence of an immune complex–mediated pathogenesis (Box 11.5).

Case 11.6 Urticarial vasculitis

A 41-year-old woman presented with itchy lumps on her legs of 5 weeks' duration. The lumps lasted 4–5 days. She had a history of asthma from childhood and was being treated with an array of drugs. As far as she knew, she had never 'reacted' to any of these drugs. On examination, her legs showed palpable, purpuric lesions and areas of urticaria. General examination was otherwise normal. The skin lesions were those of urticarial vasculitis.

Investigations showed a low haemoglobin (107 g/l) with a hypochromic blood film. Her white cell count was 12.2×10^9/l, with a raised eosinophil count of 1.56×10^9/l; the erythrocyte sedimentation rate was 45 mm/h. Serum immunoglobulins were normal but her complement levels were low: C3 was 0.55 g/l (NR 0.8–1.4) and C4 was 0.15 g/l (NR 0.2–0.4). Antinuclear and anti-dsDNA antibodies, antineutrophil cytoplasmic antibodies, cryoglobulins and rheumatoid factor were not detected. Biopsy of an acute lesion showed histological features of vasculitis, with deposition of C3 in the deep dermal blood vessels on direct immunofluorescence. She was treated empirically with prednisolone. Her vasculitis improved considerably but no underlying cause was ever found.

Box 11.5 Proof of involvement of a specific antigen in the pathogenesis of vasculitis

- The causative antigen is part of the circulating immune complex
- Antigen, as well as antibody, is fixed in blood vessels within vasculitic lesions
- Injection of preformed antigen–antibody complexes induces tissue damage

Some forms of systemic vasculitis are strongly associated with circulating **antineutrophil cytoplasmic antibodies** (ANCA). These disorders show no evidence of immune-complex deposition or complement consumption. The sensitivity of ANCA in the diagnosis of classical granulomatosis with polyangiitis (previously known as Wegener's granulomatosis) is high (75–100%), but lower in patients with limited disease (60–70%) and only 35% in patients in remission. The pathogenesis of granulomatosis with polyangiitis is largely unknown, although the clinical pattern suggests that an inhaled antigen, possibly bacterial, may be responsible. In other conditions, such as erythema nodosum, direct assault by T lymphocytes on vascular antigens may induce vessel damage (type IV hypersensitivity), since activated T lymphocytes and macrophages are the predominant infiltrating perivascular cells.

There is no entirely satisfactory classification of vasculitis. For many years, histopathologists have based their schemes on the **size** and **site** of the vessels involved or the presence or absence of **granulomas** (Table 11.4); on the other hand, clinicians have recognized clinical syndromes, such as Henoch–Schönlein syndrome or polyarteritis nodosa. The more important conditions are discussed in other chapters according to the site at which they make a major clinical impact, for example Henoch–Schönlein syndrome in renal diseases (see Chapter 9), polyarteritis nodosa and SLE in rheumatic diseases (see Chapter 10) and granulomatosis with polyangiitis in chest diseases (see Chapter 13).

Urticarial vasculitis is a cutaneous small vessel vasculitis, presenting with persistent urticarial lesions (>24 hours and fading to leave a brown stain of haemosiderin). It may occur alone or in association with SLE. Mild forms are associated with normal complement levels, but more severe forms have marked reduction in C1q, C2 and C4. Autoantibodies to C1q may be detected. Renal involvement may occur. Treatment is with

dapsone, immunosuppressive therapy and in severe cases rituximab.

11.5.3 Cryoglobulinaemia

Cryoglobulins are immunoglobulins that form precipitates, gels or even crystals in the cold. Pathological cryoglobulinaemia occurs as a primary disorder or secondary to another disease. The clinical features are caused by the vasculitis following destruction of small blood vessels, but the severity of symptoms depends on the concentrations of the relevant proteins and the temperature at which cryoprecipitation occurs. Since some cryoglobulins can precipitate at temperatures above 22 °C, blood should be collected in prewarmed (37 °C) syringes and taken directly to the laboratory in a warmed container (thermos flask filled with sand or water at 37 °C).

Immunochemical analysis of cryoprecipitates allows their classification into three types.

Type I cryoglobulins (5–25%) are monoclonal proteins, usually IgM, which have no recognizable antibody activity. They have an inherent tendency to cryoprecipitate as the paraprotein concentration increases. In most cases, there is an underlying malignant disease, usually Waldenström's macroglobulinaemia, lymphoma or myeloma. Symptoms are due to hyperviscosity and sludging of cryoprecipitates in cold extremities.

Type II cryoglobulins (25–50%) are of a mixed type in which the monoclonal protein (usually IgM) has antibody specificity directed against the Fc portion of IgG; that is, rheumatoid factor activity. Cryoprecipitation occurs when complexes of IgM–anti-IgG antibody are formed. This type is strongly associated with chronic hepatitis C infection but may occasionally be found in B-cell malignancy or SLE. As in Case 11.7, patients typically present with features of 'immune-complex disease', such as diffuse vasculitis, arthritis and glomerulonephritis.

Type III cryoglobulins (25–50%) are of mixed polyclonal type in which polyclonal or oligoclonal IgM rheumatoid-like factors react with IgG. About one-third of cases are associated with hepatitis C. The remainder are associated with rheumatoid arthritis, SLE, polyarteritis nodosa or chronic infection (e.g. hepatitis B). Small amounts of type III cryoglobulins are found in many inflammatory conditions and are usually of no particular significance.

The treatment of cryoglobulinaemia is generally directed towards management of any recognized underlying disorder. Common-sense measures such as avoidance of cold environments and wearing warm clothing are helpful, but plasmapheresis and immunosuppression may be required.

11.5.4 Lupus erythematosus

The clinical features of lupus erythematosus (LE) range from a severe disease involving many organs, including the kidney, joints, brain and skin (SLE; see Chapter 10), to a benign, chronic, purely cutaneous form, called **discoid lupus**

Table 11.4 Classification of vasculitis

Vessel size	Granuloma present	Granuloma absent
Large	Giant cell arteritis	–
	Takayasu arteritis	
Medium	Eosinophilic granulomatosis with polyangiitis (formerly Churg–Strauss syndrome)	Polyarteritis nodosa
Small	Granulomatosis with polyangiitis (formerly Wegener's granulomatosis)	Microscopic polyarteritis
		Henoch–Schönlein syndrome
		Hypersensitivity (cutaneous) vasculitis
		Urticarial vasculitis

Case 11.7 Mixed cryoglobulinaemia

A 45-year-old woman presented with ankle oedema due to nephrotic syndrome. In the preceding 5 years, she had experienced several episodes of a purpuric, erythematous, papular rash on the legs, accompanied by a bilateral arthropathy of the knees and ankles. A biopsy of the rash had shown features of vasculitis that had responded to systemic steroids. She now had a non-selective proteinuria of 10 g/day and a creatinine clearance of 74 ml/min. Serum alanine aminotransferase (ALT) was increased at 140 U/ml (NR <50). Rheumatoid factor was detectable to a titre of 1/1280 but antinuclear antibodies were negative. Hepatitis B surface antigen was absent but antibodies to hepatitis C and hepatitis C viral RNA were detected in her serum. The serum immunoglobulins, measured at room temperature, were IgG 2.10 g/l (NR 7.2–19.0); IgA 0.85 g/l (NR 0.8–5.0); and IgM 2.80 g/l (NR 0.5–2.0). Complement levels were abnormal, with a C3 of 0.80 g/l (NR 0.8–1.4) and a C4 of 0.02 g/l (NR 0.2–0.4). The very low C4 level raised the suspicion of cryoglobulinaemia. A warm sample of her serum contained a mixed cryoglobulin, composed of a monoclonal IgM and polyclonal IgG. A skin biopsy showed scattered deposits of IgM, IgG and C3 in dermal blood vessels. The histology of a renal biopsy showed membranoproliferative glomerulonephritis: on direct immunofluorescence, granular deposits of IgM and IgG were seen along the epithelial basement membrane. The final diagnosis was mixed cryoglobulinaemia secondary to chronic hepatitis C infection with cutaneous vasculitis, arthropathy and membranoproliferative glomerulonephritis. No risk factors for hepatitis C infection were identified; she was treated with a good response.

erythematosus (DLE). Between these ends of the spectrum, all variations can occur. While it may be artificial to distinguish SLE from DLE, there are important clinical, immunological and prognostic differences between these forms of LE (Table 11.5).

The skin lesions of DLE are usually distinctive but, in cases of difficulty, immunological investigations are often helpful. Direct immunohistological examination of biopsies from areas of sun-exposed, normal skin (the lupus band test; Fig. 11.5) is usually negative (Table 11.5). The prevalence of transformation from DLE to a systemic disease is around 10% or less.

A third form of clinically distinct cutaneous lupus is **subacute cutaneous lupus erythematosus** (SCLE; Case 11.8). Although SCLE and DLE have features in common, there are definite differences (Table 11.5). SCLE is non-scarring, less persistent, more widespread and more frequently complicated by alopecia than is DLE. Patients with SCLE often have a mild systemic illness characterized by joint pains and fever, but severe central nervous system and kidney disease are uncommon. Patients with this form of cutaneous LE have antibodies to the cytoplasmic antigen Ro (or SS-A) (see Chapter 19).

11.5.5 Systemic sclerosis

Systemic sclerosis is a chronic fibrosing disease of unknown aetiology. It can affect the skin, blood vessels, musculoskeletal system and many internal organs (Case 11.9). Since indurated and thickened skin is the most striking feature of the disease, the term scleroderma is often used as a synonym for systemic sclerosis. Sclerodermatous changes may be localized or generalized, and generalized scleroderma can be further classified (Fig. 11.13) into **limited systemic sclerosis**, in which cutaneous and internal involvement is relatively limited (although Raynaud's phenomenon is often severe), and **diffuse systemic sclerosis**, in which skin and visceral involvement is usually

Table 11.5 Characteristic features of the different forms of cutaneous lupus erythematosus (LE)

	Discoid LE	Subacute cutaneous LE	Systemic LE
Usual age of onset, years	30–40	<40	<40
Skin features	Oedematous plaques with scaling	Widespread	Almost anything
	and follicular plugs	Symmetrical	
	Scarring	Non-scarring erythematous plaques	
	Face, ears, scalp	Upper chest, back, shoulders	
Systemic features	None	Joint pains, fever, malaise	Almost any organ affected
Antinuclear antibodies present in	25%	80%	95%
dsDNA antibodies present in	0%	30%	70–85%
Anti-Ro antibodies present in	<5%	70%	30%
Predominant HLA type	B7	B8, DR3	B8, DR3
Positive direct immunofluorescence of			
Lesional skin	90%	40%	90%
Normal, sun-exposed skin	0%	20%	75%

Case 11.8 Subacute cutaneous lupus erythematosus

A 34-year-old woman presented with a 2-year history of a waxing and waning rash on her neck and arms. She had noticed that the rash was likely to flare following exposure to bright sunlight. Her general health was good, although in the last few months she had developed flitting pain and stiffness in the small joints of her hands. She had no history of Raynaud's phenomenon, mouth ulcers or eye trouble. On examination, there was an extensive skin rash involving the neck and arms and extending onto the face. The rash was red, raised above the surrounding skin and tended to form ring-like patterns with scaly margins (Fig. 11.11). There was no evidence of vasculitis and there were no other abnormal physical signs. The skin appearances were those of subacute cutaneous lupus erythematosus (SCLE); there was no clinical evidence of systemic involvement.

Laboratory investigations showed a normal haemoglobin, white cell count, blood creatinine and urinalysis. Antinuclear antibodies were detected at a titre of 1/100 and antibodies to Ro were detected by precipitation. Serum C3 and C4 levels were normal. A biopsy of affected skin on the neck showed typical changes of SCLE. Direct immunofluorescence demonstrated granular deposits of C3 and IgG along the basement membrane zone in the affected skin. She was treated with sunscreens, topical steroids and hydroxychloroquine. Over a period of several months, the skin lesions became less frequent but still flared after sun exposure.

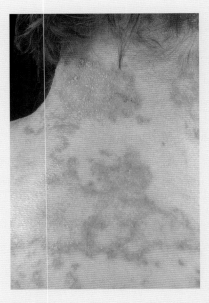

Fig. 11.11 Typical changes of subacute cutaneous lupus erythematosus on the neck.

extensive and sometimes life threatening. Limited systemic sclerosis was formerly known as the CREST syndrome (this acronym is explained in Fig. 11.14).

Systemic sclerosis usually presents between the ages of 45 and 65 years; women are affected four times more frequently than men. It is a rare disorder with a prevalence of around 1 in 10 000. The prognosis depends upon disease severity, but the overall 10-year survival rate in diffuse disease is about 40%. **Renal failure** and malignant hypertension were historically the major causes of death, but the incidence of this complication has declined with improved treatments for hypertension, particularly angiotensin-converting enzyme (ACE) inhibitors. **Pulmonary fibrosis** has now become the most feared complication in diffuse disease. Limited systemic sclerosis is a more benign disorder with a 10-year survival of 60–70%, although severe Raynaud's phenomenon is a major cause of morbidity in this group. There is also a risk of **pulmonary hypertension** developing many years into the disease, with significant associated mortality.

Diagnosis of systemic sclerosis is largely clinical, supported by biopsy of skin and other organs and assessment of the microcirculation in the hands by nailfold microscopy and thermography. Several patterns of autoantibody production are seen in systemic sclerosis, some of which are useful diagnostic or prognostic markers (Table 11.6). **Autoantibodies** to Scl-70 (an enzyme, topoisomerase 1, important in controlling coiling of DNA superhelices) are found almost exclusively in patients with systemic sclerosis, where, particularly in association with HLA-DR52a, they are associated with subsequent development of pulmonary fibrosis. Anticentromere antibodies are strongly associated with limited systemic sclerosis (sometimes also known as the CREST syndrome). Other patterns of autoantibody production are less clearly associated with different patterns of disease, although some subtypes of nucleolar autoantibodies, such as those directed against RNA polymerase types I–III, may be associated with severe disease. The presence of any of these patterns of autoantibody production is predictive of the development of scleroderma in subjects presenting with Raynaud's phenomenon and therefore useful only for prognosis if progression is suspected.

The pathology of the skin and affected organs is characterized by marked deposition of extracellular matrix, often centred around blood vessels, together with abnormalities of the vessels themselves; vessels are often obliterated by intimal proliferation. *Inflammatory changes are not severe and C-reactive protein is not raised.*

The **pathogenesis** of systemic sclerosis is poorly understood, but vascular, immunological and fibrotic abnormalities have been identified (see Fig. 11.14). There is no proof that scleroderma is primarily an immunological disease, and no evidence that any of the autoantibodies plays any direct role in the pathogenesis; i.e. they are only secondary markers.

Circumstantial evidence that T cells play a role in scleroderma comes from the observation that a scleroderma-like disorder may occur in chronic graft-versus-host disease, which is thought to be largely T cell mediated. In scleroderma itself, activated CD4$^+$ T

Case 11.9 Systemic sclerosis

The patient first developed Raynaud's phenomenon in her early 20s. In cold weather, her hands and toes became white and painful and then turned blue; when the circulation returned, it was accompanied by extreme redness and pain (see Fig. 11.12). Several years after developing Raynaud's phenomenon, she noticed some tethering and thickening of her skin, starting in the hands but eventually affecting her face and mouth. On one occasion, an ulcer on her right index finger discharged 'tiny pieces of chalk'. At the age of 54, she developed dysphagia: she could swallow food only if she took fluids with it. At the age of 56, diarrhoea became a problem. Barium studies showed pseudodiverticulae typical of systemic sclerosis, a hiatus hernia, an atonic oesophagus and stomach, and a dilated, distorted proximal jejunum.

When reassessed at the age of 59, her heart, chest and abdomen were normal. She showed marked sclerodactyly and typical skin changes of scleroderma. Soft-tissue, calcified nodules were present on her fingers, forearms and over the patellae. Telangiectasia was evident on the hands, face and lips. Over the following 2 years she became increasingly short of breath, with marked ankle oedema and worsening of the diarrhoea. Lung function tests showed a restrictive defect with a reduction in transfer factor. A computed tomography scan of the thorax showed no evidence of pulmonary fibrosis, but an electrocardiogram and echocardiogram suggested right-ventricular strain secondary to pulmonary hypertension associated with limited systemic sclerosis. There was no biochemical evidence of renal or liver disease.

She has taken part in controlled trials of new treatments for systemic sclerosis; none has worked. She has now been referred to a specialist pulmonary hypertension unit for assessment as to whether she might benefit from treatment with bosentan, an endothelin 1 antagonist to prevent progression to pulmonary fibrosis.

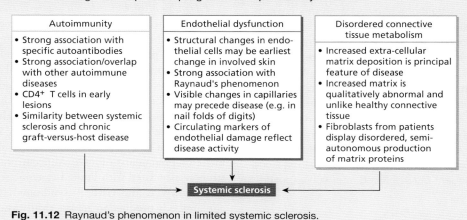

Autoimmunity	Endothelial dysfunction	Disordered connective tissue metabolism
• Strong association with specific autoantibodies • Strong association/overlap with other autoimmune diseases • CD4+ T cells in early lesions • Similarity between systemic sclerosis and chronic graft-versus-host disease	• Structural changes in endothelial cells may be earliest change in involved skin • Strong association with Raynaud's phenomenon • Visible changes in capillaries may precede disease (e.g. in nail folds of digits) • Circulating markers of endothelial damage reflect disease activity	• Increased extra-cellular matrix deposition is principal feature of disease • Increased matrix is qualitatively abnormal and unlike healthy connective tissue • Fibroblasts from patients display disordered, semi-autonomous production of matrix proteins

Systemic sclerosis

Fig. 11.12 Raynaud's phenomenon in limited systemic sclerosis.

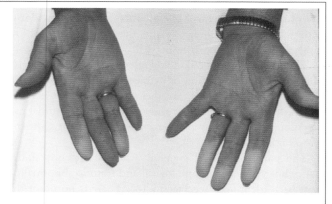

Fig. 11.13 Classification of scleroderma.

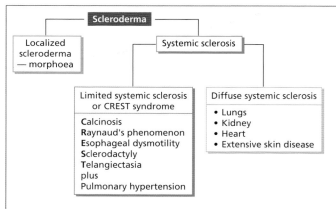

Scleroderma

Localized scleroderma — morphoea

Systemic sclerosis

Limited systemic sclerosis or CREST syndrome	Diffuse systemic sclerosis
Calcinosis Raynaud's phenomenon Esophageal dysmotility Sclerodactyly Telangiectasia plus Pulmonary hypertension	• Lungs • Kidney • Heart • Extensive skin disease

Fig. 11.14 Features of systemic sclerosis.

cells are found in early lesions and *in vitro* experiments, suggesting that these T cells may activate dermal fibroblasts (either directly or indirectly via endothelial cells or macrophages) to increase production of collagen and other matrix proteins.

Regardless of the stimulus, scleroderma fibroblasts develop marked abnormal function with a sustained increase in production of connective tissue proteins. There is some evidence that

Table 11.6 Autoantibodies in systemic sclerosis

	Frequency in patients with systemic sclerosis
Any antinuclear antibodies	80%
• Anticentromere antibody	
Limited disease	90%
Diffuse disease	5%
• Antinucleolar antibody	40%
• Anti-Scl-70 antibody	25%
• Antiribonucleoprotein (RNP) antibody	10%
• Anti-Ro antibody	<5%
• Anti-dsDNA antibody	0
Rheumatoid factor	25–33%

transforming growth factor (TGF)-β is a key mediator of fibrosis, as it is expressed at high levels in tissue from systemic sclerosis; fibroblasts from patients with the disease express abnormally high levels of TGF-β receptors. Signalling through these receptors induces synthesis of collagen and induces further production of TGF-β. This semi-autonomy of scleroderma fibroblasts may explain two puzzling features of the disease: first, the very poor response to immunosuppression, and second, the minimal evidence of inflammation in involved tissues.

The **aetiology** of systemic sclerosis is also poorly understood. Genome-wide association studies have confirmed that various HLA alleles are linked to particular complications, the strongest association being between HLA-DR52a and lung fibrosis in scleroderma (the risk of lung disease is 17 times greater in patients with this allele). Furthermore, there are associations between particular systemic sclerosis-specific autoantibodies: HLA-DQB1 and NOTCH4 with anticentromere and HLA-DPA1/B1 with antitopoisomerase I. Other immune genes identified were CD247, IRF5 and STAT4. Scleroderma tends to occur in geographical clusters, suggesting unknown environmental risk factors. A small proportion of cases have been associated with exposure to environmental toxins, particularly vinyl chloride. The similarities between systemic sclerosis and chronic graft-versus-host disease led to the development of the microchimerism hypothesis. Microchimerism develops when small numbers of fetal or maternal cells cross the placenta during pregnancy and then persist in the mother or child, respectively. Fetal cells can be detected in the blood and tissues of some normal healthy women up to decades after the birth of these children. It has been suggested that delayed onset of an immune response against these chronically engrafted cells might lead to systemic sclerosis. Some evidence exists that the burden of microchimeric cells may be higher in systemic sclerosis, but the significance of this elegant hypothesis is as yet unclear.

Treatment is largely limited to management of complications (ACE inhibitors for hypertension, vasodilators for Raynaud's, the **endothelin-1 antagonist bosentan** for pulmonary hypertension). *Immunosuppression plays no current role in management of the skin changes*, although may be of very limited use in pulmonary fibrosis. A great variety of antifibrotic drugs and immunomodulatory drugs have been used with almost uniformly negative results.

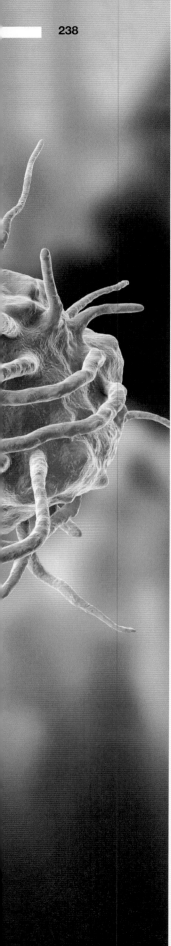

CHAPTER 12
Eye Diseases

Key topics

 Visit the companion website at **www.wiley.com/go/misbah/immunology** to download cases on these topics.

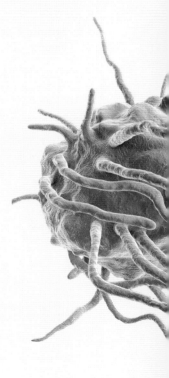

Chapel and Haeney's Essentials of Clinical Immunology, Seventh Edition. Edited by Siraj A. Misbah, Gavin P. Spickett, and Virgil A.S.H. Dalm.
© 2022 John Wiley & Sons Ltd. Published 2022 by John Wiley & Sons Ltd.

12.1 Introduction

The eye is a fragile and complex organ, whose physiological function is intolerant of any distortion in structure. Immunological defence mechanisms within the eye need to strike a delicate balance between exclusion or rapid elimination of invading pathogens and the need to minimize excessive inflammation within the eye, which might disrupt transmission of light, impair retinal processing or cause damage to ocular tissue. For this reason, the eye relies heavily upon mechanical or physical barriers to infection.

Immunologically, the eye can be divided into two major compartments: the conjunctival sac and the globe (Fig. 12.1).

12.1.1 Conjunctival sac

The conjunctival sac has similar defence mechanisms to the skin and upper respiratory tract mucosa and is affected by similar diseases (Table 12.1). The conjunctival sac is the main site for entry of antigen into the eye. The major physical barriers to antigen entry are blinking and the free flow and drainage of tears. These physical factors are supplemented by antimicrobial factors within tears such as IgA and lysozyme. The conjunctiva can respond briskly to local irritation or injury, being highly vascular and containing mast cells. As in other sites, persistence of inflammation within the eye leads to the accumulation of chronic inflammatory cells, i.e. activated T and B cells and macrophages.

12.1.2 The globe

The anatomy of the globe is summarized in Fig. 12.1. Two principal types of tissue are present: avascular tissues (cornea, lens, vitreous and sclera) and highly vascular tissues (the uveal tract, the posterior part of which is closely associated with the retina). Historically, the globe was regarded as invisible from the immune system (immunologically privileged, Chapter 5) because of a lack of lymphatic drainage, the presence of an endothelial blood–eye barrier, and the avascular nature of much of the globe's contents. This physical separation of the eye and the immune system is important in preventing autoimmune disease within the eye, but it is now known that *active suppression of immune responses is also of major importance in limiting inflammation within the globe*.

Antigens can potentially enter the globe via the sclera, cornea, optic nerve or uveal tract. The tough physical barrier of the avascular tissues can normally exclude most antigens, provided conjunctival function is normal. The uveal tract, however, is highly vascular and has the capacity for trapping blood-borne antigens or microorganisms, a property that is shared with other highly vascular structures such as the glomerulus. As in the kidney, this is limited by the presence of tight junctions between uveal endothelial cells, which usually limit extravasation of cells or plasma. This **blood–eye barrier** may, however, break down in response to injury of many kinds.

If antigen does gain access to the globe, immune responses to that antigen are likely to be reduced or inhibited. Multiple mechanisms underlie this **downregulation**: immunosuppressive cytokines such as transforming growth factor (TGF)-β are present within the eye, but cells throughout the cornea express high levels of a protein called Fas ligand (FasL), which will bind to any cells expressing its receptor, Fas, and trigger apoptosis in the Fas-bearing cells. Since Fas is richly expressed upon most cells that migrate into sites of inflammation, such as activated T cells, macrophages and neutrophils, this mechanism limits inflammation within the eye. FasL/Fas interactions also help to maintain tolerance within the eye, since autoreactive T cells entering the eye are deleted. Disruption of this process may contribute to autoimmune and hypersensitivity disease within the eye.

Immunological diseases of the eye fall into two groups: the eye may either be the sole target of local immunological mechanisms or it may be one of many tissues involved in a systemic process (Table 12.2).

The symptoms and signs of inflammation involving different parts of the eye are summarized in Fig. 12.2 and these diseases are discussed later in the chapter.

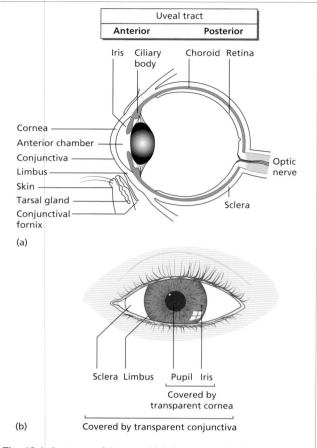

Fig. 12.1 Anatomy of the eye. (a) In lateral section (only the lower eyelid is shown). (b) Frontal view (left side).

12.2 Conjunctivitis

Conjunctival inflammation is very common. The major causes are infection and hypersensitivity reactions (see Table 12.1).

12.2.1 Conjunctival infection

Case 12.1 emphasizes the importance of mechanical barriers in protecting the eye from infection. Failure of blinking and loss of the tear film will inevitably lead to severe infection *even in the absence of any immunological defect*. **Bacterial infection** can also follow trauma to the eye and can be the sequel to other forms of ocular inflammation, such as viral infection. Local immune responses do have some role to play: patients with antibody deficiency can develop bacterial conjunctivitis, usually caused by Haemophilus influenzae (also commonly responsible for respiratory tract infections in these patients).

Infection is the most important cause of conjunctivitis worldwide. The commonest organism involved is Chlamydia trachomatis, an intracellular bacteria-like agent that causes trachoma; over 400 million people suffer from this condition. They show a profound local immune response to the organism. Specific antichlamydial antibodies are found in tears and serum, but the concentration is not related to the outcome. Treatment requires systemic and topical antibiotics and the prognosis, if treated in the early stages, is excellent. Where treatment is unavailable, trachoma commonly causes blindness, especially if accompanied by superadded bacterial infection.

Table 12.1 Conjunctivitis and types of hypersensitivity

Disease	Mechanism of hypersensitivity	Aetiology
Seasonal conjunctivitis	IgE-mediated (type I)*	Grass pollens + other antigens
Vernal conjunctivitis	IgE-mediated plus Th2 cells	Airborne allergens
Atopic keratoconjunctivitis	Atopic (probably Th2 cells)	Ocular equivalent of atopic dermatitis
Cicatrizing conjunctivitis (pemphigoid)	Antibody on conjunctival basement membrane (type II)	Autoimmune
Stevens–Johnson syndrome	Immune complex (type III)	Drug reaction or unknown
Sarcoidosis	Granuloma (type IV)	Unknown
Contact dermatoconjunctivitis	Cellular immune reactions (type IV)	Drugs, cosmetics, contact lens solutions

*Types I–IV refer to the Gell and Coombs' classification; see Chapter 1.

Table 12.2 Systemic immunological diseases and the eye

Conjunctiva	Post-infectious syndrome or arthritis urethritica (previously known as Reiter's syndrome)
	Sarcoidosis
	Pemphigus/pemphigoid
	Sjögren's syndrome
Cornea	Sjögren's syndrome
	Systemic vasculitis
Uveal tract and retina	Sarcoidosis
	Spondyloarthropathies
	Ankylosing spondylitis
	Post-infectious syndrome or arthritis urethritica (previously known as Reiter's syndrome)
	Psoriatic arthritis
	Enteropathic arthritis
	Systemic lupus
	Juvenile idiopathic arthritis
	Behçet's disease
Sclera	Systemic vasculitis
	Rheumatoid arthritis (scleromalacia perforans)
	Granulomatosis with polyangiitis (previously known as Wegener's syndrome)

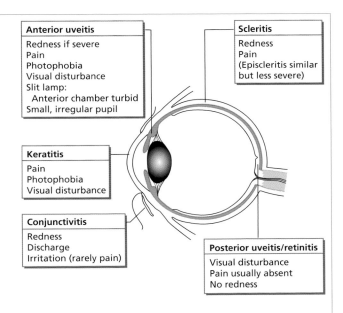

Anterior uveitis
Redness if severe
Pain
Photophobia
Visual disturbance
Slit lamp:
  Anterior chamber turbid
Small, irregular pupil

Scleritis
Redness
Pain
(Episcleritis similar
but less severe)

Keratitis
Pain
Photophobia
Visual disturbance

Conjunctivitis
Redness
Discharge
Irritation (rarely pain)

Posterior uveitis/retinitis
Visual disturbance
Pain usually absent
No redness

Fig. 12.2 Symptoms and signs of eye disease.

The commonest viral cause of conjunctivitis in adults is **adenovirus**. Another virus causing conjunctivitis is **herpes simplex**. Primary infection occurs in childhood and is usually asymptomatic; if inflammation does occur, it is usually confined to the skin, conjunctiva and superficial cornea, where the actively replicating virus causes typical herpetic ulcers. Recurrent herpes infection may result in a type IV hypersensitivity keratitis (section 12.3).

12.2.2 Allergic conjunctivitis

The various forms of allergic conjunctival disease are summarized in Table 12.1. Seasonal and perennial conjunctivitis are extremely common disorders. Allergic conjunctivitis is discussed in more detail in Chapter 4 (section 4.5, as well as Cases 4.4 and Case 4.5) and in Case 12.2.

12.2.3 Autoimmune conjunctivitis

All types of hypersensitivity may damage the conjunctiva (Table 12.1). Specific autoantibodies directed against conjunctival antigens are involved in the pathogenesis of ocular pemphigoid (cicatrizing conjunctivitis) and pemphigus (see Chapter 11, section 11.4.1).

12.2.4 Stevens–Johnson syndrome

This is a severe form of erythema multiforme, which produces ocular changes in 50% of patients with severe oral ulceration. *Early diagnosis of ocular involvement is imperative.* The syndrome is probably caused by CD8[+] T cells killing keratinocytes in a drug-specific, major histocompatibility complex (MHC) class I restricted manner, via the perforin/granzyme-mediated pathway. Levels of the cytolytic protein **granulysin**, produced by drug-specific CD8[+] T cells and natural killer (NK) cells, are high in the blister fluid and positively correlated with the clinical severity of the disease. The trigger, in genetically susceptible individuals, is usually a drug, often one given to treat infection (Table 12.1). The severe conjunctivitis leads to ulceration,

Case 12.1 Conjunctival infection

A 22-year-old man was involved in a motorcycle accident and suffered a severe closed head injury that produced diffuse cerebral injury and a fracture of the left temporal bone. He was admitted to a neurosurgical intensive care unit and required artificial ventilation for 17 days. A tracheostomy was performed to assist with ventilation. He gradually became independent of the ventilator, and regained consciousness and was eventually transferred to the neurosurgical ward. He was noted to have a left facial nerve palsy (caused by the fracture) and to be restless and confused, but no other focal neurological defect was identified. The facial nerve palsy impaired his ability to blink on the left. While he was unconscious, both his eyes had been taped shut to prevent injury and infection. Attempts were made to tape the left eye shut on the ward, but he persistently removed the dressing. Three days after his transfer to the ward, the left eye was noted to be red with crusted swollen lids. The cornea was hazy and he was photophobic. A clinical diagnosis was made of *infective conjunctivitis and keratitis* secondary to exposure. Swabs taken from the eye grew Pseudomonas aeruginosa. He was treated vigorously with topical antibiotics and the eyelids were temporarily sutured together. Despite this, he suffered considerable corneal scarring with loss of visual acuity in the left eye.

Case 12.2 Allergic conjunctivitis

A 23-year-old student vet presented with a history of intermittent redness and itching of the eyes, associated with some swelling of the eyelids. These episodes occurred only when he was involved in small-animal work, particularly when handling rabbits. Each episode lasted for several hours and several recent episodes had been associated with sneezing and running of the nose, but no wheeze. He had also noticed that large, itchy weals developed on his skin if he was scratched by a rabbit. He had a history of mild hay fever. Skin-prick testing showed a marked positive response to rabbit proteins and moderate levels of rabbit-specific IgE were found in his blood. A diagnosis of *allergic conjunctivitis and rhinitis* due to rabbit hypersensitivity was made. He was able to limit the problem by taking a non-sedative antihistamine on the days when he was likely to be exposed to rabbits.

antibiotics are used to prevent superinfection. Other treatments now being used in severe cases include ciclosporin and antitumour necrosis factor agents such as etanercept. High-dose intravenous immunoglobulin was previously used but is no longer recommended.

12.2.5 Other causes of conjunctivitis

T cell–mediated Th1 immune (type IV) mechanisms are involved in allergic contact dermatitis (see Chapter 11) and **contact dermatoconjunctivitis** (Table 12.1). This eye condition is characterized by erythematous, indurated lesions on the eyelids. There is less conjunctival injection than in immediate reactions. Ophthalmic contact sensitizers include almost all topical drugs (such as antibiotic drops or atropine-like compounds), cosmetics and especially contact lens solutions.

Conjunctivitis may also be a feature of other systemic diseases such as post-infective syndrome or **arthritis urethritica** (previously Reiter's syndrome) and **sarcoidosis**. Of patients with arthritis urethritica (see Chapter 10), 75% develop conjunctivitis (see Chapter 4, Fig. 4.2), while 15% also have an iridocyclitis. Uveitis (30%) is commoner than conjunctivitis (5%) in patients with sarcoidosis (see Chapter 13).

12.3 Keratitis

Recurrent **herpes simplex stromal keratitis** is probably due to a cell-mediated hypersensitivity reaction rather than to active virus infection. Epithelial cells may be damaged during the

Case 12.3 Stevens–Johnson syndrome

A 17-year-old girl was admitted as an emergency with a 3-day history of severe ulceration of her lips, 'sticky' eyes, sore feet, diffuse itching and an erythematous rash. Following a major epileptic fit 8 days previously, she had been put on carbamazepine. On admission, she was pyrexial with extensive haemorrhagic ulceration of the mouth, which became too sore even to take fluids. A *clinical diagnosis of Stevens–Johnson syndrome* was made and she was treated immediately with systemic corticosteroids (45 mg daily). She improved symptomatically, but when an ophthalmologist was asked to see her 3 weeks later she was found to have severe conjunctival ulceration and punctate keratitis. The conjunctival ulcerations required 'rodding' to prevent adhesion of the raw surfaces and she was also treated with topical antibiotics to prevent infection. Unfortunately, she then developed cicatricial entropion (inward-turning eyelids), with resulting corneal trauma. The lid deformity was surgically corrected and further corneal ulceration prevented by an extended-wear contact lens. Another late complication of this syndrome is obliteration of the conjunctival sac, leading to 'dry eye', corneal scarring and even blindness.

secondary keratitis and infection. Long-term ocular complications, as in Case 12.3, are common. Treatment of the ocular complications may be disappointing, although intensive, short-term, topical steroids help to reduce inflammation and prevent conjunctival ulceration, and alternative topical primary infection, so that T lymphocytes become sensitized to persistent viral antigens or virally altered corneal antigens. Topical steroids may be required to prevent permanent scarring and blindness.

Marginal ulcers are sometimes seen in response to **staphylococcal infection**, particularly in younger patients, and are thought to be due to deposited antigen–antibody complexes.

Marginal ulcers also occur in vasculitides, particularly rheumatoid vasculitis and granulomatosis with polyarteritis (GPA). An important complication is the **peripheral corneal melting syndrome**, which can lead to corneal perforation with prolapse of the uveal tissue – an ocular emergency. Systemic immunosuppression may be helpful, but corneal grafting may be necessary.

Keratoconjunctivitis sicca is inflammation resulting from insufficient lacrimal gland secretions. The patient complains of sore or gritty eyes, and tear secretion is deficient when measured by Schirmer's test (see Chapter 10). Dry eyes are common in elderly people, but in some patients the dry eyes are accompanied by a dry mouth (due to involvement of salivary glands) and by arthritis (Sjögren's syndrome). Treatment of dry eyes is difficult, as dryness is experienced only when the lacrimal glands are severely damaged. Artificial tears are usually the only option.

Damaged cornea can be replaced with a cadaveric graft (see Chapter 8). Although it is antigenic, the cornea is a poor inducer of allogeneic immune responses (see section 12.1). In avascular grafts, MHC compatibility is irrelevant, and over 90% of those that remain avascular are successful. However, rejection of a corneal graft is associated with revascularization, and MHC matching may then be important; well-matched grafts can survive despite revascularization.

12.4 Scleritis

The episcleral tissue is that between the fascia of the eyeball and the sclera itself. Inflammation of episcleral tissue, **simple episcleritis**, is common, particularly in women. It is a benign condition and resolves in 3–4 weeks. The cause is unknown, but an autoimmune process has not been excluded. **Nodular episcleritis** is a more protracted disease; about 30% of patients have an associated systemic rheumatic disease (usually rheumatoid arthritis).

Inflammation of the sclera, **scleritis**, is a severe and painful disease that can lead to blindness. It occurs in association with severe systemic vasculitic diseases, such as rheumatoid arthritis, polyarteritis nodosa, GPA, relapsing polychondritis or systemic lupus erythematosus.

12.5 Uveitis

Uveitis, or inflammation of the uveal tract, describes a common group of conditions that can be classified into **anterior, posterior and pan-uveitis**. Anterior uveitis includes iritis and cyclitis. Posterior uveitis usually refers to choroiditis, but retinitis or retinal vasculitis are often part of the same pathological process and are discussed here together with choroiditis. Since the inflammation in uveitis extends beyond the uveal tract into the lens, vitreous and retina, the more general term **intraocular inflammation** has been proposed, but this is not in widespread use.

All parts of the uveal tract can be affected by either acute or chronic inflammation, and uveitis can occur as a purely ocular process or as a manifestation of systemic disease. As outlined in section 12.1, the highly vascular uveal tract has great potential for trapping blood-borne antigen, immune complexes and microorganisms.

12.5.1 Anterior uveitis

Acute anterior uveitis can occur in association with several systemic diseases, most notably sarcoidosis and the seronegative spondyloarthropathies (see Chapter 10). Those associated with seronegative spondyloarthropathies are commonest in those individuals with the HLA allele B27. This HLA allele (found in around 5% of the healthy population) is also present in about 50% of patients with recurrent anterior uveitis with no evidence of systemic disease, suggesting that common disease mechanisms may underlie many cases of uveitis, regardless of associated systemic disease (Fig. 12.3). Over half of the UK cases of uveitis have no underlying disease, i.e. **idiopathic uveitis**.

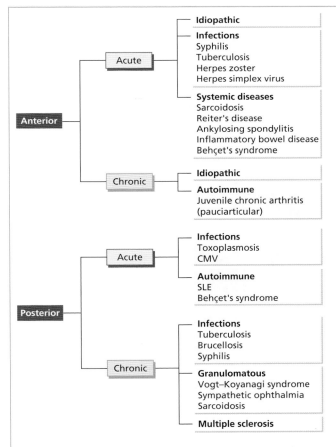

Fig. 12.3 Classification of uveitis by site and time scale of symptoms (post-trauma or surgery cases not included). CMV, cytomegalovirus; SLE, systemic lupus erythematosus.

Mild recurrent anterior uveitis is usually self-limiting and symptomatically treated with local steroids and mydriatic agents under ophthalmic supervision. However, once there is inflammation of the anterior uvea involving a breakdown of the 'blood–aqueous humour barrier', there is outpouring of serum proteins and inflammatory cells into the anterior chamber (see Fig. 12.2). The inflammatory exudate, which can be seen by slit-lamp microscopy, may form small deposits on the back of the cornea (keratic precipitates, Fig. 12.4). The back of the inflamed iris may become stuck to the lens (posterior synechiae), producing an irregularly shaped pupil and increased pressure in the posterior chamber (secondary glaucoma).

Mouse experimental allergic uveitis (EAU) is provoked by distant immunization with a well-defined retinal autoantigen and is mediated by CD4+ T cells. This model has shown that cells in both chambers of the eye can suppress activation of bystander T cells and the production of inflammatory cytokines. In the anterior segment and the aqueous humour, suppress activation of T cells is by cell-to-cell contact with corneal endothelial cells and iris pigment epithelial cells, whereas in the posterior chamber retinal pigment epithelial cells suppress the activation of T cells via soluble factors. Both can induce CD25+Foxp3+Treg cells (CD8+ and CD4+) to control activation of bystander T cells. Similar mechanisms have been described in humans, though the precise mechanisms are less well explored as yet; however, there is hope that small suppressive molecules might form the basis of immune therapy for refractive autoimmune uveitis in humans in the future.

However, once uveitis has occurred, any inflammatory agent can trigger a recurrence. Sensitized Th1 and Th17 cells, as well as macrophages, play an effector role in ocular inflammation. Slight changes in vascular permeability in the eye, like those in the kidney, encourage the deposition of immune complexes or antigen and further activate macrophages.

In contrast to acute anterior uveitis, **chronic anterior uveitis** is painless and presents with insidious loss of vision, due to a combination of raised intraocular pressure and cataract formation. This can occur without systemic disease, but most notably occurs in children with juvenile idiopathic arthritis, particularly in those with early-onset disease involving a small number of joints and who have antinuclear antibodies (about 50% of children with this pattern of arthritis have uveitis). *Ophthalmological screening of children with juvenile idiopathic arthritis is essential, as early detection and treatment can prevent blindness in this silent, insidiously progressive disease.*

12.5.2 Posterior uveitis

Posterior uveitis (or choroiditis) (Fig. 12.3) is also painless and presents with visual impairment. This can occur as one of a group of idiopathic disorders confined to the eye, but *more often occurs secondary to infection or systemic inflammatory disease.* The inflammatory process is often centred on blood vessels, particularly when acute (Fig. 12.5). It is appropriate to consider choroiditis, choroidoretinitis and retinal vasculitis under the same heading.

Acute choroidoretinitis occurs in several connective tissue diseases, most notably Behçet's disease (Case 12.4) and systemic lupus erythematosus. Vigorous immunosuppression may be sight saving in these disorders. However, similar ocular changes may be seen in infection, which should be excluded before immunosuppression is used.

A particularly devastating form of acute choroidoretinitis is caused by cytomegalovirus infection in patients with severe defects in cellular immunity, particularly in advanced human immunodeficiency virus (HIV) infection. This is difficult to treat and often blinding.

Chronic posterior uveitis can occur in a number of chronic infections, in sarcoidosis and in Vogt–Koyanagi syndrome (uveitis and vitiligo). Granuloma formation occurs in several of

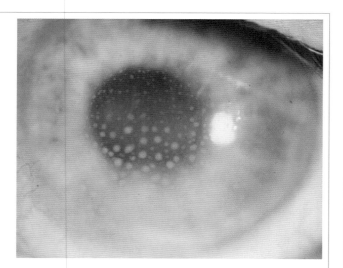

Fig. 12.4 Keratic precipitates cover the posterior surface of the cornea in a patient with granulomatous uveitis. Courtesy of Mr N. P. Jones.

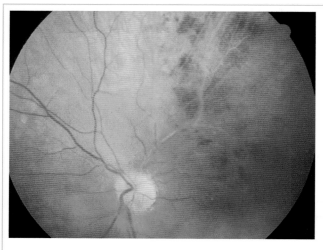

Fig. 12.5 Retinal vasculitis showing vascular occlusion and haemorrhage from damaged vessels. Courtesy of Mr N. P. Jones.

A 21-year-old man from a Turkish family presented with a painful left eye for 2 days associated with blurred vision. He also gave a 3-month history of relapsing and remitting ulceration of his mouth and scrotum. Three days later the right eye also became involved.

Ophthalmological examination showed a florid anterior uveitis of such severity that neutrophils in the anterior chamber settled out to form a fluid level visible to the naked eye: a hypopon (Fig. 12.6). There was no posterior uveitis at this stage. A clinical diagnosis of *Behçet's disease* was made. He was treated with oral and topical (ocular and mucosal) corticosteroids and a low dose of colchicine. The eye changes and ulceration gradually settled.

However, 3 months later he developed painless deterioration of vision in the left eye and was found to have a severe retinal vasculitis. This was treated aggressively with oral corticosteroids and azathioprine, with little response. Despite treatment with ciclosporin, mycophenolate mofetil and infliximab over the following year, he also developed vasculitis in the right retina. He then presented with a left hemiparesis due to cerebral vasculitis. His treatment was switched to pulsed intravenous cyclophosphamide. This gradually controlled the ocular inflammation and he has developed no further neurological symptoms. His vision remains severely impaired.

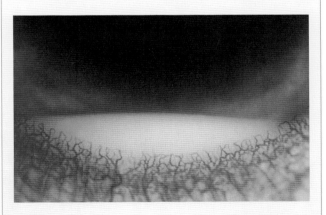

Fig. 12.6 Hypopyon due to severe anterior chamber inflammation in Behçet's disease. Courtesy of Mr N. P. Jones.

these disorders and it seems likely that Th1 cell–mediated hypersensitivity underlies their pathogenesis. A mild chronic posterior uveitis also occurs in multiple sclerosis. This is not of any clinical consequence, but is of interest in showing that the disease process in multiple sclerosis is not confined to the central nervous system.

The suspicion of an associated systemic disorder depends on the pattern of the uveitis (bilateral, granulomatous site) and on a careful clinical history and examination. *'Uveitis investigations' are unrewarding, as there are no specific laboratory tests.*

12.5.3 Uveitis following trauma

Lens-induced uveitis occurs about 2 weeks after surgery to the lens (Case 12.5) or may be seen spontaneously in eyes with mature disintegrating lenses. Lens damage may release 'hidden' antigens and the subsequent uveitis is believed to be due to the immune response to those antigens. Although injection of sterile lens antigens into the eye has a minimal effect, any natural adjuvants present (such as bacterial antigens) potentiate the immune reaction. Animal experiments suggest that lens-induced uveitis is caused by local production of specific antibodies to denatured lens antigens, which cross-react with native uveal antigens. Antibodies to lens proteins are also found in the eye and circulation in human disease. The disease is usually confined to the traumatized eye, except in elderly patients when spontaneous leakage of lens protein may provoke a bilateral reaction.

Sympathetic ophthalmia is a devastating bilateral, progressive granulomatous uveitis following penetration or perforation of one orbit. Uveitis in the non-traumatized eye is thought to be due to an autoimmune T-cell response to antigens liberated from the other eye. A severely traumatized 'blind' eye should be removed within 2 weeks of injury to avoid risk of a sympathetic reaction in the intact eye. A choroiditis is the first sign, but granulomatous inflammation eventually involves the whole tract. Animal experiments suggest that a penetrating injury releases minute doses of retinal antigens into the subconjunctival space with drainage to the local lymph node where autosensitization occurs. Treatment is difficult, but ciclosporin A and steroids may limit progression.

Sympathetic ophthalmia is often used as a striking example of how self-tolerance can break down when self-antigen from an 'immunologically privileged' site gains access to the immune system. Theoretically, sympathetic ophthalmia could complicate any invasive surgical procedure on the eye. However, the extreme rarity of this disorder after both surgery and trauma (fewer than five cases per year in the USA) emphasizes how powerfully the eye suppresses inappropriate immune responses by the mechanisms outlined in section 12.1. Sympathetic ophthalmia has been associated with similar HLA alleles to the Vogt–Koyanagi-Harada syndrome (a rare bilateral granulomatous uveitis, associated with high circulating levels of γ-interferon and antibodies to retinal S antigen), suggesting some similarities in the immunopathogenesis of these two forms of granulomatous uveitis.

A 73-year-old woman had a left-sided extracapsular cataract extraction and lens implant, although the cortical lens material was never completely removed. She made an uneventful post-operative recovery, but 2 weeks later developed a severe uveitis in the same eye. Two years after the operation, she still has to use topical steroids to suppress the uveitis. The presumed diagnosis is *lens-induced uveitis*.

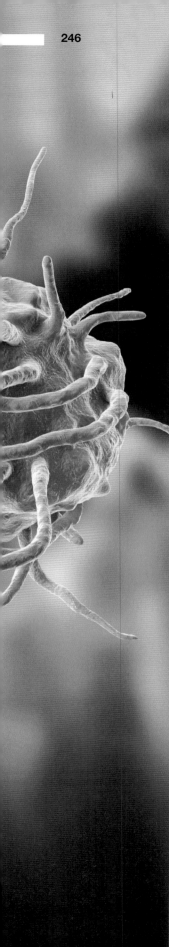

CHAPTER 13
Chest Diseases

Key topics

 Visit the companion website at **www.wiley.com/go/misbah/immunology** to download cases with additional figures on these topics.

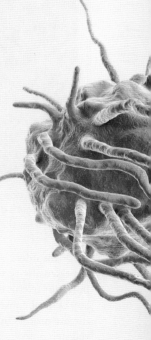

Chapel and Haeney's Essentials of Clinical Immunology, Seventh Edition. Edited by Siraj A. Misbah, Gavin P. Spickett, and Virgil A.S.H. Dalm.
© 2022 John Wiley & Sons Ltd. Published 2022 by John Wiley & Sons Ltd.

13.1 Introduction

Antigens can enter the respiratory tract either in the inspired air or via the circulation. Organisms that enter through the airways may be killed by local defence mechanisms, persist in the lungs with damaging consequences (such as granuloma formation or fibrosis) or invade the systemic circulation to cause septicaemia. Since all the blood from the right side of the heart passes through the pulmonary bed, the respiratory tract is also exposed to circulating organisms, immune complexes and toxic substances from distant sites.

The respiratory tract can be crudely but usefully divided into **two** anatomical, functional and pathological compartments: the **airways** (from the nose to the terminal bronchiole) and the **air spaces** (or alveoli). The airways are protected from inhaled microorganisms and other potentially injurious particles by multiple mechanical factors, backed up by soluble antimicrobial proteins and rapid recruitment of neutrophils and other inflammatory cells (Fig. 13.1). Access to the alveolar compartment is therefore usually limited to very small inhaled particles (<5 µm diameter; see Chapter 4, Fig. 4.4) and organisms or antigen carried via the pulmonary circulation. Particles and organisms gaining access to the alveoli encounter further protective mechanisms such as the surfactant proteins (which have a complement-like function) and alveolar macrophages. **Alveolar macrophages** are responsible for ingesting, killing and degrading foreign material, both living and dead. Although their action in removing organisms from the lower respiratory tract is crucial, their reaction to inert materials can sometimes cause pulmonary damage. Viable cells from the alveoli can be recovered by bronchoalveolar lavage (BAL). Macrophages constitute 80–85% of cells in BAL fluid, while lymphocytes (mostly T cells) constitute about 10%. **Cigarette smoking** increases the cell yield by four- to fivefold and the macrophages are filled with tars and silicates. The proportion of neutrophils (10–20%) in BAL is also increased in smokers compared with non-smokers (2–5%), and most are activated, containing a high concentration of neutrophil elastase, which may play a role in the lung destruction seen in chronic bronchitis and emphysema.

Antigen-specific immune components are also found in the respiratory tract. **Bronchial-associated lymphoid tissue (BALT)** forms part of a common mucosal immune system (see Chapter 14). Unlike gut-associated lymphoid tissue, BALT is not constitutively present in healthy subjects, but is induced in response to repeated or persistent infection or other injurious stimuli such as smoking. Under these circumstances, BALT becomes organized in follicles and consists mainly of B cells, but distinct sites of collections of T cells are found on the periphery of these follicles. Epithelium overlying the BALT is devoid generally of cilia and goblet cells, but displays membranous projections into the lumen, suited to selective antigen sampling, like the counterpart in the intestine – the M cell (see Chapter 14). Antigens are transported into the follicle where they can stimulate antigen-specific T and B cells. Subsequently, IgA precursor B cells migrate into lymphatics and thence to the blood; bronchial IgA-bearing cells recirculate through both gut and lungs, so dispersing antigen-sensitive cells.

There are also large numbers of less organized lymphocytes in the lung within the pulmonary vasculature, in the lung interstitium and in the bronchoalveolar space.

Although relatively few lymphocytes are seen on routine sections, when calculated for the whole lung lymphocyte numbers are similar to the circulating blood pool, i.e. about 10×10^9 lymphocytes.

Plasma cells producing IgE and IgG are also found in the bronchial tract. The physiological reason for the presence of IgE cells in the lung is unknown; it may even be an evolutionary accident, since the respiratory tract is a foregut derivative and IgE has a role in expulsion of intestinal parasites. While its physiological function is unclear, IgE is implicated in immediate (type I) hypersensitivity mechanisms (see Chapter 4) responsible for allergic asthma and hay fever.

We have considered respiratory diseases under four headings: infection, granulomatous disease, interstitial lung disease and vasculitis. **Allergic diseases, which constitute the major immunological airways diseases, are considered in Chapter 4.**

13.2 Respiratory infections

Infectious processes within the respiratory tract usually affect either the airways (e.g. rhinitis, sinusitis, laryngitis, bronchitis) or alveoli (pneumonia), although pneumonia can develop as a consequence of airways infection, particularly the small airways (bronchopneumonia) (Case 13.1).

Most respiratory tract infections reflect an interaction between virulent microorganisms and a relatively normal respiratory tract, whose protective mechanisms have been overcome either by the organism or by other injurious factors such as smoking or malnutrition. The respiratory tract is, however, also the most common site for infection to develop in immunodeficient subjects, and *compromised immunity must be considered in all patients who present with serious, persistent, therapy-resistant, unusual or recurrent infections.*

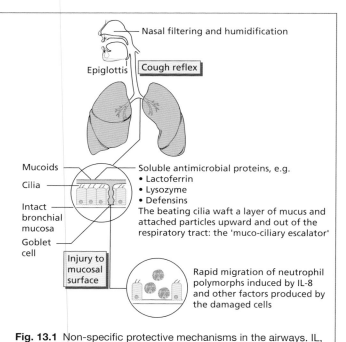

Fig. 13.1 Non-specific protective mechanisms in the airways. IL, interleukin.

Table 13.1 Respiratory infections classified according to site and pattern of infection

Site	Organism	Incidence and pattern of infection	Predisposing factors
Upper respiratory tract	Viral	Common – colds	
	Bacterial	Less common – sinusitis	Physical damage
			Viral infection
			Immune dysfunction
Lower respiratory tract	Viral	Pneumonia – rare in adults	Immune dysfunction
		Bronchiolitis due to respiratory syncytial virus common in children	
	Bacterial	Common	Age
			Smoking
			Immune dysfunction

13.2.1 Infection in the immunocompetent host

The airways are a major target for **viral infection** (Table 13.1), manifested most typically as the common cold, caused by many different viruses. These viruses usually replicate better in the cooler upper airways than at normal body temperature. Infection is probably cleared largely by virus-specific cytotoxic T cells.

Bacterial infection of the airways is less common and often occurs as a result of *suppression of defence mechanisms by prior viral infection*. The transient susceptibility of the airways to infection induced by some viral infections is only partially understood, but includes physical factors such as inhibition of ciliary function and damage to the airway epithelium (e.g. influenza), and more subtle immunological mechanisms such as reduced expression of major histocompatibility complex (MHC) molecules (adenoviruses) and inhibition of cytokine production (e.g. measles inhibits interleukin [IL]-12 production). The most striking example is **influenza A**, which can

---

Case 13.1   Pneumonia and chronic lymphatic leukaemia

A 65-year-old man was admitted with bilateral lower-lobe pneumonia. He had felt exhausted for 6 months, had lost 3 kg in weight and suffered 4 chest infections that responded to antibiotics. He did not smoke. He was clinically anaemic, but had no finger clubbing, lymphadenopathy or splenomegaly. On investigation, he had a low haemoglobin (92 g/l) and a raised erythrocyte sedimentation rate (ESR: 84 mm/h). The white cell count was very high (98 × 10⁹/l) and 95% of these were lymphocytes. The platelet count was normal. Serum immunoglobulins were all low: IgG 3.2 g/l (NR 7.2–18.0), IgA 0.6 g/l (NR 0.8–5.0) and IgM 0.3 g/l (NR 0.5–2.0); no paraprotein bands were seen.

A provisional diagnosis of pneumonia complicating chronic lymphatic leukaemia (CLL) was made and CLL was confirmed by surface marker studies, which showed that 98% of peripheral lymphocytes were monoclonal B cells (Chapter 6).

Sputum cultures grew untypable Haemophilus influenzae. Treatment with amoxycillin resulted in rapid clearing of the pneumonia but, in view of his high lymphocyte count and mild anaemia, he was started on chlorambucil to control the lymphoproliferation. He lacked detectable serum antibodies and failed to make IgG antibodies to pneumococci on immunization; furthermore, all three major classes of serum immunoglobulins were low. Prophylactic IgG replacement therapy was started at a dose of 0.4 g/kg body weight per month, and he remained well for the next 5 years.

lead to devastating pneumonia, usually caused by Staphylococcus aureus, in debilitated patients. *However, the most important causes of pneumonia in the immunocompetent host are bacterial* (Table 13.1).

Bacterial pneumonia is a common problem. It accounts for up to 10% of hospital admissions in developed countries and carries a considerable mortality: in the UK, pneumonia causes 25% of all deaths from lung disease. While most of these deaths occur as a final event in debilitated patients, some previously healthy children and adults also die of pneumonia in spite of seemingly appropriate antibiotic therapy. The most devastating consequences of pneumonia are seen in developing countries. Each year, about 5 million children die of pneumonia before they are 5 years old. In South American countries, for instance, infant mortality from pneumonia and influenza is approximately 30 times greater than in the USA. Pneumococcal infections account for the majority of bacterial pneumonias and carry a mortality rate of 6–30%. Immunization against pneumococcal infections with polyvalent conjugate vaccines has significantly reduced the invasive disease in young children. However, pneumococcal disease remains a notable cause of mortality in the developing world and community-acquired pneumococcal pneumonia is still a problem in adults in the developed world despite pneumococcal polysaccharide immunization. A recent Canadian study showed that the polysaccharide vaccine was not effective in patients with chronic obstructive airways disease who were 65 years of age or older, but it reduced the risk of acquiring pneumonia by 80% in younger patients. Hospital admission rates and lengths of stay were lower in the vaccine group.

13.2.2 Infection in the immunocompromised host

Serious or recurrent infection does not always reflect disordered immunity (Table 13.2). The abnormal mucosal environment in cystic fibrosis is a potent predisposing cause for infection, as is bronchial obstruction due to factors ranging from tumours to plugging by mucus. Recurrent bronchial inflammation from many causes, particularly when associated with obstruction, leads to the development of bronchiectasis: dilated, damaged bronchi that themselves predispose to further infection, thus

Table 13.2 Important non-immunological causes of recurrent or severe infection

Airway obstruction
- Tumour
- Foreign body (e.g. peanuts in children)
- Inflammatory/fibrotic (e.g. in tuberculosis)

Mucociliary dysfunction
- Cystic fibrosis (abnormal mucus)
- Ciliary dyskinesia (genetic defect in ciliary proteins)
- Squamous metaplasia (due to smoking)

amplifying and perpetuating the process. *However, there are certain infections or patterns of infection that should always lead to the consideration of underlying immunodeficiency* (Fig. 13.2). Some of these infections (such as Pneumocystis pneumonia) are virtually always associated with underlying immunodeficiency, whereas chronic sinopulmonary infection is associated with antibody deficiency in only 5% of cases. Nevertheless, **the highly treatable nature of many immunodeficiency states (particularly antibody deficiencies) makes investigation mandatory** (see Chapter 3).

In adults, secondary causes of immunodeficiency are more common than primary ones and should be excluded first (see Chapter 3). An insidious pneumonic illness with dry cough, dyspnoea and fever may be caused by Pneumocystis carinii, cytomegalovirus (CMV) or atypical mycobacterial infection, and should raise the possibility of acquired immune deficiency syndrome (AIDS; see Chapter 3). Opportunistic viral, fungal and protozoal infections are common in patients with **AIDS** or iatrogenic defects in cell-mediated immunity, but such patients also suffer from common bacterial infections. Patients with AIDS frequently have infections with several microorganisms simultaneously.

13.3 Granulomatous diseases

The granulomatous diseases are a heterogeneous group of disorders with differing aetiologies, clinical presentations, histological characteristics and responses to therapy.

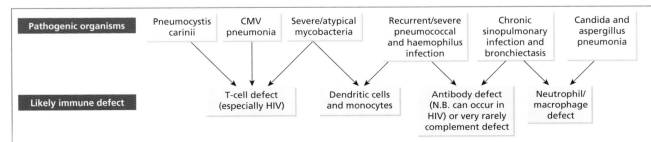

Fig. 13.2 Patterns of respiratory infection associated with specific immunodeficiencies. CMV, cytomegalovirus; HIV, human immunodeficiency virus.

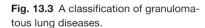

Fig. 13.3 A classification of granulomatous lung diseases.

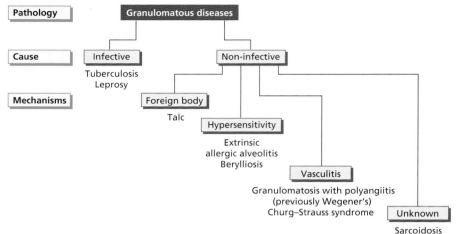

13.3.1 Formation of a granuloma

A **granuloma** is a histological structure made up largely of macrophages that have differentiated into epithelioid cells and often also fused to form multinucleate giant cells. Granulomas form in the presence of an antigen or foreign substance that cannot be easily broken down or eliminated; they can be regarded as a mechanism for containing and possibly destroying that antigen or foreign body, and may be reversible if antigen is destroyed only slowly. However, granuloma formation is frequently associated with increased deposition of fibrous tissue. This fibrosis, which is irreversible, is often the most troublesome feature of granulomatous diseases. Granulomatous diseases can be both infective and non-infective (Fig. 13.3).

The most important **immunological pathway** leading to granuloma formation involves CD4⁺ T cell–dependent activation of macrophages (type IV hypersensitivity). The presence of a suitable intracellular antigen, such as mycobacterial cell wall, induces the production of IL-12. This cytokine then stimulates the development of a Th1 T-cell response, with production of cytokines such as interferon (IFN)-γ. The process appears to be sustained and perpetuated by IFN-γ, IL-12 and other cytokines, in particular tumour necrosis factor (TNF)-α, produced by both T cells and macrophages themselves (Fig. 13.4). The key role of TNF-α in sustaining this process is shown by the reduction or resolution of granuloma by anti-TNF agents. Although useful therapeutically in the treatment of Crohn's disease and sarcoidosis, these agents also cause an increased risk of tuberculosis. Epithelioid cells also produce fibrogenic cytokines such as transforming growth factor (TGF)-β and can synthesize the active form of vitamin D from inactive precursors. Active vitamin D plays an important role in stimulating macrophage differentiation within the granuloma. In some granulomatous disorders, sufficient active vitamin D is produced to cause hypercalcaemia.

Granulomas also form in some diseases dominated by a Th2 pattern of cytokine production, such as schistosomiasis and

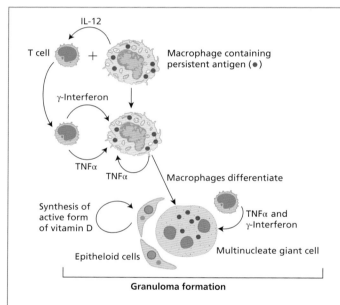

Fig. 13.4 Mechanisms of T cell–dependent granuloma formation. IL, interleukin; TNF, tumour necrosis factor.

eosinophilic granulomatosis with polyangiitis (EGPA, previously known as the Churg–Strauss syndrome), though the mechanism in these disorders is less clear.

13.3.2 Tuberculosis

The global impact of infection with Mycobacterium tuberculosis is enormous. *Around one-third of the world's population is infected with the tubercle bacillus and about 1.5 million people die every year from the consequences of this infection.* The greatest part of this burden of disease falls upon the developing world. Tuberculosis is a disease driven by poverty and poor nutrition. Immunosuppression associated with human immunodeficiency

Table 13.3 Risk factors for developing tuberculosis

1. Poverty and malnutrition
2. Close contact with patients with active infection
3. Immunosuppression (especially secondary to HIV infection or anti-TNF drugs)
4. Prolonged residence in countries with high prevalence of tuberculosis
5. Genetic predisposition

HIV, human immunodeficiency virus; TNF, tumour necrosis factor.

virus (HIV) infection has combined with these older risk factors to increase the incidence of tuberculosis (Table 13.3). The impact of tuberculosis in Western Europe and North America is minimal by comparison, and has fallen considerably over the last 50 years, though this downward trend has stopped now. This is due to a combination of HIV infection, increased mobility of populations across the world and worsening pockets of poverty even in the richest of nations. Other immunosuppressive factors should not be forgotten, particularly poor nutrition and the immunosuppressive effect of infections such as measles. Vitamin D deficiency (due to diet or lack of exposure to sunlight) may be an important co-factor, reflecting the role of this vitamin within granulomas. The outcome of exposure to M. tuberculosis depends on several factors: susceptibility genes play a significant role, as does the intensity of exposure to M. tuberculosis; high levels of exposure may overwhelm even vigorous immune responses.

Mycobacterium tuberculosis is a slow-growing bacterium with an inert, waxy cell wall. It produces no toxins and causes disease only by its stimulation of the body's immune defence mechanisms coupled with an inexorable increase in numbers. The organism is rapidly taken up by alveolar macrophages. In most individuals, activation of dendritic cells results in a brisk Th1-pattern immune response, leading to local granuloma formation in an area of lung and the draining lymph node. This contains and effectively eliminates the organism, although the immune system alone may never be able to clear M. tuberculosis completely. Once infection has occurred, the organism remains in a **latent form** if the host is untreated, even when disease does not develop. In a proportion of infected individuals, the T-cell response is less effective and the granulomatous response only partially contains the organism. An area of localized but progressive **granulomatous inflammation** develops, which slowly enlarges and often cavitates due to a necrotic process called caseation, which is typical of tuberculous granulomas and distorts surrounding structures by fibrosis. The Th1 response to M. tuberculosis may wax and wane over time: latent disease can reactivate if immunity is suppressed (by malnutrition, drugs or intercurrent infection) and become clinically evident. Treatment with anti-TNF agents specifically reduce resistance to reactivation, indicating the important role played by TNF in suppressing the infection.

If the T-cell response is defective, or skewed towards a Th2 pattern, then the organism reproduces freely in macrophages and disseminated disease may develop. This is **miliary tuberculosis**

(Fig. 13.5), where many organs are involved by small collections of macrophages packed with mycobacteria, with only partial evidence of granuloma formation. This is associated with marked systemic ill-health, due to cytokine release from macrophages. Cytokine release is driven partly by the ineffective T-cell response and partly by the direct effect of the mycobacterial cell wall on dendritic cells.

Improvement in diet and living conditions, and more recently control of HIV infection, are the major public health measures that reduce the impact of tuberculosis. The introduction of **prophylactic immunization** with an attenuated form of mycobacterium, bacillus Calmette–Guérin (BCG), had a significant role in reducing invasive disease infection due to mycobacterial species in young children. It is used to protect hospital personnel and tuberculosis contacts, though evidence for efficacy is controversial. New vaccines are needed urgently.

The presence of a T-cell response to M. tuberculosis can be established clinically by injecting mycobacterial antigen intradermally and assessing the delayed skin reaction at 48–72 h (the basis of the **Mantoux test**; Fig. 13.6). This is useful in assessing prior immunity before immunization, and may also be a helpful diagnostic pointer in active disease. However, such tests are subjective and largely superseded by the **interferon**

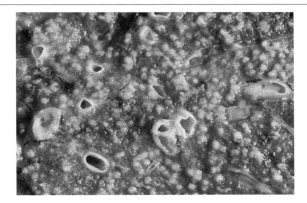

Fig. 13.5 Cut section of lung from a patient who died from miliary tuberculosis. Note the 2–5-mm nodules scattered through the lung tissue. 'Miliary' means 'resembling millet seeds'.

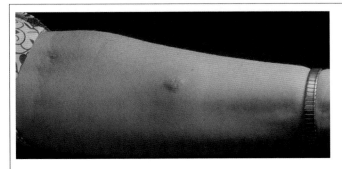

Fig. 13.6 Strongly positive Mantoux reaction 96 h after the intradermal injection of antigen from Mycobacterium tuberculosis.

Case 13.2 Pulmonary tuberculosis

A 23-year-old man presented with a 4-week history of coughing, breathlessness and malaise. He had lost 4 kg in weight, but had no history of night sweats or haemoptysis. He had returned from holiday in Pakistan 2 months earlier. On examination, he was mildly pyrexial (37.8 °C), but had no evidence of anaemia or clubbing. Crepitations were audible over the lung apices; there were no other physical signs. His haemoglobin and white cell count were normal, but the C-reactive protein (CRP) was 231 mg/l. The chest X-ray showed bilateral upper- and middle-lobe shadowing, but no hilar enlargement. Sputum was found to contain acid-fast bacilli and Mycobacterium tuberculosis was confirmed by polymerase chain reaction (PCR) and subsequently cultured. A diagnosis of pulmonary tuberculosis was made. The patient was treated with isoniazid and rifampicin for 6 months, together with pyrazinamide for the first 2 months. He was allowed home on chemotherapy when his sputum became negative on direct smear. The chest X-ray is now much improved.

Case 13.3 Sarcoidosis

A 36-year-old man complained of breathlessness on exercise for 6 months. He also had mild chest tightness and stiff joints, but no skin or eye problems. There was no family history of chest disease and he had never been abroad. He had been immunized with bacillus Calmette–Guérin (BCG) as a schoolboy. On examination, he had no clubbing and no abnormal chest signs. Investigations showed a normal haemoglobin (143 g/l), white cell count (4.4×10^9/l) and differential (27% lymphocytes, 70% neutrophils), a mildly raised C-reactive protein (CRP: 23 mg/l) and increased serum levels of angiotensin-converting enzyme (ACE). A serum biochemical profile, including serum calcium, was otherwise normal. A chest X-ray showed fine, diffuse radiological shadows, predominantly in the mid zones, and bilateral hilar lymphadenopathy. Lung function tests were normal and a Mantoux test was negative. A clinical diagnosis of sarcoidosis was made. Since he had pulmonary infiltration on X-ray, he was treated with corticosteroids to good effect.

gamma release assay (IGRA; Chapter 19). Diagnosis of active infection, however, is done by polymerase chain reaction (PCR) of induced sputum or biopsy material, still confirmed by microscopy and culture (Case 13.2).

Treatment regimens comprise a combination of several antimicrobial agents (e.g. rifampicin, isoniazid, pyrazinamide and ethambutol), often administered for a period of 6 months. Unfortunately, recent years have seen the emergence of multidrug-resistant (MDR) and extensively drug-resistant (XDR) tuberculosis strains. These resistant organisms necessitate treatment with second-line agents and are associated with high mortality rates. MDR and XDR tuberculosis loom as particularly daunting public health problems, hence the urgency for new vaccines. The BCG vaccine only partially protects against MDR and XDR; it is protective to non-tuberculous mycobacteriosis (NTM, MAC) because of BCG cross-reactivity.

13.3.3 Sarcoidosis

Sarcoidosis is a multisystem, granulomatous disorder most commonly affecting young adults of either sex (Case 13.3). It is less common after the age of 40 years.

Clinically, there are two types (Table 13.4): **acute** sarcoid and **insidious-onset** sarcoid. Bilateral hilar lymphadenopathy alone is asymptomatic and may be a chance finding on chest X-ray. Acute sarcoid presents as erythema nodosum with or without arthralgia; this form is particularly common in Scandinavia and common in the UK. Most patients, however, have a more insidious disease; this form is about 10 times more prevalent in Afro-Caribbean people than in most other ethnic groups.

Table 13.4 Systemic involvement in sarcoidosis (with incidence in either group of patients)

Acute sarcoidosis
Fever
Malaise
Arthralgia
Iritis
Erythema nodosum
Bilateral hilar nodes on chest X-ray (100%)
Radiological pulmonary infiltrates
Insidious sarcoidosis
Breathlessness due to alveolitis
Lymphadenopathy – common
Hepatic involvement – often subclinical (20–85%)
Hypercalciuria/hypercalcaemia (10–50%)
Anterior uveitis (10–35%)
Skin lesions – plaques/erythema nodosum (10%)
Pulmonary infiltrates on chest X-rays
Late stages show fibrosis only
Bilateral hilar nodes (uncommon)
Neurosarcoid

The **diagnosis** of sarcoidosis depends on the clinical and radiological picture and the histology of any lesions that can be biopsied. Historically, the Kveim test was used to establish a diagnosis of sarcoidosis, but since this involves injection of biological material derived from splenic tissue of patients with sarcoidosis, the test is now abandoned.

Tuberculosis is an important **differential diagnosis** of sarcoidosis. Curiously, the Mantoux test is nearly always negative in active sarcoidosis, even in subjects known to have a previously positive test, and then becomes positive again as the sarcoidosis goes into remission or is treated. The immunological basis for this phenomenon is unknown. Serum angiotensin-converting enzyme (ACE) is frequently used, but the test's utility is limited by frequent false positives and often misinterpreted, *so it should not be undertaken.* Soluble interleukin 2 receptor (sIL-2R) is a more sensitive biomarker that can be used to rule out sarcoidosis in patients suspected of sarcoidosis.

Other laboratory tests are of little value in diagnosis or predicting disease evolution, although it is important to exclude hypercalcaemia due to uncontrolled vitamin D synthesis. Histologically, sarcoid granulomas are no different from granulomas in many other diseases, except that no pathogens or necrosis are seen. Epithelioid and giant cells are found focally, and persistent lesions may become fibrotic and irreversible.

As no definitive diagnostic test for sarcoidosis exists, a diagnosis is made based on three criteria:

- Clinical and radiographic manifestations in keeping with sarcoidosis.
- Exclusion of other diseases with similar clinical presentations (including primary antibody deficiency).
- Identification of non-caseating granuloma on histopathological examination.

The **immunopathology** of sarcoidosis is consistent with a Th1-cell response to an unknown, persistent, non-particulate antigen. There is often evidence of B-cell activation, with a polyclonal increase in immunoglobulin production. Macrophage production of IL-12 and the expression of IL-12 receptors are increased in sarcoidosis, which seems likely to drive granuloma formation. Lung cells from patients with a better prognosis and self-limiting disease seem to produce higher amounts of the immunosuppressive cytokine TGF-β than those who progress. Sarcoidosis seems to occur on a variety of genetic backgrounds, with only weak MHC associations in HLA-B and HLA-C loci, identified in genome-wide association studies of large cohorts with sarcoidosis. The similarities between sarcoid and tuberculosis have led to speculation that sarcoid is due to some form of mycobacterium, but no consistent evidence has yet been found to support an infective process.

Inhalation of beryllium dust can produce lung disease (berylliosis), which is histologically identical to sarcoidosis. Berylliosis is strongly associated with the possession of a specific amino acid (glutamate) at position 69 in the β chain of HLA-DP. This amino acid lies within the antigen-binding groove and may affect binding of beryllium ions, possibly complexed with a self-peptide. There is no evidence that sarcoidosis is caused by beryllium exposure, but berylliosis does provide an instructive example of how a granulomatous disease can develop in response to a simple inert antigen, without invoking an infectious process.

The **prognosis** of sarcoidosis depends on whether or not granulomas or fibrosis develop in vital organs. Those who present with acute disease have an excellent prognosis after treatment and 90% recover within 3 months, although the chest X-ray changes may take a further 3 months to resolve. Insidious-onset sarcoid can proceed to generalized sarcoidosis; those who present with exertional dyspnoea or non-productive cough often have a better prognosis than asymptomatic cases, because they receive treatment. About 5% of patients with sarcoidosis die from their disease.

Treatment depends upon the severity of disease. Many patients improve spontaneously, but those with pulmonary infiltrates and evidence of granulomata in vital organs, such as the nervous system or lungs, should receive steroid therapy. Corticosteroids also correct the hypercalcaemia. For patients with refractory disease or requiring steroid-sparing therapies, other immunosuppressive agents can be added, including methotrexate and azathioprine. The release of TNF from activated alveolar macrophages led to trials evaluating different anti-TNF agents. Although these studies have yielded mixed results in pulmonary sarcoidosis, initiation of a TNF antagonist can be considered. Other investigational treatment strategies include the use of golimumab, ustekinumab, rituximab and JAK/STAT inhibitors.

13.4 Interstitial lung disease

There are many causes of non-infectious inflammation of the airspaces and connective tissue of the lung, which can be classified under the general banner of interstitial lung disease (or parenchymal lung disease) (Table 13.5). Many of these disorders have a strong immunological contribution to their pathogenesis. Although this classification usually excludes specific infection, *infection can both mimic and complicate interstitial lung disease, and should be considered part of the differential diagnosis.*

Almost all forms of interstitial lung disease can lead to a common endpoint, **pulmonary fibrosis** (see Table 13.5), an end stage of disease that is effectively irreversible and associated with severe disability and significant mortality. *Regardless of the initial cause, the pathogenesis of the fibrotic process may be similar in many disorders characterized by pulmonary fibrosis.* Injury and/or stimulation of alveolar macrophages leads to production of cytokines such as TGF, which induces fibroblasts both to proliferate and to synthesize large amounts of extracellular matrix proteins (such as collagens), and chemotactic chemokines recruit bone marrow–derived fibrocytes from the blood.

In some interstitial lung diseases, for example sarcoidosis, it is thought that the fibrotic process is driven by immunologically mediated chronic inflammation. Immunosuppressive and antiinflammatory treatment is therefore effective in limiting progression of lung fibrosis. The assumption that chronic inflammation precedes fibrosis led to widespread use of immunosuppressive treatment in some forms of pulmonary fibrosis, usually with little or no clinical response. However, it is now

Table 13.5 Major causes of interstitial lung disease and pulmonary fibrosis

Systemic autoimmune diseases

Inorganic dusts
- Asbestos
- Silica

Hypersensitivity to known inhaled antigens
- Extrinsic allergic alveolitis
- Berylliosis

Drug hypersensitivity/toxicity
- Cytotoxic drugs (e.g. bleomycin)
- Paraquat poisoning
- Drugs associated with eosinophilic pneumonia (e.g. nitrofurantoin)
- Methotrexate

Pulmonary eosinophilia

Granulomatous diseases
- Sarcoidosis
- Tuberculosis

Idiopathic interstitial pneumonias

clear that *pulmonary fibrosis can develop and progress without any evidence of preceding chronic inflammation.* Similar patterns of fibrosis without inflammation may be seen in other diseases in which there is strong evidence for an autoimmune pathogenesis, especially systemic sclerosis. Potential strategies for limiting fibrosis therapeutically include inhibition of fibrogenic cytokines such as TGF-β or, since recruitment of circulating fibrocytes plays a dominant role in fibrosis, inhibition of chemokine action and cell recruitment. Very recently, tyrosine kinase inhibitors have been introduced for treatment of pulmonary fibrosis. Until such strategies are widely available, *severe established pulmonary fibrosis can be treated only by lung transplantation.*

13.4.1 Pulmonary eosinophilia

The pulmonary eosinophilias are a group of disorders characterized by lung pathology (manifest as fleeting shadowing on the chest X-ray) accompanied by blood eosinophilia ($>0.4 \times$ 10^9/L). These can be further divided into bronchopulmonary and pneumonic types (Fig. 13.7). Bronchopulmonary eosinophilia is usually due to infection with Aspergillus fumigatus in asthmatic patients, but the pneumonic type, which consists of pneumonia and a blood eosinophilia, has several causes.

Allergic bronchopulmonary aspergillosis (ABPA) typically occurs in chronic asthmatics, but is also increasingly recognized to complicate cystic fibrosis (Case 13.4). Inhaled spores of A. fumigatus germinate and grow in the bronchi, behaving as an insoluble, particulate immunogenic stimulus that triggers specific antibody production and Th2-dependent release of IL-4, IL-5 and IL-13; these recruit eosinophils into the airways and adjacent alveoli to cause eosinophilic consolidation. Attacks are characterized by paroxysms of coughing, with the production of large, well-formed casts. There may be areas of lung collapse and bronchiectasis due to plugging of a bronchus by casts. A typical cast contains inspissated mucus, often with fungal hyphae; the production of fungal casts is diagnostic. In their absence, however, skin testing with Aspergillus antigen shows immediate (type I) and late (type III) reactions in 90% of cases and precipitating and RAST antibodies to Aspergillus are detectable in the serum (see Chapter 19).

The aim of **treatment** is to treat the infection and inflammation and ensure that these plugs are removed, otherwise bronchiectasis can ensue. If the plugs are not expectorated,

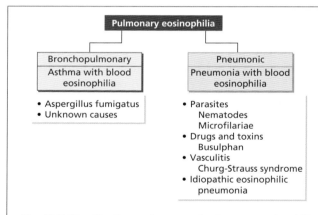

Fig. 13.7 Classification and causes of pulmonary eosinophilia.

🔍 Case 13.4 Allergic bronchopulmonary aspergillosis

A 54-year-old woman presented with a 5-year history of a cough productive of mucopurulent sputum. On several occasions she had coughed up plugs of mucus. Courses of antibiotics had proved ineffectual. She had suffered from asthma for over 20 years and had a daughter with asthma. On examination, a few crepitations were audible in the left axillary region, but the chest X-ray was apparently normal. She had a blood eosinophilia (1.05 × 10⁹/l; normal < 0.4 × 10⁹/l). The total serum IgE was 325 IU/ml (normal <125 IU/ml). Skin tests showed immediate (type I) hypersensitivity to cat fur, grass pollen and Aspergillus fumigatus. Her serum also contained strong precipitating antibodies ('precipitins') to this mould. At bronchoscopy, the left lingular bronchus was plugged with golden, tenacious mucus. This was aspirated and sent for culture; Aspergillus fumigatus was subsequently grown. Her allergic bronchopulmonary aspergillosis was treated with itraconazole and a 10-day course of oral corticosteroids. She has subsequently remained symptom free on a low-dose steroid inhaler and the antifungal agent in the spore season (September–December).

bronchoscopy is required to remove them. Systemic steroids may be needed to suppress the inflammatory and immunological response to A. fumigatus; they cause rapid clearance of shadows and reduce the rate of recurrence. Antifungal therapies, particularly the newer ones, are used to speed recovery and reduce the risk of relapse, though as yet no inhalable formulation of antifungal therapy is available to enable local treatment of aspergillosis. Several case reports have shown promising results when the anti-IgE monoclonal antibody omalizumab is used alongside systemic steroid therapy.

Pneumonic eosinophilias, which are not associated with asthma, are of gradual onset and characterized by lassitude, night cough, shortness of breath and chest X-ray shadowing. With this insidious onset, many cases do not present until irreversible pulmonary fibrosis is established. There are several causes, but globally helminth infection is the most common cause (Fig. 13.7). A Th2 response against the parasitic worm drives the development of eosinophilia, with IL-5 playing a central role in eosinophil production. There are two major patterns of pneumonic eosinophilia associated with parasitic infection: first, an acute form, which occurs soon after infection as helminths migrate through the lung – this is known as **Loefler's syndrome**. Second, a more chronic syndrome known as **tropical pulmonary eosinophilia**. This occurs in filariasis, presents insidiously and may lead to pulmonary fibrosis. The serum IgE level is raised in those with parasitic eosinophilic pneumonia, and specific IgE against the infecting helminth may be present.

Acute and chronic **idiopathic eosinophilic pneumonia** may occur in the absence of any triggering infection or other external trigger. Treatment is with corticosteroids (Fig. 13.8).

In the rare **hypereosinophilic syndrome**, eosinophilic infiltration of tissues seems uncontrolled and occurs without evidence of preceding inflammation or allergy. Men aged 20–50 years are affected predominantly, and tissue damage is most obvious in the heart (producing a cardiomyopathy) and in the central nervous system. The eosinophil proliferation is usually polyclonal, although eosinophilic leukaemia can sometimes develop. In some cases, a clonal proliferation of Th2 cells may cause hypereosinophilia.

13.4.2 Extrinsic allergic alveolitis

Extrinsic allergic alveolitis (EAA) results from immune reactions in the alveoli to a variety of inhaled organic **materials** (Table 13.6). In the USA, the condition is known as 'hypersensitivity pneumonitis'. The clinical presentation may be acute, subacute or chronic. Patients exposed to high concentrations of the inhaled antigen usually present with acute disease (as in Case 13.5), whereas those who are chronically exposed to relatively small doses of antigen over a prolonged period are more likely to develop insidious disease (Case 13.6). In the UK, the commonest cause of EAA is budgerigar fanciers' lung; in the USA, humidifier lung.

Early **histological** lesions show a mononuclear cell infiltration in the alveoli. This often proceeds to granuloma formation

Table 13.6 Common antigens involved in some varieties of extrinsic allergic alveolitis*

Antigen	Source	Disease
Microorganisms		
Micropolyspora faeni	Mouldy hay	Farmers' lung
Thermactinomyces candidus	Contaminated humidifiers	Humidifier lung
Thermactinomyces sacchari	Mouldy sugar cane	Bagassosis
Aspergillus clavatus	Mouldy barley	Malt workers' lung
Animal proteins		
Pigeon serum proteins	Pigeon droppings	Pigeon breeders' disease
Budgerigar or parrot serum proteins	Budgerigar or parrot droppings	Bird fanciers' lung
Chicken proteins	Chicken droppings and urine	Feather pluckers' disease
Rat serum proteins	Rat urine	Rodent handlers' lung

* This list is not intended to be exhaustive: there are many other examples.

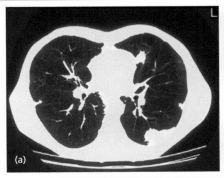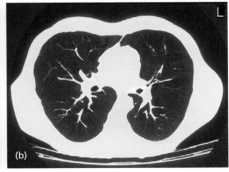

Fig. 13.8 High-resolution computed tomography scans of the lungs of a patient with chronic eosinophilic pneumonia. (a) Scan on the left shows patchy ground-glass shadowing indicating active disease. (b) Scan on the right taken 3 months later after corticosteroid treatment shows resolution of most of the changes.

Case 13.5   Extrinsic allergic alveolitis: farmers' lung

A 36-year-old farmer was admitted as an emergency with headache, fever, shortness of breath, a non-productive cough and myalgia. These symptoms came on suddenly. He had no features of upper respiratory tract infection, although he had had similar symptoms 3 weeks previously and had been treated with antibiotics. On examination, he had a tachycardia of 120/min, a temperature of 38 °C and bilateral widespread crepitations. His chest X-ray showed faint mottling in the middle and lower zones of both lung fields, but no hilar enlargement. He had a high white cell count (15 × 10⁹/l). A Mantoux test was negative. Lung function studies showed a restrictive defect.

His serum contained precipitating antibodies (see Chapter 19) to Micropolyspora faeni and Aspergillus fumigatus. The probable diagnosis was farmers' lung, a variety of extrinsic allergic alveolitis caused by hypersensitivity to antigens found in mouldy hay. In retrospect, his earlier bronchial 'infection' was almost certainly a similar episode. His symptoms and X-ray changes gradually improved, although he continued to have exertional dyspnoea for 3 weeks. This man depended on his farm for his livelihood and was therefore reluctant to consider changing his job. He was strongly advised to dry his hay before storage or to let someone else handle the hay! Six weeks after discharge, he returned with acute symptoms after feeding hay to his cattle. He had had no immediate shortness of breath, but 5 h later had again experienced acute fever, malaise, shortness of breath, a cough and myalgia. This episode convinced him that there was a relationship between hay and his illness; his wife has fed the animals and handled the hay for the last 6 years and the patient (and his wife!) have remained well.

 Case 13.6   Extrinsic allergic alveolitis: bird fanciers' lung

A 41-year-old woman presented with gradual weight loss, lethargy and breathlessness on exertion of 4 months' duration, with intermittent mild wheezing and a cough. She was a non-smoker who bred budgerigars as a hobby. On examination, there were scattered crepitations throughout both lung fields, but finger clubbing was absent. On investigation, she had a normal haemoglobin, white cell count and C-reactive protein (CRP). A chest X-ray showed a diffuse, generalized haziness in both lower zones, but pulmonary function tests were normal. A Mantoux test was negative. Precipitating antibodies to budgerigar antigens were present in her serum.

A laboratory diagnosis of extrinsic allergic alveolitis due to hypersensitivity to budgerigar serum proteins (bird fanciers' lung) was made. The patient gave away her birds, and her symptoms regressed over a few months. Eight years later, her serum still contains antibodies to budgerigar serum proteins, but she is asymptomatic – and birdless.

with surrounding infiltration by macrophages, plasma cells and CD8⁺ T lymphocytes. *EAA is therefore a differential diagnosis in any granulomatous or infiltrative condition of the lungs.* In the subacute stage, obliterative bronchiolitis may also be present and permanent lung damage due to interstitial fibrosis may occur after repeated exposure. The precise **pathogenesis** is unclear, but immunofluorescent studies of lung biopsies during the early stages have shown deposits of antigen, IgG, IgM, IgA and C3 in the lesions, consistent with an immune complex–mediated (type III) mechanism. Activated T cells (both CD4⁺ and CD8⁺) are also present and it seems likely that type IV hypersensitivity is involved, particularly in cases with granuloma formation and fibrosis.

The clinical features of **acute EAA** often resemble infection (as in Case 13.5) and this possibility should be considered in all patients who present with an 'acute atypical pneumonia'. Systemic symptoms are typical and occur about 6 h or more after exposure to the dust. The attacks can subside rapidly, but recur on further exposure. In many cases, the causal agent may not be appreciated. It is only by careful charting of the relationship between jobs and symptoms that work-related hypersensitivities are suspected. **Chronic EAA** is more common and

often presents with gradual exertional dyspnoea and a dry cough, accompanied by anorexia, weight loss and malaise. It is seen most commonly with low but near-continuous exposure, for instance where a single caged bird is responsible. Interstitial diffuse pulmonary fibrosis may have already developed in these patients at the time of presentation. Management is focused on avoidance of the triggering antigen. However, systemic steroids are often used in severe cases.

13.4.3 Idiopathic interstitial pneumonias

The **idiopathic interstitial pneumonias** (IIPs) are a group of disorders characterized by varying degrees of inflammation and fibrosis of the lung interstitium (i.e. between the epithelial and endothelial basement membranes). The classification of these conditions is becoming increasingly complex and there is little international consensus.

They are diagnoses of exclusion, made only when EAA and other causes of pulmonary fibrosis (see Table 13.5) have been ruled out. The IIPs are often considered as autoimmune disorders, although the evidence for autoimmunity is largely circumstantial (Table 13.7). There are several distinct patterns of

Table 13.7 Evidence that the idiopathic interstitial pneumonias (IIPs) may be immunological disorders

Association with autoimmune diseases

All patterns of IIP may occur in rheumatoid arthritis and systemic sclerosis

Circulating autoantibodies

50% of patients have:

Antinuclear antibodies (but no significant dsDNA binding)

Rheumatoid factor (often low titre)

Bronchoalveolar fluid may contain

Lymphocytes (up to 15%)

Macrophages – often 'activated' and containing ingested 'immune complexes'

Histology

Lymphocytic infiltration involving $CD4^+$ > $CD8^+$ T cells

Expression of major histocompatibility complex class II antigens on alveolar epithelial cells

Immunoglobulin and complement deposition in early stages only

IIP (Table 13.8). All present with a similar clinical picture of progressive exertional breathlessness and dry cough, with the commonest age of onset being 40–50 years. Examination reveals widespread inspiratory fine crackles, and clubbing is often present. The various forms of IIP are defined histologically and **biopsy is the best way to make a definitive diagnosis**. Making a correct diagnosis is critical, since the response to therapy and prognosis vary enormously. The various types of IIP can also be distinguished on high-resolution computed tomography (HRCT) scanning, although this is less reliable than histology. One of the most important prognostic features on HRCT is **'ground-glass' shadowing**, the presence of which may predict a response to corticosteroids.

The **aetiology** of the IIPs is unclear. Genetic factors do not appear to make a major contribution, as these conditions do not seem to run in families. The risk of IIP is increased two- to fivefold by exposure to environmental factors that may injure the lung, such as smoking and occupational exposure to wood, stone and metal dusts, and there is some evidence that infection (for example, Epstein–Barr virus) may act as a trigger. Two rarer forms of IIP, desquamative interstitial pneumonia and respiratory bronchiolitis with interstitial lung disease, occur almost exclusively in smokers, and improve with smoking cessation.

Idiopathic pulmonary fibrosis (IPF), sometimes called cryptogenic fibrosing alveolitis in the UK, is the most common and serious of the IIPs, with a prevalence in the UK of around 1 in 5000 adults (Case 13.7). The presentation is usually with insidiously progressive breathlessness. The mean survival following diagnosis is very poor at 3–5 years. HRCT typically shows patchy, peripheral basal fibrosis *with no ground-glass shadowing*. **Histology** shows damaged alveoli and patchy fibrosis, becoming more extensive and developing a 'honeycomb' appearance as the disease progresses. There is some evidence that the underlying process is due to inadequate autophagy. Autophagy is a process that helps maintain homeostatic balance between the synthesis, degradation and recycling of organelles and proteins. The importance of this function in mammals is being unravelled slowly and may well play a part in conditions resulting in **fibrosis without preceding inflammation**.

Given the lack of inflammation, it is perhaps not surprising that **IPF should show little or no response to conventional immunosuppression**. Nevertheless, given the bleak prognosis, patients with IPF are often subjected to a period of

Table 13.8 Epidemiology, histology, treatment and outcome in the idiopathic interstitial pneumonias

	Relative frequency, %	Histology	Response to immunosuppression	Outcome
Idiopathic pulmonary fibrosis	55	Fibrosis	Minimal	50–70% mortality at 5 years
Non-specific interstitial pneumonia	25	Cellular infiltrate with some fibrosis	Reasonable (better if less fibrosis on biopsy)	Reasonable. 10% mortality at 5 years
Smoking-associated interstitial pneumonia	15	Mainly cellular infiltrate, little fibrosis	Usually good (key intervention is smoking cessation)	Good with treatment
Cryptogenic organizing pneumonia	3	Mainly cellular infiltrate, little fibrosis	Good	Good with treatment
Lymphocytic organizing pneumonia	<1	Mainly cellular infiltrate, little fibrosis	Good	Good with treatment
Acute interstitial pneumonia	<1	Fibrosis	Poor	>50% mortality. Survivors may recover completely

Case 13.7   Idiopathic pulmonary fibrosis

A 57-year-old man complained of malaise, anorexia and increasing exertional breathlessness for 4 months. When pressed, he admitted that the dyspnoea had been present for 2 years, but he had attributed this to smoking 30 cigarettes a day. He had been treated for two episodes of 'bronchitis' in the preceding winter. On examination, he had finger clubbing and widespread crepitations in his chest, but no arthropathy, cyanosis or skin lesions. Investigations showed a normal haemoglobin, C-reactive protein (CRP) and white cell count, but a raised erythrocyte sedimentation rate (ESR: 80 mm/h).

All serum immunoglobulin levels were raised; IgG was 24 g/l (NR 6.8–19.0), IgA 9.7 g/l (NR 0.8–5.0) and IgM 12.0 g/l (NR 0.5–2.0). No paraprotein was detected. His serum contained antinuclear antibodies (titre 1/160) and rheumatoid factor (titre 1/64). A chest X-ray showed diffuse fine shadowing throughout both lung fields, especially in the lower zones, consistent with diffuse pulmonary fibrosis. A high-resolution computed tomography (HRCT) scan showed extensive established fibrosis with no evidence of ground-glass shadowing (Fig. 13.9). This was supported by results of lung function tests. A video-assisted thorascopic lung biopsy showed extensive non-uniform fibrosis and minimal inflammation. Since no other cause was found, a diagnosis of idiopathic pulmonary fibrosis was made. The histology, CT findings and the rapid clinical progression suggested a poor prognosis. A trial of oral corticosteroids, ciclosporin and azathioprine had no beneficial effect. He was referred for lung transplantation, but died from respiratory failure before a suitable organ became available. If this patient had presented nowadays, a trial with one of the novel tyrosine kinase inhibitors would probably have been commenced.

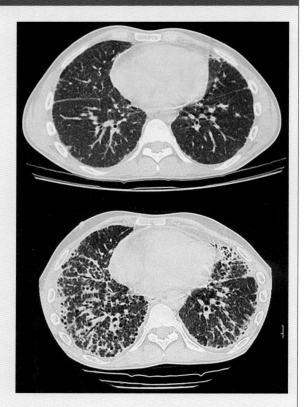

Fig. 13.9 High-resolution computed tomography scan showing (top) established fibrosis at diagnosis with relentless progression over 1 year despite aggressive immunosuppressive therapy (bottom).

intense immunosuppression with high-dose corticosteroids and drugs such as azathioprine. *If a good response occurs, this may indicate that the diagnosis of IPF is wrong* and the patient has a more treatable disorder such as non-specific interstitial pneumonia.

In Europe and Asia, a milestone has recently been reached with the licensing of the first IPF-specific drug, pirfenidone. *In vitro* pirfenidone **inhibits TGF-β–stimulated collagen synthesis**, decreases synthesis by fibroblasts of extracellular matrix proteins, and blocks the proliferative effects of platelet-derived growth factor (PDGF) on fibroblasts isolated from IPF lung. A Cochrane review of clinical trials has shown improved progression-free survival. More recently, the triple tyrosine kinase inhibitor nintedanib, targeted at the PDGF receptor, fibroblast growth factor (FGF) receptor and vascular endothelial growth factor (VEGF) receptor, was shown to be effective in IPF and in patients with systemic autoimmune diseases complicated by pulmonary fibrosis, including systemic sclerosis. **Single-lung transplantation** is now an effective treatment in selected patients with relentlessly progressive disease. Patients receiving a transplant are 75% less likely to die than equivalent

patients on the transplant waiting list. The disease does not recur in the transplanted lung.

Non-specific interstitial pneumonia (NSIP) accounts for around a quarter of patients with IIP and is a more benign, treatment-responsive disorder than IPF (Table 13.8). This responsiveness to immunosuppressive drugs correlates with significant inflammatory changes on biopsy, and the presence of ground-glass shadowing on HRCT. Although the overall prognosis of NSIP is much better than that of IPF, there is considerable heterogeneity in outcome: histologically, more fibrosis and less inflammation signifies a poorer prognosis. NSIP is the pattern of IIP most strongly associated with connective tissue disease.

13.5 Connective tissue disease and the lung

Systemic autoimmune diseases frequently involve all parts of the respiratory system: pleura, airways, lung parenchyma and pulmonary vessels (Table 13.9). Although lung disease causes symptoms in a significant minority of these patients, subclinical

Table 13.9 Patterns of lung disease in the major connective tissue diseases

	Rheumatoid arthritis	SLE	Myositis	Systemic sclerosis
Pleural disease	Common	Common	No	Rare
Interstitial lung disease	Yes – NSIP and IPF pattern	Rare	Yes – NSIP and IPF pattern	Yes – usually IPF pattern
Isolated pulmonary hypertension	No	No	No	Yes
Intrapulmonary nodules	Common	No	No	No
Respiratory muscle weakness	No	Yes – usually diaphragm	Yes	No
Vasculitis/pulmonary haemorrhage	No	Yes but rare	No	No

IPF, idiopathic pulmonary fibrosis; NSIP, non-specific interstitial pneumonia; SLE, systemic lupus erythematosus.

pleural disease and/or mild pulmonary fibrosis are present in more than 50% of patients with rheumatoid arthritis (RA). Although NSIP and IPF are the two most common patterns of interstitial lung disease in systemic autoimmune disorders, all forms of IIP can occur. The response to treatment and prognosis mirrors, in general, that seen in IIP occurring in isolation. 'Isolated' pulmonary hypertension (that is, not secondary to interstitial lung disease or pulmonary thromboembolism) occurs particularly in limited systemic sclerosis (see Chapter 11). Lung disease secondary to treatment of systemic autoimmune diseases is also common. Infection may complicate all forms of immunosuppressive treatment, with the pattern of infection reflecting the nature of the immunosuppressive drug: for example, bacterial, viral and Pneumocystis infection with the T and B cell–suppressing drug cyclophosphamide, tuberculosis with anti-TNF agents. *Methotrexate, the most commonly used drug for the treatment of RA, can cause interstitial lung disease, usually with a picture resembling NSIP.*

13.6 Pulmonary vasculitis

The lungs are a major site of involvement in systemic vasculitis, reflecting the highly vascular nature of the pulmonary bed. Pulmonary vasculitic syndromes often produce alveolar inflammation (particularly when the vasculitis involves small blood vessels at the alveolar level) and can cause pulmonary fibrosis.

The most devastating form of pulmonary vasculitis involves small vessels at the alveolar level and presents with diffuse and often overwhelming **pulmonary haemorrhage**. This life-threatening emergency occurs particularly in **Goodpasture's syndrome**, **microscopic polyarteritis** and occasionally in **systemic lupus erythematosus** (SLE). Pulmonary haemorrhage usually occurs in parallel with rapidly progressive glomerulonephritis (reflecting small-vessel involvement in the kidney). These disorders are discussed in more detail in Chapter 9. In the granulomatous vasculitides, granulomatosis with polyangi-

itis (GPA) and EGPA, the respiratory tract is a major target organ; these disorders are discussed in section 13.6.1.

13.6.1 Granulomatosis with polyangiitis (previously Wegener's)

The characteristic feature of this condition is a **necrotizing granulomatous vasculitis**. It is one of many forms of vasculitis involving the lung.

Although most patients have pulmonary involvement, this can be asymptomatic; multiple nodules are sometimes seen on HRCT scan taken for other reasons. The clinical features can be divided into those caused by local granuloma formation (such as the changes in the lungs, the paranasal sinuses and the nasopharynx) and those due to vasculitis in other organs (namely glomerulonephritis, keratoconjunctivitis/episcleritis, polyarthralgia and cutaneous vasculitis) (Fig. 13.10).

The **diagnosis** of GPA depends on the clinical features and histopathological identification of the typical necrotizing vasculitis and granuloma. Nasal mucosa is easily biopsied, but occasionally open lung biopsy is required. A renal biopsy should be performed if there is evidence of kidney involvement. Antibodies directed against a neutrophil cytoplasmic antigen (cANCA, see Chapter 19) are found in over 90% of patients with active GPA and in about 40% of patients in remission. cANCA in GPA usually have specificity for a cytoplasmic enzyme called proteinase 3 (PR3). The finding of ANCA in sputum and BAL fluid suggests that these antibodies are produced in the respiratory tract of such patients. ANCA antibodies and raised C-reactive protein (CRP) levels are helpful in diagnosis and assessment of disease activity.

Untreated GPA is rapidly fatal, with a mean survival of 5 months and a 5-year survival of <10%. The treatment of choice was prednisolone plus cyclophosphamide, for which the remission rate was approximately 90%, and about 50% of patients sustained this remission for over 5 years. Now rituximab

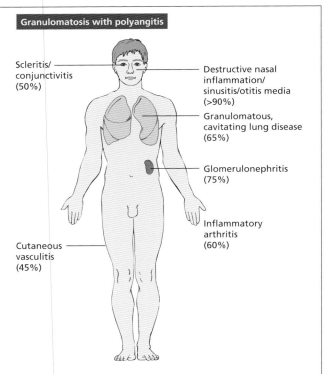

Fig. 13.10 Major clinical features of granulomatosis with polyangiitis.

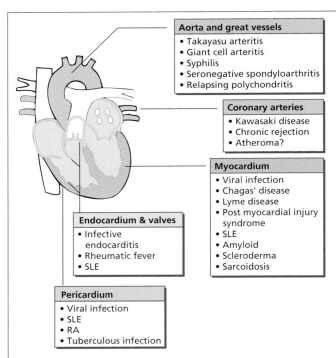

Fig. 13.11 Immunological diseases affecting the heart and great vessels. RA, rheumatoid arthritis; SLE, systemic lupus erythematosus.

has been shown to be a safe alternative to cyclosphosphamide and is used for remission induction in patients presenting with severe disease flares; it has become the standard care for patients with chronically relapsing or refractory GPA.

EGPA refers to a related but rare multisystem disorder in young adults with a diagnostic triad of asthma and systemic vasculitis associated with marked peripheral eosinophilia. ANCA reactivity is found less frequently and is of less diagnostic value. Without treatment, the mortality of EGPA may be as high as 50% within 3 months of diagnosis. Fortunately, the condition usually responds well to corticosteroid therapy and there are reports on the beneficial use of rituximab and anti-IL5 agents in EGPA.

13.7 Cardiac disease

Immunological disease processes involving the heart and great vessels can be classified according to either their cause or the anatomical structures involved (Fig. 13.11). Some disorders selectively involve one tissue within the heart, whereas others can involve all structures, i.e. **pancarditis** (e.g. in rheumatic fever or SLE).

13.7.1 Pericarditis

Inflammation of the pericardium presents primarily with pain, but sometimes with the haemodynamic consequences of a pericardial effusion or pericardial fibrosis. The pericardium is structurally very similar to the pleura and *these two tissues are often involved by the same disease processes (e.g. in RA and SLE)*. Chronic inflammation of the pericardium can be asymptomatic: over 40% of patients with RA have evidence of pericardial disease at post mortem, but symptomatic pericarditis occurs in less than 10% during life.

13.7.2 Myocarditis

Myocardial inflammation presents primarily with heart failure or disruption of the cardiac rhythm due to damage to the conducting system. Worldwide, the most important immunological disease process affecting the myocardium is **Chagas' disease**, caused by Trypanosoma cruzi.

Although autoimmune mechanisms lead to myocardial involvement in rheumatic fever, bacterial infection hardly ever causes myocardial disease directly, with the notable exception of the carditis associated with **Lyme disease**, due to direct invasion of the myocardium by the spirochaete Borrelia burgdorferi. Recognition of this condition is important, as there is an excellent response to antibiotics.

Viral infection may also cause myocarditis, particularly viruses that have a tropism for muscle such as the Coxsackie family. This is usually transient. The involvement of viruses in the most common form of chronic myocardial disease, dilated cardiomyopathy, is less certain. Plausible hypotheses and animal models have been developed implicating viral infection in triggering a chronic T cell–mediated autoimmune process directed against myocardial antigens. However, evidence that this mechanism plays a role in most patients with dilated cardiomyopathy is lacking.

Autoimmune processes have a more clearly defined role in the post-myocardial injury syndromes (e.g. Dressler's syndrome), which may occur 1–2 weeks after cardiac surgery or myocardial infarction. An autoimmune response occurs to sequestered cardiac antigens released as a result of cardiac damage (analogous to the development of sympathetic ophthalmia after eye injuries, Chapter 12), though this is rare nowadays.

13.7.3 Endocarditis

Endocardial inflammation presents principally with cardiac valve dysfunction: usually valvular incompetence, but sometimes stenosis or embolism from the damaged valve. The most significant long-term consequence of **rheumatic fever** (see Chapter 2) is valve damage due to endocardial involvement. The likelihood of endocardial inflammation is greatly increased by factors that lead to endothelial damage within the heart, in particular turbulent flow around a structurally abnormal heart valve, damaged by previous rheumatic endocarditis. This endothelial damage allows antigen (including bacteria) and antibody to gain access from the circulation.

Colonization of heart valves by bacteria leads to **infective endocarditis**. This can be a devastating acute infection leading to rapid valve destruction (usually associated with infection with Staphylococcus aureus), but more often occurs in a subacute form where an antibody response against organisms of low virulence leads to a multisystem immune complex disease associated with glomerulonephritis, vasculitis and complement consumption.

13.8 Coronary artery disease

Vasculitis of the coronary arteries can occur as a rare feature of many forms of systemic vasculitis affecting medium-sized or large arteries (e.g. polyarteritis nodosa, giant cell arteritis), but occurs most notably as the most serious clinical feature of **Kawasaki's disease**. The cause of Kawasaki's disease is unknown, but there is some evidence that bacterial superantigens play a pathogenic role. Prompt treatment with aspirin and intravenous immunoglobulin abates the systemic symptoms but, more importantly, reduces morbidity and mortality from the coronary artery disease (Case 13.8).

A very different pattern of immunologically mediated coronary artery disease occurs in the recipients of heart transplants. Progressive intimal fibrosis occurs, which can occlude the coronary arteries. This process of **chronic rejection** is more likely to occur if there is substantial HLA mismatch between donor and recipient and if episodes of acute rejection have occurred. There is some evidence that CMV infection may act as a cofactor in this process. A comparable process occurs in vessels in transplanted kidneys, and there are also similarities with chronic graft-versus-host disease and scleroderma. *In all these disorders immunological mechanisms appear to lead to fibrosis without significant evidence of inflammation.* The underlying mechanisms are unknown.

The most common cause of coronary artery disease is **atherosclerosis**. Increasingly, it is understood that the pathogenesis of atherosclerosis involves inflammatory mechanisms as well as lipid accumulation and thrombosis. Lipid-laden macrophages have been shown to secrete numerous inflammatory mediators, and systemic markers of inflammation (such as CRP at very low levels) have been shown to correlate with atherosclerotic disease. It has been hypothesized that these inflammatory changes could result from an immune response against sequestered bacterial or viral antigens in the vessel wall, or an autoimmune response against lipoproteins damaged by free radicals. There is only weak evidence to support these hypotheses at present.

Although the evidence that atherosclerosis itself is an autoimmune disease is somewhat limited, there is clear evidence that *some chronic immunological diseases increase the risk of developing atherosclerosis and its consequences.* In patients with SLE, the risk of myocardial infarction may be increased as much as 50 times above that of age- and sex-matched controls.

Case 13.8 Kawasaki's disease

A 2-year-old girl became unwell and feverish. She was seen by her GP, who felt she had a chest infection and prescribed a broad-spectrum antibiotic. She remained persistently unwell over the next 2 days and was admitted to hospital. On admission she was febrile (38.2 °C), looked ill and had enlarged lymph nodes in her neck and a blotchy red rash on her limbs. Her chest was clear and ear drums normal. Systemic infection was suspected. Investigations showed a raised white cell count (24 × 10^9/l, 90% neutrophils), a platelet count of 600 × 10^9/l and a C-reactive protein (CRP) of 143 mg/l; however, a chest X-ray was clear, urine and cerebrospinal fluid (CSF) contained no cells on microscopy and subsequent blood, urine and CSF cultures were sterile. She remained unwell over the next 4 days and over this time developed marked swelling and redness of the hands and feet. Kawasaki's disease was suspected and this diagnosis was confirmed by an echocardiogram, which demonstrated aneurysms of the right and left anterior descending coronary arteries. She was treated with high-dose (2 g/kg) intravenous immunoglobulin (IVIG) and oral aspirin and her fever subsided over the next 48 h. Over the next 2 weeks she developed striking peeling of the skin over the hands and feet. A repeat echocardiogram showed that the coronary arteries had improved but localized dilation was still apparent. The best results of IVIG treatment are seen when given early in the course of disease, before aneurysms have developed. She remains under long-term cardiological follow-up.

Case 13.9 Takayasu's arteritis

A 23-year-old typist was referred to a rheumatologist with a 3-month history of cramp-like discomfort, which occurred reproducibly with any task involving the left arm. She was otherwise well, smoked five cigarettes per day and her only medication was a combined oral contraceptive. Examination revealed no abnormality in the neck or arm. A provisional diagnosis of tendonitis was made and she was treated with physiotherapy without benefit. Her erythrocyte sedimentation rate (ESR) was found to be mildly elevated at 30 mm/h (normal <10), but no cause was identified for this.

Two months later she was admitted to hospital following an episode of right-sided weakness associated with speech disturbance. She had a very mild right hemiparesis (which resolved over the next 6 h), a left-sided carotid bruit and a mild fever (37.7 °C). Her blood pressure was 165/90, taken from the right arm. Investigations included a C-reactive protein (CRP) of 31 mg/l, normal creatinine, cholesterol 4.8 mmol/l (normal <5.7), negative antinuclear antibody (ANA), antineutrophil cytoplasmic antibody (ANCA), cardiolipin antibodies, lupus anticoagulant and normal immunoglobulins. An electrocardiogram (ECG) and echocardiogram were also normal. Three days after admission she asked why the nurses had such great difficulty measuring her blood pressure in the left arm, and used the right instead. Further assessment revealed that the radial and brachial pulses were almost impalpable on the left. Doppler ultrasound studies indicated an arterial systolic pressure of 80 mmHg in the left arm. An aortogram showed long, tapering tight stenoses of the left common carotid and subclavian arteries, with less severe lesions in the left renal artery. A diagnosis of Takayasu's arteritis was made and she was treated with high-dose corticosteroids. Her ESR returned to normal and subsequent ultrasound studies showed partial resolution of the carotid and subclavian stenoses.

This increase in risk is not wholly attributable to conventional risk factors such as hypertension and serum cholesterol, or treatments such as corticosteroids. The risk seems to be higher with increased activity and severity of the underlying disease. The mechanisms are unknown, but plausible hypotheses argue that the increased production of cytokines in these disorders upregulates adhesion molecules and procoagulant factors on endothelial cells, which facilitates the process of atherogenesis.

13.9 Diseases of the great vessels

Inflammation of the aortic wall or **aortitis** can occur as a feature of a number of disorders (see Fig. 13.11). Most of these disorders affect principally the proximal aorta with a variable amount of distal disease. The consequences of aortitis are twofold: first, aortic dilation and even aneurysm formation may occur, leading to stretching and incompetence of the aortic valve, and more rarely aortic rupture or dissection. Second, stenotic lesions may develop in the branches of the aorta, either at their junction with the aorta or more diffusely along the length of the branching vessels.

Takayasu's disease is a granulomatous vasculitis of the aorta and its branches, usually occurring under the age of 40 years and more commonly in women (Case 13.9). It presents with the consequences of occlusion or stenosis of the aortic branches: neurological symptoms, vascular insufficiency in the arms, hypertension due to renal artery stenosis and features of systemic illness including fever, malaise, weight loss, arthralgia and myalgia. CRP and erythrocyte sedimentation rate (ESR) are typically elevated, but blood tests are of no specific help in making the diagnosis, which is often delayed. Aortography and magnetic resonance imaging can be used to confirm the diagnosis. The response to steroids is often reasonable, but surgery or angioplasty may be required where structural changes do not respond to immunosuppression.

CHAPTER 14
Gastrointestinal and Liver Diseases

Key topics

Visit the companion website at **www.wiley.com/go/misbah/immunology** to download cases with additional figures on these topics.

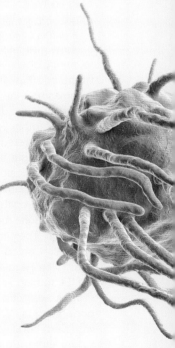

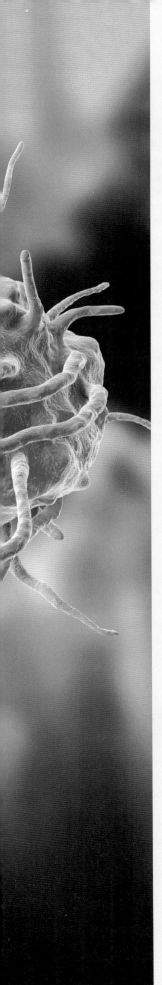

Chapel and Haeney's Essentials of Clinical Immunology, Seventh Edition. Edited by Siraj A. Misbah, Gavin P. Spickett, and Virgil A.S.H. Dalm.
© 2022 John Wiley & Sons Ltd. Published 2022 by John Wiley & Sons Ltd.

14.1 Introduction

14.1.1 Normal immune mechanisms

The gastrointestinal tract is the largest immunological organ in the body. Over 90% of the exposure of the human body to microorganisms occurs at the mucosal surface of the gastrointestinal tract and over 400 bacterial species inhabit the average human gut. The gut is protected by several **non-specific mechanisms** (Fig. 14.1). Epithelial cells form an important physical barrier via their intercellular tight junctions and turn over rapidly (every 24–96 h). Any injury to the epithelial barrier results in rapid migration of adjacent viable epithelial cells to cover the denuded area, a process called 'restitution', while lymphocytes and macrophages migrate out through pores in the basement membrane to provide temporary host protection. The acid pH of the stomach is a formidable chemical barrier to many organisms and bacterial overgrowth is a consequent complication in patients with achlorhydria due to atrophic gastritis. Any change in the normal microflora of the intestine also allows pathogenic bacteria to flourish: an example is pseudomembranous colitis caused by the toxin-producing bacterium Clostridium difficile in patients given certain antibiotics.

Mucosal immune responses involve the gut-associated lymphoid tissue (GALT). Lymphocytes are found at three sites within the mucosa (Fig. 14.2 and Box 14.1).

GALT is divided into two functional compartments: an afferent arm – Peyer's patches – where interaction occurs between luminal antigen and the immune system; and an effector arm – the diffusely distributed intraepithelial and lamina propria lymphocytes.

Peyer's patches are covered by specialized epithelium (follicle-associated epithelium). Some of these epithelial cells have surfaces that seem folded under the scanning electron microscope (Fig. 14.3). These microfold, or M, cells sample and actively transport particulate antigens from the lumen into the 'dome' area, where priming of both T and B lymphocytes occurs. Within Peyer's patches are specialized T cells that induce antigen-activated IgM-bearing B lymphocytes to switch isotype to IgA, as well as immature IgA+ cells that are probably independent of T cells.

Primed B lymphoblasts, committed mainly to producing IgA class antibody, migrate from Peyer's patches, via the lymphatics and mesenteric lymph nodes, to the thoracic duct and hence into the circulation (Fig. 14.2). These cells return preferentially to the lamina propria, a process called 'homing'. Once back in the gut, they mature into IgA plasma cells and are responsible for local and secretory immune defences. The number of IgA-producing cells in the lamina propria far exceeds the numbers producing IgM, IgG or IgE.

The IgA coating the epithelium is specially adapted for its function. IgA plasma cells produce monomeric IgA, which is converted into a dimer by a smaller 'joining' peptide (J chain), also produced by the plasma cells. The polymeric immunoglobulin receptor is synthesized by epithelial cells and is essential for transport of **secretory IgA** into the lumen of the gut (Fig. 14.4). The receptor binds the dimeric IgA, the complex is endocytosed and transported through the cytoplasm to the luminal surface of the cell, where proteolysis of the polymeric Ig receptor occurs. As a result, the IgA dimer is released into the gut attached to a 70-kDa proteolytic fragment of the receptor, called the secretory component. Secretory component stabilizes the secretory IgA molecule and protects it from proteolytic attack by enzymes in the gut. Secreted dimeric IgA neutralizes viruses, bacteria and toxins, prevents the adherence of pathogenic microorganisms to gut epithelium and so blocks the uptake of antigen into the systemic immune system – a role termed 'immune exclusion'.

There is a similar **migration pathway for T lymphocytes** whereby activated T cells from mesenteric nodes 'home' both to the epithelium and to the lamina propria. **Intraepithelial lymphocytes** (IELs) express both non-rearranged innate immune receptors and rearranged adaptive immune receptors and have been conserved throughout vertebrate evolution. Their importance is underlined by the fact that they populate the gut before birth, unlike conventional T cells. Peripheral blood T cells rarely express the human mucosal lymphocyte antigen 1 (HML-1), but nearly all IELs do (Fig. 14.5). HML-1 (CD103) is an adhesion molecule of the β_7-integrin family. It is important in the homing of IEL, allowing IEL to bind via HML-1 to its ligand, E-cadherin, expressed on epithelial cells.

IELs are not a homogeneous population: they comprise at least **three different T-cell phenotypes**. The major population is CD8+ and shows increased expression of the γ/δ form of the T-cell receptor (TCR) when compared with peripheral lymphocytes. In contrast to the epidermis, where TCR-$\gamma\delta$ T cells are the sole population of lymphocytes, there are also TCR-$\alpha\beta$ T cells in the respiratory and intestinal tracts; the third subset expresses neither

CD4 nor CD8 and is not found elsewhere in lymphoid organs. IELs of the $\gamma\delta$ T-cell type have limited TCR diversity, but are able to respond immediately, in a manner similar to innate cells, avoiding a priming step before secreting cytokines.

Some IELs are cytotoxic and some have natural killer (NK) cell activity, functions important in the control of gut viruses, particularly enteroviruses. IELs also seem to have a role in controlling epithelial cell barrier function, i.e. 'restitution'.

Large numbers of lymphocytes, NK cells, mast cells, macrophages and plasma cells are seen in the **lamina propria**. T and B lymphocytes are both found, but T cells predominate in a ratio of about four to one. These T cells do not proliferate well after stimulation of the TCR, yet produce large amounts of the cytokines interleukin (IL)-2, IL-4, interferon (IFN)-γ and tumour necrosis factor (TNF)-α. Such lymphocytes express at least two molecules essential for homing to the gut: $\alpha_4\beta_7$ integrin and the chemokine receptor CCR9. MAdCAM-1 (see Chapter 1, section 1.2.5). The ligand for $\alpha_4\beta_7$ is expressed widely in gut mucosal vessels and is the predominant adhesion molecule in the intestinal lamina propria.

Many similarities exist between the mucosal lymphoid tissues of the gut and organs such as the bronchus, breasts, salivary glands and uterine cervix. Lymphoblasts from any of these sites will repopulate all mucosa-associated lymphoid tissue in irradiated animals, with a selective preference for the organ of origin. If antigen is fed to lactating females, specific IgA antibodies appear in the milk, and gut-derived lymphoblasts home to breast tissue, lungs and parotid glands as well as back to the gut. There is evidence, therefore, of a **common mucosal immune system as well as site-specific lymphocyte homing**. This has at least one important implication: it may eventually prove possible to provide immune protection at one mucosal site by immunization at another.

14.1.2 Spectrum of the intestinal immune response

Ingestion of antigens can lead to a local or systemic immune response, or oral tolerance (specific immune unresponsiveness).

The gut can mount a **local immune response** to an antigen independent of a systemic response. For example, immunization against poliomyelitis with oral attenuated Sabin vaccine typically gives better protection than the injected killed Salk vaccine, even though both induce serum antibodies of IgG and IgA class. Local IgA antibody, produced in response to the oral vaccine, partly blocks uptake of pathogenic virus into the circulation. However, the disadvantage of the oral vaccine was that the attenuated (but still living) virus can revert to wild type and cause poliomyelitis in immunocompromised recipients, so this is no longer used in the World Health Organization (WHO) programme to eradicate poliomyelitis worldwide.

A range of macromolecules and particles are absorbed by the intestine into the portal or systemic circulations, via either the glandular epithelium covering the villus or the specialized M cells. Up to 2% of a dietary protein load can appear antigenically intact in the circulation. Sinusoidal phagocytes (Kupffer cells) of the liver destroy much of the antigen, but enough passes through the liver to stimulate **systemic antibody production**, particularly in the spleen. Antibody formed in the spleen goes directly into the portal circulation to complex with incoming antigen. Circulating immune complexes of IgA with dietary antigens are regularly found in normal people after meals.

A unique feature of the mucosal immune system is its ability to downregulate immune responses to dietary antigens – **oral tolerance**. In animal models, oral feeding of an antigen followed by systemic antigenic challenge results in marked reduction of antibody levels and cell-mediated immunity compared with animals not fed the antigen first. This has led to attempts to treat autoimmune diseases in humans by feeding autoantigens to patients (see Chapters 5 and 7).

Normally the intestinal immune system steers a delicate course between the undesirable extremes (Table 14.1) of immune incompetence, with resulting vulnerability to ingested pathogens (e.g. infective diarrhoea due to other non-pathogenic bacteria) and hypersensitivity, with damage each time the relevant antigen is eaten (e.g. coeliac disease). **Beneficial homeostasis is achieved by IELs** responding to epithelial stress signals to maintain the balance of the intestinal bacterial load and IELs are directly involved in epithelial cell growth and repair. Most of the data are obtained from mouse studies and supported by observations in humans, but experimental data on human tissue are being developed and initial studies show similar results.

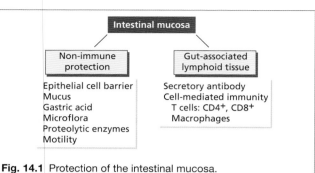

Fig. 14.1 Protection of the intestinal mucosa.

Box 14.1 Sites of lymphocytes in the gut

- Organized lymphoid aggregates (Peyer's patches) beneath the epithelium of the terminal small intestine
- Lymphocytes within the epithelial cell layer (intraepithelial lymphocytes)
- Lymphocytes scattered, with other immunocompetent cells, within the lamina propria

Fig. 14.2 Organization and structure of gut-associated lymphoid tissue (GALT).

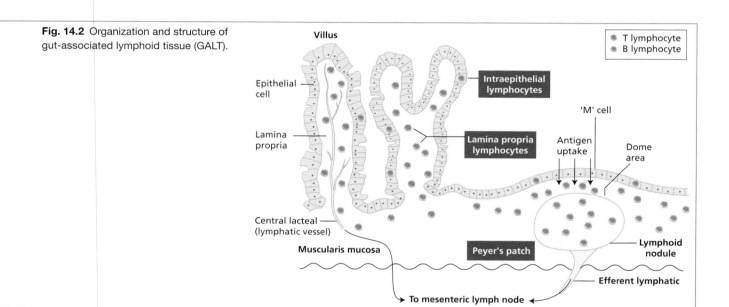

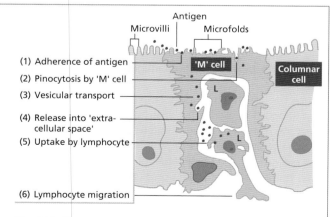

Fig. 14.3 The stages involved in the transport of antigen by the M cell from the intestinal lumen into the extracellular space, where it is taken up by dendritic cells and T lymphocytes (L).

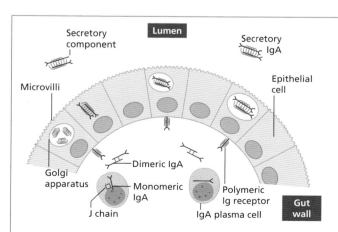

Fig. 14.4 Synthesis and transport of secretory IgA through the gut epithelial cells into the gut lumen.

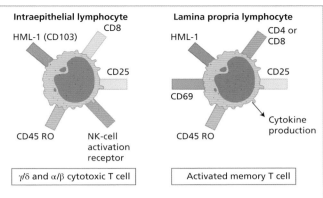

Fig. 14.5 Typical phenotypes of gut lymphocytes. CD25, activation marker; CD45 RO, memory cell marker; CD69, activation marker; NK, natural killer.

Table 14.1 Some examples of immunological involvement in intestinal disease

1 Infection with virulent organism	Gastroenteritis (e.g. Campylobacter, Salmonella)
2 Immunodeficiency, e.g. primary or secondary	Chronic infection with enteropathogens (enteric bacteria and parasites [Giardia, Cryptosporidium] enteroviruses, including Norovirus); nodular lymphoid hyperplasia, lymphoma
3 Autoimmunity, e.g. gastric atrophy	Pernicious anaemia
4 Hypersensitivity to dietary antigen	Coeliac disease
	Food allergy
	Eosinophilic enteritis

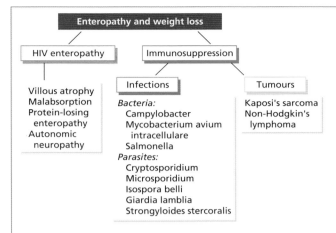

Fig. 14.6 Gastrointestinal manifestations of human immunodeficiency virus (HIV) infection.

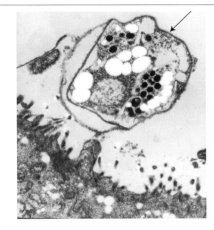

Fig. 14.7 Scanning electron micrograph of Cryptosporidial infestation (arrowed) of the intestine.

14.2 Infection and the gut

Infections of the gastrointestinal tract range from infectious diarrhoea that can be life threatening, especially in immunodeficient children and elderly people with co-morbidities, to mild food poisoning in otherwise healthy individuals. In addition, systemic viruses can cause gastrointestinal lesions as well as enteropathogens.

An important example is the involvement of the intestinal tract in human immunodeficiency virus (HIV) infection. About half of all patients with **HIV infection have gastrointestinal involvement** that causes serious morbidity. Diarrhoea, malabsorption and weight loss are the most common manifestations and, in Africa, this wasting syndrome is called 'slim disease'. HIV infects lymphocytes and macrophages within the gut as well as the intestinal cells. Impairment of the intestinal immune response, with consequent chronic infection with enteropathogens and the development of intestinal tumours such as lymphoma or Kaposi's sarcoma (Fig. 14.6), adds to the considerable morbidity. The principal change in the small intestine is a partial villous atrophy detectable early in the natural history of HIV infection. Breastfeeding may transmit HIV in humans, suggesting that the intestine is an important portal of entry for HIV. Enteropathogens causing intestinal infections in HIV patients are of the same types as in immunocompetent subjects (Fig. 14.7), but the clinical symptoms produced by these infections are chronic, lasting for the duration of the patient's life. Treatment of the bacterial infections remains a major problem, since some of the organisms (such as Cryptosporidia) cannot be eradicated by available antibiotics. Furthermore, viral causes (such as rotavirus) are important too.

Gut infections in otherwise healthy individuals are usually **self-limiting** unless the pathogen, such as Salmonella, is particularly virulent. However, in children with T-cell defects (such as severe combined immunodeficiency) or particular susceptibility to given organisms (such as interferon defects; see Chapter 3), such infections may be life threatening. Premature neonates and elderly people are also vulnerable, especially if invasive interventions or broad-spectrum antibiotics have been administered, resulting in Group B streptococcal infection in the former or Clostridium difficile in the latter.

14.3 Gastritis

14.3.1 Atrophic gastritis and pernicious anaemia

The gastric mucosa contains several cell types: parietal cells producing acid and intrinsic factor, chief cells producing pepsinogen, epithelial cells, mucus neck cells and endocrine cells. Chronic inflammation of the gastric mucosa (gastritis) is relatively common, and associated with atrophy of gastric glands and loss of specialized secretory cells (Fig. 14.8). Two main types of gastritis are recognized (Table 14.2). Type A is immunologically mediated; type B gastritis is not autoimmune and is usually caused by Helicobacter pylori infection. Autoimmune gastritis is associated with other organ-specific autoimmune disease, both in a given patient and in families (Table 14.3).

Pernicious anaemia (PA) is characterized by megaloblastic anaemia due to malabsorption of vitamin B_{12}, itself secondary to deficiency of intrinsic factor secretion and gastric atrophy. Most patients are over 60 years old and women are affected more often than men (ratio 3: 2) (Case 14.1). About 2% of people over 60 years old have undiagnosed PA. The most common presenting features are tiredness and weakness (90%), dyspnoea (70%), paraesthesia (30%) and a sore tongue (25%). Although neurological features due to B_{12} deficiency are relatively rare (about 5%), involvement of the posterior and lateral columns of the spinal cord (subacute combined degeneration) is a serious complication, as the degeneration may not reverse on vitamin B_{12} treatment.

Over 90% of patients with PA produce an antibody to a parietal cell antigen independent of intrinsic factor. This antibody, **gastric parietal cell (GPC) antibody**, is commonly detected by indirect immunofluorescence (see Fig. 14.8) and its molecular target is the gastric proton pump (H^+K^+ATPase) contained within the membranes of the secretory canaliculi. These antibodies are unlikely to be pathogenic *in vivo* because gastric H^+K^+ATPase is not accessible to circulating autoantibodies. GPC antibodies are found in nearly all patients with PA and provide a useful screening test, but because they can be present in other diseases and in healthy individuals, diagnosis depends on the demonstration of intrinsic factor antibodies or **low serum B_{12} levels** (Table 14.4). However, because intrinsic factor antibodies are only found in 70% of cases, a negative result does not exclude the disease.

Evidence from mouse models suggests that Th1 type CD4+ T cells initiate the autoimmune gastritis. Transfer of CD4+

Table 14.2 Types of gastritis

Feature	Type A	Type B
Association	Pernicious anaemia	Helicobacter pylori infection
Antral inflammation	Antral sparing (fundus and body affected)	Antritis (fundus and body also affected)
Antral gastrin cell counts	High	Low
Serum gastrin level	High	Low
Intrinsic factor production	Low	Normal
Acid production	Low (achlorhydria)	Normal or low
Gastric autoantibodies:		
Parietal cell	Present	Absent
Intrinsic factor	Present	Absent
Other autoimmune disease	Often present	Absent
Risks of malignant disease	Gastric carcinoma	Gastric carcinoma
	(3× risk)	(2–6× risk)
	B-cell gastric lymphoma	

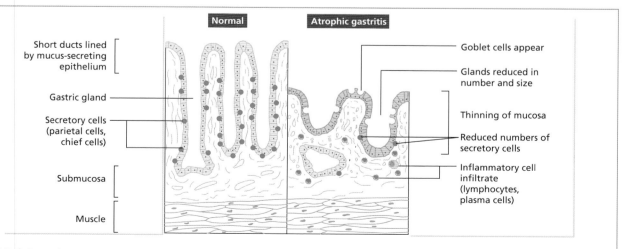

Fig. 14.8 Schematic representation of normal gastric mucosa and the histological changes seen in atrophic gastritis.

Table 14.3 Features of pernicious anaemia (PA) consistent with an autoimmune aetiology

1 Presence of autoantibodies to:
- Gastric parietal cell canaliculi (90%)
- Intrinsic factor (70%)
- Thyroid antigens (50%)

2 *In vitro* inhibition of parietal cell function and inhibition of intrinsic factor by autoantibodies

3 Association with other autoimmune disorders:
- Autoimmune thyroid disease
- Thyrotoxicosis
- Hashimoto's thyroiditis
- Myxoedema
- Autoimmune adrenalitis (Addison's disease)
- Insulin-dependent diabetes mellitus
- Primary ovarian failure
- Vitiligo
- Idiopathic hypoparathyroidism
- Myasthenia gravis

4 Occurrence of PA/other autoimmune conditions in relatives:
- First-degree relatives, especially females (30% have PA)
- Concordance in monozygotic twins

5 Good experimental response to immunosuppressive drugs (not used clinically):
- Increased absorption of vitamin B
- Some regeneration in parietal cells

T-cell clones that recognize the β subunit of gastric $H^+K^+ATPase$ into naive mice results in gastritis and serum antibodies to the target antigen. However, this may not be the initial **pathogenesis**, since transfer of autoantibodies and $CD8^+$ T cells has no such effects. The immunopathology responsible for gastritis of PA in humans is not known. Gastrin acts to stimulate gastric acid secretion and is a known growth factor for human gastrointestinal cancer, including stomach cancer, for which PA is a recognized risk factor. Autoantibodies to gastrin receptors have been detected in patients with PA, but the precise pathogenesis and the role of stimulating or blocking antibodies have yet to be worked out.

Intrinsic factor (IF) is a 60-kDa glycoprotein produced by gastric parietal cells. It binds avidly to dietary vitamin B_{12} and the B_{12}–IF complex is carried normally to the terminal ileum, where it is absorbed after binding to intrinsic factor receptors on ileal cells. *Malabsorption of vitamin B_{12} in patients with PA is due to intrinsic factor deficiency* and two mechanisms are responsible. First, the progressive destruction of parietal cells leads to failure of IF production. The severity of the gastric lesion correlates with the degree of impairment of IF secretion. Second, patients with PA produce autoantibodies that impair absorption of the B_{12}–IF complex in the ileum. **Two types of IF antibody** are recognized (Fig. 14.10). Blocking antibody is directed towards the combining site for vitamin B_{12} on IF. Binding antibody reacts with an antigenic determinant on IF distinct from the B_{12} combining site; this antibody

Case 14.1 Pernicious anaemia

A 67-year-old widow presented with gradually increasing tiredness, exertional dyspnoea and ankle swelling. Two years earlier she had been found to be anaemic and had been treated with oral iron without symptomatic improvement. She had lost 6 kg in weight, but denied any history of anorexia, dyspepsia or blood loss. On examination, she was very pale and had signs of congestive cardiac failure.

Laboratory investigations showed a very low haemoglobin of 54 g/l with a reduced white cell count of $3.7 \times 10^9/l$ (and a platelet count of only $31 \times 10^9/l$). A blood film showed marked macrocytosis with a mean cell volume of 112 fl. Bone marrow examination revealed marked megaloblastic erythropoiesis with abundant iron stores. Serum vitamin B_{12} was 40 ng/l (NR 170–900), but serum folate, serum iron and total iron-binding capacity were normal. Her serum contained strongly positive gastric parietal cell antibodies of IgG class (Fig. 14.9) and blocking antibodies to intrinsic factor. Antibodies to thyroid peroxidase were also found, although the patient was clinically and biochemically euthyroid.

The patient had pernicious anaemia and was therefore started on intramuscular injections of hydroxycobalamin at 3-monthly intervals. Four days after the first injection, her reticulocyte count rose to 16%.

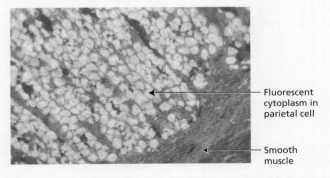

Fluorescent cytoplasm in parietal cell

Smooth muscle

Fig. 14.9 Gastric parietal cell antibodies detected by indirect immunofluorescence (see Chapter 19).

Table 14.4 Occurrence of gastric autoantibodies

Condition	Parietal cell antibody	Intrinsic factor antibody
Pernicious anaemia	*Serum* 90%	
	IgG – 65%	Blocking type 70%, IgG
	IgA – 25%	Binding type 35%
	Gastric juice 70%	
Relatives of patients with PA	IgA 30%	Blocking type 85%, IgA <1%
Other autoimmune disease:		
Thyroid disease		
Diabetes mellitus	20%	5%
Addison's disease		
Iron-deficiency anaemia	25%	<1%
Healthy adults		
Females >60 years	10%	<1%
Females <20 years	2%	<1%
Clinical value	*Screening test*	*Diagnostic test – though not essential, since low serum B12 levels can act as a surrogate and not all cases are positive*

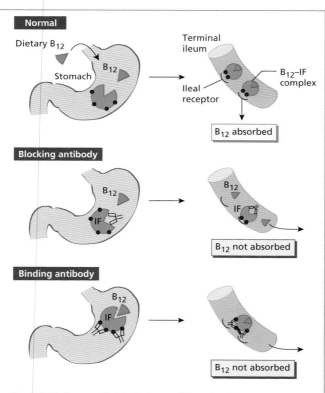

Fig. 14.10 Types of intrinsic factor (IF) antibody and their effect on vitamin B_{12} absorption.

can react either with free IF or with the B_{12}–IF complex to inhibit absorption (Fig. 14.10). Binding antibody rarely occurs without blocking antibody. Blocking antibody is readily detected in serum by radioimmunoassay or enzyme-linked immunosorbent assay (ELISA), but large amounts of free B_{12} in the circulation (e.g. after B_{12} injection) can produce a false-positive result.

Although IF antibodies are found more frequently in the gastric juices than in the sera of patients with PA (Table 14.4), it is more convenient to test sera. Antibodies to IF are specific and rarely occur in the absence of overt or latent PA.

14.4 Food-induced gastrointestinal disease

14.4.1 Food allergy

Doctors and the public have different perceptions of food allergy. Up to 20% of 'food-allergic' adults believe their symptoms to be food dependent, although the objective confirmation of prevalence is nearer 1%. A limited number of foods are responsible for true food allergy; the patient's history provides most of the diagnostic clues. Some patients have acute, life-threatening anaphylactic reactions, e.g. peanut allergy, while others have localized gastrointestinal reactions with diarrhoea, bleeding and failure to thrive, e.g. children with 'cow's milk protein intolerance'.

There are circumstances where patients experience distressing food-related symptoms that cannot be confirmed by objective tests or food challenge. Many of these cases have atypical or non-specific symptoms and involve foods rarely implicated in allergic reactions. It is inappropriate to label such patients as having food allergy without evidence of an immunological reaction to a food.

Food allergy and intolerance are discussed more fully in Chapter 4.

14.4.2 Coeliac disease

Coeliac disease, or gluten-sensitive enteropathy, is a relatively common small bowel enteropathy resulting from immunological hypersensitivity to ingested gluten (the storage protein of wheat and related cereals) in genetically susceptible individuals. Coeliac disease is most prevalent in Europeans and rare in Chinese or Afro-Caribbean people. Population screening surveys based on autoantibody testing have suggested a prevalence of 2% in the UK and 1% by biopsy; worldwide prevalence is probably twice these rates.

The characteristic **histological lesion** in untreated cases is the loss of normal villi with a marked increase in the numbers of IELs, particularly those expressing the γ/δ TCR (Figs 14.11 and 14.12); the infiltrate resolves following elimination of gluten from the diet, suggesting that the intestinal damage may be caused by a local cell-mediated reaction to gluten or a derivative. Within the lamina propria there is a mixed-cell infiltrate of plasma cells, stimulated CD4⁺ lymphocytes, macrophages, mast cells and basophils.

Coeliac disease runs in families: 10–20% of first-degree relatives, 40% of HLA-identical siblings and around 75% of monozygotic twins are affected. In Europeans, coeliac disease is strongly associated with inheritance of the histocompatibility antigens HLA-DQ2 and HLA-DQ8: most coeliac patients carry these risk alleles, but they are also found in 20% of the general population. Together, the HLA-DQ2 and HLA-DQ8 alleles are estimated to account for 40% of the **genetic risk** in coeliac disease. Consequently, it is likely that at least one other, non-HLA-linked gene, maybe on the long arm of chromosome 5, is involved in disease susceptibility. The absence of complete concordance in identical twins implies that other factors are involved, presumably environmental. Whatever these factors are, patients with coeliac disease remain sensitive to gluten for the rest of their lives.

Two factors are obviously important in the **pathogenesis** of coeliac disease (Fig. 14.13): exposure to gluten and a genetic predisposition to react to it. A unique 33 amino acid gluten peptide (33mer) is thought to initiate the disease because it encloses several, in part overlapping, HLA-DQ2–binding and T cell–stimulating epitopes that are resistant to intestinal proteinases. This peptide undergoes deamination by an enzyme – tissue transglutaminase (TTG) – in the small intestine. The deamination of glutamine residues to glutamic acid results in a negative charge that potentiates gluten binding to HLA-DQ2 and HLA-DQ8. The deaminated glutens are then endocytosed

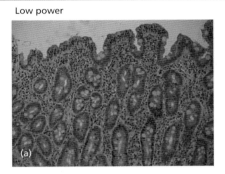
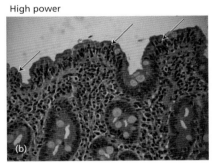

Fig. 14.11 Typical histological features of coeliac disease shown in (a) low and (b) high power. Intraepithelial lymphocytes are arrowed.

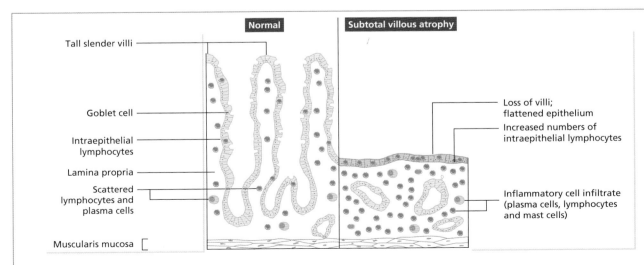

Fig. 14.12 Schematic representation of normal jejunal mucosa and histological changes in patients with coeliac disease.

Fig. 14.13 Proposed pathogenesis of coeliac disease. IFN, inferferon; TCR, T-cell receptor.

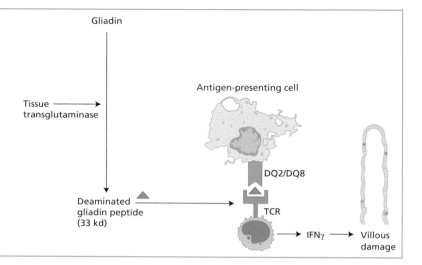

and processed by antigen-presenting cells to three epitopes that are subsequently recognized by T-cell receptors of CD4⁺ T cells. These activated T cells generate IFN-γ and other cytokines that are believed to cause the villous atrophy and crypt hyperplasia characteristic of coeliac disease. There are several strands of supporting evidence: (i) the mucosal damage is similar to that seen in experimental animal models involving T cell–mediated injury and in the enteropathy of graft-versus-host disease (see Chapter 8); (ii) gluten-specific, HLA-DQ2 and -DQ8–restricted T cells have been isolated from the small intestines of coeliac patients; and (iii) T-lymphocyte infiltration of the small bowel epithelium is seen in biopsies within hours of gluten exposure. TTG is a target of autoantibodies in coeliac disease, enabling reliable serological diagnostic tests, though it is not clear whether these autoantibodies are actually pathogenic or secondary to intestinal damage. New drugs are being investigated that block the action of tissue transglutaminase and therefore prevent the toxic effect of gluten in patients with coeliac disease.

Patients with coeliac disease and gluten sensitivity can **present** in many ways (Fig. 14.14) and only a relatively few present with typical intestinal features of diarrhoea or malabsorption; the diagnosis may be overlooked for months or years, as in Case 14.2. A jejunal biopsy is the only essential diagnostic test of coeliac disease. However, there are **two immunological tests that are extremely useful**: (i) measurements of serum IgA levels *with* (ii) IgA antibodies against 'endomysium' of primate oesophagus or human umbilical cord; these are in fact detecting TTG, so that screening with an ELISA to detect antibodies to TTG is used for screening prior to confirmation with endomysial antibodies.

The diagnostic specificity and sensitivity of IgA antibodies to endomysium or TTG are well above 95%. Consequently, they are used to screen populations at risk as a result of heredity, extraintestinal features or associated disorders (Table 14.6). These tests show that coeliac disease is underdiagnosed. Fatigue is often an early and persistent symptom. While immunological

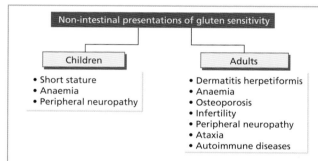

Fig. 14.14 Non-intestinal but increasingly common clinical presentations of coeliac disease.

tests cannot substitute for a diagnostic biopsy, they can be used to select those patients in whom a biopsy is needed, and may come to be used in children without a biopsy if the cut-off can be clarified and an international consensus reached.

The prevalence of selective IgA deficiency is increased approximately 10-fold in coeliac disease patients. The role of IgA deficiency is important, since the autoantibodies are of the IgA class – so if serum IgA is absent (<0.07 g/L), there is no chance to detect the diagnostic autoantibodies; tests for IgG antibodies to TTG or endomysium are used, though less specific and so less useful.

Coeliac disease is a **premalignant condition**: the risk of T-cell lymphoma is 50-fold higher than in the general population. There is also an increased frequency of carcinoma of the jejunum, oesophagus and pharynx. Treatment with a gluten-free diet reduces significantly the likelihood of subsequent small-intestinal malignant disease. It is not known why malignancy occurs, but the oncogene c-myc is found in maturing jejunal enterocytes, particularly in untreated coeliac disease. Persistent stimulation by gluten may therefore lead to malignant proliferation of lymphoid tissue.

Dermatitis herpetiformis (DH) is a bullous skin eruption that is associated with a coeliac-like lesion in the jejunum in

Case 14.2 Coeliac disease

A 35-year-old school cook presented to her dentist with a 30-month history of a sore mouth and tongue; she was treated with triamcinolone oral paste without improvement. Three months later she developed loose stools and generalized but vague abdominal pain. On questioning, she had felt tired for 2 years and had lost 8 kg in weight during the preceding 6 months despite a good appetite. During her second and third pregnancies she had developed moderate folic acid–deficiency anaemia. There was no family history of gastrointestinal disease and no abnormalities were found on examination.

Laboratory investigations showed a macrocytic anaemia but normal white cell, platelet and reticulocyte counts. The blood film showed many Howell–Jolly bodies (fragments of nuclear material within red blood cells; Fig. 14.15), suggestive of hyposplenism. Bone marrow examination revealed active erythropoiesis with early megaloblastic features but no stainable iron. The appearances were those of a combined deficiency of iron and folate/vitamin B_{12}; laboratory tests confirmed this (Table 14.5). In view of the blood film and the malabsorption of fat, coeliac disease was the most likely diagnosis. Her serum was positive for IgA antibodies to endomysium and to tissue transglutaminase, strongly supporting the clinical diagnosis. A jejunal biopsy was performed: this showed a convoluted pattern of stunted villi under the dissecting microscope, and subtotal villous atrophy with marked increase in intraepithelial lymphocytes and chronic inflammation in the lamina propria (Fig. 14.11).

The patient was started on a strict gluten-free diet with folic acid, iron and calcium supplements. One year later, she had put on 4.8 kg. A repeat jejunal biopsy showed improvement in villous architecture. This improvement following gluten withdrawal confirmed the diagnosis of coeliac disease and the patient will continue her gluten-free diet for life.

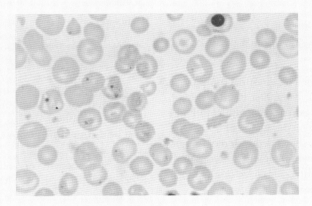

Fig. 14.15 Howell–Jowell bodies in a blood film (purple dots in red cells).

Table 14.5 Laboratory investigation in Case 14.2

Investigations of anaemia			Investigations of malabsorption		
Analyte	**Value**	**NR**	**Analyte**	**Value**	**NR**
Hb	107 LOW	120–160 g/l	Serum albumin	27	35–50 g/l
Mean cell volume	102 HIGH	80–90 fl	Serum calcium	2.22	2.33–2.60 mmol/l
Serum iron	5.9 LOW	14–29 µmol/l	Serum phosphate	0.74	0.80–1.45 mmol/l
Iron-binding capacity	85 HIGH	45–72 µmol/l	Serum alkaline phosphatase	70	20–85 IU/l
Serum folate	1.0 LOW	2–13 µg/l	Serum IgG	8.2	7.2–19.0 g/l
Red cell folate	52 VERY LOW	165–600 µg/l	Serum IgA	3.9	0.8–5.0 g/l
Serum vitamin B_{12}	197 NORMAL	160–900 ng/l	Faecal fat excretion	25	<17 mmol/day
			Serum endomysial antibodies (IgA class)	Positive	
			Anti-tissue transglutaminase (IgA class)	Positive	

Table 14.6 Immunological features of coeliac disease

Circulating antibodies

IgA antibodies to tissue transglutaminase and endomysium

IgA/IgG antibodies to gliadin (not measured routinely as poor diagnostic sensitivity and specificity)

Mucosal lesion

Infiltration by immunocompetent lymphoid cells

Genetic factors

Positive family history

Associated with HLA-DQ2 or -DQ8

Associated autoimmune disorders

Dermatitis herpetiformis

Extrinsic allergic alveolitis

Endocrine disorders: thyroid disease, Addison's disease, diabetes mellitus

Rheumatic disorders: systemic lupus erythematosus, rheumatoid arthritis, Sjögren's syndrome

Immunological complications

Hyposplenism due to splenic atrophy

Development of lymphoma (especially intestinal)

Table 14.7 Some differences between ulcerative colitis and Crohn's disease

	Ulcerative colitis	Crohn's disease
Disease site	Colon	Any part of gastrointestinal tract
Inflammation	Mucosal	Transmural, granulomatous
Cytokine profile	Th2	Th1
DNase-sensitive ANCA positivity	50–80%	5–20%
Genetic factors	HLA-DR2	Chromosome 16: NOD2
		Chromosome 12: IFN-γ
		Other loci on chromosomes 6 and 14
Concordance in monozygotic twins	6–14%	45%
Risk in first-degree relatives	×10	×30
Smoking	Protective	Harmful

ANCA, antibodies to neutrophil cytoplasmic antigens; IFN, interferon; NOD, nitric oxide dismutase.

almost all patients (see Chapter 11). The intestinal morphology improves on a gluten-free diet and, if the diet is strict enough, the skin lesion may also remit. The genetic background of DH is similar to coeliac disease; there is a high prevalence of HLA-DQ2 or -DQ8. Biopsy of the skin lesions shows deposition of IgA and C3 below the epithelial basement membrane; these lesions probably represent damage by IgA immune complexes originating in the intestinal mucosa following gluten ingestion.

14.5 Autoimmune enteropathy

Rare children have a severe and extensive enteropathy that is not due to coeliac disease, cow's milk protein intolerance or other recognized forms of food-related intestinal disease. Some of these individuals have an autoimmune enteropathy, characterized by protracted diarrhoea, often associated with organ-specific autoantibodies and a family history of autoimmune disease. This condition may be related to the immune deficiencies of IPEX (immunodysregulation polyendocrinopathy enteropathy X-linked syndrome) and APECED (autoimmune phenomena, polyendocrinopathy, candidiasis, and ectodermal dystrophy) (see Chapter 3)

14.6 Inflammatory bowel disease

14.6.1 Crohn's disease and ulcerative colitis

Ulcerative colitis and Crohn's disease are chronic inflammatory disorders of the gastrointestinal tract, with a tendency to remit and relapse (Table 14.7). Ulcerative colitis affects only the colon, and is confined to the mucosal layer. Crohn's disease, on

the other hand, may affect any part of the gastrointestinal tract from mouth to anus, although the ileocaecal region is most frequently involved. It can affect the colon alone and then must be distinguished from ulcerative colitis and other diseases causing segmental colitis, such as tuberculosis, intestinal lymphoma, lymphocytic or collagenous colitis, the latter being associated with long-term use of non-steroidal antiinflammatory drugs (NSAIDs). The diagnosis of both conditions is made by endoscopy, biopsy and radiology. **Immunological tests** have little part to play in the routine assessment of inflammatory bowel disease (IBD), although acute-phase proteins, such as C-reactive protein (CRP; 19-h half-life) and orosomucoid (5-day half-life) are useful in monitoring disease activity and the response to treatment, particularly in Crohn's disease. Faecal calprotectin is now used routinely as a screen to distinguish IBD from irritable bowel syndrome (IBS). However, the sensitivity and specificity of the test range from 70–80% to >90% in different studies. It may be more useful in Crohn's disease than ulcerative colitis, and may perform better in children and young adults. DNase-sensitive antineutrophil cytoplasmic antibodies, with perinuclear highlighting that is distinct on immunofluorescence from pANCA and cANCA (Chapter 19), have been shown in the sera of around 60% of ulcerative colic patients and 20% of Crohn's patients (Table 14.7). The target antigen is a nuclear histone, but this may be a secondary marker and not involved in pathogenesis. However, several clinical features of IBD suggest that the immune system is involved in the pathogenesis, including the occurrence of aphthous ulceration, iritis, erythema nodosum and arthritis, the association with disorders such as ankylosing spondylitis or primary sclerosing cholangitis, and the response to immunosuppressive drugs.

Histologically, Crohn's disease and ulcerative colitis are distinct, though the common finding is inflammation – as suggested in the term 'inflammatory bowel disease'. Transmural inflammation in **Crohn's disease involves lymphocytes, plasma cells and eosinophils, and there is granuloma formation** (Fig. 14.16). The **mucosa in ulcerative colitis is infiltrated with neutrophils as well as plasma cells and eosinophils**. With increasing severity of disease, there is ulceration with loss of goblet cells and formation of crypt abscesses. Compared with normal intestine, inflamed bowel shows intense expression of major histocompatibility complex (MHC) class II antigens on epithelial cells, and on lymphatic and vascular endothelium, while T lymphocytes and macrophages infiltrating the diseased lamina propria express activation markers such as CD25 (IL-2 receptor), as in other types of inflammation. The **pathogenesis** of Crohn's disease is complex, but is related to three interacting factors: genetic susceptibility, gut microflora and immune-mediated tissue injury (Fig. 14.17). Intestinal inflammation arises from abnormal immune reactivity to bacterial flora in the intestines of patients who are genetically susceptible. There is considerable evidence that **genetic factors** contribute to the pathogenesis of Crohn's disease and have a more dominant role than in ulcerative colitis, since siblings of patients have a much higher risk of developing Crohn's disease than the general population (Table 14.7). Even so, in Crohn's disease the concordance in monozygotic twins is only 45%, so environmental factors must also operate, and indeed most (70%) patients with Crohn's disease are smokers, while those with ulcerative colitis (5%) are not. Crohn's disease is a polygenic disorder (Table 14.7) and mutations in the nitric oxide dismutase (NOD)2 genes on chromosome 16 have been conclusively linked to about a fifth of cases of Crohn's disease. NOD2 is a cytosolic receptor for pathogenic components of gut bacteria and defective NOD2 makes its bearer susceptible to Crohn's disease, but this is only one of several genes linked to this condition (Fig. 14.17). The variants of NOD2 associated with Crohn's disease give a reduced response to lipopolysaccharide in dendritic cells, so reduced signalling through this innate immune pathway and activation of other inflammatory pathways, particularly in neutrophils.

The **pathogenesis of Crohn's disease** remains a puzzle. Genetic manipulation of cadherins in mice disrupts intercellular tight junctions and leads to chronic intestinal inflammation, while deletion of specific cytokine genes (IL-10 'knockout' mice) results in a Crohn's-like disease in the presence of normal luminal flora. Crohn's disease is driven by activated Th1 cells secreting IL-12, TNF-α and IFN-γ with an important role for Th17 cells, in response to commensal bacterial exposure. In response to these cytokines, the main mediators of tissue damage are matrix metalloproteinases generated by neutrophils. T-effector cells also show increased resistance to apoptosis, and with reduced regulatory T cells (Tregs), this allows the inflammatory process to continue. The role of intestinal microflora in Crohn's disease is undisputed (an elemental diet is successful in extreme cases), but claims that infection by Mycobacterium

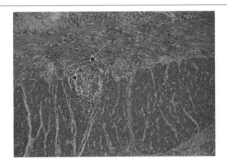

Fig. 14.16 A typical granuloma (arrowed) in the muscular layer of the bowel in Crohn's disease shown in low power.

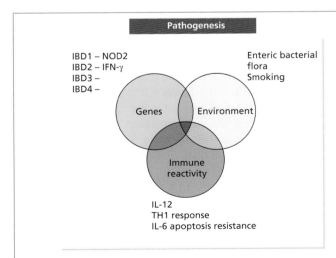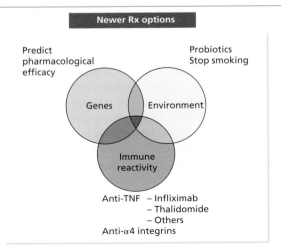

Fig. 14.17 Current understanding of the aetiology and pathogenesis of Crohn's disease and new approaches to treatment. IBD, inflammatory bowel disease; IFN, interferon; IL, inleukin; NOD, nitric oxide dismutase; TNF, tumour necrosis factor.

tuberculosis or measles virus triggers the disease have not been substantiated.

Studies of intestinal inflammation in humans and animals suggest that **ulcerative colitis results from environmental factors triggering a loss of tolerance to intestinal flora in genetically susceptible individuals**. Several pieces of evidence implicate environmental factors: cigarette smoking or early appendectomy seems to be protective, while lack of breastfeeding and treatment with NSAIDs increase the risk of developing ulcerative colitis. The retrograde gradient of lesions mirrors the bacterial concentration gradient in the colon and inflammation can occur in the ileal pouch after surgical anastomosis, 'pouchitis', which responds to treatment with metronidazole. In ulcerative colitis, the mucus layer in the ascending colon to the rectum is thinner than in a healthy mucosa and partly denuded, and the number of mature goblet cells is decreased in inflamed ulcerative colitic lesions and mucin synthesis is decreased. Whether this represents a primary failure of goblet cell function or differentiation or whether these findings are secondary remains to be determined.

Better understanding of the likely pathogenesis of Crohn's disease has led to changes in **management** (Fig. 14.17). The traditional therapeutic approach is based on a step-up strategy, using less toxic drugs, but often less efficacious in mild disease, while reserving more efficacious (but potentially more toxic) drugs for severe disease later or patients unresponsive to first-line therapy. However, the natural course of the disease has not been altered by conventional treatments. **Monoclonal antibodies to TNF-α** such as infliximab and adalimumab are proven to be safe and effective treatment for severe, resistant or fistulating Crohn's disease (Case 14.3). About 50–65% of patients respond beneficially to infusion of infliximab and 20–30% of patients go into remission, allowing infliximab to be used as maintenance therapy in some cases. The **monoclonal antibody, vedolizumab, binding to the $\alpha_4\beta_7$ integrin (LPAM-1, lymphocyte Peyer's Patch adhesion molecule)** can block T-lymphocyte migration into inflammatory foci, while cytokine-targeted treatment with the anti-IL12/IL23 monoclonal antibody **ustekinumab** is now also licenced for Crohn's disease; this antibody blocks T-cell activation via the cytokines. Alteration of the gut microbial environment by probiotics and cessation of smoking are also beneficial in some patients. Ulcerative colitis is treated in the first instance with derivatives of 5-aminosalicylic acid. Azathioprine and topical steroids are used for moderate disease. Resistant disease can be treated sequentially with an anti-TNF agent (infliximab or adalimumab), followed by vedolizumab. **Tofacitinib, a Janus kinase (JAK) inhibitor**, is now licenced for use in ulcerative colitis, the first new oral treatment for many years.

Surgery may be required. In Crohn's disease, this needs to be considered with caution as the disease is usually multifocal. In contrast, total colectomy in ulcerative colitis is curative, and abolishes the long-term risk of colonic cancer.

Monitoring remission and relapses has involved invasive procedures such as colonoscopy, but measuring CRP in serum and faecal calprotectin levels may reduce this. Calprotectin is a 36-kDa calcium- and zinc-binding protein that accounts for about 60% of total proteins in the cytosol fraction in neutrophil granulocytes and indicates an excess of

---

🔍 Case 14.3 Crohn's disease

A 30-year-old woman was admitted with a 4-week history of increasing bloody diarrhoea and abdominal pain; she had lost 3 kg in weight. She smoked 25 cigarettes a day. On examination, she was not clinically anaemic but had a temperature of 37.8 °C. She was tender over the right iliac fossa, and had a number of hypertrophic tender anal skin tags, which she thought were haemorrhoids. Sigmoidoscopy to 15 cm showed a red, granular mucosa with mucopus and contact bleeding. Laboratory investigations showed a low haemoglobin (108 g/l) with a raised C-reactive protein (CRP: 67 mg/l), but a normal white cell count. Urea and electrolytes, serum vitamin B$_{12}$, folate, iron, ferritin and iron-binding capacity were normal. Her total serum proteins were 54 g/l (NR 62–82) with a serum albumin of 29 g/l (NR 35–50). Antibodies to neutrophil cytoplasmic antigens (ANCA) were not detected. Faecal examination and culture revealed no ova or Campylobacter. Clostridium difficile toxin was absent from the stools.

The rectal biopsy taken at sigmoidoscopy showed a small area of ulceration of the surface epithelium with considerable mucopus. Many crypt abscesses were present. The lamina propria contained a heavy infiltrate of lymphocytes, plasma cells and macrophages. Several non-caseating granulomas (Fig. 14.16) were present in the muscular layer. The appearances were those of Crohn's disease affecting the colon. A small bowel barium examination showed extensive areas of fissuring ulceration interspersed with areas of apparently normal mucosa – skip lesions. She was treated with corticosteroids and a 3-month course of metronidazole, with symptomatic improvement. She was strongly advised to stop smoking, but refused to heed this advice.

Over the next 2 years her symptoms worsened, with an anal fistula, persistent diarrhoea and colicky lower abdominal pain despite prednisolone 15 mg per day. She was weaned off prednisolone and started on budesonide, but then developed spondyloarthropathy of the left hip, both knees and her left wrist. Because of her limited response to steroids, she was given an intravenous infusion of a monoclonal antibody to tumour necrosis factor – infliximab (see Chapter 7). Clinically she improved and her bowels were open two or three times each day, without nocturnal diarrhoea. This remission lasted nearly 3 months before her profuse diarrhoea and abdominal pain returned. She has now had four infusions of infliximab, each inducing symptomatic improvement of several months' duration. She still smokes.

neutrophils in the bowel. It is a valuable non-invasive test, but is not a replacement for surveillance colonoscopy in extensive ulcerative colitis, where there is a significant long-term cancer risk.

14.7 Viral hepatitis

Viral hepatitis is an infection of the liver caused by one of a range of specific liver viruses (Table 14.8), though other viruses, such as Epstein–Barr virus, CMV, herpes simplex virus and rubella, also cause hepatitis.

14.7.1 Hepatitis A

Hepatitis A (HAV; Table 14.8) is caused by a small RNA picornavirus that replicates in the gut and liver. HAV causes a mild or unnoticed illness in children or young adults. The **diagnosis** can be confirmed either by demonstrating virus in the faeces or by detecting a rise in specific antibodies (Fig. 14.18). Antibody tests are usually more reliable because the virus has often been eliminated completely before the patient seeks medical attention. Sera collected within a few weeks of the onset of symptoms contain antihepatitis A antibody that is almost exclusively IgM; its presence indicates recent infection. Later, IgG antibodies to HAV merely indicate previous exposure (Case 14.4).

The **pathogenesis** of liver cell damage in viral hepatitis is due to the immune response by infiltrating CD8 T lymphocytes and NK cells, which may result in the destruction of infected hepatocytes, as postulated for hepatitis B (HBV). The younger the patient, the milder the infection tends to be. Most patients with HAV make a full recovery, and progression to chronic hepatitis or cirrhosis is extremely rare.

Epidemiological control of HAV is largely dependent on high standards of personal hygiene and proper disposal of sewage. Person-to-person spread is common in close communities. In countries where disposal of sewage is primitive, HAV is endemic, as shown by a major outbreak involving 1.2 million people in China in 1988. For travellers or non-immunized close contacts of affected patients, human normal immunoglobulin provides about 90% protection against HAV for a period of 4–6 months. For long-term protection, HAV vaccine

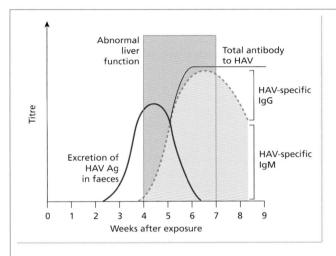

Fig. 14.18 Humoral immune response in acute hepatitis A virus (HAV) infection. Ag, antigen.

Table 14.8 Comparison of major features of hepatitis A, B, C and E

	Hepatitis type			
	A	**B**	**C**	**E**
Type of virus	RNA	DNA	RNA	RNA
Incubation period (days)				
Average	30	70	50	40
Range	15–45	50–180	15–150	15–60
Transmission				
Blood inoculation	+	+++	+++	–
Faecal–oral	+++	+	–	+++
Sexual	–	++	+	–
Vertical (transplacental)	–	+++	+	–
Age of patient	Any – usually young	Any	Any	Any – usually young adults
Severity of infection	Mild	Occasionally severe	Mild	Mild, but can be fulminant in pregnancy
Chronicity	Very rare	Common	Very common	Rare
Extrahepatic features	Rare	Common	Rare	Rare
Development of hepatoma	Very rare	Common	Common	Rare

Case 14.4 Hepatitis A

An 18-year-old man presented with a 10-day history of anorexia, nausea and upper abdominal discomfort. Two weeks earlier, he had experienced some mild arthralgia in his fingers, which lasted for 2 days. He normally smoked 20 cigarettes and drank 2–3 pints of beer each day, but had done neither for several days. He had noticed that his urine was much darker than normal. There was no significant medical history. On examination, he was afebrile but jaundiced. There were no needle tracks on his arms. His liver was just palpable and tender.

Hepatitis was diagnosed and confirmed by routine investigations. His serum bilirubin was 48 µmol/l (NR 1–20), with raised liver enzyme levels – aspartate transaminase 895 IU/l (NR 5–45); alanine transaminase 760 IU/l (NR 5–30) – and an alkaline phosphatase of 128 IU/l (NR 20–85). A monospot test for infectious mononucleosis was negative. Hepatitis B surface antigen (HBsAg) was also negative, but he had detectable IgM antibodies to hepatitis A virus. He was managed conservatively at home. There is no active treatment for hepatitis A infection, although rest may be beneficial. The clinical and biochemical evidence of hepatocellular damage subsided over the next 4 weeks, but he continued to feel vaguely unwell for several months. A further blood sample after 6 months showed IgG antibody to hepatitis A. Antibody to core antigen (IgM anti-HBcAg) appears early on and is a reliable marker of current acute infection, whereas IgG anti-HBcAg merely indicates previous infection. Clinical recovery and clearance of the virus are associated with the disappearance of HBeAg and then HBsAg, with subsequent detection of their respective antibodies during convalescence (Fig. 14.20). In practice, the diagnosis of hepatitis B infection is usually confirmed by detecting HBsAg in sera collected during the acute phase of the illness, or by showing a rising titre of antibody to HBcAg. Patients with acute hepatitis B do not need treatment.

gives over 97% protection against infection and lasts at least 10 years; this is recommended for all travellers to countries in which HAV infection is endemic.

14.7.2 Hepatitis B

HBV is one of the most widespread infections in humans and the commonest cause of worldwide liver disease. In general, the prevalence is low in cold, developed countries and high in hot, developing countries. HBV may be spread by several routes (see Table 14.8), and **transmission** has occurred in minute quantities of infected blood or blood products by the use of shared or unsterile syringes, unsterile needles in tattooing and acupuncture, or by surgical or dental procedures. The rate of transmission by needlestick injury may be as high as 20–30% compared with a transmission rate of 3% for hepatitis C (HCV) and 0.3% for HIV. HBV is also transmitted sexually, particularly in those with multiple sexual partners. Mothers positive for HBV have a high risk of infecting their infants in pregnancy (see Chapter 18). The earlier in life a person is infected, the more likely he or she is to become a carrier: virtually all babies infected in the neonatal period become chronic carriers and this is the predominant route of transmission in countries where HBV is endemic. It has been estimated that there are about 300 million carriers in the world. In the UK, about 0.1–0.3% of the general population are believed to be carriers, but in tropical Africa, China and South-East Asia, this proportion rises to 8–35%.

Electron microscopy of serum infected with HBV reveals three types of particle: spheres, filaments and virions (Dane particles; Fig. 14.19). HBsAg is found on the surfaces of all three types of particle. A second antigen is associated with the core (HBcAg), while a third, HBeAg, is located within the core of the virus particle.

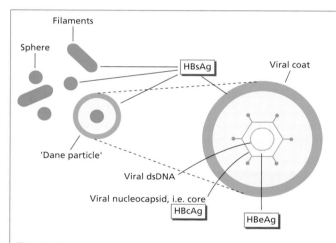

Fig. 14.19 Schematic diagram of the three morphological types of particle found in hepatitis B. Only the Dane particle is infective.

Acute HBV infection may go unnoticed or be associated with vague symptoms only. Typically, however, infection leads to the appearance of HBsAg in the blood 2 or more weeks before abnormal tests of liver biochemistry or the onset of symptoms (Fig. 14.20). HBsAg remains detectable usually until the convalescent phase. HBeAg is a good measure of infectivity because it appears soon after HBsAg and is closely associated with the inner core (HBcAg) and viral DNA. IgM antibody to core antigen (IgM anti-HBcAg) appears early on and is a reliable marker of current acute infection, whereas IgG anti-HBcAg merely indicates previous infection. Clinical recovery and clearance of the virus are associated with the disappearance of HBeAg and then HBsAg, with subsequent detection of their respective antibodies during convalescence (Fig. 14.20). In practice, the diagnosis of HBV infection is

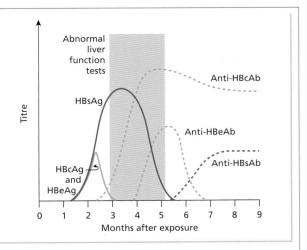

Fig. 14.20 Humoral immune responses in acute hepatitis B infection.

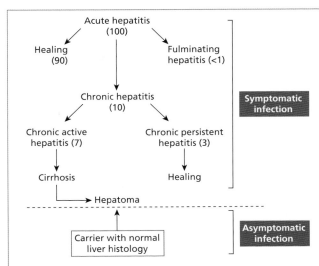

Fig. 14.21 Outcome of hepatitis B infection. Percentages of patients shown in brackets.

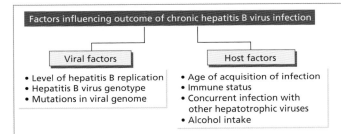

Fig. 14.22 Factors influencing outcome of chronic hepatitis B virus infection.

usually confirmed by detecting HBsAg in sera collected during the acute phase of the illness, or by showing a rising titre of antibody to HBcAg. Patients with HBsAg persisting in the serum for over 6 months are defined as carriers. They may be of high or low infection risk to others depending on the presence or absence, respectively, of HBeAg. Overall, the **transmission** rate following inoculation injury with HBsAg-positive material is about 3–5%. If the patient/donor is also HBeAg positive, the transmission rate rises to over 20%, but is only 0.1% if the patient/donor is HBe antibody positive. These risks are important to healthcare workers: in the UK, workers who are HBeAg positive cannot carry out invasive 'exposure-prone' procedures on patients. Consequently, all healthcare workers in developed countries are immunized with HBV vaccine.

Natural elimination of infection in acute HBV involves immunological lysis of infected cells and removal of infective virus particles. Cytotoxic CD8+ T cells are responsible for destroying the infected hepatocytes, while antibody-dependent mechanisms neutralize extracellular virus particles and so prevent the spread of infection to other liver cells. HBV is not directly cytopathic; as with HAV, liver injury is the result of the immune responses of the host to these antigens on the cell surface.

Acute fulminant hepatitis is associated with abnormally rapid clearance of HBsAg and HBeAg, implying an excessive, self-damaging immune response. In contrast, immunocompromised patients usually develop subclinical disease associated with viral persistence if the deficiency involves T-cell immunity.

As HBV is not cytopathogenic, HBV-specific T cells are responsible for **chronic HBV hepatitis**. HBV-specific CD8+ and CD4+ cells infiltrate the liver and produce IL-17, IL-22 or both, attracting Th17 cells with low levels of inhibitory receptors, resulting in inflammation in the liver. The precise immunopathology of chronic hepatitis and mechanisms of progression to cirrhosis, depending on the balance between HBV-specific CD4 and CD8, Th17 and NK cells, are still to be worked out.

Three main forms of **chronic carriage of HBV** are recognized: chronic active hepatitis, chronic persistent hepatitis and carriage with relatively normal liver histology. About 10% of previously symptomatic adults and over 90% of babies born of HBeAg-positive mothers become chronic carriers (Fig. 14.21). Most show chronic active hepatitis on liver biopsy. Those HBsAg carriers who give no history of previous symptomatic hepatitis usually have chronic persistent hepatitis or relatively normal liver histology. These groups of carriers were probably infected during the neonatal period, when the relative immaturity of the immune system can lead to tolerance of HBsAg (Fig. 14.22). Their response to other organisms, met at a later age, is completely normal.

Extrahepatic complications are probably the result of deposition of circulating immune complexes composed of viral antigens and host antibodies. Some complexes, particularly those formed in antigen excess, can be deposited in the kidney and cause glomerulonephritis. Complexes formed in antibody excess are large and usually present as vasculitic lesions. Chronic HBV surface antigenaemia is a risk factor, particularly in the

Far East, for the development of polyarteritis nodosa (see Chapter 10) or mixed essential cryoglobulinaemia (see Chapter 9).

Primary hepatocellular carcinoma (hepatoma) is a common tumour in countries with a high prevalence of HBV carriers. Carriers are about 100 times more likely to develop hepatoma than non-carriers. A raised level of serum α-fetoprotein (AFP) is found in 30–95% of hepatoma patients (depending on the series) and provides a useful diagnostic marker because of its negative predictive value (see Chapter 19).

The aims of **therapy** are a reduction in the level of viraemia and improvement in hepatic function. In contrast to HCV (see section 14.7.3), nucleotide analogues (NUCs) are safe and effective in HBV patients and can even be given at the stage of hepatic decompensation, unlike IFN-α therapy; liver failure can be reversed in a significant proportion of patients, and for those that require liver transplantation (see Chapter 8) NUCs are used pre and post transplantation to prevent reinfection. Lamuvidine, adefovir and entecavir are commonly used nucleoside analogues that inhibit the viral enzyme reverse transcriptase and so lower concentrations of HBV DNA in most patients in association with an improvement in liver histology, a fall in liver enzymes to normal and reduction of long-term complications including hepatocellular carcinoma. Viral replication commonly returns when NUCs are stopped

Long-term NUC therapy prevents disease progression and reverses liver fibrosis and cirrhosis.

The outcome of liver transplantation with NUCs in patients with HBV cirrhosis has improved long-term survival: the 5-year survival rate is about 80%. For those with hepatocellular carcinoma, patient survival and disease-free survival at 3 years after liver transplantation are also round 80%.

Several preventative measures have been taken to **reduce the incidence of HBV infection**:

- High-risk carriers are prevented from performing 'exposure-prone' procedures.
- The incidence of post-transfusion HBV has been greatly reduced by screening potential blood donors for HBsAg.
- 'HBV immunoglobulin', obtained from convalescent patients, is of prophylactic value for individuals following single acute exposure to blood from HBsAg-positive patients.
- Active immunization is recommended.

HBV vaccine is available as a genetically engineered surface antigen introduced into a yeast vector (see Chapter 7). The vaccine is safe and effective; the protection rate is over 80% in adults and 90% in neonates, although several factors are associated with a suboptimal response (Box 14.2). The duration of protection is now >15 years in most people, but depends on the antibody titre attained. If HBV and its consequences are to be eradicated, worldwide immunization is needed. In some endemic countries, all newborn babies are immunized with HBV vaccine and given HBV immunoglobulin simultaneously – so-called active/passive immunization. The cost of the

> **Box 14.2 Factors associated with a suboptimal response to hepatitis B vaccine**
>
> - Age
> - Genetic predisposition – low response in HLA-B8, -DR3
> - Alcoholism
> - Renal failure
> - Obesity – higher protection if vaccine given into deltoid rather than buttock
> - Immunosuppression – including human immunodeficiency virus infection
> - Virus 'escape' mutants – natural virus may differ from vaccine

vaccine is an impediment to global vaccination schemes, but the WHO recommends routine HBV vaccination for countries that can afford to buy the vaccine and have a carrier rate of over 2.5% of the population. A proportion of patients (<5%) do not respond to the vaccine after the standard three doses, as judged by the development of protective antibody levels. It is unclear whether they have T-cell immunity and are protected. Usually a further three doses of a different vaccine are given. The higher dose (40 μg) used for patients with renal failure can be used. If obtaining protection is essential (certain occupations), then the vaccine can be given with IFN-γ.

14.7.3 Hepatitis C

During the 1970s, it was established that many cases of post-transfusion hepatitis were due neither to HAV nor to HBV infection. The viruses responsible were initially called non-A, non-B (NANB) hepatitis viruses, but it is now known that nearly all cases of post-transfusion hepatitis are caused by HCV, an RNA virus. HCV is a highly variable agent that **undergoes rapid mutations, with six major genotypes** and over 100 subtypes, many of which are grouped geographically.

Although HCV was first identified and characterized in association with blood transfusions, this route of **transmission** now accounts for only a small proportion of cases of HCV in the UK since screening of blood and blood products was introduced in the 1990s (compare with Chapter 16, Case 16.7). A history of parenteral drug abuse is the most common risk factor, with about 70% of drug abusers being positive for HCV antibody, compared with about 0.2% of blood donors. Healthcare workers appear to have a slightly increased risk. Sexual and perinatal transmission has been described, but these are comparatively inefficient routes, with a 5% risk of infection from a partner or mother with HCV.

HCV infection is **characterized clinically** (see Table 14.8) by an incubation period of around 50 days. Acute infection is usually mild and asymptomatic. Only 10% of patients become jaundiced and it is rarely a cause of fulminant hepatic failure. HCV infection has a complex natural history, not yet fully defined (Fig. 14.23). Without treatment, about 60–80% of patients develop chronic hepatitis and 10–20% are at risk of developing cirrhosis, often 20–30 years following infection, and hepatocellular carcinoma after a further 10 years. Chronic HCV is frequently associated with extrahepatic features such as mixed cryoglobulinaemia, glomerulonephritis, seronegative arthritis and cutaneous vasculitis.

HCV uses several strategies to evade the host immune response: (i) the high HCV replication rate can outpace the normal immune response; (ii) studies suggest that CD8⁺ T cells become 'anergic' and unable to produce IFN during the peak of viraemia; and (iii) HCV 'counterattacks' several components of the cellular immune response by promoting CD95 (Fas)-induced apoptosis of virus-specific cytotoxic T cells.

Typical **histological features** of HCV include lymphoid aggregates in portal areas, reactive epithelial changes of bile ducts and moderate lymphocytic infiltration of hepatic parenchyma. Although the cellular immune response of the host is rather weak in the chronic phase of HCV, the balance of liver-infiltrating, HCV-specific CD4⁺ and CD8⁺ Th1, Th17 and NK cells determines the development of liver fibrosis and cirrhosis.

The **diagnosis** of HCV infection depends on demonstrating viral RNA by polymerase chain reaction (PCR), though serological testing is still used in countries with limited resources. HCV infection is usually not diagnosed until a patient has symptoms of liver failure or liver function tests are done for unrelated reasons. The long-term prognosis following **successful treatment with antiviral therapy** is excellent, though the risk of hepatocellular carcinoma persists. Treatment with IFN-α restores transaminase levels to normal and improves liver histology in 50% of patients in the short term; several factors may contribute to a favourable response (Box 14.3). Pegylated interferon, interferon coupled to polyethylene glycol, has a long half-life and needs to be given only once a week rather than three times weekly for interferon. The combination of pegylated interferon and ribavirin clears HCV infection, resulting in a good response in patients with HCV genotypes 2 and 3. Triple therapy with IFN-α, ribavirin and a NUC (such as boceprevir or telaprevir) is used for genotype 1 infection and those with decompensated cirrhosis, since the response is less satisfactory (Case 14.5).

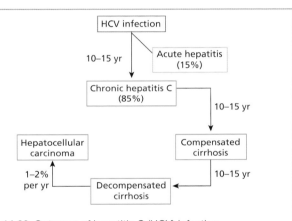

Fig. 14.23 Outcome of hepatitis C (HCV) infection.

Box 14.3 Factors contributing to a sustained beneficial response to interferon-α in hepatitis C patients

- Age <40 years
- Duration of infection <10 years
- Low body weight <70 kg
- Absence of cirrhosis
- Low level of viraemia
- Hepatitis C virus genotypes 2 or 3

🔍 Case 14.5 Hepatitis C-induced liver disease

A 29-year-old man was noted to have abnormal liver function tests on routine 'well-man' medical screening in the private health sector. Apart from an episode of cellulitis and septic arthritis aged 24 years, he had been fit and well. He had no symptoms of liver disease and his GP notes showed no record of jaundice. Liver function testing, subsequently repeated twice, showed a mild chronic hepatitis with serum alanine transaminase levels of 140–210 IU/l (NR 0–50), and normal serum levels of alkaline phosphatase, bilirubin and albumin. He had no detectable antibodies to smooth muscle or mitochondria. Virus serology showed no evidence of exposure to hepatitis A or B. However, he was positive for hepatitis C antibody, but negative for hepatitis C virus RNA by polymerase chain reaction (PCR). He underwent a liver biopsy, which showed normal liver architecture. There was mild non-specific portal tract inflammation, but no piecemeal necrosis or fibrosis.

The source of his chronic hepatitis C liver disease was uncertain. He denied any use of intravenous drugs and had received no transfusions of blood or blood products. However, he was adorned with tattoos on his limbs and trunk. Tattooing carries a risk of transmitting hepatitis C of up to 3% in countries in which hepatitis C is not endemic. It has been suggested that up to 40% of current carriers were infected by tattooing. The risk is increased by multiple tattooing, work by an amateur tattooist, and if the tattooist is hepatitis C positive.

He was told that his chronic hepatitis was likely to progress only slowly and over decades provided he abstained from alcohol, but that his liver biopsy would need to be repeated every 2 years or so, as an indicator of the potential need for antiviral therapy.

HCV recurs in patients following **liver transplantation**, but appears to progress less rapidly than HBV in this situation. Now that the genome has been cloned, the development of a protective **vaccine** is a realistic goal. The antigenic differences imply that a polyvalent vaccine will be needed.

14.7.4 Other hepatitis viruses

Hepatitis D (delta) virus is an incomplete RNA virus that can only replicate in the presence of HBV. Hepatitis D is found wherever HBV is endemic and is spread by the same routes. Simultaneous co-infection with HBV and hepatitis D is usually self-limiting, but can be associated with more severe acute hepatitis and increased morbidity. Superinfection of an HBsAg-positive, chronically infected person with hepatitis D virus leads to an increased prevalence of chronic active hepatitis and cirrhosis compared with HBV infection alone.

Hepatitis E virus is an enterically transmitted RNA virus (see Table 14.8). It is endemic in Asia, Africa, the Middle East and Central America. Outbreaks in China and India have affected many thousands of people, usually young adults. Hepatitis E runs a self-limiting course in most people, but fulminant hepatitis can occur in pregnant women with fatality rates of 25% in women infected in the third trimester. Surviving infants seem to be unaffected and chronic hepatitis does not occur.

Hepatitis G virus – or GB virus (GBV), from the initials of an American surgeon infected with a non-A, non-B, non-C, non-D virus – is a parenterally transmitted agent. Co-infection with HBV and HCV can occur, but hepatitis G does not cause clinical hepatitis on its own. It is found in about 2% of blood donors and around 20% of patients who receive regular blood products.

Seronegative hepatitis is the term for remaining cases of non-ABCDEG hepatitis and accounts for up to 10% of acute

hepatitis. Such cases often have more severe jaundice and higher levels of serum transaminases, but usually recover completely. The route of transmission is unknown.

14.8 Autoimmune liver diseases

14.8.1 Chronic active hepatitis

By definition, chronic hepatitis is a chronic inflammation of the liver that lasts for more than 6 months. On the basis of the liver biopsy appearances, two broad categories are recognized: chronic persistent hepatitis and chronic active hepatitis.

Chronic persistent hepatitis is characterized by non-specific inflammation of the portal zones of the liver only. Some cases complicate viral hepatitis (particularly HBV and HCV), alcohol, drug hypersensitivity or chronic IBD. In contrast to chronic active hepatitis, immunological investigations are normal, progression to cirrhosis is rare, treatment is unnecessary and the overall outlook is excellent.

Chronic active hepatitis (CAH) is also marked by the presence of a mononuclear cell infiltrate in the portal areas, but this also extends into the parenchyma to produce necrosis of individual periportal hepatocytes ('piecemeal necrosis'). As the disease progresses, piecemeal necrosis extends from the portal tracts to the central veins ('bridging necrosis'), eventually causing cirrhosis. CAH also has several, widely different aetiologies, such as HBV, HCV, alcohol, drugs (minocycline, isoniazid, nitrofurantoin), Wilson's disease and α_1-antitrypsin deficiency. In cases where no aetiological agent is found, an autoimmune basis is suspected. Autoimmune hepatitis and CAH associated with HCV infection are the major recognized forms in Western countries (Case 14.6).

Characteristically, **autoimmune hepatitis** (Table 14.9) affects young to middle-aged women, 60% of whom have associated autoimmune disorders such as haemolytic anaemia,

---

Case 14.6 Chronic active hepatitis

A 43-year-old woman presented with a 5-month history of weight loss (6 kg), anorexia, irritability and generalized pruritus. On examination, she was icteric with numerous spider naevi, scratch marks, palmar erythema and hepatosplenomegaly. Investigations showed a low haemoglobin (95 g/l) with a normal white cell count, but an erythrocyte sedimentation rate of 140 mm/h. The prothrombin time was prolonged, but urea and electrolytes, calcium and phosphate concentrations were normal. Although the serum albumin was normal (41 g/l), the total serum proteins were raised at 93 g/l (NR 62–82), with a raised serum bilirubin of 34 μmol/l (NR 1–20), alanine transaminase of 152 IU/l (NR 5–30), and aspartate transaminase of 164 IU/l (NR 5–45). The alkaline phosphatase level was normal (83 IU/l). Her serum immunoglobulins showed an increased IgG level of 44 g/l (NR 7.2–19.0) with normal IgA and IgM levels. No paraprotein was present on serum electrophoresis.

Antinuclear antibodies (IgG class) were strongly positive to a titre of 1/10 000 and antibodies to dsDNA were positive (60% binding; normal <30%). Her serum was positive for antibodies to smooth muscle (Fig. 14.24) to a titre of over 1/1000 (see Chapter 19). HBsAg and hepatitis C antibody were absent and alpha-fetoprotein (AFP) was not detected. The immunological picture strongly favoured a diagnosis of autoimmune hepatitis. She was therefore started on prednisolone (30 mg/day) and vitamin K, with dramatic improvement. Her serum bilirubin, transaminases and prothrombin time returned to normal over the next fortnight. A diagnostic liver biopsy was performed: this showed chronic active hepatitis with cirrhosis. She was continued on prednisolone (15 mg/day) and is fully reassessed every 6 months, including a repeat liver biopsy as appropriate.

Table 14.9 Major features of autoimmune chronic active hepatitis and primary biliary cirrhosis

Feature	Autoimmune hepatitis	Primary biliary cirrhosis
Sex	Female > male (6: 1)	
Age at onset	10–30 years	40–60 years
Family history	Uncommon	5%
Associated autoimmune disease	Common	Unusual
Smooth-muscle antibodies	Positive 85% – high titre	Not present
Antinuclear antibodies	Positive in 80%	Unusual
Anti-DNA antibodies	Often positive	Rare
Antimitochondrial antibodies	Positive 5%	95%
Antibodies to liver and kidney microsomes	Positive 40% (higher in children)	
Serum immunoglobulins	IgG level raised	IgM level raised
HLA type	HLA-B8: aggressive disease in younger patients	None known
	HLA-DR4: extrahepatic features	
Response to steroids	Good	Poor
Risk of hepatoma	Low	Very low

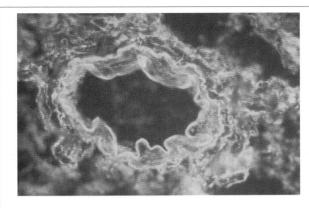

Fig. 14.24 Smooth muscle antibodies staining actin in a blood vessel (indirect immunofluoresence using patient serum and rat liver sections – see Chapter 19).

Liver injury results from T cell–mediated damage to genetically predisposed hepatocytes. Aberrant expression of MHC class II molecules on the surfaces of hepatocytes facilitates expression of normal liver cell membrane constituents to antigen-processing cells, which stimulate the clonal expansion of autoantigen-sensitized cytotoxic T cells; these infiltrate liver tissue and release tissue destructive cytokines. Aberrant HLA expression is associated with inflammation triggered by viral infection or drugs.

Treatment of autoimmune hepatitis is currently aimed at suppressing the effector mechanisms of this self-damaging response. Randomized controlled trials have shown that prednisolone induces clinical remission and prolongs life, and that liver histology shows less inflammatory activity, though cirrhosis cannot be reversed. The addition of azathioprine enables lower doses of prednisolone to be used or even withdrawn, while maintaining the patient in remission. The 10-year survival rate is 90% for autoimmune hepatitis patients without cirrhosis, but only 50% when cirrhosis is present.

For patients with cirrhosis, liver transplantation gives good survival rates (>90% at 5 years), although milder disease may recur in the graft despite intensive immunosuppression.

14.8.2 Primary biliary cirrhosis

Primary biliary cirrhosis (PBC) is a chronic progressive disease characterized by progressive destruction of small intrahepatic bile ducts with portal inflammation leading to fibrosis and cirrhosis. About 25–50% of patients are asymptomatic at diagnosis, and this phase can last for many years. Symptomatic patients usually present with pruritus (50%), right upper quadrant pain (25%) or symptoms of hepatic decompensation (20%) (Fig. 14.25). Characteristically, the disease affects middle-aged women; 5% have affected relatives. Clustering of cases has also been reported. The reported incidence ranges from 5 to 20 per million people per year and seems to be increasing.

type 1 diabetes mellitus, thyroiditis, fibrosing alveolitis or glomerulonephritis. Smooth-muscle antibodies (SMAs) are not specific for autoimmune hepatitis and are found as a temporary phenomenon in many patients with viral infections, particularly adenovirus and infectious hepatitis. Classically, high-titre IgG antibodies to smooth muscle are a marker of autoimmune hepatitis, the target antigen being actin, a cytoskeletal protein (Fig. 14.24). However, **antibodies to liver and kidney microsomes** (LKMs) also occur in a proportion of CAH patients, mainly children. The antigen recognized by LKM antibodies is a human cytochrome P450, also found in a recombinant antigen – cytochrome mono-oxygenase CYP2D6 – which demonstrates molecular mimicry with a component of HCV. Similar antibodies, directed against different isoenzymes of the cytochrome, have been found in cases of drug-induced hepatitis. A distinct form of LKM-positive autoimmune hepatitis has been recognized in association with APECED (Chapter 15). LKM antibodies are not thought to be pathogenic and their titres do not correlate with severity or treatment response. However, as markers they are helpful indicators of a potential autoimmune pathogenesis and can be of use in guiding therapy.

As in Case 14.7, the diagnosis of PBC may be overlooked at first. However, **antimitochondrial antibodies** (AMAs) provide a vital diagnostic test. About 95% of patients with PBC have circulating AMAs by either immunofluorescence (Fig. 14.26) or ELISA; the test is specific 98% for PBC. Several AMA staining patterns are recognized on indirect immunofluorescence: the M2 type is the most important marker of PBC and the target antigen is the E2 component of pyruvate dehydrogenase (PDC-E2), a mitochondrial enzyme. There is no evidence that AMAs are responsible for the pathogenesis of PBC. In animals at least, experimental induction of antibodies to the pyruvate dehydrogenase complex fails to trigger PBC, while in humans there is no correlation between serum antibody titre and liver damage; AMAs are therefore secondary to the damage and only act as a marker of PBC. Mitochondrial antibodies are also found in a small proportion of patients with CAH or cirrhosis of unknown aetiology.

The characteristic **histological lesion** in the early stages is the presence of granulomas in the portal tracts with destruction of middle-sized bile ducts (Fig. 14.27). The damaged ducts are surrounded and infiltrated typically by CD4⁺ T lymphocytes, with a further surrounding infiltrate of CD8⁺ T cells at the periphery of the portal tract, the site at which cirrhosis develops eventually. Infiltrating CD4⁺ and CD8⁺ T cells are also specific for PDC-E2. Copper is retained in the liver in chronic cholestasis and its demonstration is useful in diagnosing late-stage PBC.

The **pathogenesis** of bile duct damage in PBC is unclear. Bile ducts in PBC patients express increased densities of adhesion molecules, MHC class II antigens, IL-2 receptor and

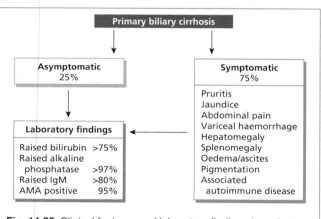

Fig. 14.25 Clinical features and laboratory findings in patients with histologically proven primary biliary cirrhosis. AMA, antimitochondrial antibody.

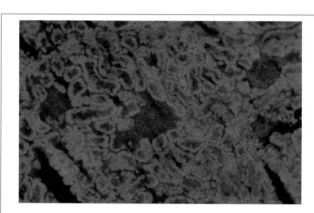

Fig. 14.26 Antimitochondrial antibodies by indirect immunofluorescence using patient serum and rat liver sections (see Chapter 19).

Case 14.7 Primary biliary cirrhosis

A 62-year-old woman presented with a 6-week history of generalized itching and progressive shortness of breath. She also had a dragging feeling in the right upper quadrant of her abdomen. There was no history of weight loss, anorexia or jaundice. She smoked 25 cigarettes a day. On examination, she had many scratch marks but no xanthomas, xanthelasmas or jaundice. A large right-sided pleural effusion was present, with smooth, firm moderate enlargement of the liver. She was thought to have a bronchial carcinoma with hepatic secondaries.

Investigations showed a haemoglobin of 131 g/l, a normal white cell count and an erythrocyte sedimentation rate of 93 mm/h. Prothrombin time, urea and electrolytes, calcium, phosphate, total proteins, serum albumin and serum bilirubin were normal. However, the alkaline phosphatase was 1050 IU/l (NR 20–85), aspartate transaminase 166 IU/l (NR 5–45) and alanine transaminase 121 IU/l (NR 5–30). HBsAg and hepatitis C antibody were not detected. A chest X-ray confirmed the right pleural effusion, but showed no evidence of malignancy or tuberculosis. The pleural effusion was aspirated three times; on each occasion malignant cells were absent, culture was non-contributory, the fluid had the characteristics of a transudate and pleural biopsies were normal.

During her stay in hospital, however, the patient became obviously jaundiced, with a rise in serum bilirubin from 8 to 32 μmol/l. She also developed ascites and a palpable spleen. In view of her progressive obstructive jaundice, she underwent a laparotomy; no surgically correctable cause could be found, but a liver biopsy was taken. This showed the typical changes of primary biliary cirrhosis. Immunological tests were first performed at this stage – rather late! Antimitochondrial antibodies were present (Fig. 14.25) to a titre of 1/10 000. Serum immunoglobulins showed a polyclonal rise in IgM to 6.20 g/l (NR 0.5–2.0) with normal IgG and IgA levels. She was given cholestyramine to control her itching and ursodeoxycholic acid therapy. In the 4 years since diagnosis, she has been reasonably well.

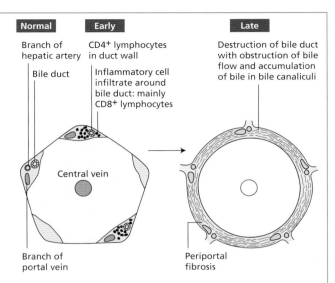

Fig. 14.27 Schematic representation of histological features of early and late stages of primary biliary cirrhosis.

pyruvate dehydrogenase compared with normal ducts, and so represent potential targets for the infiltrating activated T cells (CD4⁺ and CD8⁺). It is not clear why the autoimmune response in PBC is restricted to the biliary tree, when target mitochondrial antigens are present in all cells. There are similarities between PBC and chronic graft-versus-host disease (see Chapter 8). Graft-versus-host disease is known to be mediated by cytotoxic T cells. PBC has been associated with HLA-DR7 and -DR8, while -DR11 and -DR13 appear to be protective. Other genes may be involved. 'Clustering' of reported cases implies that an environmental agent is somehow involved. A Gram-negative environmental bacterium, Novosphingobium aromaticivorans, has been suggested as a potential trigger, with possible cross-reactivity between bacterial antigens and mitochondrial proteins in the liver. PBC is also strongly associated with recurrent urinary tract infections with Escherichia coli. Smoking is strongly associated with the development of PBC.

The course of PBC is characterized by insidious progression to almost invariably fatal hepatic cirrhosis. In asymptomatic patients with positive antimitochondrial antibodies and normal liver enzyme concentrations but histological features of early PBC, 75% become symptomatic and 40% show histological progression over a 10-year follow-up period. In symptomatic people with abnormal liver function tests, the median survival time from diagnosis to death is about 10–15 years, and less (5–7 years) in those with advanced histological disease. Despite this poor prognosis, the long natural history makes adequate prospective studies of **therapy** difficult to do. Patients are treated symptomatically: for instance, pruritus usually responds to cholestyramine. Several randomized controlled trials have shown that ursodeoxycholic acid (UDCA), an endogenous tertiary bile acid, is effective in improving liver biochemistry and reducing AMA titres. The drug reduces the risk of developing oesophageal varices and cirrhosis, but a meta-analysis of eight placebo-controlled trials reported no difference in overall death rates between UDCA-treated and placebo-treated patients. The mechanism of action of UDCA and its effect on long-term progression seem multifactorial: it appears to reduce aberrant MHC class II expression on hepatocytes, reduce cytokine progression and induce apoptosis. Standard immunosuppressive drugs such as corticosteroids, azathioprine, methotrexate, mycophenolate and ciclosporin are ineffective in PBC.

Obetocholic acid, a farnesoid-X receptor antagonist, reduces bile acid synthesis and has shown promise in several trials, with reductions in liver enzymes. Rituximab (anti-CD20) and ustekinumab (anti-IL12/IL23) have been trialled, with variable benefit.

Liver transplantation remains the only effective therapy for patients with end-stage PBC, though with better management in the last decade fewer patients are reaching this stage. Indications for transplantation are either symptomatic disease or signs of end-stage liver disease. Results are good, with 5-year survival in excess of 80%. PBC recurs in the allograft with a cumulative risk of 20–30% at 10 years, but recurrent PBC does not affect long-term patient or graft survival, perhaps due to long-term immunosuppression with ciclosporin.

14.8.3 Associated syndromes

About 80% of patients with PBC have associated autoimmune disorders (Box 14.4). Most have **Sjögren's syndrome** (see Chapter 8). This combination of cholestasis, dry eyes, dry mouth and pancreatic hyposecretion classifies PBC as a 'dry gland' or 'sicca' syndrome. Some patients show a **mixed picture of PBC with CAH**. These hybrids are histologically similar to CAH, but are positive for AMA and have raised serum transaminase and alkaline phosphatase levels. About one in three patients with cryptogenic cirrhosis is positive for smooth muscle, mitochondrial or nuclear antibodies. It has been suggested that these cases represent an end stage of autoimmune liver disease, where the destruction of liver cells or bile duct epithelial cells has 'burnt out', leaving the patient with cirrhosis.

Sclerosing cholangitis is a chronic cholestatic liver disease characterized by an obliterative inflammatory fibrosis of the biliary tract. It can lead to biliary cirrhosis, liver failure and carcinoma of the bile ducts. Primary sclerosing cholangitis (PSC) usually presents insidiously with jaundice and hepatosplenomegaly in young adults. The cause is unknown, but there is a close association with IBD, especially ulcerative colitis (Box 14.5); about 5% of patients with ulcerative colitis develop PSC, typically those with pancolitis. Conversely, 50–75% of patients with PSC have colitis. Chronic infection with Cryptosporidia can also cause sclerosing cholangitis and it may be secondary to bile duct stones or bile duct surgery. There is no specific treatment. Liver transplantation is the only option and PSC is now the second most common indication for liver transplantation in the UK.

Box 14.4 Associated syndromes in patients with primary biliary cirrhosis

- Sjögren's syndrome
- Sicca syndrome
- Autoimmune thyroid disease
- Systemic lupus erythematosus
- Scleroderma
- CREST syndrome
- Rheumatoid arthritis
- Fibrosing alveolitis
- Renal tubular acidosis

Box 14.5 Immunological features in primary sclerosing cholangitis

- Associated with HLA-B8, -DR3/-DR52
- Hypergammaglobulinaemia
- Positive atypical antineutrophil cytoplasmic antibodies in 70% of patients – associated with a more severe course
- Increased expression of HLA class II antigens on biliary epithelial cells
- Associated with other immune diseases: ulcerative colitis; primary antibody deficiency

Box 14.6 Limited evidence for immunological involvement in alcoholic liver disease

- The mononuclear cell infiltrate is composed mainly of T lymphocytes
- Reports of an increased prevalence of circulating autoantibodies, including antibodies to dsDNA, in patients with alcoholic hepatitis and/or cirrhosis; probably secondary antibodies to damage
- Antibodies reacting with acetaldehyde-altered liver cell membrane antigens are present in some patients
- Lymphocytes from these patients are cytotoxic to hepatocytes *in vitro*
- Women who are HLA-B8 positive are especially susceptible

Table 14.10 Basic distinctions between directly toxic and hypersensitivity drug reactions

	Directly toxic	Hypersensitivity
Susceptibility	All subjects	Some subjects
Dose related?	Yes	No
Onset following first exposure	Immediate (hours–days)	Delayed (days–weeks)
Onset following second exposure	Immediate	Less delayed (days)

14.8.4 Alcohol-induced liver disease

Alcoholic liver disease is common and found in 15–20% of those who abuse alcohol. Several factors contribute to the liver damage. Alcohol and its metabolites are directly hepatotoxic and cause ultrastructural changes within hours of ingestion. Progression to hepatitis and cirrhosis occurs in some subjects even after cessation of intake, implying that a host factor(s) influences susceptibility. Many of the immunological features of alcohol-induced disease (Box 14.6) are common to other types of liver injury and probably result from dysfunction of the mononuclear phagocytes of the liver (Kupffer cells).

14.8.5 Drug-induced liver disease

A number of drugs can damage the liver; some drugs (or their metabolites) are directly hepatotoxic, while others induce a hypersensitivity reaction (Table 14.10).

Hypersensitivity reactions occur in only a minority of patients exposed to these drugs and the severity of the reaction is not dose related. The drug or a metabolite may combine with a component of the liver cell membrane or denature a 'self' antigen; in either case a 'new' antigen may be formed that is no longer tolerated as 'self'. However, successful attempts to prove immunological hypersensitivity to a drug are rare. The immunological features are usually non-specific, for example oxyphenisatin (a constituent of many laxatives) and isoniazid may induce hepatitis. Although the reaction usually subsides when the drug is stopped, some patients progress insidiously to a form of CAH that is indistinguishable from the 'autoimmune' type and is often accompanied by circulating (presumably secondary) antibodies to nuclei, smooth muscle or LKMs (as in Case 14.6). Deliberate rechallenge would clearly be unethical. In cases of halothane hepatitis, rechallenge has been inadvertent and pyrexia and eosinophilia may precede the appearance of jaundice. Some patients, exposed to halothane on a number of occasions, have eventually lost their hypersensitivity; it is not known whether this was due to faster handling of the toxic metabolite (enzyme induction) or to the development of immunological tolerance.

CHAPTER 15
Endocrinology and Diabetes

Key topics

Visit the companion website at **www.wiley.com/go/misbah/immunology** to download cases with additional figures on these topics.

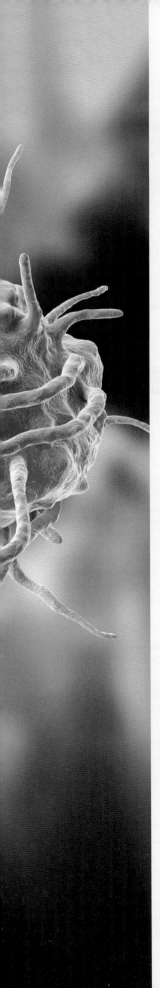

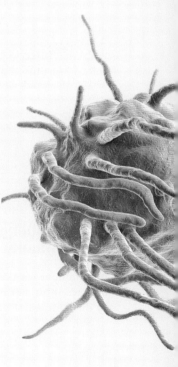

Chapel and Haeney's Essentials of Clinical Immunology, Seventh Edition. Edited by Siraj A. Misbah,
Gavin P. Spickett, and Virgil A.S.H. Dalm.
© 2022 John Wiley & Sons Ltd. Published 2022 by John Wiley & Sons Ltd.

15.1 Introduction

Endocrine cells may be localized in a defined glandular structure such as the adrenal gland, or distributed throughout a non-endocrine organ such as the stomach. Functional disorders of endocrine glands result from **overactivity**, with excessive production of the hormone, or from **atrophy**, with failure to produce the relevant hormone. There are many causes of glandular dysfunction, but autoimmunity to endocrine tissues is one of the commonest.

Most autoimmune endocrine disorders are clinically silent until they present with features of insufficiency of the affected organ. *At this stage the gland is often irreversibly damaged, with little prospect of recovery even if the autoimmune process were arrested.* Current treatment of many of these diseases therefore centres on replacement of hormones. The long period of silent inflammation and glandular destruction, which can last for many years, offers a window during which progress of these diseases could potentially be reversed, if they were detected. However, detection and treatment of preclinical endocrine autoimmunity is currently confined to experimental studies involving small numbers of first-degree relatives of subjects with polyendocrine syndromes or autoimmune diabetes, to define those who are at increased risk of developing the condition.

Fig. 15.1 Examples of autoantibodies in endocrine and other organ-specific autoimmune diseases. TSH, thyroid-stimulating hormone.

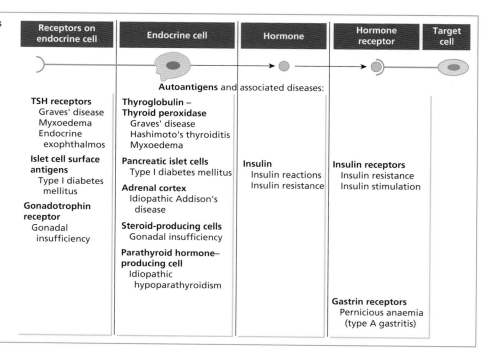

15.2 Mechanisms of endocrine autoimmunity

Autoimmune reactions may be directed against endocrine cells, their receptors, hormones or the receptors on the cells targeted by the hormone (Fig. 15.1).

Since the first report of autoimmune thyroid disease in 1957, autoimmune diseases of every endocrine organ and virtually all endocrine cells have been described.

Autoantibodies to endocrine cells are organ specific and detected only by tests using antigen from the specific endocrine gland involved (Chapter 19). This contrasts with non-organ-specific diseases (such as systemic lupus erythematosus), where

non-organ-specific antigens (such as nuclear antigens) are present in all organs and tissues of the body. A feature of **organ-specific autoimmunity** is that several autoantibodies to endocrine glands may be found in a single patient; this patient may have clinical evidence of one or many endocrine disorders or may be asymptomatic – in other words, *the presence of autoantibodies does not necessarily indicate autoimmune disease.*

There are several mechanisms of autoimmune damage (Fig. 15.1) and more than one mechanism may occur in a given disease. Evidence suggests that both T cells and antibodies often work in parallel to produce autoimmune endocrine disease. As a broad generalization, T cells (both CD4 and CD8) are responsible for glandular destruction and antibodies act via mechanisms discussed in section 15.10 to disturb the physiological function of the gland. Primary autoantibodies are pathogenic and act on surface receptors of the target cells; those autoantibodies that are secondary to glandular destruction acting as markers of disease. Alternatively, neutralization of enzymatic activity by autoantibodies may be pathogenic too.

Antibodies can influence the function or growth of an endocrine gland. Primary stimulating and blocking antibodies against receptors are well recognized, as are antibodies that selectively influence cell growth. Patients may have a mixture of receptor antibodies, some of which stimulate and some of which block the receptor. Shifts from one type to the other explain why some patients fluctuate from overactivity to underactivity of the gland.

15.3 Thyroid disease

Several thyroid antigens are recognized, including the thyroid-stimulating hormone (TSH) receptor, thyroglobulin, thyroid peroxidase (thyroid microsomal antigen), sodium/iodide symporter (the transporter responsible for iodine uptake by thyroid cells), as well as other surface and cytoplasmic thyroid antigens. The most widely available and clinically useful antibody tests are those for **thyroid peroxidase** (secondary or marker antibodies) and the TSH receptor (primary pathogenic antibodies) (Table 15.1).

15.3.1 Thyrotoxicosis

Thyrotoxicosis is a common condition with a prevalence of about 20 per 1000 of the population. It can occur at any age, but the incidence peaks in the third and fourth decades. It is about 5–10 times more common in women than in men. Thyrotoxicosis is most commonly due to **Graves' disease**

(autoimmune hyperthyroidism) or to local hyperactive nodules in the thyroid gland. The diagnosis is made by biochemical thyroid function tests (see Case 15.1). Serum **autoantibodies to thyroid peroxidase** confirm Graves' disease, but these antibodies occur in other autoimmune thyroid conditions too (see Table 15.1). Those patients who have high titres of these autoantibodies are the ones most likely to proceed to thyroid failure, known as myxoedema.

The pathogenesis involves IgG **autoantibodies to the TSH receptor** on the surface of human thyroid cells (Fig. 15.2). Almost all patients with Graves' disease have TSH receptor antibodies that stimulate the thyroid cell (thyroid-stimulating antibodies; Figs 15.2 and 15.3), resulting in thyrotoxicosis or overactive thyroid; however, it is not necessary to measure these autoantibodies routinely for diagnosis.

The autoimmune thyroid is characteristically infiltrated by T lymphocytes: both CD8+ and CD4+ cells are present. These T cells express a more limited number of T-cell receptor genes (see Chapter 1) than do peripheral blood T cells from the same patient; the implication is that intrathyroid T cells are less diverse because they are enriched for T cells specific for thyroid-derived peptides.

Two of every 1000 pregnant women are thyrotoxic and occasionally such pregnancies result in **neonatal Graves' disease**. This is due to transplacental transfer of thyroid-stimulating IgG autoantibodies from mother to fetus. The neonatal disease can be severe: affected babies have goitre, exophthalmos, feeding problems, pyrexia and tachycardia and may develop heart failure unless treated promptly. Spontaneous recovery gradually occurs over 2–3 months, as the maternal

Table 15.1 Prevalence and relative strength of antibodies to thyroid peroxidase commonly detected in various thyroid diseases

Clinical presentation	Antibodies to thyroid peroxidase
Thyrotoxicosis	
Graves' disease	Positive (low titre)
Hot nodules	Negative
Goitre	
Hashimoto's thyroiditis	Positive (high titre)
Simple goitre	Negative
De Quervain's thyroiditis	Transient positive
Carcinoma	Negative
Thyroxine deficiency	
Primary myxoedema	Positive
Normal population	Positive (5–10%)

Case 15.1 Graves' disease

A 29-year-old woman presented with a 3-month history of increased sweating and palpitations with weight loss of 7 kg. On examination, she was a nervous, agitated woman with an obvious, diffuse, non-tender, smooth enlargement of her thyroid, over which a bruit could be heard. She had a fine tremor of her fingers and a resting pulse rate of 150/min. She had no evidence of exophthalmos. A maternal aunt had suffered from 'thyroid disease'.

On investigation, she had a raised serum T3 of 4.8 nmol/l (NR 0.8–2.4) and a T4 of 48 nmol/l (NR 9–23). Measurement of her thyroid-stimulating hormone showed that this was low normal, 0.4 mU/l (NR 0.4–5 mU/l). The biochemical findings pointed to primary thyroid disease rather than pituitary overactivity. Circulating antibodies to thyroid peroxidase (titre 1/3000; 200 IU/ml) were detected by agglutination. A diagnosis of autoimmune thyrotoxicosis (Graves' disease) was made. She was treated with an antithyroid drug, carbimazole, to control her thyrotoxicosis, and surgery was not required.

Fig. 15.2 Surface of a thyroid cell showing actions of the primary antibodies in autoimmune thyroid diseases. LATS, long-acting thyroid stimulator.

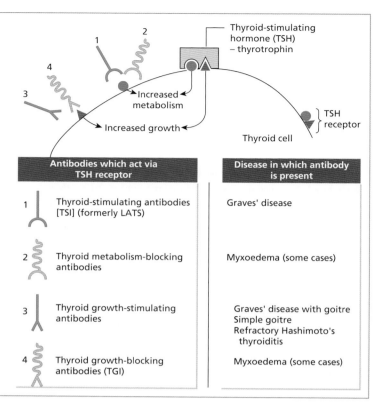

Antibodies which act via TSH receptor	Disease in which antibody is present
1 Thyroid-stimulating antibodies [TSI] (formerly LATS)	Graves' disease
2 Thyroid metabolism-blocking antibodies	Myxoedema (some cases)
3 Thyroid growth-stimulating antibodies	Graves' disease with goitre Simple goitre Refractory Hashimoto's thyroiditis
4 Thyroid growth-blocking antibodies (TGI)	Myxoedema (some cases)

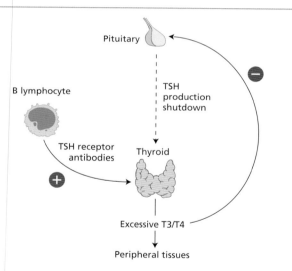

Fig. 15.3 Pituitary–thyroid axis in Graves' disease. TSH, thyroid-stimulating hormone.

IgG is metabolized at a rate consistent with its half-life (i.e. 3–4 weeks) (see Chapter 18).

The degree of thyrotoxicosis in Graves' disease is not related to the size of the goitre; indeed, 10% of patients do not have an enlarged thyroid. **Thyroid growth-stimulating immunoglobulin (TGI)** has been demonstrated in the sera of patients with Graves' disease with goitre, as well as in some patients with toxic multinodular goitres or non-toxic goitres. In contrast to the thyroid-stimulating immunoglobulins (TSI) that cause hyperthyroidism, *these antibodies correlate with goitre size* but not with the overproduction of T3 and T4.

Half of the patients with Graves' disease develop **exophthalmos**; this may precede, coincide with or follow the hyperthyroid phase. It may even occur occasionally in euthyroid patients or in association with Hashimoto's thyroiditis or primary myxoedema. Smoking is a strong risk factor. Exophthalmos results from myositis affecting the eye muscles and a proliferation of retroorbital tissue. The myositis is accompanied by infiltration of lymphocytes – particularly CD4+ T cells. Retroorbital fibroblasts secrete hydrophilic glycosaminoglycans (GAGs) in response to T-cell cytokine signalling, altering the osmotic pressure and resulting in fluid accumulation. The sera from affected patients contain antibodies that bind to eye muscle extract; some of these antibodies cross-react with other orbital antigens as well as thyroid antigens. The TSH receptor seems to be aberrantly expressed in the inflamed orbital tissue, suggesting that an immune response to this antigen may also contribute to the eye disease. In patients with severe exophthalmos and optic nerve compression ('**malignant exophthalmos**'), high-dose steroids are of value, sometimes coupled with other immunosuppressive drugs. If there is deterioration, surgical decompression is indicated.

A few (3–5%) patients with Graves' disease develop **pretibial myxoedema**; they tend to have exophthalmos as well. Pretibial myxoedema refers to well-demarcated, subcutaneous thickening of the anterolateral aspects of the legs; these areas do not pit on pressure, and are shiny and reddish brown in appearance. The development of pretibial myxoedema is not related to the duration or extent of the hyperthyroidism. Its pathogenesis is not well understood, although, as in thyroid eye disease, aberrant expression of the TSH receptor has been described in the affected tissue and secretion of GAGs by cytokine-stimulated fibroblasts is believed to play a role.

Genetic factors are important in the aetiology of Graves' disease. A positive family history of hyperthyroidism is found in around 50% of patients and there is 20–40% concordance in monozygotic twins, but less than 5% in dizygotic twins. As with several other organ-specific autoimmune diseases, HLA-DR3 and polymorphisms of the CTLA-4 gene (see Chapter 1) are both strongly associated with Graves' disease in Caucasians, but genetic associations in other ethnic groups are less well defined. **Environmental** triggers of Graves' disease remain obscure. Some limited evidence exists for infection with several viruses in thyroid tissue in patients with the disease. There is also an association between the onset of Graves' disease and psychological stress. Treatment of multiple sclerosis with the lymphocyte-depleting monoclonal antibody Campath-1H can induce Graves' disease in around 10% of those treated, possibly by depleting an inhibitory T-cell population (see Chapter 5).

Graves' disease can be treated successfully by antithyroid drugs or surgery. *Although trials with immunosuppressive drugs are ongoing to reduce levels of the causative antibodies in selected patients, these are not generally required in treatment of Graves' disease* (Box 15.1).

15.3.2 Hashimoto's thyroiditis

Hashimoto's disease is much more common in women than in men and is probably the commonest cause of goitre in the UK (Case 15.2). At presentation, 75% of patients are euthyroid, 20% are hypothyroid, and the remaining 5% are hyperthyroid and have a disease that closely resembles Graves' disease (known as 'Hashitoxicosis'). *About 50% of patients eventually become hypothyroid due to destruction of the thyroid gland.* Hashimoto's thyroiditis is familial and associated with other organ-specific autoimmune diseases. The close relationship and familial association with Graves' disease, combined with the fact that Hashimoto's thyroiditis may sometimes evolve into Graves' disease (and vice versa), imply a linked pathogenesis.

The **pathogenesis** (Box 15.2) of Hashimoto's thyroiditis involves T cells specifically sensitized against thyroid antigens, with an uncertain contribution from thyroid growth-stimulating antibodies. There are two major clinical forms of the disease: goitrous and atrophic autoimmune thyroiditis. The goitre results from a combination of marked lymphocytic infiltration of the gland together with some degree of hypertrophy of thyroid tissue. The cellular infiltrate consists mainly of CD8+ and CD4+ T cells and some B cells, which can form lymphoid follicles. These cells display activation markers and a range of cytokines can be detected in the inflamed tissue. Destruction of thyroid cells probably occurs by Fas-mediated apoptosis triggered by cytotoxic T cells (see Chapter 5). T cells

Box 15.1 Indirect evidence implicating immunological mechanisms in the pathogenesis of Graves' disease

- Thyroid infiltration by T lymphocytes (both CD4+ and CD8+ cells) and plasma cells
- The presence of circulating autoantibodies to thyroid antigens, especially the thyroid-stimulating hormone (TSH) receptor. Antibodies to the TSH receptor cause stimulation of cultured thyroid cells
- An increased risk of thyroid disease in first-degree relatives of patients with Graves' disease
- Associations with other autoimmune diseases, including myasthenia gravis, pernicious anaemia and rheumatoid arthritis
- Transient Graves' disease in the neonates of pregnant women with Graves' disease

Case 15.2 Hashimoto's thyroiditis

A 39-year-old woman presented with a large, painless swelling in her neck. The enlargement had been a gradual process over 2 years. She had no other symptoms and felt generally well. On examination, her thyroid was diffusively enlarged and had a rubbery consistency. There were no signs of thyrotoxicosis or of thyroid failure on clinical examination.

Thyroid function tests showed that she was euthyroid; T3 was 1.2 nmol/l (NR 0.8–2.4), T4 was 12 nmol/l (NR 9–23) and thyroid-stimulating hormone (TSH) was 6.3 mU/l (NR 0.4–5 mU/l). However, her serum contained high-titre antibodies to thyroid peroxidase (1/64 000; 4000 IU/ml).

This patient had Hashimoto's thyroiditis. The goitre was huge, and she was treated by partial thyroidectomy; the goitre did not recur, and the patient has remained euthyroid for 12 years.

Box 15.2 Evidence for an autoimmune pathogenesis in Hashimoto's thyroiditis

- T cells specific for thyroid antigens are present in the circulation. T-cell clones derived from these cells can kill cultured thyroid cells
- Demonstration of serum autoantibodies that stimulate or block the growth or division of thyroid cells
- Thyroid infiltration by T lymphocytes (both CD4+ and CD8+ cells) and plasma cells
- Induction of experimental, cell-mediated autoimmune thyroiditis by injection of thyroid antigens
- Association of other autoimmune diseases in given individuals and in families

responsive to thyroid antigens (particularly thyroid peroxidase and thyroglobulin) can be detected in both blood and thyroid tissue.

The **differential diagnosis** of Hashimoto's thyroiditis includes simple goitre and subacute (de Quervain's) thyroiditis. The latter usually presents with bilateral painful tender enlargement of the thyroid gland, a low-grade fever and general malaise. Hyperthyroidism is often detectable and is transient. It may be followed by a period of hypothyroidism. Recovery is almost always complete; **De Quervain's thyroiditis** may be of infective origin, since the condition often follows a viral illness. Antibodies to thyroid antigens are usually transient and of low titre; high-titre antibodies to thyroid peroxidase suggest considerable thyroid damage, and the patient may ultimately develop myxoedema. About 70% of the patients with this rare subacute thyroiditis have the HLA antigen B35, suggesting that susceptibility to this disease is also partly governed by the major histocompatibility complex (MHC), but by a different region from other autoimmune endocrine diseases.

The levels of thyroid autoantibodies in patients with Graves' disease and Hashimoto's thyroiditis tend to fall during pregnancy and rebound afterwards. Many pregnant women without overt thyroid disease develop fluctuations in thyroid autoantibodies, with transient disturbances of thyroid function – **post-partum thyroiditis**. The prevalence of the disorder is about 5–10% of all pregnancies. Thyroid dysfunction in the year following pregnancy should be treated cautiously, although the proportion of women with post-partum thyroiditis who later develop overt autoimmune thyroid disease is unknown.

15.3.3 Idiopathic thyroid atrophy (myxoedema)

The term myxoedema describes the severe form of hypothyroidism in which deposition of mucinous substances leads to thickening of the skin and subcutaneous tissues, but it is often used as a label for hypothyroidism in general (see Case 15.3). There are several causes (Fig. 15.4). **Idiopathic thyroid atrophy**, like Hashimoto's thyroiditis, is more commonly found in women. Thyroid biopsies (done for research purposes) show a lymphocytic infiltration, fibrosis and atrophy. Conventional antithyroid antibodies are present in roughly the same proportion of patients as in Hashimoto's thyroiditis (see Table 15.1).

The **pathogenesis** of idiopathic thyroid atrophy is interesting. Just as there are antibodies that stimulate thyroid cell metabolism (in Graves' disease) and those that stimulate growth (in simple and Hashimoto's goitre), so there are antibodies in idiopathic thyroid atrophy that block both growth and metabolism (see Fig. 15.2). Growth-blocking antibodies can occur in the absence of function-blocking antibodies. These appear to be primary antibodies, which react with TSH receptors or other membrane sites; the reason for their production is unknown. Maternal growth-blocking antibodies may play a part in the failure of the thyroid to develop *in utero*, so leading to athyreotic cretinism.

Like Graves' disease, the **genetic predisposition** to autoimmune hypothyroidism and Hashimoto's thyroiditis is linked to

Case 15.3 Primary myxoedema

A 41-year-old woman complained to her doctor that she 'always felt cold', and that she had become increasingly clumsy. Although she made no other complaint, her husband had noticed increasing physical and mental lethargy in his wife in recent months. One of her sisters had thyroid disease and her mother suffered from pernicious anaemia. On examination, her skin was dry, her voice was hoarse and her hair was coarse and brittle. Her pulse rate was 58/min, with a blood pressure of 140/70. Her tendon reflexes showed a markedly delayed relaxation phase.

Clinically, she had hypothyroidism and this was confirmed by thyroid function tests; her serum T3 was 0.4 nmol/l (NR 0.8–2.4), T4 was 4 nmol/l (NR 9–23), and thyroid-stimulating hormone (TSH) was 12.1 mU/l (NR 0.4–5 mU/l). High titres of autoantibodies to thyroid peroxidase were found in the patient's serum to a titre of 1/128 000 (6400 IU/ml). This patient therefore had primary myxoedema and she was treated with replacement doses of L-thyroxine.

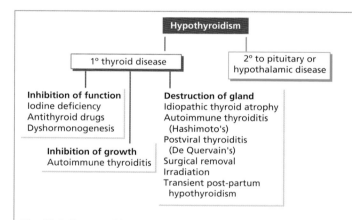

Fig. 15.4 Causes of hypothyroidism.

polymorphism within the HLA locus and the CTLA-4 gene. Unlike Graves' disease, there is no strong association with HLA-DR3, but instead a range of relatively weak associations with various HLA polymorphisms, which differ with ethnic group.

Environmental triggers are uncertain. Smoking, infection and exposure to high and low levels of iodine have all been linked to hypothyroidism. Treatment with certain drugs (for example, lithium or interferon-α) can induce autoimmune hypothyroidism. Exposure to environmental radiation (e.g. following the Chernobyl disaster) has been associated with an increased incidence of thyroid autoimmunity. The high prevalence of subclinical thyroid autoimmunity in Western populations (see Table 15.1) suggests that environmental triggers

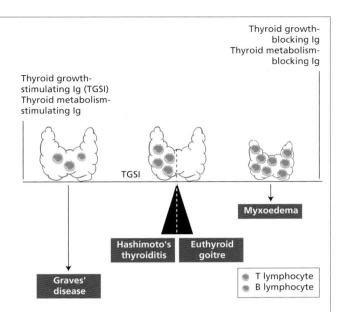

Fig. 15.5 Autoimmune thyroid disease. The clinical state depends on the balance between immunological mechanisms operating at any one time.

Table 15.2 Types of diabetes mellitus		
Features	Type I	Type II
Prevalence	1: 3000 population	3: 100 population (and rising)
Age at onset	Usually <30 years	Usually >40 years
Speed of clinical onset	Acute	Insidious
Associated with autoimmune disorders	Yes	No
Islet-cell antibodies	Yes	No
Other autoantibodies	Sometimes	No
Percentage of cases of diabetes mellitus	10–20%	80–90%
HLA association	DR3 and DR4	No

must either be very widely distributed, that these populations are particularly susceptible or that no specific external trigger exists. Current models of autoimmunity suggest that autoimmune responses can potentially develop after disruption of a target organ by many different inflammatory processes.

Autoimmune thyroid disease shows that the clinical state depends on the balance between the effects of sensitized T cells and autoantibodies against target antigens (Fig. 15.5). In this respect, autoimmune thyroid disease serves as a model for other autoimmune endocrine states.

15.4 Diabetes mellitus

15.4.1 Classification of diabetes mellitus

Diabetes mellitus is divided into **insulin-dependent diabetes mellitus (IDDM or type 1)** and **non-insulin-dependent diabetes mellitus (NIDDM or type 2)** (Table 15.2). Type 2 is not discussed further. Type 1 diabetes can be subdivided into two main forms: type 1A, usually of childhood onset and characterized by immunologically mediated destruction of the β cells of pancreatic islets, and type 1B, where severe β-cell destruction occurs in the absence of any obvious immune response directed against the pancreas. Antibodies against islet cells can be detected in type 1A but not type 1B diabetes (see Case 15.4).

15.4.2 Immunopathogenesis of type 1 diabetes mellitus

Like thyroid disease, type 1 diabetes mellitus is an organ-specific autoimmune disease and is associated with other organ-specific autoimmune diseases such as thyrotoxicosis or

Case 15.4 Diabetes mellitus

A 26-year-old pregnant woman attended the antenatal clinic regularly. She had no family history of diabetes. At 24 weeks' gestation she was found to have asymptomatic glycosuria. A glucose tolerance test showed that not only was her fasting blood glucose raised, but she had poor glucose tolerance. Gestational diabetes was diagnosed and the patient was admitted for diabetic control. This was achieved on oral hypoglycaemic agents alone and the patient was instructed to check her urine daily. The pregnancy was uneventful and a normal, 3.8 kg baby was born. The patient's glucose tolerance returned to normal in the puerperium; however, her serum, which was found to contain antibodies to pancreatic islet cells at the time of diagnosis, remained positive. Nine years later, after yearly checks, the patient developed overt diabetes mellitus.

myxoedema. *Insulin production fails in autoimmune diabetes because of a specific immune response directed against the insulin-producing β cells in the pancreatic islets of Langerhans.* Histological studies show extensive immune infiltration of the islets by activated CD8 and CD4 T cells and macrophages, reduction in the number of β cells and relative sparing of the glucagon-producing cells. β cells show expression of both class II MHC and co-stimulatory molecules, indicating that they may present autoantigens to CD4+ T cells. Cellular infiltration of the islets, and consequent β-cell damage, may precede overt diabetes by many years, sometimes decades; the presence of subclinical β-cell destruction is suggested by the presence of circulating islet-cell antibodies (ICAs), activated T cells and impaired glucose tolerance long before clinical diabetes develops (Fig. 15.6).

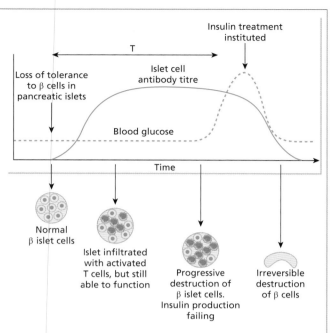

Fig. 15.6 Relationship between immunologically mediated damage to islet cells, islet-cell antibodies as a marker of this process and blood glucose. The time interval '*t*' represents the window of opportunity for immunological intervention to prevent diabetes.

Numerous **autoantigens** have been identified in autoimmune diabetes. Antibody responses, and to a lesser extent T-cell responses, against these antigens have been studied in detail. Those antigens most closely linked to diabetes include islet-cell cytoplasmic enzymes, particularly glutamic acid decarboxylase (**GAD**) and **IA-2** (a tyrosine phosphatase), **ZnT8** (a zinc transporter in β cells) and **insulin** itself. **ICAs** detected by immunofluorescence are probably made up of a mixture of antibodies reacting against GAD and several other cytoplasmic antigens. The relationship between these autoimmune responses and islet-cell damage is not well defined, but the recurrence of diabetes following pancreatic transplantation between IDDM-discordant identical twins, histological studies and evidence from animal models suggest that β cells are probably killed by cytotoxic T cells, with autoantibodies playing a more minor role. The description of type I diabetes in a 14-year-old boy suffering from X-linked agammaglobulinaemia suggests that B cells are not necessary in the development of this condition, though B cells or antibodies may facilitate early presentation. This is supported by a mouse model of type 1 diabetes in which depletion of B cells results in reduced incidence and delayed onset of pancreatic failure.

Among the numerous potential autoantigens, GAD has been the subject of particular interest. Antibodies to GAD were first described in the neurological condition called '**stiff man syndrome**', which is often associated with IDDM and ICA. Antibodies to GAD are highly predictive of subsequent development of IDDM, and T- and B-cell responses to GAD have

been shown to be of major pathogenic importance in an animal model of diabetes.

Genetic factors make a considerable contribution to the risk of developing type 1A IDDM. An unaffected identical twin of a newly diagnosed diabetic has an approximately 45% chance of subsequently developing the disease, compared with a risk of 0.4% in the general population. Associations with specific MHC polymorphisms can account for a substantial proportion of this genetic predisposition. Around 95% of diabetics from north European ethnic groups possess HLA-DR3 or -DR4 (compared with around 45% of healthy subjects), and around 40% of Caucasian type 1A diabetics are DR3/DR4 heterozygotes (compared with only 2.5% of healthy subjects). Studies of HLA genes at the molecular level showed that this association with HLA-DR is secondary to a stronger link with certain HLA-DQ variants, particularly the DR3, DQ2 or DR4, DQ8 haplotypes. A critical factor seems to be the amino acid at position 57 in the HLA-DQβ chain. Genetic variants of DQB that encode the amino acid aspartate at this position seem to confer protection against IDDM, whereas variants encoding other amino acids increase the risk. The HLA-DR3 and -DR4 association arises because, in north European populations, these DR alleles are linked to DQβ alleles that do not encode aspartate. The mechanism behind this very specific molecular association is not known, but amino acid 57 in HLA-DQβ lies in the 'antigen-binding groove' and could potentially influence binding of a critical autoantigenic peptide. No genetic associations have been identified for type 1B diabetes.

Although this is the strongest and most clearly defined association between a gene and risk of diabetes, detailed studies of large numbers of families suggest that interactions between **10 and 15** genes are important in controlling the onset of IDDM. The locus with the second strongest linkage to IDDM is a noncoding region of the insulin gene; polymorphisms in this region may influence how strongly the insulin gene is expressed in the thymus. Other associations have been identified, including polymorphisms in the CTLA4 gene and interleukin (IL)-2 receptor gene. It is not surprising that type 1 diabetes is therefore a polygenic disease, as with other autoimmune conditions with particular susceptibilities and increased risk associated with a positive family history.

The observation that more than 50% of non-diabetic identical twins of newly diagnosed diabetics do not ultimately develop diabetes shows that **environmental** factors also play a role in triggering this disease. This is further emphasized by a marked global increase in incidence of IDDM over the last decade, and the seasonal variation in diagnosis, with autumn and winter peaks. Models of environmental causation of IDDM have centred on infectious agents, although exposure to cow's milk or other food proteins has also been suggested as a risk factor. A small number of cases of diabetes can be temporally linked to specific infections, particularly with viruses that are known to have a tropism for the pancreas such as mumps and Coxsackie. Similarities have been noted between the sequence of certain Coxsackie virus proteins and antibodies to

GAD, suggesting a potential for autoimmunity triggered by molecular mimicry (see Chapter 5). However, the only infection that has been unequivocally linked to type 1 diabetes is congenital rubella, which is now very rare. Most newly diagnosed diabetics show no consistent relationship with any specific infection; autoimmune diseases can potentially follow a variety of inflammatory insults to the target organ, not just infections.

15.4.3 Treatment of diabetes mellitus

Treatment of IDDM is replacement insulin only, though attempts have been made to prevent IDDM or stop β-cell destruction involving intensive immunosuppressive therapy (e.g. ciclosporin, azathioprine). Since probably less than 10% of functioning β-cell mass remains at diagnosis, not surprisingly success in inducing remission of diabetes has been limited. Several other potential early immunomodulatory therapies are under investigation, including T-cell depletion with monoclonal antibodies, tumour necrosis factor (TNF)-α inhibition and co-stimulation blockade.

An alternative approach would be to induce specific tolerance to major islet-cell antigens. It is not known whether this could be achieved in human IDDM, but animal experiments suggest that administration of autoantigen by particular routes (especially via mucosal surfaces) can alter the immune response to that antigen, and both prevent and arrest the course of IDDM.

Pancreatic transplantation has become successful in the last decade. The outlook is relatively good for patients with a pancreas transplant, especially for those that receive a simultaneous kidney transplant for associated renal failure, most transplanted pancreases functioning well for 10 years.

Type II diabetes is not associated with ICA. This type of diabetes shows a strong familial tendency, but no association with autoimmunity or with any particular HLA type. However, over 10% of adult patients initially treated by diet or oral hypoglycaemic drugs do have ICAs in their sera at presentation. Often these patients eventually require insulin therapy to achieve satisfactory diabetic control; therefore, they are latent type 1 diabetics.

15.4.4 Complications of diabetes mellitus

Infection is a major complication of diabetes mellitus. The pattern of infection in poorly controlled diabetes is consistent with a neutrophil defect, with a high incidence of staphylococcal and fungal infection. Patients with poorly controlled diabetes have defects in neutrophil function that reverse following adequate insulin therapy.

The long-term complications of diabetes mellitus involve diseases of **major arteries** (leading to atheroma) or of **capillaries** (microangiopathy). Microangiopathy is responsible for the retinal and glomerular lesions of diabetes. In developed countries, diabetic retinopathy accounts for much of the acquired blindness in young and middle-aged adults. Retinopathy is rarely found within 5 years of diagnosis, but more than one-third of patients are affected 15–20 years after diagnosis. Long-term control of blood glucose and other cardiovascular risk factors (such as hypertension and serum cholesterol) reduces the incidence and severity of these complications. Renal failure is a common cause of death in those with poorly controlled type 1 diabetes.

15.4.5 Are immunological tests useful?

Immunological tests have no part to play in the clinical diagnosis of type 1 or type 2 diabetes mellitus. The autoantibody response to islet-cell antigens does, however, powerfully predict the risk of developing IDDM in first-degree relatives (Fig. 15.7): the risk of diabetes increases dramatically with the number of antigens targeted by the antibody response. If antibodies are detected against three major antigens, development of diabetes is virtually certain to develop over the next few years. The titre of ICAs is also important in determining outcome: among relatives of patients with IDDM, over 50% of those with high-titre ICAs develop IDDM compared with less than 10% of those with low-titre antibodies. In a population sample of school children, those positive for ICA were about 500 times more likely to develop IDDM over a 10-year period than children negative for serum ICA. At present, there are no safe and effective immunological interventions to prevent islet-cell destruction in those individuals at high risk of diabetes. However, once such therapies are available, the case for clinical screening programmes will become very strong. Furthermore, in a recent study of the prevalence of organ-specific autoantibodies in type 1 diabetic patients, there was a considerably higher prevalence of autoantibodies that would predict other autoimmune conditions, or even polyendocrine disorders (see section 15.10), compared to healthy controls.

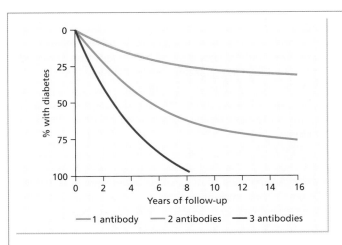

Fig. 15.7 The relationship between the number of autoantibody specificities directed against insulin, IA-2 and/or glutamic acid decarboxylase (GAD) detected in the serum of first-degree relatives of patients with type 1 diabetes, and subsequent development of diabetes. Those patients with three antibodies develop diabetes fastest.

15.5 Adrenal disease

Primary adrenocortical hypofunction, or **Addison's disease**, is an uncommon disease that affects 6 in every 100 000 of the population. Some cases of Addison's disease are due to destruction of the adrenal cortex by tuberculosis, other granulomatous diseases or carcinoma (primary or secondary); the majority (75–80%) of cases, called idiopathic Addison's disease, are autoimmune in origin, i.e. autoimmune adrenalitis.

15.5.1 Autoimmune adrenal disease

Autoimmune adrenalitis affects the adrenal cortex but spares the adrenal medulla. Like other autoimmune endocrinopathies, it is more common in women and reaches a maximum incidence between 40 and 50 years of age. Patients' sera should be tested for all organ-specific autoantibodies, as 40% of patients have at least one other autoimmune endocrinopathy (Table 15.3). The presence of autoantibodies may predict future onset of the associated disease, so that replacement therapy (or other relevant treatment) can be started promptly (see Case 15.5).

Evidence for immune involvement in idiopathic Addison's disease is shown in Box 15.3. The presence of antibodies to cytoplasmic adrenal cortex antigens suggests immune involvement, since fewer than 5% of patients with adrenal damage due to tuberculosis have this antibody. Cell-mediated immunity to adrenal tissue can be demonstrated in about 60% of patients with 'idiopathic' Addison's disease. Antibodies to corticotrophin receptors have also been detected; these block adrenocorticotrophic hormone (ACTH)-induced adrenal cell growth

in vitro. As in Graves' disease, where autoantibodies to the TSH receptor are pathogenic, such antibodies are primary and pathogenic with or without secondary cytoplasmic antibodies.

One of the key enzymes in steroid biosynthesis, 21α-hydroxylase, seems to be the major target autoantigen in adrenal autoimmunity. Autoantibodies to other endocrine tissues can often be detected. For example, 60% of patients have elevated serum antithyroid peroxidase antibodies. As with other organ-specific autoimmune conditions, autoimmune adrenalitis is strongly associated with HLA B8, DR3 and DR4 alleles.

15.6 Parathyroid disease

Some cases of parathyroid failure, usually in childhood, are due to organ-specific autoimmunity. These are often accompanied by Addison's disease, premature ovarian failure or pernicious anaemia. Vitiligo (another autoimmune condition affecting the skin – see Chapter 11) may precede autoimmune hypoparathyroidism. Autoantibodies to cytoplasmic parathyroid tissue are detected in 30–70% of patients with idiopathic hypoparathyroidism.

15.7 Gonadal disease

15.7.1 Oophoritis

Primary amenorrhoea or premature menopause is often described in women with autoimmune disease, particularly 'idiopathic' Addison's disease, hypothyroidism or hypoparathyroidism. Histologically, the ovaries show lymphocytic

---

Case 15.5 Addison's disease

A 12-year-old girl presented with vague abdominal discomfort for 6 months. She had noticed occasional diarrhoea but had not passed any blood. She admitted to weight loss (6 kg) and anorexia. On examination, she was obviously pigmented, although she thought this was sun induced; however, her buccal mucosa and gums were also brown. There were no other physical signs.

She had a low cortisol level and her response to the adrenocorticotrophic hormone in a Synacthen test was poor. A diagnosis of adrenal cortical failure was made. X-ray of her abdomen showed no calcified areas in either adrenal gland, and her serum contained antibodies to adrenal cortex, consistent with a diagnosis of Addison's disease due to autoimmune adrenalitis. Her serum also contained antibodies to pancreatic islet cells and thyroid microsomes. In view of her young age at presentation and these serum antibodies, she will be followed at yearly intervals to see if she develops other autoimmune endocrinopathies.

Table 15.3 Association of 'idiopathic' Addison's disease with other endocrine diseases

Associated autoimmune disease	Patients (%) with other organ involvement
Thyroid diseases	19
Diabetes mellitus	15
Ovarian failure	8
Hypoparathyroidism	4
Pernicious anaemia	2

Box 15.3 Evidence for immune involvement in idiopathic Addison's disease

- Association with other autoimmune diseases
- Presence of autoantibody to steroid cells of adrenal cortex, especially to 21α-hydroxylase, and high incidence of other organ-specific autoantibodies
- Diffuse lymphocytic infiltration of adrenal cortex
- Evidence of cell-mediated immunity to adrenal cortex antigens
- Adrenal failure produced experimentally in animals by immunization with adrenal tissue, with transfer by lymph node cells

infiltration (oophoritis), as do the other target organs in auto-immune endocrinopathies. These women sometimes have **steroidal cell antibodies** that react with Leydig cells, ovarian granulosa and theca interna cells. The presence of such antibodies predicts ovarian failure, especially in patients who have Addison's or other autoimmune disease and yet still have normal menstrual function. Sera from other women with premature menopause inhibit the binding of follicle-stimulating hormone (FSH) to its receptor. The pathogenic significance of ovarian antibodies in autoimmune oophoritis remains to be determined.

15.8 Infertility

15.8.1 Immunology of infertility

Between 5% and 15% of infertile couples show evidence of sperm antibodies. These antibodies may be produced by the man, the woman or both.

Experimental male animals can be made sterile by active or passive immunization with testicular or seminal antigens. In humans, damage to the seminal tract by surgery, accidental trauma, occlusion or infection may trigger autoimmunity to testicular and seminal antigens. For example, antisperm antibodies appear in the serum in 50% of vasectomized men within 6–12 months of surgery. Antisperm antibodies seldom appear in seminal plasma following vasectomy, as local antibody production occurs proximal to the operation site. High titres of antisperm antibodies may appear in the semen after reversal by vasovasostomy and so reduce or annul the success of the reversal (see Chapter 18).

15.9 Pituitary disease

Compared with other endocrine organs, autoimmune disease of the pituitary is rare. Patients who have multiple autoimmune endocrine diseases occasionally have antibodies that stain normal human pituitary gland, but the significance of these is unclear.

15.10 Autoimmune polyendocrine disease

The close relationship between different autoimmune endocrine diseases is clear from preceding discussions. They may overlap not only in individual patients but also in other members of a family. The association of at least two autoimmune endocrinopathies in a single patient is known as **autoimmune polyendocrine disease**.

Three principal patterns of autoimmune polyendocrine disease have been identified, although not all cases fit neatly into this pattern. These syndromes show a strong tendency to aggre-

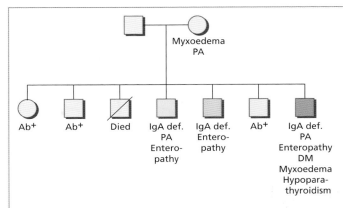

Fig. 15.8 A family study in type 3 autoimmune polyendocrinopathy. Ab+, Autoantibody positive but no clinical disease; DM, diabetes mellitus; IgA def., IgA deficiency; PA, pernicious anaemia.

gate within families, although sporadic cases do occur. Families with so-called type I polyglandular syndromes have autoimmune failure particularly of the parathyroids, adrenal cortex and gonads, together with chronic mucocutaneous candidiasis. This autosomal recessive syndrome, also known as **APECED (autoimmune polyendocrinopathy, candidiasis and ectodermal dysplasia)**, is caused by mutations in the AIRE gene (see Chapter 5). Families with type 2 polyglandular syndromes have adrenal failure together with thyroid and/or islet-cell autoimmunity. Type 3 polyendocrine disease consists of the combination of thyroid autoimmunity with at least two other autoimmune disorders, particularly pernicious anaemia, IDDM and non-endocrine immunological disorders such as IgA deficiency, autoimmune enteropathy or myasthenia gravis. Type 2 and Type 3 autoimmune syndromes are genetically heterogeneous, although both have been linked to the A1 B8 DR3 haplotype and tend to have a dominant pattern of inheritance (Fig. 15.8). An X-linked syndrome has also been described, characterized by diarrhoea, diabetes, hypothyroidism and eczema. This syndrome, known as **IPEX (immune dysregulation, polyendocrinopathy and X-linked inheritance)**, is caused by mutations in a gene encoding a transcription factor that is expressed at high levels in CD4 CD25 regulatory T cells (Tregs). Affected infants have absent Tregs and require human stem cell transplantation to prevent an neonatal death, so early diagnosis is particularly important.

There is a strong link between coeliac disease (Chapter 14, section 14.4.2) and type 1A diabetes. Approximately 10% of patients with type 1 diabetes have tissue transglutaminase and/or endomysial IgA antibodies, and about half of these patients have histological evidence of coeliac disease on small bowel biopsy, which is usually clinically silent. There is overlap between the genetic predispositions to these two diseases, with the DR3, DQ2 haplotype being strongly associated with both.

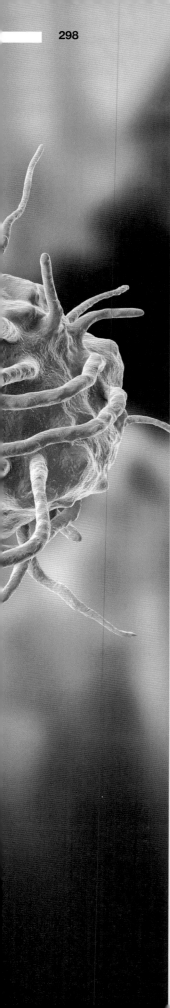

CHAPTER 16
Non-malignant Haematological Diseases

Key topics

 Visit the companion website at **www.wiley.com/go/misbah/immunology** to download cases with additional figures on these topics.

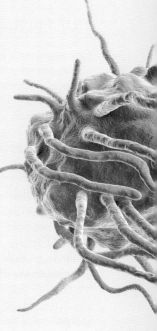

Chapel and Haeney's Essentials of Clinical Immunology, Seventh Edition. Edited by Siraj A. Misbah, Gavin P. Spickett, and Virgil A.S.H. Dalm.
© 2022 John Wiley & Sons Ltd. Published 2022 by John Wiley & Sons Ltd.

16.1 Introduction

In this chapter, those haematological diseases in which the immune response plays a pathogenic role are considered. For example, anaemia, thrombocytopenia, neutropenia or disordered blood clotting can all be due to **antibodies directed against components of blood**. In most cases, these antibodies are autoantibodies. However, disease also results from the stimulation of alloantibodies (isoimmune antibodies) by repeated blood transfusions or pregnancy. Direct activation of complement by erythrocytes and the role of the immune system in bone marrow failure (such as aplastic anaemia) are also discussed here. Malignancies of lymphocytes, namely leukaemias and lymphomas, are discussed in Chapter 6.

Reductions in circulating cells in general may be due to **either failure of production or excess immune destruction** (as illustrated for anaemia in Fig. 16.1). Before considering an immune cause, other causes of haemolysis should be excluded, for example sickle cell disease, thalassaemia and G6PD deficiency.

16.1.1 Mechanisms of immune destruction

The immune system can destroy mature erythrocytes, platelets and neutrophils as well as some haematological precursors in the bone marrow. Immune destruction of red cells is used as the model shown later, though the **mechanisms are common** to all forms of destruction of cellular blood components resulting in cytopenias (Box 16.1).

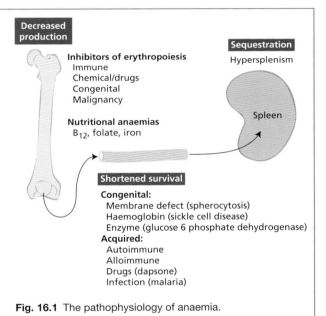

Fig. 16.1 The pathophysiology of anaemia.

Box 16.1 Mechanisms of immune destruction in cytopenias

- Antibodies attach to antigen on cell surfaces prior to phagocytosis in spleen – most common (extravascular)
- Complement-mediated lysis following antibody binding – less common (intravascular)
- Direct complement lysis without antibody involvement – rare
- Soluble immune complexes binding via CR1 (C3b) receptors (immune adherence) prior to phagocytosis
- Soluble immune complexes binding via Fc receptors (innocent bystander destruction) prior to phagocytosis

16.2 Autoimmune haemolytic anaemias

The common **causes** of anaemia are given in Fig. 16.1, which shows that the immune system is not often involved; nutritional deficiencies account for many more cases of anaemia than autoimmune processes. Autoimmune haemolytic anaemia (AIHA) is the commonest cause of shortened survival of red cells in Caucasians, though hereditary defects (such as sickle cell anaemia) are more common in other racial groups.

AIHA may be **primary** (idiopathic, with no known cause) or **secondary** to preexisting disease. Autoantibodies formed in the secondary cases do not appear to be any different, either serologically or immunochemically, from those in primary AIHA. Fig. 16.2 shows the different types of AIHA.

The **diagnosis** of AIHA depends on the demonstration of autoantibodies attached to the patient's red cells or free in the serum. The screening test used is the Coombs' test (Fig. 16.3); antibodies and complement components are detected on the surface of red cells by means of an antiglobulin reagent. This is a mixture of antibodies that reacts with IgG, IgM or C3, but cannot distinguish between specific antibodies directed against red cells and immune complexes attached to the surface by Fc or C3b receptors. In practice, the only immune complexes that are adsorbed sufficiently firmly to be a problem are drug–antibody complexes. Therefore, if the patient has signs of increasing haemolysis and no history of medication, a positive Coombs' test is good presumptive evidence for AIHA due to

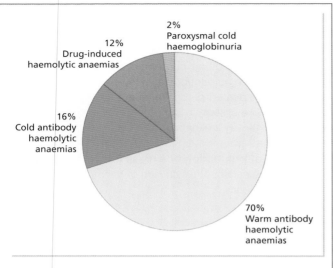

Fig. 16.2 Frequencies of different types of haemolytic anaemias.

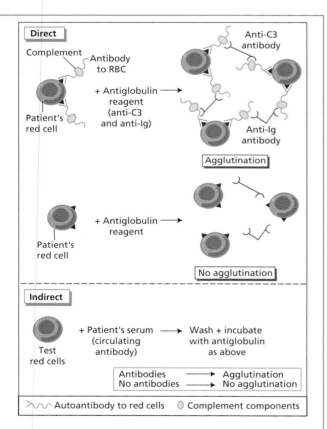

Fig. 16.3 Principles of the direct and indirect Coombs' tests. RBC, red blood cells.

autoantibodies. Specific antibodies to IgG, IgM and C3 can be used at different incubation temperatures to type the AIHA (Box 16.2) and antibodies eluted off the red cell surface to enable typing of their specificity.

Box 16.2 Antibodies in autoimmune haemolytic anaemia

- Warm-reactive IgG autoantibodies, which are best detected at 37 °C
- Cold-reactive IgM autoantibodies, which are detected at temperatures between 4 °C and 37 °C
- Drug-provoked immune haemolytic anaemias
- Complement-activating IgG of paroxysmal cold haemoglobulinuria (Fig. 16.4)

Table 16.1 Comparative features of warm and cold autoimmune haemolytic anaemia (AIHA)

	Warm AIHA	Cold AIHA
Age (in years)	30+	60+
Cause of symptoms	Chronic haemolysis	Peripheral microvascular obstruction, e.g. Raynaud's phenomenon
Mechanism of anaemia	Opsonization and phagocytosis	Intravascular haemolysis related to cold
Jaundice	Common	Uncommon
Splenomegaly	Common	Uncommon
Underlying disease	Present in approx. 50%	Uncommon but accompanying Raynaud's phenomenon
Response to steroids	Good	Poor
Response to splenectomy	50% of cases improve	Poor
Usual class of antibody + type of response	IgG – polyclonal	IgM – monoclonal/polyclonal
Commonest specificity of antibody	Usually non-specific	Anti-I antigen

16.2.1 Warm antibody haemolytic anaemias

The **warm antibody type** of AIHA (Table 16.1) affects all ages and both sexes, although most patients are over 30 years old. It is of varying severity and may be transient or persist for years. About one-half of the patients have idiopathic disease (Table 16.1), but in the remainder the anaemia is secondary to lymphoma or autoimmune disease, especially systemic lupus erythematosus (SLE) (see Fig. 16.4). The aetiology of primary idiopathic AIHA is unknown, although there are sporadic reports of familial occurrences of AIHA.

Usually, warm antibody AIHA is caused by IgG antibodies that react to protein antigens on the surface of red blood cells at body temperature.

Red cells from AIHA patients are **direct Coombs' test positive**. The commonest reaction pattern (50%) on red cells is to have both IgG and C3 fixed on their surfaces; IgG only is found in 40% of cases. In the remaining 10%, complement alone is detected, nearly always in the form of C3d (see Chapter 1). The immunoglobulin is nearly always polyclonal, i.e. of mixed κ and λ light chain types.

Free autoantibodies can also be demonstrated in the serum of about one-third of patients by an indirect antiglobulin test (Fig. 16.3). A positive test for free autoantibody is associated with more severe haemolysis (as in Case 16.1). In most cases, IgG autoantibodies are non-agglutinating (and therefore called 'incomplete' by haematologists), but they are nevertheless destructive. If enzyme-treated cells are used, the sensitivity of the test is increased due to a reduction of surface charge, making the cells more 'agglutinable'.

Many antibodies can be **eluted** from the red cells' surfaces even if there is no free antibody in the serum. These polyclonal autoantibodies may have specificity against a particular red cell antigen or represent a mixture of antibodies against common erythrocyte surface antigens.

The commonest pathogenesis in warm antibody haemolytic anaemia is coating of red cells by opsonizing antibody alone or with complement components (including C3b). Such opsonized cells are removed from the circulation by **splenic macrophages** (Box 16.1).

Management consists of attempts to reduce antibody production as well as excessive red cell destruction. Corticosteroids are the mainstay of treatment and have reduced mortality considerably. Other immunosuppressive drugs, such as cyclophosphamide and azathioprine, have been used as steroid-sparing agents. Unfortunately, the condition tends to relapse when azathioprine is stopped. There is now good evidence that the anti-CD20 monoclonal antibody rituximab (Chapter 7) is useful in managing AIHA resistant to conventional treatments. Removal of the B cells producing the autoantibodies by rituximab is successful in approximately 70% of AIHA patients, but at the cost of destroying all mature B cells and resulting transient antibody deficiency for up to 1 year or so.

Splenectomy is nearly always beneficial if steroids fail; as well as removing the site of phagocytosis, a source of autoantibody production is eliminated. This has to be balanced against the increased risk of infection (see Chapter 3, section 3.5.1). *Blood transfusion is contraindicated unless anaemia is life threatening.*

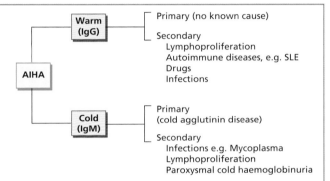

Fig. 16.4 Causes of different types of haemolytic anaemias. AIHA, autoimmune haemolytic anaemia; SLE, systemic lupus erythematosus.

Case 16.1 Primary autoimmune haemolytic anaemia (AIHA)

A 32-year-old man gradually noticed that he had 'yellow eyes' and dark urine, felt continually tired and was short of breath when climbing stairs. He had no other symptoms; in particular, there was no itching, fever or bleeding; he was not taking any drugs. On examination, he was anaemic and jaundiced but afebrile, with no palpable lymphadenopathy, hepatosplenomegaly, rash or arthropathy.

On investigation, his haemoglobin was very low at 54 g/l. The white cell count appeared raised (40 × 10⁹/l), but this was due to nucleated red cells being counted as leucocytes by the automated counter. The blood film showed gross polychromasia with nucleated red cells and spherocytes; the reticulocyte count in the blood was 9%. His serum bilirubin (47 mmol/l), aspartate transaminase (90 IU/l) and lactate dehydrogenase levels (5721 IU/l) were raised. Further tests showed that his red cells had IgG and C3 on their surfaces by the direct Coombs' test. Serum contained warm non-specific autoantibodies (i.e. reactive with all the red cells in the test panel). Antinuclear antibodies and rheumatoid factor tests were negative and immunoglobulin levels were normal; there were no paraprotein bands in his serum or urine. Large amounts of urinary haemosiderin were detected.

A laboratory diagnosis of primary AIHA due to warm antibodies (leading to haemolysis and jaundice) was made. He failed to respond to high-dose corticosteroids and had a splenectomy 3 weeks later. Although impalpable, the spleen was twice the normal size; histology did not reveal a malignancy. He made a good post-operative recovery; his haemoglobin rose rapidly and the reticulocyte count fell. He took prophylactic penicillin for at least 2 years after surgery to prevent severe Streptococcus pneumonia infection.

16.2.2 Cold antibody haemolytic anaemias

Cold antibody haemolytic anaemias may be primary or secondary (Fig. 16.4). Patients with **cold haemagglutinin disease (CHAD)** present with chronic haemolytic anaemia (anaemia, haemoglobinuria and jaundice) and severe Raynaud's phenomenon on exposure to cold (see Table 16.1). Idiopathic CHAD is the most common form and is a disorder of elderly people; secondary cases occasionally occur in association with non-Hodgkin's lymphoma, Mycoplasma pneumoniae infection or infectious mononucleosis. Rarely, a patient who has had 'idiopathic' CHAD for years develops a lymphoma.

Usually, cold antibody AIHA is caused by IgM antibodies that bind to polysaccharide antigens on the surface of red blood cells in the **patient's cold extremities**. As the blood warms up again, complement is activated and intravascular haemolysis results. This is one of few known examples of a direct haemolytic role of complement *in vivo*. Red cells from all patients with CHAD have detectable IgM on their surfaces at 4 °C; on warming, the antibody detaches from the erythrocyte surface, but fixed C3d can still be detected by a Coombs' test. The temperature levels between which the antibody reacts with the red cell antigens is termed the **thermal range**.

Free cold autoantibodies (**cold agglutinins**) are also present in the patient's serum. Ninety per cent of pathological cold antibodies are specific for I antigen (Case 16.2). This antigen occurs only on adult red cells and the 'i' antigen, by contrast, only on cord blood cells. Of cold antibodies, 8% are anti-i;

such cases are usually associated with infectious mononucleosis. In contrast to warm agglutinins (see Table 16.1), the cold antibodies found in idiopathic CHAD or in association with a lymphoma are monoclonal, though the amount of monoclonal antibody is usually far too small to be detectable as a paraprotein by serum electrophoresis; those that develop after an infection are polyclonal.

Treatment is usually unnecessary provided that the patient keeps the extremities warm. Steroid treatment and splenectomy are relatively ineffective since red cell destruction is predominantly intravascular. Treatment of an underlying lymphoma may stop the haemolysis, especially if rituximab is used. Plasma exchange removes circulating IgM rapidly in severe cases.

16.2.3 Drug-induced autoimmune haemolytic anaemias

Drugs can provoke an AIHA (Case 16.3) by three mechanisms (Box 16.3). Not all patients with a positive Coombs' test develop overt haemolysis; *only those affected clinically need to have the drug withdrawn.*

16.2.4 Paroxysmal nocturnal haemoglobinuria

Paroxysmal nocturnal haemoglobinuria (PNH) is a rare acquired clonal mutation of the pig-A gene of stem cells. resulting

---

🔍 Case 16.2 Cold haemagglutinin disease

A 77-year-old man presented one winter with malaise and very cold hands and feet. He admitted to a tendency to bruise easily, and to passing dark urine in cold weather. He was not on any medication and was a non-smoker. On examination, he had some bruising on the shins and was mildly jaundiced. His fingers and toes were cold, but not ischaemic. He had small but palpable lymph nodes in both axillae and groins but no hepatosplenomegaly.

His haemoglobin was low (100 g/l) and the blood film showed rouleaux formation (autoagglutination) and polychromasia; neutrophil, lymphocyte and platelet counts were normal. He had raised serum bilirubin and lactate dehydrogenase levels: serum iron, folate and vitamin B$_{12}$ measurements were normal. He had normal IgG (8.3 g/l) and IgA (1.2 g/l) levels and a slightly raised IgM (4.2 g/l); electrophoresis of serum and urine showed no paraprotein bands. He had a normal level of serum β$_2$-microglobulin. There were cold antibodies in his serum that agglutinated red cells of 'I' specificity. A laboratory diagnosis of cold haemagglutinin disease leading to haemolysis and mild jaundice was made. He was advised to keep as warm as possible at all times. He has been seen regularly over the last 8 years, but has not required active treatment or developed an overt lymphoid malignancy.

🔍 Case 16.3 Cephalosporin-induced haemolytic anaemia

A 72-year-old woman with osteoarthritis suffered acute haemolysis after her right hip was replaced. She had no evidence of splenomegaly and no lymphadenopathy to suggest an underlying malignancy. No explanation was found for the episode; warm and cold antibody tests were negative. She remained well until she had the other hip replaced 2 years later, when she again developed haemolysis soon after the anaesthetic, as well as after the revision 7 months later. Her serum was found to react with red cells coated with the cephalosporin used at the time of anaesthetic induction. She was advised that she had cephalosporin-induced haemolytic anaemia and to avoid this antibiotic in the future. She invested in a MediAlert bracelet to ensure that she was not given cephalosporins even if unconscious and was tested for cross-reactivity to penicillin.

Box 16.3 Mechanisms of drug- and infection-induced haemolytic anaemias

- Most antibodies against drugs causing autoimmune haemolytic anaemia (AIHA) are warm and have cross-reactive specificity for rhesus antigens for an unknown reason, e.g. dapsone
- Some drugs can act as haptens, after active or passive binding to the red cell; antibodies against the drug then opsonize the red cells, which are subsequently phagocytosed
- Immune complex of drug and antibody, can be adsorbed onto red cells by immune adherence
- Some drugs trigger an AIHA indistinguishable from idiopathic warm AIHA
- Most warm antibodies recognize the Rhesus antigens or the band 3 anion transporter
- Cold antibodies induced by *Mycoplasma* recognize the I antigen
- Cold antibodies in children or after syphilis (Donath-Landsteiner antibody) recognize the P antigen (the receptor for Parvovirus)

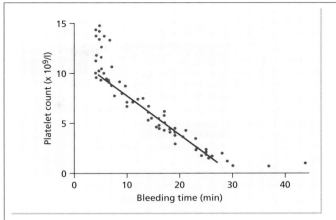

Fig. 16.5 Relevance of platelet level to bleeding time using platelets from normal individuals. Source: Harker LA, Slichter SJ (1972). The bleeding time as a screening test for evaluation of platelet function. *New England Journal of Medicine*, 287(4), 155–159.

in the **production of an abnormal anchor protein (GPI)** in red cells, granulocytes and platelets. This affects CD55 (decay-accelerating factor, DAF), and CD59 (homologous restriction factor 20, HRF-20). The haemolytic manifestations are due to failure to inhibit ongoing complement activation on the surface of the abnormal erythrocytes. Although the name suggests that haemolysis occurs at night, it can occur at any time, intermittently, and is particularly associated with intercurrent infections, surgery or immunization.

The proportion of abnormal cells in a given patient is **highly variable**. Some patients have fewer than 2% PNH clones, whereas others have over 90%. Patients with only a small proportion of abnormal cells may show no overt haemoglobinuria and yet develop chronic haemolytic anaemia. Some patients have a thrombotic tendency due to abnormal platelets, while others seem prone to infections, presumably due to defective neutrophil function.

The basic abnormalities lie in the cell membrane protein, GPI; abnormalities of this protein allow the alternate complement pathway to proceed once activated, resulting in lysis. This formed the basis of the Ham's test, in which lysis of the patient's red cells was produced by serum acidified to activate the alternate pathway. Normal red cells are protected by the presence of **two complement-inhibitory proteins (CD55 and CD59)** on their surface; these **are missing** in PNH. Ham's test has now been replaced by flow cytometric analysis of CD55 and CD59. Using flow cytometry, the relative size of the abnormal clone can be derived.

Treatment of mild PNH is largely symptomatic. Most patients take iron and folate supplements, and blood transfusions are administered when required. Anticoagulation may be required for the thrombotic tendency. Glucocorticoids have

been used, but with limited efficacy. More recently, eculizumab – a humanized monoclonal antibody that binds to C5 and blocks activation by the C5 convertase – has been licensed for the treatment of PNH. Eculizumab-mediated inhibition of terminal complement activation has been shown to reduce haemolysis, reduce transfusion requirements and improve quality of life. Some patients with severe PNH, particularly if associated with myelodysplasia, are good candidates for bone marrow transplantation.

16.2.5 Alloantibodies causing anaemia

Alloantibodies are, by definition, directed against antigens not found in the host (see Chapter 1). They can cause anaemia in only two situations: transfusion of incorrectly matched blood (see section 16.7); or in pregnancy, when maternal antibodies (IgG) cross the placenta and react with 'foreign' fetal red cell antigens (see Chapter 18 and later Case 16.5).

16.3 Immune thrombocytopenia

Thrombocytopenia is defined as a blood platelet count of <150 × 10^9/L, though it may not be symptomatic until the platelet count drops to <10 × 10^9/L (Fig. 16.5).

Thrombocytopenia may be caused by decreased production, shortened survival, increased consumption or sequestration in the spleen (Fig. 16.6), processes similar to those of anaemia. **Autoimmune thrombocytopenia** can also be considered in the same way as AIHA: idiopathic (Case 16.4) or secondary to autoimmune diseases (e.g. SLE), infection (e.g. human immunodeficiency virus, HIV), malignancy or drugs (e.g. quinine). Alloantibodies may also cause thrombocytopenia *in utero* (Case 16.5). Unlike haemolytic anaemia, the antibodies are not temperature dependent. Autoantibodies are directed against platelet-specific antigens.

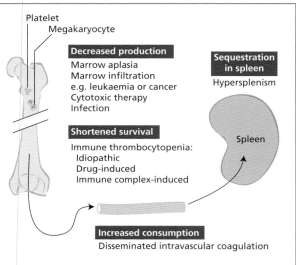

Fig. 16.6 Known causes of thrombocytopenia.

Immune thrombocytopenia (ITP) differs from thrombocytopenia due to circulating immune complexes with 'bystander involvement'. **Bystander involvement**, in which the antigen is unrelated to platelets, occurs in acute immune thrombocytopenia of childhood (which follows infection and is transient) and in some drug-induced thrombocytopenias; these involve Fc (IgG) receptors on platelets (Box 16.1). However, classic 'immune-complex' diseases other than SLE are rarely associated with thrombocytopenia, which suggests that circulating platelet-specific antibodies are probably responsible for low platelet counts in SLE.

Alloantibodies can also cause thrombocytopenias. Those provoked by pregnancy can cause neonatal thrombocytopenia (see Case 16.5), while those induced by transfusion cause post-transfusion purpura.

16.3.1 Autoimmune immune thrombocytopenia

As with other idiopathic diseases, the *diagnosis of ITP is one of exclusion* of the known causes of thrombocytopenia (Fig. 16.6).

Case 16.4 Autoimmune immune thrombocytopenia

A 29-year-old man presented with spontaneous bruising of his legs and arms. He had had three recent epistaxes but no other bleeding. He was not taking any drugs and had no risk factors for human immunodeficiency virus (HIV). There were no physical signs apart from bruises and scattered petechiae on the legs. The spleen was not palpable. On investigation, he had a normal haemoglobin (138 g/l) and white cell count, but a low platelet count of $10 \times 10^9/l$ (normal $>150 \times 10^9/l$). His serum C-reactive protein (CRP) and immunoglobulin levels were normal; direct Coombs' test was negative; antinuclear and DNA-binding antibodies and rheumatoid factor were absent. His bone marrow contained an increased number of normal megakaryocytes but was otherwise normal. A diagnosis of immune thrombocytopenia was made and he was started on a high dose of prednisolone. His platelet count rose rapidly over the next few days and the steroids were tailed off over 4 weeks. He relapsed 10 months later with further bruising, but again responded to a short course of oral steroids.

Case 16.5 Neonatal alloimmune diseases

A 32-year-old woman undergoing a twin pregnancy had been given a blood transfusion for a post-partum haemorrhage in her first pregnancy 3 years earlier. The current pregnancy and delivery were normal and *non-identical* twin boys were born, both with Apgar scores of 10. Four hours later, both infants had extensive purpura on their abdomens, arms and legs, but neither was jaundiced.

Twin 1 had a platelet count of $30 \times 10^9/l$ and his haemoglobin was 176 g/l. He did not become jaundiced and his platelet count gradually rose without treatment over several weeks. His platelet count was normal ($400 \times 10^9/l$) at 2 months.

Twin 2 had a platelet count of $46 \times 10^9/l$ and a normal haemoglobin (190 g/l). However, he rapidly developed anaemia (Hb 84 g/l) and jaundice (bilirubin 300 mmol/l) at 48 h. A Coombs' test was positive and his red cells were found to be group A, whereas his mother's cells were group O. In view of the rising serum bilirubin, an exchange transfusion was performed. Following this, his haemoglobin and platelet count returned to normal and he was discharged 6 days later with a platelet count of $213 \times 10^9/l$ and a haemoglobin of 132 g/l.

The mother's serum was found to contain IgG antibodies to the father's platelets and to some, but not all, of a panel of platelets from normal, unrelated donors. These antibodies were typed as specific anti-HPA-1a antibodies and had been provoked by the previous pregnancy and transfusion. These antibodies crossed the placenta to cause alloimmune thrombocytopenia in both twins. Twin 2 also had a red cell incompatibility and so needed an exchange transfusion to compensate for haemolysis. It is unusual for an ABO incompatibility to require an exchange transfusion (see Chapter 18, section 18.4.5). His platelet count returned to normal more quickly than that of twin 1 because the antibodies to platelets were removed by the exchange.

Low platelet numbers are due to autoantibodies, demonstrable by routinely available assays, using recombinant platelet antigens in enzyme-linked immunosorbent assay (ELISA). The term 'immune thrombocytopenia' is applicable in adults and in the *chronic* disease in children, since in both cases circulating **autoantibodies to platelets** have been shown to have platelet specificity. The platelet antigen HPA-1 (GPIIIa, CD61) is the major target antigen.

Acute ITP is characterized by the rapid appearance of generalized purpura in a previously healthy child or, less commonly, adult. Large bruises follow minor trauma. Haemorrhagic bullae may occur in the mouth, epistaxis and conjunctival haemorrhages are common, and gastrointestinal haemorrhage and haematuria are less frequent. Other physical signs may be absent.

Acute ITP is the commonest form of **ITP in children** (Table 16.2), with a peak incidence about the age of 7 years. In over 50% of the children it follows immunization or a common viral infection 1–3 weeks previously. Most children (85%) have a benign course, do not require treatment and recover spontaneously within 3 months. Treatment is reserved for life-threatening haemorrhage (such as cerebral haemorrhage), though this is extremely rare, as the platelets are functional and only a few platelets are required to prevent severe haemorrhage (Fig. 16.5). *Fewer than 10% of children progress to chronic ITP.*

Chronic ITP usually has an insidious onset with minor bruising and scattered petechiae (Table 16.2). Significant episodes of bleeding may be separated by months or years, during which the platelet counts are normal. This is mainly a disorder of adults, affecting women more than men. ITP can be a feature of HIV-related disease, so this should be considered in the differential diagnosis, especially if there are other clinical features (see Chapter 3, section 3.5.4). **Investigations** show a low platelet count, usually $<40 \times 10^9$/L, for more than 3 months. A blood film may show large platelets and minute platelet fragments. Bone marrow examination may show an increased number of megakaryocytes, suggesting that the

thrombocytopenia is due to increased platelet destruction rather than decreased production (Fig. 16.6). The spleen is not enlarged.

Tests for platelet antibodies are of two types: the direct test on platelets themselves, detected by flow cytometry (a platelet Coombs' test); and the indirect (serum) test for free antibodies against platelet antigens. The direct test is positive in 90% of adult patients with chronic ITP. The remainder may constitute a separate disease, since the bone marrow shows decreased megakaryocytopoiesis and the patients are refractory to therapy. Free serum antibodies with specificity for the platelet antigens, glycoprotein IIb/IIIa, can be assayed by an ELISA using purified antigens on a plate, but this is only positive in 30% of patients with chronic ITP; the particular specificity appears to have no clinical significance.

The **pathogenesis** of ITP has been well studied. The spleen is a major site of autoantibody synthesis. Platelets with IgG on their surfaces are sequestered in the red pulp of the spleen (Fig. 16.6), where circulating platelets with surface IgG are rapidly removed by phagocytosis. This has been shown with radiolabelled platelets sensitized with IgG, which are removed from the circulation in a few hours, compared with a normal half-life of a few days.

The object of **management** is to restore the platelet count to normal, but active therapy is not indicated unless there is acute bleeding. The vast majority of children recover spontaneously without sequelae. Adults whose platelet counts are between 40 and 100×10^9/L and who only have occasional bruising rarely do not require active treatment.

Children or adults with **active bleeding** require corticosteroids to prevent further destruction of platelets, and about 60% of patients respond within 2 weeks. Corticosteroids may work by suppressing phagocytosis of antibody-coated platelets by macrophages in the spleen and liver. Patients who fail to respond, or who have a transient response but relapse into fresh bleeding after a month of steroids, may need splenectomy after intravenous immunoglobulin has raised the platelet count (Chapter 7, section 7.2.3). **Splenectomy** removes both the major site of phagocytosis and that of autoantibody production and is successful in most patients. It carries the risk of overwhelming post-splenectomy sepsis and prophylactic antibiotics and immunization against capsulated organisms are required. High-dose intravenous immunoglobulin is useful in refractory patients. Large doses of IgG transiently block Fc (IgG) receptors on phagocytic cells as well as reducing platelet binding of autoantibodies by idiotypic neutralization. The anti-CD20 monoclonal antibody **rituximab** has been used successfully to treat ITP and can be employed as second-line treatment with glucocorticoid therapy. Cytotoxic drugs (such as azathioprine) may be used in adults if these measures fail, or as last-line treatment in those unfit for splenectomy. For the 5% of patients with refractory ITP, treatment with **thrombopoietin receptor agonists (romiplostim, eltrombopag)** to increase the megakaryocyte count is proving to be effective and safe.

Table 16.2 Comparison of acute and chronic immune thrombocytopenia

	Acute	Chronic
Age of onset	Childhood	20–50 years
Sex	Both	F: M = 3: 1
Preceding infection	Usual	Not associated
Bleeding	Sudden	Insidious
Platelets*	Low (20)	Variable (10–40)
Spontaneous resolution	Most patients	Rare
Duration	Few weeks	Months to years
Treatment	Nil usually	Corticosteroids ± splenectomy

* $\times 10^9$/l.

Pregnancy in women with ITP is usually uneventful, but the newborn infant may have neonatal thrombocytopenia. This is due to transplacental passage of IgG autoantibodies that then fix to fetal platelets. If bleeding or purpura develops, or the platelet count is very low, intravenous immunoglobulin can be given to raise the number of circulating platelets. Alternatively, the mother may receive intravenous immunoglobulin prior to delivery. In untreated infants, the platelet count gradually rises over the next 3 months as the maternal autoantibody is catabolized. Such neonatal thrombocytopenia is similar to that due to haemolytic alloantibodies, also produced by the mother (see section 16.3.3 and Chapter 18).

16.3.2 Drug-induced thrombocytopenia

The pathogenesis of drug-induced thrombocytopenia is similar to that of drug-induced AIHA (Box 16.3). Many drugs have been implicated, including quinine and *p*-aminosalicylic acid. There is clinical improvement and an increase in the platelet count when the drug is stopped.

16.3.3 Neonatal thrombocytopenia

Neonatal thrombocytopenia may be due to **antibodies that cross the placenta**. These may be autoantibodies in mothers with chronic ITP, or alloantibodies formed by the mother to paternal antigens present on fetal platelets. The immunopathology is similar to that of haemolytic disease of the newborn (see Chapter 18, section 18.4.5). Several platelet iso-antigen systems are recognized; the most important is the HPA-1a system. Sera from women who have an obstetric history of a bruised or thrombocytopenic baby should always be tested against their husbands' platelets (Case 16.5). The treatment of an infant with 'neonatal alloimmune thrombocytopenia' is the same as for those whose mothers have ITP.

16.4 Immune neutropenia

Neutropenia may be due to failure of production in or, rarely, export from the bone marrow (Fig. 16.7); alternatively, increased consumption or sequestration (usually in the spleen) can also cause neutropenia (Chapter 3, Fig. 3.10). The traditional definition of neutropenia is $1.5 \times 10^9/L$, but *clinical effects are unusual unless the count drops below $0.5 \times 10^9/L$.*

Antibodies to neutrophils can cause syndromes that parallel AIHA and ITP, such as autoimmune neutropenia, alloimmune neonatal neutropenia and drug-induced immune neutropenia. As for other blood components, neutropenia may be idiopathic or secondary to diseases such as SLE and other immune-complex diseases. The commonest causes of neutropenia are drugs and infections; rare genetic causes of neutropenia are discussed in Chapter 3.

Autoimmune **antibodies to neutrophils** react with surface neutrophil antigens and are difficult to detect on cells, which rapidly ingest the complex formed by their membrane antigen and the autoantibody. Recombinant antigens in ELISA are

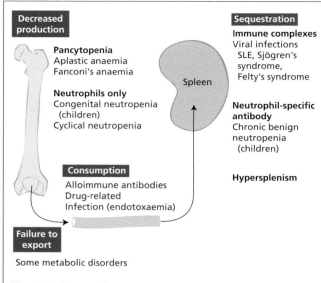

Fig. 16.7 Causes of neutropenia. SLE, systemic lupus erythematosus.

used, though autoantibodies are difficult to distinguish from immune (IgG) complexes reacting with IgG Fc receptors.

Neutropenia secondary to SLE may be due to immune complexes or to antineutrophil IgG antibodies. **Felty's syndrome** describes a complex of neutropenia accompanied by splenomegaly, high-titre rheumatoid factor and rheumatoid arthritis (see Chapter 10, section 10.4). Most patients are HLA-DR4 positive. There is increased granulocyte production by the bone marrow as well as increased granulocyte turnover. It is thought that neutrophils coated with IgG are sequestered in the spleen, eventually resulting in splenomegaly. However, splenectomy does not always cure the problem, suggesting that this mechanism operates in only some of the patients. Antibodies to an elongation factor eFIA-1 have been detected.

Antineutrophil antibodies have also been detected in **drug-induced neutropenia**; these antibodies appear to be autoantibodies, which disappear when the drug is discontinued.

Neonatal neutropenia due to allogeneic antibodies is an extremely rare but sometimes fatal syndrome, as although such antibodies are commonly found in multiparous women, they rarely result in neonatal disease. These antibodies may also be responsible for mild transfusion reactions that are poorly understood (see section 16.7).

16.5 Haematopoietic progenitor cells

Aplastic anaemia is the term given to pancytopenia due to reduced numbers of pluripotent stem cells. It may be genetic (e.g. Fanconi's anaemia), secondary (to infection, drugs or thymoma) or, in 60% of cases, idiopathic (acquired with no known cause). Parvovirus may cause a severe but transient aplastic anaemia.

Suppression of erythropoiesis in the bone marrow involves **autoantibodies (IgG) to erythroblast progenitors or to**

erythropoietin, excessive **suppression by autologous CD8⁺ T** lymphocytes, or both. The response to antilymphocyte globulin or ciclosporin in 50% of patients suggests variable aetiologies. Stem cell transplantation is the treatment of choice and the 5-year survival is >90%. For those for whom there is no suitable donor, ciclosporin with antilymphocyte globulin offers 90% survival at 5 years. However, non-transplanted patients remain at risk of developing marrow malignancies in the longer term, as with other forms of marrow dysplasia. Many patients may develop PNH (see above).

16.6 Immune disorders of coagulation

16.6.1 Primary antiphospholipid antibody syndrome

A stroke in a young person (under 50 years), recurrent fetal loss or recurrent thrombosis (arterial/venous) may indicate an underlying primary antiphospholipid antibody syndrome (Table 16.3; see Chapters 10 and 18). The vastly increased risk of cerebral thrombosis or embolism in these patients makes it important to measure these antibodies in all **young stroke patients** (Case 16.6), as well as those with major arterial or venous thrombosis (Fig. 16.8). Patients with high-titre antiphospholipid antibodies alone (commonly called anticardiolipin antibodies, as this is the major phospholipid involved)

should be anticoagulated for life, since devastating, acute vasculopathy can occur, involving major vessels to vital organs.

16.6.2 Other antibodies to coagulation factors

Antibodies to circulating coagulation factors occur in treated haemophiliacs and in association with SLE and other autoimmune states. **Factor VIII antibodies** are the commonest and develop in 20–30% of patients with severe haemophilia treated with human factor VIII concentrates. Treatment with very high doses of intravenous immunoglobulin has been used successfully for patients with catastrophic bleeding. Factor VIII autoantibodies are also found in rare patients with SLE, or in elderly persons without overt underlying disease, in whom bleeding is difficult to stop.

Antibodies to the prothrombin converter complex (factors Xa, V, phospholipid and calcium) are found in up to 40% of patients with SLE, provided a sensitive assay is used. These are usually patients who have had thrombotic episodes or renal involvement. They have prolonged kaolin–cephalin clotting time and failure to correct the clotting defect with normal plasma implies that an antibody is present. The current test of choice is the dilute Russell Viper venom test (dRVVT). Such

Table 16.3 Comparison of primary antiphospholipid antibody (APA) syndrome and systemic lupus erythematosus (SLE)

	Primary APA	SLE
Female: male	2: 1	9: 1
Age (years):		
range	20–60	15–60
mean	38	24
Antinuclear antibody	45%	>90%
Antibodies to double-stranded DNA	Nil	80%
Antiphospholipid antibodies	100%	40%
Lupus anticoagulant	60%	10%

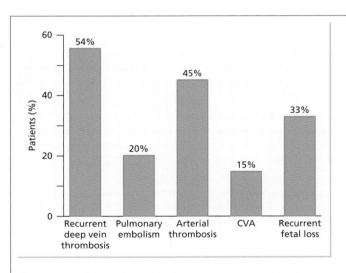

Fig. 16.8 Clinical presentations in the primary phospholipid antibody syndrome. CVA, cerebrovascular accident.

🔍 Case 16.6 Primary antiphospholipid antibody syndrome

A 28-year-old woman was admitted with a stroke due to a cerebral vascular thrombosis. She had had four spontaneous abortions in the past. She was a non-smoker. Cerebral angiography confirmed the thrombosis, but showed normal vasculature otherwise. Haemoglobin, platelet and white cell counts were normal, as were her serum immunoglobulins, C3 and C4 levels. Antibodies to nuclei, extractable nuclear antigens and double-stranded DNA were negative, but she did have high-titre antiphospholipid antibodies. Coagulation tests showed a prolonged kaolin–cephalin clotting time that did not correct with normal plasma, i.e. lupus anticoagulant. A diagnosis of primary antiphospholipid antibody syndrome was made, so she received long-term anticoagulant therapy. She made a good recovery from the stroke.

an antibody is known as the **lupus anticoagulant**. It is paradoxical that this 'anticoagulant' usually results in thrombosis *in vivo*. These antibodies are distinct from those to cardiolipin with different specificities, although they usually occur together and have related immunopathologies (see Table 16.3). There is considerable overlap between the clinical features associated with both the lupus anticoagulant and antiphospholipid antibodies. Patients with abnormal thrombosis may have either or both, so it is important to test for both.

16.7 Blood transfusion

Blood transfusion must be safe, i.e. immunologically compatible and free of infection (Box 16.4).

16.7.1 Principles of blood transfusion

The ABO red cell system is unique because **naturally occurring antibodies** (IgM) are found in human sera. For example, if group A blood was given to a group B patient whose blood contains natural anti-A antibodies, these antibodies would lyse the donated cells, causing a potentially fatal transfusion reaction. Blood is always matched for ABO antigens.

To prevent sensitization to rhesus antigens (and the risk of a subsequent transfusion reaction), donor and recipient are also tested for compatibility for the immunologically strongest rhesus antigen, D antigen. Other minor red cell antigens occur only infrequently or are poorly immunogenic.

Matching for ABO and rhesus antigens alone should **prevent major incompatibilities**. In addition, recipients' sera are screened for rare preexisting antibodies, produced as a result of a pregnancy or previous transfusion, which may destroy donor red cells, since transfusion reactions due to preexisting antibodies can be fatal. A test panel of red cells, containing most antigens of known blood group systems, is used as well as cells from selected donors. Sera are screened for 'complete' (IgM) antibodies, which will agglutinate red cells in saline, and 'incomplete' antibodies (IgG), which are detectable by an

Table 16.4 Potential complications of blood transfusion (fortunately rare)

Complication	Cause
Red cell destruction	ABO mismatch
	Antibodies to other red cell antigens previously undetected in recipient's plasma
	Boost of low-level antibody to significant level by transfusion
Febrile reactions (rarely anaphylaxis)	Anti-leucocyte antibodies
	Anti-platelet antibodies (e.g. HLA, HPA-1a)
	Anti-IgA antibodies in selective total IgA deficiency
Infection	Hepatitis C
	HIV
	Cytomegalovirus
	Malaria

indirect antiglobulin (Coombs') test. It is not necessary to identify donor antibodies because these are rapidly diluted on transfusion.

Despite these precautions, red cells are sometimes destroyed by a **haemolytic transfusion reaction** (Table 16.4). Unfortunately, *the commonest cause of a severe transfusion reaction is still a human error*, either in handling blood samples or mistaken patient identity. Haemolytic transfusion reactions due to ABO incompatibility usually result in massive haemolysis, haemoglobinuria, shock and disseminated intravascular coagulation. A mismatch due to rhesus incompatibility usually results in gradual haemolysis, which does not interfere with renal function, but the patient's haemoglobin fails to rise following transfusion. Mild transfusion reactions (fever, drop in blood pressure) are common, around 1%, but not clinically significant provided patients are monitored carefully.

Occasionally, transfusion reactions occur 5–10 days after transfusion. The delay is due to the time lag required for the production of antibodies by the patient. This alloimmune response means that the patient's own cells are negative in a direct Coombs' test, but the transfused cells are positive for IgG and complement. This type of **delayed transfusion reaction** occurs after multiple blood transfusions, such as those required in open-heart surgery or severe gastrointestinal bleeding.

16.7.2 Risks of blood transfusion

A variety of **blood-borne infections** can be transmitted by blood transfusion, though measures to screen donors and treat blood products with antiviral agents have reduced the risks

---

Box 16.4 Steps taken to ensure the safety of blood for transfusion

- Screening the recipient's serum for antibodies that react with donor red cells
- Ensuring that the transfused red cells will not stimulate any unwanted antibodies in the recipient
- Screening all units of blood for hepatitis B antigen, antibodies to human immunodeficiency virus (HIV) and hepatitis C, and syphilis antigens (though polymerase chain reaction [PCR] will be used soon)
- Blood used for babies is also screened for antibodies to cytomegalovirus (though PCR will be used soon)

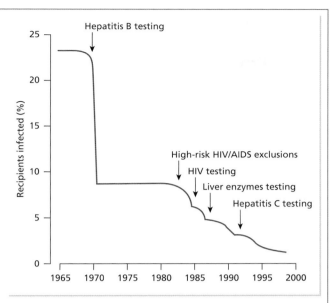

Fig. 16.9 Reduction of risk of hepatitis following multiple blood transfusions. AIDS, acquired immune deficiency syndrome; HIV, human immunodeficiency virus.

considerably. Donors likely to have been exposed to malaria, hepatitis viruses or HIV are discouraged from giving blood. Together with increased screening, these measures have dramatically reduced transmitted infection in the last decades (Fig. 16.9) – see Case 16.7.

Currently, whole blood is given rarely. Haemorrhage requires plasma expanders to maintain blood volumes and red cell concentrates to raise the haemoglobin. Concentrated platelets are used to prevent bleeding in marrow failure (aplastic anaemia, acute leukaemia); a failure to increase the platelet count suggests destruction by recipient's alloantibodies and potential platelet donors and the recipient may have to be HLA class I matched. The advent of granulocyte colony-stimulating factors (G-CSF) has made granulocyte transfusions largely unnecessary. **Plasma products** currently include immunoglobulin, fresh frozen plasma, factor VIII and albumin, though recombinant products have replaced the last two in many countries. Polyclonal immunoglobulin and fresh frozen plasma, however, will continue to be made from human blood and measures such as solvent/detergent treatment against lipid-coated viruses, ultrafiltration and pasteurization, have improved the safety of these agents.

🔍 Case 16.7 Transmission of hepatitis C by a blood product in the early 1990s

David was diagnosed as having a common variable immune deficiency disorder aged 28 years, after developing bronchiectasis over the preceding 5 years. He had also suffered from episodes of urethritis, eventually found to be due to Ureaplasma urealytica (a common organism known to cause significant infections in antibody-deficient patients). He received 25 g of intravenous immunoglobulin at 3-week intervals, with regular monitoring of his liver function tests (6-weekly). After 3 years of uneventful infusions, he developed raised alanine transaminase levels and rapidly became jaundiced. His serum was now positive for hepatitis C virus by polymerase chain reaction (HCV-PCR). He had iatrogenic hepatitis C. He was admitted for assessment and the jaundice and liver enzyme levels reversed spontaneously; he received 6 million units of interferon (IFN)-α subcutaneously three times a week for 6 months. The PCR became negative within 4 weeks and has remained so over the next 20 years, as have his liver function tests.

This type of transmission of hepatitis C is thankfully very rare nowadays, since blood products are treated routinely with solvent/detergent or other methods to inactivate lipid-coated viruses. Such a patient would now receive a directly acting agent, as the results of such treatment are superior.

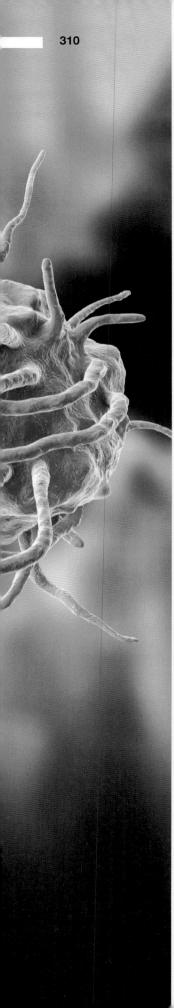

CHAPTER 17
Neuroimmunology

Key topics

Visit the companion website at **www.wiley.com/go/misbah/immunology** to download cases with additional figures on these topics.

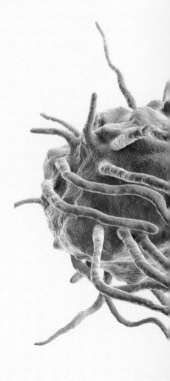

Chapel and Haeney's Essentials of Clinical Immunology, Seventh Edition. Edited by Siraj A. Misbah, Gavin P. Spickett, and Virgil A.S.H. Dalm.
© 2022 John Wiley & Sons Ltd. Published 2022 by John Wiley & Sons Ltd.

17.1 Introduction

The central and peripheral nervous systems are not excluded from immune disease. The immune system participates actively in nervous tissue to counteract infection, and so, as elsewhere, cells can enter these tissues in **inflammation**. T and B lymphocytes, as well as neutrophils, monocytes and macrophages, can invade inflamed nervous tissue. In infections and multiple sclerosis (MS), intrathecal B cells are responsible for locally synthesized immunoglobulin found in the cerebrospinal fluid (CSF). T cells and macrophages, while protecting against infection, can also cause direct damage, as in chronic viral infection, post-infective states and demyelination.

The **blood–brain barrier** normally excludes intravascular proteins, including immunoglobulin (Ig)G, and this must be breached before extrathecal circulating autoantibodies reach the central or peripheral nervous systems. In this way, circulating autoantibodies can be responsible for the pathogenesis of several antibody-mediated neuropathies, such as the Lambert–Eaton myasthenic syndrome (LEMS). This disease is an excellent example of the way in which an autoimmune pathogenesis has been proven by following clinical clues over many years (Box 17.1). Other autoimmune diseases selectively damage central or peripheral nervous tissue itself (e.g. MS and Guillain–Barré syndrome, respectively) or the muscle end-plates (e.g. myasthenia gravis). On the other hand, involvement of nervous tissue may be part of a systemic disorder (e.g. in systemic lupus erythematosus, SLE).

Box 17.1 Evidence for autoimmune aetiology of Lambert–Eaton myasthenia (LEMS)

1953	Clinical description of disease
1972	LEMS associated with other organ-specific autoimmune diseases in patients – suggesting autoimmune cause
1984	Plasma exchange – successful therapy for affected patients, suggesting pathogenic autoantibodies in plasma
1987	Human plasma from patients causes characteristic changes (electrophysiological + electron-microscopical) in mice, proving humoral pathogenesis
1991	Autoantibodies to calcium channels detected in 20% of patients
1991	Autoantigen in small cell cancer present in 50% of LEMS patients
1994	Additional epitopes for antibodies to voltage-gated Ca^{2+} channels (VGCC) defined; now disease-specific antibodies detected in 100% of patients
1995	Randomized, placebo-controlled, cross-over study showed improved muscle strength with intravenous immunoglobulin therapy and associated reduction of autoantibody titres (i.e. immunomodulation reduced pathogenic antibodies)
1999	Active immunization with calcium channel peptides caused mild LEMS-like disease in rats
2006	Passive transfer of disease from an affected mother to baby, causing transient neonatal weakness
2007	Mice transfected with mutated VGCC gene showed electrophysiological changes of LEMS

17.2 Infections

The incidence of bacterial meningitis in infants has been reduced dramatically by means of immunization against the encapsulated organisms that are the major causes of these diseases. Normal children under the age of 2 years are unable to make antibodies to the carbohydrate capsules of Haemophilus influenzae type b (see Case 17.1), Streptococcus pneumoniae or Neisseria meningitidis and these pathogens accounted for 90% of meningitis seen in children until the early 1990s. Since the introduction of new vaccines against most of these pathogens, in which carbohydrate antigens have been coupled to protein carriers in order to provoke protective antibodies in infants and young children (see Chapter 7, section 7.7), the incidence of meningitis due to Haemophilus influenzae type b and Neisseria meningitides type C has fallen dramatically in many countries (see Chapter 7, Figure 7.8). However, **routine immunization** is only given at the age of 2 months and infants are susceptible until then (as in Case 17.1) if their mothers were not immunized. Now that these vaccines have been in use for >25 years, such infections in infants should now

lead to suspicion of a primary immune deficiency in the mother. Disease in immunized children should also raise alarm bells!

Infections of the central nervous system (CNS), meningitis and encephalitis are relatively uncommon in immunocompetent adults. Severe, unusual or recurrent brain infections should raise the possibility of an immune defect (see Chapter 3 and section 17.5), particularly an antibody or complement defect.

Another important example is human immunodeficiency virus (HIV), which leads to opportunistic microorganisms – viruses, fungi, parasites or intracellular bacteria – that infect the CNS (Table 17.1). The signs of inflammation in **HIV-positive patients** may be modified; fever and meningism are often absent and CSF may contain few cells, little protein and no detectable antibodies to the organisms involved, making diagnosis more difficult before the routine use of polymerase chain reaction (PCR) to detect infective agents directly.

In addition, the causative virus, HIV, can itself infect the brain to produce a range of problems, including **acquired immune deficiency syndrome (AIDS) dementia**. Neurological abnormalities occur clinically in about 50% of HIV-infected

Case 17.1 Haemophilus influenzae type b meningitis

Alice was a normal, full-term baby who was breast-fed and gained weight appropriately in the first 6 weeks of life. At 7 weeks she became acutely miserable, stopped feeding and her mother felt that she was very warm; when she took her temperature, it was 40 °C. In the surgery, the doctor found that she had neck stiffness and Alice then vomited all over the couch. There was no rash or bruising, but the left eardrum was inflamed. Meningitis was suspected; the doctor gave Alice an intramuscular injection of penicillin and instructed her mother to take her straight to the hospital where the on-call paediatrician was waiting. The clinical diagnosis of meningitis was confirmed and blood and cerebrospinal fluid (CSF) samples were taken immediately and intravenous antibiotics started. The CSF showed increased numbers of neutrophil leucocytes (131×10^6/L) and a few Gram-negative coccobacilli, despite the initial dose of penicillin. Three days later these were shown to be Haemophilus influenzae and serotyping showed them to be Haemophilus influenzae type b. The full blood count showed a circulating neutrophilia (29×10^9/L) and the C-reactive protein level was 230 mg/L. Alice made a rapid recovery with intravenous and subsequently oral antibiotics, with supportive management to ensure adequate ventilation and fluids. There were no long-term sequelae and she was immunized with childhood vaccines (including Hib) once she was fully recovered at 6 months (4 months later than healthy children).

Table 17.1 Important neurological complications of human immunodeficiency virus (HIV) infection

Primary HIV infection

Dementia

Atypical meningitis

Myelopathy

Opportunistic infections

Cerebral toxoplasmosis

Meningitis – cryptococcal, tuberculous

Encephalitis due to cytomegalovirus/herpes simplex virus

Progressive multifocal leucoencephalopathy (papovavirus, also known as JC virus)

Cytomegalovirus retinitis

Tumours associated with viruses

Kaposi's sarcoma (human herpes virus-8)

B-cell lymphoma (Epstein–Barr virus)

adult patients and in many HIV-infected children. Subclinical disease may be even more common, since up to 75% of brains of AIDS patients are found to be affected post mortem. Pathological changes range from white matter pallor and mild lymphocytic infiltration to macrophage abnormalities (including multinucleate giant cells) associated with macrophage activation. Computed tomography (CT) may show cerebral atrophy.

Infections can result in damage even after the causative pathogen has been eliminated. **Parainfectious encephalitis** occurs some time following a childhood viral illness (rubella, measles, chicken pox). This is due to demyelination following bystander activation of T cells or molecular mimicry resulting in specific T cells mistaking myelin for virus (see Chapter 5, section 5.5). Although the condition is usually self-limiting, permanent damage or death may result.

In contrast, **subacute sclerosing panencephalitis (SSPE)** is a rare, progressive disease of children, who present with insidious dementia. The disease follows measles infection several years earlier, and high levels of specific antimeasles antibody as well as measles virus are found in the brain, blood and CSF. The intrathecal IgG is

not only oligoclonal, but also can be absorbed out with measles virus itself. There is no obvious defect in the adaptive immune responses to measles virus; such children may have defective innate immunity, in particular abnormal Toll-like receptors (TLRs) that are important in early protection against many viruses.

Progressive multifocal leucoencephalopathy is a rare demyelinating disease that can be induced by papoviruses and typically occurs in immunosuppressed patients, such as those with AIDS or those receiving immunosuppressive treatment, including therapeutic monoclonal antibodies, particularly natalizumab, which blocks anti-α4-integrins required for migration of leucocytes that would control the papovavirus.

17.3 Demyelinating diseases of the central nervous system

17.3.1 Multiple sclerosis

MS is common in Caucasians, with a prevalence of 1 case per 2000 population (see Chapter 3, Table 3.1). It is an **inflammatory disease of white matter** in the CNS. It is a hugely variable disease, in terms of disability, rate of progression and prognosis. The clinical diagnosis of MS can be difficult, as definite histopathological confirmation by biopsy is not done in life. The **clinical features** depend on the site of the pathological lesion in the brain (as in Case 17.2); many plaques are clinically silent. The rate of new lesions is unpredictable and also variable. Subgroups of MS depend on the rate of progression and recovery between attacks; relapsing and remitting MS is quite distinct from progressive disease.

Optic neuritis is a similar inflammatory, demyelinating disease of one or both optic nerves, with recovery in 75–90% of patients. An oligoclonal pattern of IgG is found in CSF from most patients with optic neuritis and nuclear magnetic resonance imaging (MRI) shows silent lesions elsewhere in the brain. It can be due to many causes, but approximately 50–80% of these patients will develop MS within 15 years, as in Case 17.2. Clinical diagnosis of MS depends on evidence of at least two attacks separated in time and sites of lesions, with exclusion of all other causes, as in Case 17.2. **Confirmatory tests** are required. Poor nerve conduction can be demonstrated by prolonged responses on evoked potential testing. MRI of

Case 17.2 Multiple sclerosis

A 38-year-old woman presented with tingling, numbness and clumsiness of both hands for one week, with a band of numbness from the umbilicus to the axillae. Six months earlier, following an upper respiratory tract infection, she had experienced a short episode of blurred vision that she put down to tiredness. She was now anxious because her maternal grandmother had suffered from multiple sclerosis (MS).

On neurological examination, she had absent abdominal reflexes with brisk tendon jerks and bilateral extensor plantar responses. Blood investigations were normal, including a full blood count, C-reactive protein, vitamin B$_{12}$ and folate levels and syphilis serology. A lumbar puncture was carried out. The cerebrospinal fluid (CSF) investigation results are shown in Table 17.2. Oligoclonal IgG bands (see Chapter 19, Fig. 19.8) are not found in normal CSF, but are found in 90% of patients with MS; in the absence of clinical signs of infection, this test is almost diagnostic of MS (see Box 17.2).

The clinical diagnosis was MS; other possible diagnoses, such as neurosyphilis or subacute combined degeneration of the cord, were excluded by investigation. Magnetic resonance imaging (MRI) showed some silent lesions; the patient asked to be followed carefully without specific therapy at this stage in view of her mild symptoms.

Table 17.2 Cerebrospinal fluid investigations for multiple sclerosis in Case 17.2

Protein concentration	0.4 g/L (NR 0–0.4 g/L)
Red blood cells	None
Lymphocytes	3 × 10⁶/L (NR < 5 × 10⁶/L)
IgG/albumin ratio	26% (NR 4–22%)
Isoelectric focusing	Oligoclonal bands present

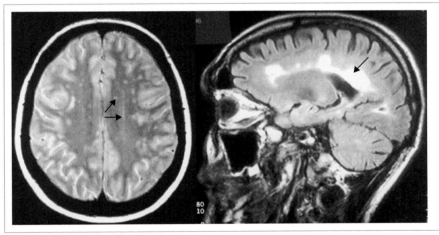

Fig. 17.1 Magnetic resonance imaging (MRI) of brain of multiple sclerosis patient showing white matter changes due to demyelination (arrows). Source: Axford J & O'Callaghan C (eds) *Medicine*, 2e (2004). Reproduced with permission of John Wiley & Sons Ltd.

the brain (Fig. 17.1) shows lesions in 90% of affected individuals but, like all imaging, is non-specific and can be unreliable, especially in elderly people. International protocols are available to neuroradiologists to standardize their interpretations of MRI scans in these patients.

The pathological lesion in MS, seen at post-mortem brain biopsy, is a '**plaque**'; this is an area of the white matter in which myelin and oligodendrocytes are absent. Myelin is a protein–phospholipid material that surrounds axons in a multilayered, dense spiral. Myelin sheaths in the CNS are formed by compacted membranes of oligodendrocyte extensions. The integrity of the myelin sheaths depends on the maintenance of normal oligodendrocyte function. Axons without myelin sheaths are poor conductors of nerve impulses, resulting in a neurological deficit. In the early stages of a plaque, there is tissue oedema, apoptotic oligodendrocytes and infiltrating cells; lymphocytes and macrophages are seen around

the venules in the area. B cells are involved in the local production of immunoglobulin, while others, including T cells and macrophages, are part of the acute inflammatory process (Fig. 17.2).

Routine examination of CSF is not enough. It is essential to look at the nature of the immunoglobulin (Box 17.2). Immunoglobulin present in CSF may have been synthesized in the CNS or passively transferred from serum. The concentration of CSF IgG is best expressed in relation to another serum protein that is not synthesized in the brain, as this level will indicate the integrity of the blood–CSF barrier. Most formulae are based on the ratio of IgG/albumin measured by the same technique (see Chapter 19, section 19.4). Intracerebral synthesis of IgG will produce a rise in the IgG/albumin ratio. However, if the raised CSF IgG concentration is due to a 'leaking' blood–brain barrier, then the albumin content will be similarly elevated and the resulting IgG/albumin ratio will remain constant.

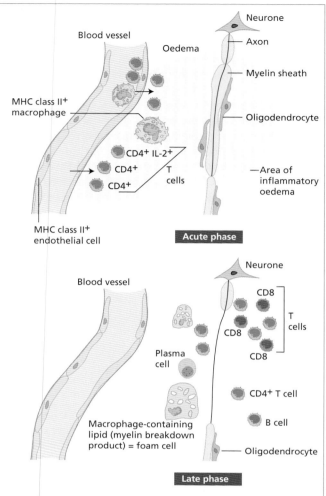

Fig. 17.2 Immunopathogenesis of multiple sclerosis. IL, interleukin; MHC, major histocompatibility complex.

The cause of MS is unknown, but **environmental and genetic factors** are important. In first-degree relatives of MS patients, the disease is 30 times more common than in the general population. There is also a greater concordance rate for monozygotic (30%) than dizygotic (3%) twins – indicating a high degree of heritability. MS is common in Caucasians, with a prevalence of 60 cases per 100 000 population (see Chapter 3, Table 3.3). There is a well-documented association with human leucocyte antigen (HLA)-DR2, DR1 and DQ1 antigens in northern Europeans and North Americans, but the susceptibility of an individual will be **multifactorial**, including exposure to environmental agent(s). Genome-wide association studies with almost 10 000 cases have identified over 50 non-major histocompatibility complex (MHC) susceptibility loci and the challenge now is to prove which genetic changes are functionally important, though clearly the MHC region genes are crucial.

Several epidemiological observations link MS to an exogenous environmental agent (Box 17.3), but **extensive efforts to isolate a specific agent in MS have failed**. Infection with Epstein–Barr virus has received particular attention, but there is no definitive evidence of particular viral specificity, either humoral or cellular. Recent attempts have involved the production of recombinant antibodies prepared from clonally expanded plasma cells from CSF, as used successfully in the detection of pathogenic autoantibodies in neuromyelitis optica. However, such antibodies have failed to react with brain antigens, including myelin basic protein, so the question of the aetiology remains controversial.

Box 17.2 Immunological findings in cerebrospinal fluid (CSF) from patients with definite multiple sclerosis (MS)

Finding	Percentage of positive MS patients
Oligoclonal bands by isoelectric focusing	>95
Increased CSF IgG index	70–80
Increased cell count	50
Raised IgG/albumin ratio	50

Box 17.3 Epidemiological observations in multiple sclerosis (MS) that suggest an infective organism may be the aetiological agent

- MS is a disease of temperate climates, with a well-recognized north/south gradient in the USA and Europe
- Migrants assume the risk of the region to which they migrate if they go before the age of 15; if they go later, they retain the risk associated with their country of origin
- Occasional epidemics of MS have occurred
- 40% of new clinical events follow viral infections
- Raised titres of cerebrospinal fluid (CSF) antibodies to measles virus in many MS patients

but

- CSF IgG from patients with MS reacts with a variety of viruses
- CSF IgG shows a variety of different idiotypes
- IgG shows different specificities and isoelectric points, even within plaques from the same brain
- No herpes simplex (HSV 1/2), Epstein–Barr virus, cytomegalovirus (CMV), varicella zoster virus, human herpes virus-6 or -7 or enteroviruses within plaques by polymerase chain reaction
- Using random peptide libraries, huge number of possible reactivities within a single IgG oligoclone (brain proteins, HSV, CMV and human papilloma virus sequences)

The IgG synthesized in the brain is restricted in nature, has a narrow range of isoelectric points and appears as **typical oligoclonal bands** on isoelectric focusing (Chapter 19, Fig. 19.8). This pattern is seen in over 95% of patients with MS, *although it is not confined to MS*. CSF from patients with cerebral infections, such as neurosyphilis or subacute sclerosing panencephalitis, shows a similar pattern, although such conditions rarely cause diagnostic difficulty.

The original suggestion of myelin basic protein being important in the aetiology came from the animal model of experimental autoimmune encephalitis (EAE) in mice, induced by immunizing susceptible mice with myelin proteins, from whom transfer of activated T cells was able to induce disease in non-immunized animals. These T cells, like those in affected humans, have restricted T-cell receptors (TCRs); attempts to block these TCRs in mice have been successful in limiting the progress of the relapsing and remitting disease. However, **EAE is an imperfect model of MS**. Treatments that target particular T cells have shown efficacy in animal models, but have failed to consistently translate to benefits in MS patients, other than for Campath-1H, a humanized therapeutic monoclonal antibody against CD52 that depletes all mononuclear cells from the blood, including dendritic cells (DCs), monocytes and macrophages.

The precise immunopathogenesis of demyelination is not clear. Many inflammatory cells are present in the local lesions, known as plaques (see Fig. 17.2). Whether cells injure the oligodendrocytes directly or whether the damage results from viral or toxic agents remains controversial. New data suggest that **apoptosis of oligodendrocytes** may precede inflammation and demyelination. $CD4^+$ and $CD8^+$ T cells, with specificity for the human brain component, myelin basic protein, are present in the blood and brain of patients with MS. Whereas previously $CD4^+$ cells were thought to be most important, newer data favour **CD8 T cells** as the cause of oligodendrocyte death and the $CD4^+$ cells as responsible for inflammation. Roles are emerging for more recently defined cellular subsets, such as Th17 cells. However, a clinical trial of ustekinumab, a therapeutic monoclonal antibody against the common subunit of interleukin (IL)-12 and IL-23, which was hoped to block Th1 and Th17 to prevent intrathecal inflammation, showed no benefit.

Activated macrophages are seen in close proximity to myelin-stripped axons and are probably involved too. Autoreactive T cells are found in healthy people, but are activated only in patients with MS. Human CD4-regulatory T cells (CD4/CD25hi) can prevent activation and function of other T cells. Whereas the same numbers of CD4/CD25hi suppressor cells were found in healthy individuals and MS patients, those CD4/CD25hi from patients with MS were less able to inhibit specific activation of CD4/CD25⁻ cells, suggesting that impairment of these regulatory T cells may contribute to the breakdown of immune tolerance in patients with MS.

Targeted **immunotherapy with humanized antibodies** has proved successful. Natalizumab, a monoclonal antibody to $\alpha_4\beta_1$ integrin (VLA4), has been shown to be clinically effective. It is thought to act by preventing the entry of damaging cells into the white matter, but serious side effects (including progressive multifocal leucoencephalopathy) limit its use. Humanized anti-CD25⁺ antibody (daclizumab) inhibits interleukin-2 signalling and was licensed for patients with relapsing–remitting MS (RRMS) in 2016. However, it was withdrawn in 2018 on account of serious adverse effects, including fatal autoimmune encephalitis and hepatitis. Other recent clinical studies have implicated B cells as a therapeutic target, with ocrelizumab now being licensed for RRMS. In short, there is currently *no single specific treatment for MS*. There are no therapies that will reverse demyelination, although each episode is usually associated with some recovery as the initial oedema subsides. Corticosteroids (intravenously in severe relapse) have been used in an acute attack to suppress the inflammatory response, but elimination of the inflammatory component does not stop disease progression. The short-term efficacy of interferon (IFN)-β has been demonstrated in clinical trials, but long-term data are either unavailable or much less compelling. Thus, despite the considerable effort that has gone into MS drug discovery and development, both the pathogenesis and treatment options are limited. Other treatments currently available include Copolymer 1, comprising four amino acids antigenically similar to myelin basic protein, which has shown some promise in RRMS. Fingolimod is a novel compound produced by chemical modification of a fungal precursor and was approved as the first oral treatment for relapsing forms of MS. Its active metabolite, formed by *in vivo* phosphorylation, modulates sphingosine 1-phosphate (S1P) receptors by acting as an agonist and so altering lymphocyte migration and keeps autoreactive lymphocytes away from sites of inflammation. Prompted by two fatal cases of herpes virus infections, assessment of varicella zoster virus (VZV) status is advised prior to therapy. In seronegative patients, inoculations of VZV vaccine are indicated before fingolimod treatment occurs. Other oral therapies that have been licensed for RRMS include small molecules such as dimethyl fumarate and teriflunomide.

New evidence points to a possible inverse association of MS with inflammatory bowel disease (IBD); treatment with anti-tumour necrosis factor (TNF) monoclonal antibodies has led to exacerbation of MS or triggered demyelination in IBD patients. Conversely, IFN-β treatment for MS may worsen IBD. Antilymphocyte trafficking strategies such as α-4-integrin blockers are effective in both these diseases. It is known from mouse work that TNF receptor 1 mediates demyelination and that TNF receptor 2 mediates remyelination, suggesting that differential therapies involving small molecules to block the first and enhance TNF receptor 2 might work in MS, although previous trials of immune stimulation have been disappointing and IFN-γ made the disease worse.

The prognosis of MS depends on the subtype of disease. Overall, 20% of patients have died 20 years after diagnosis and >60% are significantly disabled.

Neuromyelitis optica (**NMO**) is a recently described condition characterized by severe optic neuritis and transverse myelitis. The relationship between this and MS has been controversial, though there are some obvious differences: the absence of oligoclonal IgG bands, the female preponderance and particular involvement of extensive spinal cord lesions involving at least three vertebrae. Once autoantibodies to aquaporin-4, the dominant water channel expressed on end-feet of astrocytes, were demonstrated in patients with NMO, it has been accepted as an autoimmune disease affecting astrocytes. The autoantibodies are pathogenic and treatment is methyl prednisolone, with or without plasma exchange, followed by rituximab.

17.4 Autoimmune diseases of the neuromuscular junction

17.4.1 Myasthenia gravis

Myasthenia gravis is an uncommon disease (prevalence 9 per 10^5 population) characterized by weakness and fatigue of voluntary muscles, including those of the eye (see Case 17.3 and

Case 17.3 Myasthenia gravis

A 67-year-old man, complaining of double vision, was found to have bilateral ptosis, covering most of the pupil on the right side and partially obscuring that on the left. The ptosis was worse in the evening and almost absent in the morning. He admitted to tiredness in the arms and legs on exercise, which recovered with resting. A clinical diagnosis of ocular myasthenia gravis was made. A Tensilon test, involving intravenous injection of edrophonium, a short-acting cholinesterase inhibitor to abolish the symptoms, was positive, but electromyography was inconclusive.

His serum contained antibodies to thyroid microsomes and to acetylcholine receptors (see Chapter 19, section 19.7). The patient improved on treatment with pyridostigmine, which prolongs the action of acetylcholine by inhibiting the breakdown.

This case is not typical of myasthenia gravis, but demonstrates that myasthenia may affect mainly ocular muscles (although only 60% have detectable antibodies to acetylcholine receptors). Myasthenia gravis is more commonly a disease of young women, who present with increasing systemic muscle fatigue (see Chapter 5, Case 5.2).

Chapter 5, Case 5.2); patients presenting with only ocular symptoms may not necessarily progress. The weakness results from impaired transmission from nerve to muscle at the neuromuscular junctions. Neurotransmission is impaired by **autoantibodies to the acetylcholine receptors** (AChRs) in the postsynaptic membrane of the muscle (Fig. 17.3). These antibodies reduce the number of receptors, by complement-mediated lysis and accelerated internalization, and possibly by blocking the receptors.

At least **four subgroups** of patients are recognized (Table 17.3), suggesting different aetiologies. Myasthenia gravis in young women (early-onset myasthenia gravis) is an organ-specific autoimmune disease (see Box 17.4), with HLA associations (HLA-B8 and HLA-DR3) that are commonly linked to such conditions. A recent genome-wide association study using strict criteria and a homogeneous population of early-onset autoimmune cases confirmed the strong association with HLA-B*08, but found that changes in the gene, PTPN22, and in TNFAIP3-interacting protein 1 (TNIP1) conferred an even stronger risk, implicating dysregulation of nuclear factor kappa B (NFκB) signalling. The involvement of HLA-B*08 suggests that CD8(⁺) T cells may play a key role in disease initiation. The aetiology of myasthenia is unknown, though dog experiments suggest an infectious cause in the early-onset autoimmune group.

As in other autoimmune diseases, there are **hyperplastic thymic changes** in early-onset myasthenia gravis, in contrast to those with a thymic tumour (Table 17.3), which include prominent formation of lymphoid follicles, germinal centres and increased numbers of mononuclear and plasma cells; the latter are one source of receptor antibodies. Myoid cells, present in myasthenic thymus and thymoma, act as a source of antigen for the production of acetylcholine receptor antibodies and antigen-specific T cells. It is essential to check for underlying thymoma by CT scanning of the chest, not only to ascertain the group but so that the enlarged thymus is removed surgically for histology, as it is not possible to distinguish hyperplasia from thymoma otherwise.

Myasthenia gravis may also be induced by D-penicillamine therapy, but reverses on discontinuation of the drug. The idiotypes of the receptor antibodies provoked by D-penicillamine are very limited, in contrast to the wide heterogeneity seen in these antibodies in 'idiopathic' myasthenia gravis.

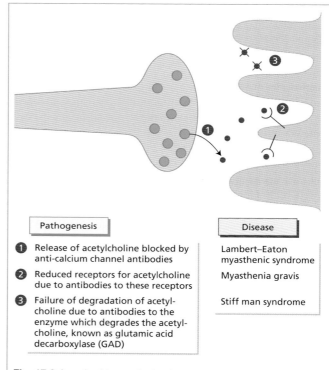

Pathogenesis	Disease
① Release of acetylcholine blocked by anti-calcium channel antibodies	Lambert–Eaton myasthenic syndrome
② Reduced receptors for acetylcholine due to antibodies to these receptors	Myasthenia gravis
③ Failure of degradation of acetylcholine due to antibodies to the enzyme which degrades the acetylcholine, known as glutamic acid decarboxylase (GAD)	Stiff man syndrome

Fig. 17.3 Impaired transmission from nerve to muscle at the neuromuscular junctions in myasthenia gravis and other muscle end-plate diseases.

The receptor autoantibodies were discovered when a known neuromuscular toxin was injected into rabbits, causing the production of circulating antiacetylcholine antibodies and resultant paralysis due to neuromuscular block, similar to that found in myasthenia gravis. Such antibodies (see Chapter 19, section 19.7) are **diagnostic** for myasthenia; nearly 90% of younger patients with systemic myasthenia have this antibody, whereas only 60% of patients with myasthenia confined to the ocular muscles are positive. Acetylcholine receptor antibodies of IgG class cross the placenta. However, only 10% of babies of myasthenic mothers develop neonatal myasthenia, since the receptor antibodies are neutralized by fetal production of antiidiotypic antibodies, presumably IgM. Around 10% of myasthenic

Table 17.3 Heterogeneity of myasthenia gravis (MG)

	Young women (early-onset MG)	Older men (late-onset MG)	Thymoma	No AcChR antibody
Proportion of patients	40–50%	15–30%	15–20%	15%
Thymic changes	Hyperplasia	Atrophy	Tumour	Unknown
Antibody titre to acetylcholine receptors	High	Low	Intermediate	None MuSK/other antibodies
Muscle weakness	Systemic	Systemic/ocular	Systemic	Systemic/ocular
Immunological therapy	Thymectomy (recover in two years) plus immune suppression	Prednisolone ± azathioprine	Thymectomy for tumour; if little improvement in weakness, important to use immune suppression as well	Prednisolone ± azathioprine
Human leucocyte antigen (HLA) associations	A1 B8 DR3	B7 DR2	None	None

---

Box 17.4 Evidence that early-onset myasthenia gravis is an autoimmune disease

- Strong association with organ-specific autoimmune diseases, such as myxoedema or diabetes, in an individual patient
- Increased incidence of organ-specific autoimmune diseases in close family members
- Thymic hyperplasia, including B cells forming follicles
- Occurrence of a transient form of myasthenia gravis in 10% of newborn babies of myasthenic mothers
- Association with human leucocyte antigen (HLA)-B8
- Identification of autoantibodies to several autoantigens (AcChRs, MuSK and Lrp4)

---

patients who are seronegative for anti-AChR antibodies will instead have autoantibodies to muscle-specific receptor tyrosine kinase (MuSK) and other autoantibodies are being discovered such as anti-Lrp4 autoantibodies, which may also be pathogenic. If early-onset myasthenia gravis is triggered by infection, it may

be no surprise that multiple antigens can act as triggers and cause disease, as in type I diabetes (Chapter 15, section 15.4.2).

Symptomatic management of myasthenia gravis is achieved using acetylcholinesterase inhibitors (see Case 17.3). Longer-term **treatment** involves suppression of production of acetylcholine receptor antibodies (e.g. with prednisolone and azathioprine; see Table 17.3), as well as prevention of stimulation. Patients with severe myasthenia gravis respond well to plasmapheresis (or high-dose intravenous immunoglobulin [IVIg] in extreme cases), in addition to immunosuppressive therapy (such as corticosteroids, azathioprine, mycophenolate mofetil or cyclosporine). Thymectomy in those with an enlarged thymus or thymoma (Fig. 17.4) removes not only some of the plasma cells producing the antibodies, but also at least one source of antigen.

17.4.2 Other autoimmune diseases of muscle end-plates

A similar **mechanism** of action by autoantibodies is seen in the Lambert–Eaton myasthenic syndrome, in which antibodies to calcium channels, related to the release of acetylcholine from

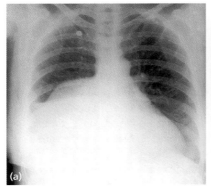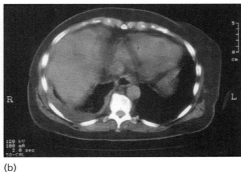

Fig. 17.4 X-ray and computed tomography (CT) scan of chest in a patient with a thymoma and myasthenia gravis. (a) X-ray shows mass in right chest and pleural effusion. (b) CT scan shows this mass pushing heart and large vessels to left (and enlarged lymph nodes and a pleural effusion due to a chest infection).

vesicles, result in weakness (see Box 17.1). The association between Lambert–Eaton myasthenic syndrome and small cell lung cancer makes full investigation and follow-up of all cases imperative. In contrast, the Stiff Man syndrome is caused by autoantibodies to the intracellular enzyme glutamic acid decarboxylase (GAD), which results in inability to relax muscles by breaking down the transmitter. This neurological syndrome is typically associated with type 1 diabetes mellitus, in which such antibodies are also pathogenic (see Chapter 15, section 15.4.2 on diabetes mellitus and cross-reactive antibodies).

17.5 Immune-mediated neuropathies

Peripheral neuropathy can be a complication of some common immune-mediated diseases, such as rheumatoid arthritis or diabetes mellitus (Table 17.4), or a common feature of rare diseases, such as polyarteritis nodosa (see Chapter 10, section 10.9) or amyloidosis (see Chapter 9, section 9.7.3). Those known to be directly mediated by immune components, including paraproteins, are listed in Table 17.5.

17.5.1 Acute idiopathic polyneuritis (Guillain–Barré syndrome)

Guillain–Barré syndrome (GBS) is an uncommon disease of subacute onset in which the peripheral nervous system is infiltrated with lymphocytes and macrophages, and myelin is destroyed as a result. There are subtypes that depend on clinical features, abnormalities found in nerve conduction studies and autoantibodies.

Half the cases of this rare condition occur in relation to an infectious illness, often a diarrhoeal illness due to Campylobacter jejuni, as in Chapter 5, Case 5.5, though 10% follow a surgical procedure and the rest are idiopathic. There is evidence that the **pathogenesis** involves the production of

Table 17.4 Common associations of peripheral neuropathies

	Percentage of patients who develop a peripheral neuropathy
Common conditions	
Rheumatoid arthritis	3
Diabetes mellitus	5–10
Myxoedema	1
Lymphoma	1
Infection (e.g. Lyme disease)	1
Pernicious anaemia	1
Uncommon conditions	
Systemic vasculitis	40
Amyloid	10
Cryoglobulinaemia	10

Table 17.5 Immune-mediated peripheral neuropathies (with associated autoantibodies if known)

Acute	Chronic
Guillain–Barré syndrome (anti-ganglioside autoantibodies)	Chronic inflammatory demyelinating polyneuropathy
Miller–Fisher syndrome (anti-GQ1 antibodies)	Multifocal motor neuropathy (anti-GM1 antibodies)
Systemic vasculitis	Paraproteinaemic neuropathy (anti- myelin-associated glycoprotein antibodies)
	Subacute sensory neuropathy (anti-Hu antibodies)

autoantibodies to peripheral nerve tissue gangliosides, triggered by infection (Box 17.5). These antibodies to known gangliosides, such as GM1, GD1a, GT1a and GQ1b, can be demonstrated in 70% of patients. There is evidence for molecular mimicry between gangliosides and the infectious agents, particularly with Campylobacter infection, that precede these conditions. Early complement activation, based on antibody binding to the outer surface of the Schwann cell, results in deposition of activated complement components and this seems to initiate the damage to myelin. Infiltration by macrophages occurs a few days after complement-mediated myelin damage. Patients undergo a lumbar puncture to rule out infectious diseases, such as Lyme disease, or malignant conditions, such as lymphoma.

Most patients improve within a few weeks of onset; their recovery is usually complete and therapy is avoided, as in Case 17.4. In severely affected patients, recovery times to unaided ventilation and walking are shortened considerably by the use of *large doses of IVIg given as soon as the diagnosis is made*, as in Chapter 5, Case 5.5. Plasma exchange is equally efficacious to IVIg in Guillain–Barré syndrome by removing pathogenic

Box 17.5 Evidence for the autoimmune nature of Guillain–Barré syndrome

- Association with preceding infection – often Campylobacter
- Cross-reactive epitopes between pathogen and autoantigen gangliosides
- IgG and C1q deposited in nerves – seen on biopsies
- Antiganglioside antibodies and antimyelin antibodies detectable in serum
- Correlation of antibodies with clinical disease course
- Oligoclonal IgG in cerebrospinal fluid
- Successful therapy with plasma exchange or high-dose intravenous immunoglobulin (immune modulation)

autoantibodies. Treatment with corticosteroids does not improve outcomes and their use is no longer advocated.

17.5.2 Chronic inflammatory peripheral neuropathies

Chronic conditions differ from the Guillain–Barré syndrome and may be relapsing and remitting or have a progressive course. The main chronic autoimmune neuropathies include chronic inflammatory demyelinating polyneuropathy (CIDP), multifocal motor neuropathy (MMN) and anti-myelin-associated glycoprotein (MAG) demyelinating neuropathy. **Treatment** with prednisone and/or plasma exchange is partially successful in some groups of patients. Regular infusions of IVIg are successful in others, but a trial of therapy is needed before embarking on long-term therapy.

Chronic inflammatory demyelinating polyneuropathy

CIDP patients are usually middle-aged and symptoms present gradually. The prevalence is around 4–8 cases per 10^5 population. A history of a preceding illness is uncommon and the aetiology remains obscure. Sensory or motor symptoms or both are accompanied by conduction block. Demyelination is multifocal, affecting spinal roots, plexuses and proximal nerve trunks, so that the clinical picture is variable.

Pathogenesis is thought to be mixed, cellular and humoral. Though there are autoantibodies in serum, the target antigens of the aberrant immune responses are unknown. A significant proportion of infiltrating γδ T cells are able to recognize glycolipid and carbohydrate moieties, suggesting involvement of natural killer (NK) T cells, which are thought to activate resid-

ing macrophages, leading to phagocytosis and production of proinflammatory cytokines. Randomized controlled trials have shown benefit from corticosteroids, high-dose IVIg and plasmapheresis, though this is patient dependent and there are no predictors to indicate which therapy will be beneficial in any given patient. Long-term therapy is required, usually with immunoglobulin, either intravenously or subcutaneously, with the dose intervals adjusted to maintain reasonable function.

Multifocal motor neuropathy

MMN is a distinct disease that should be recognized early, because it is treatable. It presents with progressive weakness, atrophy and loss of reflexes that usually begin in the hands, and is prominent in distal muscle groups. In its early stages it is frequently confused with motor neurone disease, which in contrast to MMN is not treatable. It differs from vasculitic neuropathy, because it is slow and painless and affects only motor nerve fibres. Patients with this condition have purely motor symptoms, which are usually symmetrical (see Case 17.5). The pathogenesis of MMN is poorly understood. **Autoantibodies** against **GM1 gangliosides** (GM1, GD1a and GD1b) are present in up to 60% of patients. The condition is exacerbated by steroid therapy, and high-dose IVIg (immunomodulation) is now the treatment of choice, since >70% of patients respond to a trial of high-dose IVIg therapy. Maintenance therapy with immunoglobulin, either intravenously or subcutaneously, then enables them largely to be functionally independent.

Monoclonal gammopathies

Sensory or motor neuropathies have been described in patients with monoclonal gammopathies. Of patients with sensory neuropathies, 50% have monoclonal antibodies to **MAG** – a major component of peripheral nerves (see Tables 17.5 and 17.6). These antibodies have been shown to cause demyelination in animals. Patients often present with sensory ataxia and have a distinctive pattern on nerve conduction studies. Sural nerve biopsy can be helpful, as it shows splitting of the outer myelin lamellae, probably caused by IgM deposits. Plasmapheresis, with or without immune suppression, is frequently used for disease control. Peripheral neuropathy is also found in 10% of patients with cryoglobulinaemia (see Chapter 11, section 11.6.3).

17.6 Paraneoplastic syndromes

Inappropriate expression of tumour-associated antigens that cross-react with those on normal tissues can be caused by a number of mechanisms in tumours, including mutations, rearrangements of the genome and viral insertions. Paraneoplastic syndromes can affect any organ or system. Most classic paraneoplastic syndromes are associated with antibodies to intracellular (onconeuronal) antigens, appear to be mediated by cytotoxic T-cell responses and have limited response to treatment. These patients nearly always have a

Case 17.4 Guillain–Barré syndrome

A 14-year-old boy awoke one morning two weeks after an episode of influenza with a mild weakness in his legs; his sceptical parents wondered if this was a ploy to avoid school, but during the day he developed pain in his back and 'pins and needles' in his feet. He was considerably worse the next day and complained of weakness in his arms as well, and he was admitted to hospital that evening with suspected acute idiopathic inflammatory polyneuropathy. Lumbar puncture showed no cells but a slightly raised protein level in the cerebrospinal fluid. Peripheral nerve conduction studies the next day revealed demyelination, confirming a diagnosis of Guillain–Barré syndrome. Antibodies to ganglioside GD1 were present in his blood. His condition was by now stable and so he was not treated with high-dose intravenous immunoglobulin but monitored carefully; he made a complete recovery in eight days.

Case 17.5 Multifocal motor neuropathy

A 48-year-old man presented with gradually increasing weakness in his arms. Leg weakness followed after two weeks and he experienced steady but slow downhill progression over four weeks. He had no consistent sensory symptoms. On examination, he was found to have a motor tetraparesis, most marked in the arms. Sensation was normal. Nerve conduction studies showed a demyelinating motor neuropathy in upper and lower limbs, with motor conduction velocities of 26 m/s. Antibodies to GM1 ganglioside were present in the serum, confirming the diagnosis of chronic multifocal motor neuropathy. He was treated initially with prednisolone, but this provoked further deterioration.

Intravenous immunoglobulin (IVIg, 2 g/kg body weight) was initially instituted every eight weeks, with an initial excellent response after five days that gradually deteriorated after four weeks, returning to pretreatment levels by eight weeks, in keeping with the half-life of IgG in the serum. This response to therapy was confirmed by a further infusion, after which changing the interval between infusions to three weeks and infusing IVIg (at a dose of 0.8 g/kg) resulted in sustained improvement. This condition is unusual in young children.

Table 17.6 Selected paraneoplastic neurological syndromes

Condition	Signs	Cancer	Autoantibodies to
Lambert–Eaton myasthenia (LEMS)	Fatiguability of muscles causing weakness	Small cell lung cancer	Voltage-gated calcium channels
Neuromyelitis optica	Relapsing optic neuritis, transverse myelitis, encephalopathies	Breast cancer	Aquaporin-4
Cerebellar degeneration	Ataxia, brainstem encephalitis,	Small cell lung cancer	Voltage-gated calcium channels
Limbic encephalitis	Behavioural changes, cognitive impairment, seizures	Small cell lung cancer, thymoma, adenocarcinoma of breast, prostate	Neuronal antigen – Hu
Paraneoplastic sensory neuropathy	Sensory loss and reflexia	Small cell lung cancer	Neuronal antigen – Hu
Sensorimotor neuropathy	Mononeuritis multiplex	Cancer or vasculitis	Neuronal antigen – Hu
Paraproteinaemic polyneuropathies	Motor and sensory loss	Lymphoid malignancies	Myelin-associated glycoprotein

malignancy, often covertly. The autoimmune synaptic disorders, such as LEMS, are associated with antibodies against extracellular epitopes, appear to be directly mediated by antibodies and are responsive to immunotherapy, and patients may or may not have an associated cancer, such as small cell lung cancer (Table 17.6). The neurological syndrome may predate an overt malignancy by many years, so it is always important to search for a resectable cancer, especially in the lung.

17.7 Cerebral systemic lupus erythematosus

Up to 60% of patients with SLE suffer neuropsychiatric episodes at some time (see Chapter 10, section 10.7). Most patients experience only mild but fluctuating symptoms. In some patients, spontaneous improvement occurs with time; others have irreversible changes. Cerebral thrombosis is not infrequent and is associated with antibodies to clotting factors and phospholipids (see Chapter 16, section 16.6).

Cerebral involvement in SLE remains very much a clinical diagnosis. It can be the presenting feature of SLE in an otherwise undiagnosed patient, as in Case 17.6, but this is unusual. Serological tests for systemic lupus are important, although there is no test that is specific for cerebral lupus. Antiribosomal P protein antibodies and antibodies directed against the N-methyl-D-aspartate glutamate receptor have been promoted as diagnostic markers of cerebral SLE, but lack sufficient sensitivity to make them useful in clinical practice.

17.8 Autoimmune encephalitis

There have been major advances over the past decade in delineating autoimmune encephalitis as a distinct disorder amenable to treatment with immunotherapy. The observation that autoimmune encephalitis, with a range of demonstrable autoantibodies (see Table 17.8), may possibly be as common as acute infectious encephalitis (prevalence 13/100 000) has

Case 17.6 Systemic lupus erythematosus

A 45-year-old woman presented with acute disorientation so severe that she was unable to dress herself. On neurological examination there were no abnormal findings, and routine laboratory investigations, including examination of the urine, were normal. Nuclear magnetic resonance imaging (MRI) showed three frontal lobe lesions with the characteristic appearances of vasculitis, so a detailed search for a cause was undertaken.

A laboratory diagnosis of systemic lupus erythematosus (SLE) was made (Table 17.7). Prednisolone was given with a dramatic improvement in the patient's mental state; within a week she was able to dress herself, and 10 days after admission she was able to go home. Serological tests nine months later showed only a weakly positive antinuclear antibody (ANA) at 1/160, a normal C3 level of 0.77 g/L, a low C4 level of 0.14 g/L, and persistent elevated DNA binding (68%).

Table 17.7 Investigations for cerebral systemic lupus erythematosus in Case 17.6

Antinuclear antibody (ANA)	Positive: 1/80
Antineutrophil cytoplasmic antibodies	Negative
dsDNA binding	High, 91% (normal <30%)
DNA antibodies (IgG)	Positive on Crithidia luciliae (titre 1/120)
Serum IgG	16.5 g/L (NR 6.0–12.0)
C3	0.54 g/L (NR 0.65–1.25)
C4	0.03 g/L (NR 0.2–0.5)

Table 17.8 Selected autoantibodies associated with autoimmune encephalitis

Autoantibody	Syndrome	Cancer association
NMDA-R	Limbic encephalitis	10–50% (ovarian teratoma)
LGI-1	Limbic encephalitis	<10–20% (bronchial carcinoma, thymoma)
AMPA-R	Limbic encephalitis	70% (bronchial, breast, thymoma)
CASPR2	Neuromyotonia, Morvan's syndrome	<20–40% (bronchial)
GAD65*	Stiff person syndrome, limbic encephalitis	25% (thymoma, small cell lung cancer)
DPPX	Encephalitis, diarrhoea	<10% lymphoma)
MOG	Acute disseminated encephalomyelitis	0%
Hu*, Ri*, Yo*	Cerebellitis	>50%

*Antigens located intracellularly; all other autoantibodies are directed against cell surface or synaptic antigens.
AMPA-R, α-amino-3-hydroxy-5-methyl-4-isoxazolepropionic acid receptor; CASPR2, Contactin-associated protein-like 2; GAD-65, glutamic acid decarboxylase 65; LGI-1, leucine-rich glioma inactivated; MOG, myelin oligodendrocyte glycoprotein.

transformed the outlook for these patients who were hitherto treated inappropriately for presumed infection.

A range of presenting clinical features are seen, reflecting the anatomical location of brain inflammation. Diagnosis is dependent on early recognition of clinical features supplemented by cranial imaging, CSF analysis and testing for a panel of neuronal autoantibodies. Over 37 different antibodies have been described. Differentiating between antibodies to intracellular antigens and antibodies to synaptic and surface antigens is useful, because some disorders associated with the former (classical onconeuronal antibodies) are poorly responsive to immunosuppressive therapies.

CHAPTER 18
Immunological Diseases in Pregnancy

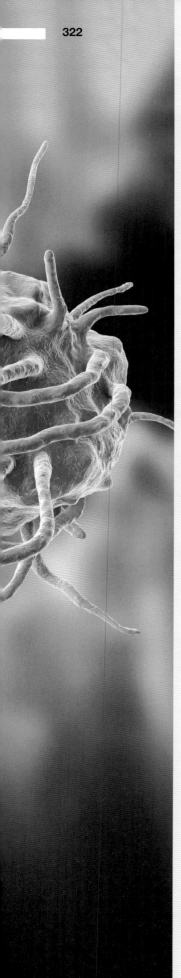

Key topics

 Visit the companion website at **www.wiley.com/go/misbah/immunology** to download cases with additional figures on these topics.

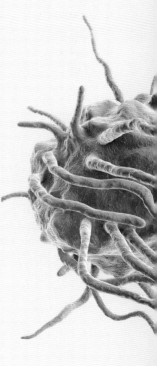

Chapel and Haeney's Essentials of Clinical Immunology, Seventh Edition. Edited by Siraj A. Misbah, Gavin P. Spickett, and Virgil A.S.H. Dalm.
© 2022 John Wiley & Sons Ltd. Published 2022 by John Wiley & Sons Ltd.

18.1 Introduction

In pregnancy, one-half of the transplantation antigens of the fetus are of paternal origin and, in an outbred species such as humans, these are different from those of the mother. The mother therefore carries a 'mismatched' fetus but, despite this, the fetus is not rejected. The reasons for this remain controversial and so the relationship between the local active recognition process (which allows successful implantation of the embryo and development of the placenta) and those systemic mechanisms that help maintain the pregnancy are not discussed here. However, protection of the fetus against infection is covered, as well as immunological disorders of pregnancy itself.

18.2 Pregnancy and maternal infection

Maternal mortality figures for the UK show that infection is the second most common cause of maternal death within 1 year of pregnancy, a figure that is consistent across the northern hemisphere. Worldwide, pregnancy is associated with a greatly increased risk of infection, particularly with malaria, toxoplasma or mycobacterial infections (tuberculosis and leprosy), which are particularly common in countries where malnutrition may be a major factor. However, the risk still persists, as illustrated in Case 18.1. Listeria is a risk, as are toxoplasmosis and human immunodeficiency virus (HIV), suggesting that there is **reduced Th1 cell activity** against intracellular pathogens during pregnancy. Pregnant women are advised to avoid unpasteurized dairy products. In addition, all pregnant women are checked routinely for antibodies to sexually transmitted diseases.

Women should check their own **immunization status** for common viral infections (especially rubella, measles and polio) prior to pregnancy and avoid exposure to chickenpox if they are not immune. The more severe risks to the fetus are discussed in the next section.

18.3 Protection of the fetus and neonate against infection

The fetus and neonate are susceptible to both bacterial and viral infections by transplacental transfer and during vaginal delivery. The extent and nature of the infection depend not only on the type of infection, but also on the immune maturity of the fetus at the time of infection. This, in turn, depends on the gestational age of the fetus (Box 18.1).

18.3.1 Development of fetal immune responses

The fetus becomes partially immunocompetent early in **intrauterine life** (Box 18.1), for example intrauterine infection with rubella virus provokes the production of fetal IgM antibodies against the virus as early as week 11. However, *T-cell development is slow* and this may account for the particular susceptibility of the fetus to viruses and intracellular bacteria. Plenty of T cells are detectable early in gestational life and T-cell numbers in blood are much higher at birth than in adults. However, their functional capacity develops late in fetal life, is still reduced at birth and increases in early life to reach adult levels in the first 2 months.

At term, although CD4+ cell numbers are high and interleukin (IL)-2 production is normal, production of other important cytokines, interferon (IFN)-γ, tumour necrosis factor (TNF) and TH2 cytokines, is low. Cytotoxic T-cell function is only one-third of that of adults and natural killer (NK) cell cytolysis is reduced also. These findings may account for the severity of neonatal infections with herpes simplex virus (HSV), cytomegalovirus (CMV), Listeria and Toxoplasma. Listeria, a facultative intracellular bacterium, is killed as a result of CD8+ cytotoxic T cells recognizing listerial antigen and major histocompatibility complex (MHC) class I antigens on the surface of the infected histiocyte or hepatocyte. With reduced cytotoxic T cells and Th1 cytokine production, the fetus is more susceptible to intracellular and viral infections than the mother, as in Case 18.1.

The fetus is protected against bacterial infection by active transfer of **maternal IgG** across the placenta (see section 18.3.2). Fortunately, neutrophil leucocytes and macrophages are fully competent and plentiful in the circulation within a few days of birth.

18.3.2 Placental transfer of IgG

IgG is transferred across the placenta by means of specific receptors in the trophoblast for the Fc region of IgG, known as FcRn; these are the same receptors used for recycling IgG, albumin and probably IgA in mucosal cells (see Chapter 1, section 1.2.4 and Chapter 7, Fig. 7.18). Transfer begins at about 12 weeks, but most of the maternal immunoglobulin is transferred after 32 weeks of intrauterine life. Extremely premature babies therefore lack circulating maternal IgG at birth (Chapter 3, Fig. 3.3) and are susceptible to bacterial as well as intracellular infections.

Infants with poor fetal growth also have lower levels of IgG at birth, due to poor placental transfer. Infants of very low birth weight (<1.5 g) have a high prevalence (up to 20%) of late-onset infections related to invasive procedures, with an infection-related mortality of 5–10%. Such infections are bacterial (involving staphylococci, enterococci, Klebsiella and Pseudomonas) and are notably those infections against which antibodies play an important protective role. Intravenous immunoglobulin (IVIg) infusions (0.5 g/kg per week) have

Case 18.1 A mother infected with Listeria

A 22-year-old primagravida stayed on a small-holding in France for the last 3 months of the pregnancy. She had been well, apart from morning sickness during the first 4 weeks of gestation. In France, she had been drinking fresh unpasteurized milk and eating home-made cheeses for 3 weeks when she developed fever, vomiting and diarrhoea, followed by headache, myalgia and low back pain that persisted for 5 days. Four weeks later, at 28 weeks' gestation, she went into premature labour and a still-born, jaundiced child was delivered after 36 h. At the baby's post mortem, there was evidence of hepatitis, purulent pneumonia, conjunctivitis and meningitis. Listeria monocytogenes was cultured from several sites and a diagnosis of fatal neonatal Listeria monocytogenes infection was made. The organism was sensitive to ampicillin and gentamycin and since there was no longer a teratogenic risk (the pregnancy being over), the mother was given a 4-week course of both antibiotics in case organisms were silently sequestered in her deep tissues. Pregnant women are now all advised to avoid unpasteurized products throughout pregnancy.

Box 18.1 Development of immune responsiveness in the fetus

- At 6 weeks of gestational age first appearance of a blood centre with macrophages in the yolk sac
- At 6–7 weeks of gestational age natural killer (NK) cells present in liver
- At 7 weeks of gestational age thymic epithelium develops, followed shortly by lymphocytes and macrophages in blood
- At 11 weeks of gestational age lymphocytes in thymus are CD3+, 4+, 8+, TCR+
- At 20 weeks of gestational age serum IgM detectable in infection (e.g. rubella) at 11 weeks and specific IgG
- **At full term**, i.e. 40 weeks of gestational age:
  - Normal B cell numbers, but these are naive and many are immature, i.e. CD5+, CD27−
  - IgM antibodies are detectable to specific proteins but not to carbohydrate antigens
  - Classical complement components are 90% of adult levels at term and those of the alternative system are at 60% of adult levels, with C8 and C9 at only 20% of adult levels
  - Although T-cell numbers are high, T-cell function at term is reduced, with normal interleukin (IL)-2 production but low levels of interferon (IFN)-γ, and tumour necrosis factor (TNF) at only 20% of adult levels; TH$_2$ cytokines are also very low and there is poor T-cell help for B cells due to low CD40 ligand (CD40L) levels. Cytotoxic T cells are only 30–60% of adult levels
  - NK cell activity normal numbers, with >50% being good cytokine producers (CD56++); reduced NK cytolysis
  - Neutrophils in normal numbers, but reduced adhesion and migration for a few days

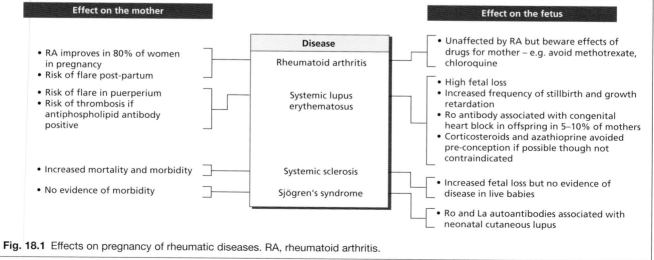

Fig. 18.1 Effects on pregnancy of rheumatic diseases. RA, rheumatoid arthritis.

🔍 Case 18.2 Hypogammaglobulinaemia of prematurity

A normal infant girl was delivered by caesarean section at 30 weeks of gestation as her 35-year-old primagravida mother had severe preeclampsia. The infant weighed 0.75 kg, had no obvious congenital abnormalities and respiration was established quickly. In view of her young gestational age, cord blood immunoglobulin measurements and amniotic fluid lecithin/sphingomyelin ratio were obtained. Her gestational age was actually 26 weeks; her serum IgG level was 0.1 g/l (NR at birth is equivalent to that of the mother, i.e. 7.2–19.0 g/l). A diagnosis of hypogammaglobulinaemia of prematurity was made and her mother's serum levels were checked and found to be normal.

Nutritional support was given and an intravascular catheter inserted to enable blood sampling. On day 10, the infant developed apnoea, bradycardia and abdominal distension. Investigations showed a neutrophilia and raised C-reactive protein (CRP) and blood cultures grew Staphylococcus aureus. Intravenous antibiotic therapy was started for this neonatal staphylococcal infection; intravenous immunoglobulin therapy was considered too, but the infant made a good recovery on antibiotics alone; she was discharged after 8 weeks (rather than on day 14 as hoped).

---

been shown to reduce late-onset infections (like that in Case 18.2) in placebo-controlled studies in the USA. IVIg is not used routinely in the UK, since the rate of serious late-onset infections is <1%; this is probably due to avoidance of invasive procedures whenever possible.

In a full-term baby, the serum level of IgG in the neonate is equivalent to that of the mother, due to transfer of maternal IgG. However, there is little active neonatal synthesis of IgG or IgA at this stage. The result is a fall in the IgG level as the maternal IgG is catabolized. The half-life of IgG is 3–4 weeks, resulting in a period of relative IgG deficiency in the blood (**physiological trough**) between 3 and 6 months (Chapter 3, Fig. 3.3).

The gradual increase of IgG thereafter is associated with expression of CD40 ligand on an increasing number of T cells, **isotype switching** from IgM to IgG and IgA production by the infant. The immaturity of B cells at birth, i.e. their CD5$^+$ nature, results in low-affinity antibody production; later the provision of the molecules involved in **somatic hypermutation** (as well as switching) results in the maturation of antibody production to high-affinity antibodies. This is accomplished by 2 months of age when routine immunizations with protein antigens begin. IgG levels rise to approach adult levels by the age of 4 years (see Chapter 3, Fig. 3.3), by which time antibodies to carbohydrate antigens can be produced too. Replacement immunoglobulin is not usually needed in the physiological trough, since specific IgM can be made. However, if the trough is prolonged (transient hypogammaglobulinaemia of infancy), IVIg can be used in the rare children who suffer from serious recurrent infections that are not preventable with prophylactic antibiotics (see Chapter 3, section 3.2.2). However, a diagnosis of a primary immunodeficiency, particularly severe combined immune deficiency (SCID), must be excluded (see Chapter 3).

18.3.3 Immunological value of breastfeeding

The **antiinfective properties** of breastfeeding have been established for many years. An array of factors in breast milk helps to reduce the incidence of neonatal infections (Box 18.2). The

---

Box 18.2 Protective factors in breast milk

- *IgA* – mainly secretory IgA – resists digestion in fetal gut. These antibodies include those against bacteria and viruses
- *Cells* – macrophages, polymorphonuclear leucocytes, lymphocytes
- *Complement components* – may be involved in opsonization by alternate pathway
- *Lysozyme* – can attack bacterial cell walls
- *Lactoperoxidase* – antistreptococcal agent
- *Lactoferrin* – inhibits growth of bacteria

---

principal immunoglobulin in human colostrum and breast milk is secretory IgA, which is resistant to the proteolytic effects of enzymes in the neonatal gut. The protective role of IgA includes virus neutralization, bactericidal activity, aggregation of antigen and prevention of bacterial adherence to epithelial cells. In contrast to some mammals, there is no evidence that significant amounts of these antibodies can be absorbed from the human neonatal gut to provide systemic protection.

The **cells in milk** are important in phagocytosis and their phagocytic ability is equal to that of blood leucocytes. Necrotizing enterocolitis is caused by bacterial penetration of the gut and occurs in infants with poor local defences; the condition is relatively uncommon in breastfed infants. Immunocompetent **lymphocytes** are also present in human milk and, although there is no evidence that these react against the neonate in a harmful way, CD4$^+$ cells will carry HIV in an HIV+ mother. *Transmission of HIV from mother to baby* has been documented in this way. Breastfeeding by HIV+ mothers is therefore discouraged in developed countries, although this is inappropriate in areas of malnutrition. With the introduction of human milk banks, the effect of sterilization (for safe storage) is important. Freezing milk reduces the number of viable cells, and autoclaving and pasteurization destroy some antibodies as well as the cells, although the nutritional properties are unaffected by these processes.

18.3.4 Reducing particular risks to the fetus/neonate from maternal infection

There are particular infection risks to the fetus or neonate. These include viruses such as hepatitis B (HBV), hepatitis C (HCV), HIV as well as CMV and HSV; bacteria, including staphylococci, enterococci, Klebsiella and Pseudomonas; and superficial fungal infections. Vaccinations in pregnancy are important in prenatal care for improving maternal health and neonatal outcomes. Maternal immunization in pregnancy has been used useful to reduce neonatal tetanus and inactivated influenza and acellular pertussis vaccines are recommended during pregnancy in some countries, as influenza affects pregnant women disproportionately and pertussis infection rates are rising; maternal immunization is projected for group B streptococcus eventually. In a pilot study with 23-valent pneumococcal polysaccharide vaccine (PPV), elevated antibody concentrations after maternal vaccination persisted in infants until 4 months of age and infants subsequently immunized responded to revaccination to provide protection in the first few years of life.

For those mothers with active HBV viraemia, infants are particularly at risk even if the mothers are immunized; the new oral antiviral therapies can be given safely in pregnancy to reduce the risk to the infant.

18.4 Disorders of pregnancy

Some diseases, such as recurrent abortions, preeclampsia or alloimmunization, are disorders of pregnancy itself. Diseases not restricted to pregnancy may also have profound effects on the pregnant woman and her baby.

18.4.1 Recurrent abortions

About 20% of all pregnancies abort spontaneously and *two-thirds of fetuses are lost even before the woman realizes that she is pregnant*. Many factors cause abortion: these include infections, congenital defects, anatomical abnormalities, endocrine abnormalities, non-immune thrombophilic states and autoimmune states, such as uncontrolled thyroid disease, systemic lupus erythematosus (SLE; see Chapter 10, section 10.7) and the antiphospholipid syndrome (see Chapter 16, section 16.6.1). Recurrent spontaneous abortions (RSAs) are defined as three or more losses in clinically identified pregnancies prior to 20 weeks, and account for about 1% of all pregnancies. *Only 20% of women probably have an immunological cause* for RSA.

The most important role for the immunology laboratory is to exclude SLE (see Cases 18.3 and 18.4) and the antiphospholipid syndrome (see Chapter 16, Case 16.6). The role of

---

🔍 Case 18.3 Recurrent spontaneous abortion

A 32-year-old woman, who had had three previous spontaneous miscarriages in the first trimester, sought advice from a specialist obstetrician. There was no history of infections in these pregnancies. Examination of the fetal products had not been done, but there was no family history of genetic disease or recurrent fetal loss in close female relatives. She had been extremely well, but she and her husband were anxious. She had no obvious rash, arthritis or bruising and appeared to have a normal uterus and cervix.

Blood tests were negative for cardiolipin, thyroid and antinuclear autoantibodies, and C-reactive protein (CRP) and immunoglobulin measurements were normal. She was advised that she had no underlying cause for the recurrent abortions and that the chance of a successful pregnancy was 30%; she delivered a healthy, live female infant 11 months later.

🔍 Case 18.4 Systemic lupus erythematosus (SLE)

A 19-year-old girl had been diagnosed as having SLE 15 months earlier, following presentation with arthritis in her hands, a rash (livido reticularis) on her arms and considerable spontaneous bruising. She had had antinuclear antibodies of 1/320, C3 of 450 mg/l, C4 of 70 mg/l and a platelet count of 54×10^9/l at that time. Renal function was normal, but she had both low-titre anticardiolipin antibodies and a lupus anticoagulant, though no antibodies to double-stranded DNA (dsDNA) at presentation. She consulted an obstetrician at 16 weeks into an unexpected pregnancy while in disease remission and on 5 mg of prednisolone daily; she had taken the message about possible difficulties in achieving a pregnancy too literally! She was seen every 2 weeks throughout the pregnancy to monitor activity of the SLE; regular full blood counts, C3, C4, creatinine, anticardiolipin and dsDNA antibody measurements were done as well as urine and blood pressure monitoring. These tests were unchanged throughout the pregnancy. A live, normal, male infant was delivered uneventfully by caesarean section at 38 weeks in view of her low platelet count. In the puerperium, she had a mild exacerbation of arthritis and rash for 6 weeks, but without proteinuria, increase in serum creatinine or DNA antibodies. The infant remained well.

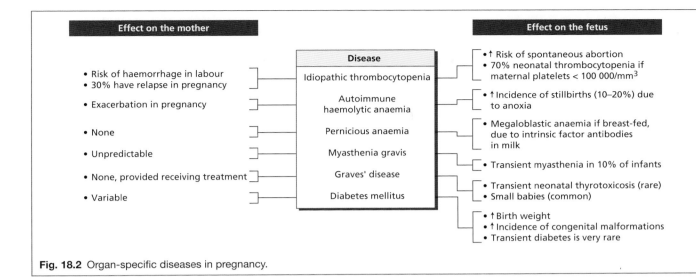

Fig. 18.2 Organ-specific diseases in pregnancy.

anticardiolipin and antiphospholipid antibodies in recurrent abortions is clear, although there is still a good deal of controversy over effective therapies. The overall prevalence of IgG and IgM antiphospholipid antibodies in healthy women varies from 2% to 7%, but only high-titre IgG antibodies are associated with recurrent fetal loss. Since 85% of women with these antibodies will have a normal pregnancy, screening women prior to pregnancy is not cost-effective. However, those who present with three or more spontaneous abortions and are found to have high-titre IgG antibodies are most at risk of further fetal loss, so these women are treated with aspirin and/or low-dose heparin in pregnancy, even though the pathogenesis is obscure. Corticosteroids are reserved for those with evidence of SLE. Intravenous immunoglobulin is not used routinely. The role of NK cells in RSA is unclear. There is a reported increase of NK cells in the placenta, and a suggestion that NK cell depletion may preserve trophoblast and spiral artery function, reducing pregnancy loss.

There is now a strong body of evidence (several clinical trials and a meta-analysis) that suggests that immunotherapy, i.e. *immunization* of the woman with her partner's lymphocytes in an attempt to suppress specific cell-mediated immunity, is *not successful* in women with recurrent abortions and has been abandoned, due to the risks of transmissible diseases.

18.4.2 Outcome of pregnancy in systemic lupus erythematosus

SLE (see Chapter 10, section 10.7, and Chapter 11, section 11.5.4) is predominantly a disease of young women who may want to have children. There is no evidence that women with lupus are subfertile, although there is undoubtedly **increased fetal loss** (abortion >10 weeks of gestation/stillbirth).

Human placental explants cultured in sera from untreated, non-pregnant women with SLE/antiphospholipid syndrome (APS) demonstrated a significant **decrease in the trophoblas-**tic cell proliferation rate and an **increase in apoptosis** compared with non-pregnant women and those with treated SLE/APS, suggesting a role for serum antibodies in the pathogenesis of failed pregnancy. Furthermore, drugs used in the treatment of SLE can affect the fetus very early in pregnancy. It is therefore important *to control the disease pre conception* in order to achieve a better outcome for mother and baby.

Women with SLE have a **70% rate of successful** pregnancies, although 1–2% of mothers with the Ro antibody will have infants with congenital heart block. Successful pregnancies are often complicated by preeclampsia, intrauterine growth retardation or prematurity.

Fetal loss has been associated with the presence of antiphospholipid antibodies and/or lupus anticoagulant, an antibody to the activated clotting factor X (see Chapter 16, section 16.6.2). Patients with these antibodies are treated with low-dose aspirin to reduce platelet aggregation. Although high doses of IVIg are sometimes used to reduce autoantibody levels prophylactically during pregnancy in APS women, this can exacerbate the disease in those with SLE. In patients whose lupus presents in pregnancy, both the morbidity risk to the mother and mortality risk to the fetus are greatly increased.

Women with other rheumatic diseases unrelated to pregnancy may become pregnant and require close medical supervision (Fig. 18.1).

18.4.3 Preeclampsia

Preeclampsia is a **disease of implantation**, in which the symptoms are expressed late in pregnancy once the complications of placental ischaemia due to poor implantation are apparent. The precise aetiology of preeclampsia is unknown, but inadequate trophoblast invasion and a failure to modify the structure of the spiral arteries result in an inadequate blood supply and hence placental ischaemia, leading to fetal anoxia. The maternal syndrome, characterized by hypertension, oedema and proteinuria, results from systemic maternal endothelial damage

---

Case 18.5 Transient neonatal Graves' disease

A 32-year-old primagravida was seen in the obstetric clinic at 16 weeks of gestation, having suffered from severe morning sickness until the 14th week. She was now complaining of heat intolerance, weight loss, palpitations and fatigue. There was no past history of thyroid disease and no family history. On examination she had a marked tachycardia, was thin and there was a bruit over the thyroid. Thyroid function tests showed undetectable thyroid-stimulating hormone (TSH) and high levels of free T3 and T4. Levels of autoantibodies to thyroid microsomes were extremely high (1/400 000) and antibodies to TSH receptors revealed that she had Graves' disease. She was treated with carbimazole and the dose was kept to a minimum to keep the T3 in the high-normal range. Surgery was not required.

As the level of TSH receptor antibodies was still high at 36 weeks, it was no surprise when the cord blood from a female infant with normal-sized thyroid (delivered at 37 weeks) was found to have high T3 and T4 levels and positive TSH receptor antibodies. The neonatologist judged that no treatment was required and the parents were reassured that neonatal Graves' disease is transient. At 3 months the baby had normal thyroid function.

---

and inflammation caused by factors released into the maternal circulation from the **ischaemic placenta**. It may be complicated, if severe, by the HELLP syndrome (haemolysis, elevated liver enzymes and low platelets). Since preeclampsia and cardiovascular diseases involve endothelial dysfunction, metabolic changes and oxidative stress and they share the same risk factors (obesity, kidney disease and diabetes), it is suggested that these vascular diseases may share aetiological factors. Low-dose aspirin has been recommended by the World Health Organization in high-risk pregnancies.

18.4.4 Fetal diseases due to alloimmunization

Alloimmunization (sensitization) of a woman against **fetal antigens** can occur when fetal red cells pass into the mother's circulation. This happens at delivery and even following minor uterine events during pregnancy. These antibodies then cross the placenta to react with fetal erythrocytes. The opsonized fetal red cells are sequestrated and destroyed by macrophages in the fetal spleen and liver, resulting in **haemolytic disease of the newborn (HDN)** (see Chapter 16, Case 16.5).

 See also Case 18.6 on the companion website, **www.wiley.com/go/misbah/immunology**

The commonest cause of HDN remains **rhesus incompatibility** between mother and fetus. Routine blood grouping of all antenatal women and their spouses detects those rhesus D-negative women who may be at risk. HDN is now prevented by administration of anti-D antibodies antenatally and immediately after delivery. These antibodies destroy any rhesus-positive fetal cells in the maternal circulation and prevent the mother from becoming sensitized. HDN may also be due to ABO incompatibility, but this is rarely severe enough to require an exchange transfusion at birth, probably because ABO antigens are less well developed in the fetus than rhesus antigens.

Alloimmunization with fetal platelets may induce the mother to produce specific **antiplatelet antibodies** (see Chapter 16, Case 16.5). The placental transfer of such antibodies results in **alloimmune neonatal thrombocytopenic purpura**; this is relatively rare (1: 1000 births), as the antigen to which these antibodies are directed (HPA-1a) is common in the general population and so most mothers are positive for the antigen and do not produce antibodies. This condition should be distinguished from idiopathic thrombocytopenic purpura (ITP), in which the mother has circulating autoantibodies to her own platelets (see section 18.4.5). *The risk of severe intracerebral bleeding in the infant is extremely rare, as the function of the platelets is not reduced.*

Maternal antibodies to the histocompatibility antigens of her fetus are found in >60% of multiparous women; they are weak in the first pregnancy but become stronger with successive pregnancies. There is *no* evidence that these antibodies, which are often IgG and thus cross the placenta, are detrimental to the fetus.

18.4.5 Organ-specific autoimmune diseases in pregnancy

The mother and/or fetus can be affected by a maternal organ-specific autoimmune disease in pregnancy (Fig. 18.2). **Haemolytic anaemia** can worsen during pregnancy, probably due to raised levels of hormones; the fetus may be affected by immunological complications of the pregnancy such as anoxia.

In those autoimmune disorders associated with **circulating IgG autoantibodies**, these antibodies may directly damage the fetus once they have crossed the placenta, as in Case 18.5 (see also Chapter 5, Table 5.2). However, this may be infrequent, as in the 10% of babies born to myaesthenic mothers (see Chapter 17, section 17.4.1).

In **ITP** the mother has thrombocytopenia due to circulating autoantibodies to her own platelets. It is rare for this to cause problems at delivery but, if so, prompt treatment with high-dose IVIg will result in a rapid rise in platelets. Autoantibodies to platelets cross the placenta, to induce neonatal thrombocytopenia in 50% of infants. Testing of the mother's and the baby's platelets will detect platelet-bound antibody. If this is present on platelets from both individuals, they are autoimmune as in ITP, or if restricted to the neonate, they are alloimmune (see section 18.4.4). The management of immune neonatal thrombocytopenia is discussed in Chapter 16 (see Case 16.5). A similar mechanism has been detected in which anti-neutrophil antibodies can cause neonatal neutropenia, but this is extremely rare.

18.5 Clinical relevance of antibodies to reproductive components

18.5.1 Antibodies to hormones

Antibodies against human chorionic **gonadotrophin** are able to prevent implantation and can be used to extend the time interval after emergency contraception with levonorgestrel. Since IgG has a half-life of 3–4 weeks, passive immunization is effective for a few weeks and active immunization can provoke adequate titres of neutralizing antibodies in sexually mature individuals, rendering the vaccinee infertile for the duration of these antibodies. Vaccines against human sperm for use in men have been tested in male monkeys, but have not been sufficiently immunogenic and have failed as yet to result in aspermia.

18.5.2 Antibodies to sperm

Fertilization is reduced or inhibited by antibodies present on the sperm surface; such antibodies are produced by the male following sterilization or by plasma cells in the female genital tract. The exact significance of such antibodies remains unclear; sperm testing has become the role of specialist andrology laboratories and is no longer part of a routine clinical laboratory repertoire.

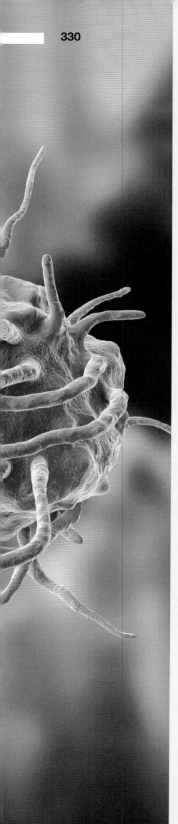

CHAPTER 19
Techniques in Clinical Immunology

Key topics

Visit the companion website at **www.wiley.com/go/misbah/immunology** to download cases with additional figures on these topics.

Chapel and Haeney's Essentials of Clinical Immunology, Seventh Edition. Edited by Siraj A. Misbah, Gavin P. Spickett, and Virgil A.S.H. Dalm.
© 2022 John Wiley & Sons Ltd. Published 2022 by John Wiley & Sons Ltd.

19.1 Introduction

There are clinical immunology laboratories across the world that not only provide numerical and qualitative data, but also expert clinical understanding for physicians and paediatricians for whom there is little training in laboratory techniques or interpretation. In order to provide a clinically relevant service, only those tests that are actually useful are included in the repertoire. However, requesters often ask for a test described in a recent paper or available in a research laboratory, so it is important to understand why particular tests are done as well as not done. Laboratory tests can be graded according to their value in the care of patients. Some tests are **essential** for diagnosis or monitoring, some are **useful** in subclassifying disorders with varying complications or outcomes, and others are of current **research** interest, but may provide added diagnostic insight in future. Unfortunately, tests are **useless** if requested in inappropriate circumstances and this applies particularly to uncritical requests such as 'autoantibody screens'. Nobody highlighted the problem better than the late Dr Richard Asher over 50 years ago (Box 19.1).

Laboratory tests differ in their sensitivity and specificity (Fig. 19.1). For optimal results, the **cut-off** point for any assay – the point above which results are considered positive – is set so that virtually no diseased patients are test-negative (false-negative results) and the fewest possible individuals without the disease are test-positive (false-positive results). The **sensitivity** of a test is defined as the proportion of diseased individuals in whom the test is positive. A negative result in a very sensitive test can be used to exclude the relevant disease ('rule out'). Test results should be negative not only in healthy people, but also in individuals with diseases with similar clinical features but different natural histories. The **specificity** of a test is the proportion of individuals without a given disease in whom the test is negative. A positive test is then virtually restricted to the disease in question ('rule in') and tests of high specificity, such as antimitochondrial antibody (AMA; Fig. 19.1), can be used to confirm the clinical diagnosis. Another way of assessing the utility of a test is to calculate the positive and negative predictive values, which are derived from the sensitivity and specificity.

Of the assays described in this chapter, some are quantitative and others are qualitative. Quantitative assays produce precise results. In general, such assays can be automated and international reference preparations are available to standardize results. Qualitative assays provide answers of normal/abnormal or positive/negative type. They can involve considerable technical expertise and interpretation of results can be subjective. Both types of assays are subject to internal **quality control**, as all laboratories have to ensure the quality and accuracy of results or a result is useless for an individual patient. **Quality assurance** (QA) is achieved by participation in External Quality Assessment Schemes (EQASs), which may be organized on a regional, national or international basis. Without these assurances, any clinical laboratory might as well toss a coin to gain a result.

All diagnostic laboratories should undergo inspection to ensure that they meet an acceptable standard of testing. This is defined in the **International Standard ISO 15189**. Every country will have an approved inspection service (in the UK this is the UK Accreditation Service – UKAS). Inspection approves a 'scope of practice' for the laboratory. Before adding a new test to the scope, a laboratory must undertake a process of verification and validation to confirm that the test performs as expected. The laboratory will have documentation on the performance of the test and will maintain appropriate internal quality control and external QA. Research tests do not necessarily meet this standard.

Box 19.1 Why does a clinician order a test?

- I order this test because if it agrees with my opinion I will believe it, and if it does not I shall disbelieve it
- I do not understand this test and am uncertain of the normal figure, but it is the fashion to order it
- When my chief asks if you have done this or that test I like to say yes, so I order as many tests as I can to avoid being caught out
- I have no clear idea what I am looking for, but in ordering this test I feel in a vague way (like Mr Micawber) that something might turn up
- I order this test because I want to convince the patient there is nothing wrong, and I don't think he will believe me without a test

Source: Asher R (1954) Straight and crooked thinking in medicine. *British Medical Journal*, ii, 460–462.

19.2 Investigation of immunoglobulins

19.2.1 Quantitation of immunoglobulins

Serum immunoglobulin measurements are essential in patients with repeated or severe infections and those with myeloma and some other lymphoproliferative disorders. They are sometimes useful in the differential diagnosis of hypergammaglobulinae-mic states (Table 19.1).

The classical techniques used for measurement involve immune-complex formation with antisera specific for the protein, in this case the human immunoglobulin isotype, to be measured. These antisera may be raised in animals by injection of the relevant antigen. Animals respond by making **polyclonal antibodies**, i.e. the resultant sera contain mixtures of antibodies from different B-cell clones and all the antibodies react with the relevant antigen, but vary in the precise nature of their variable regions. In contrast, **monoclonal antibodies** are the product of

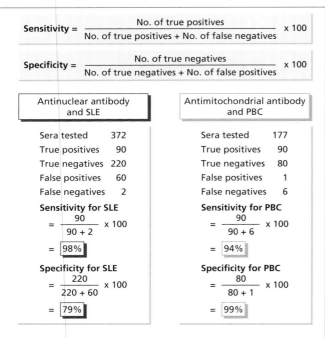

$$\text{Sensitivity} = \frac{\text{No. of true positives}}{\text{No. of true positives} + \text{No. of false negatives}} \times 100$$

$$\text{Specificity} = \frac{\text{No. of true negatives}}{\text{No. of true negatives} + \text{No. of false positives}} \times 100$$

Antinuclear antibody and SLE	
Sera tested	372
True positives	90
True negatives	220
False positives	60
False negatives	2

Sensitivity for SLE
$$= \frac{90}{90 + 2} \times 100$$
$$= \boxed{98\%}$$

Specificity for SLE
$$= \frac{220}{220 + 60} \times 100$$
$$= \boxed{79\%}$$

Antimitochondrial antibody and PBC	
Sera tested	177
True positives	90
True negatives	80
False positives	1
False negatives	6

Sensitivity for PBC
$$= \frac{90}{90 + 6} \times 100$$
$$= \boxed{94\%}$$

Specificity for PBC
$$= \frac{80}{80 + 1} \times 100$$
$$= \boxed{99\%}$$

Fig. 19.1 Sensitivity vs specificity of assays illustrated by antinuclear antibody testing for systemic lupus erythematosus (SLE) and antimitochondrial antibody (AMA) testing for primary biliary cirrhosis (PBC).

Table 19.1 Examples* of major polyclonal elevations in immunoglobulin levels

Immunoglobulin	Example
IgM	Primary biliary cirrhosis
IgA	Alcoholic liver disease
IgG	Primary Sjögren's syndrome
	Human immunodeficiency virus (HIV) infection
	Systemic lupus erythematosus
Mixed isotypes	Tuberculosis
	Hepatic cirrhosis
	Chronic bacterial infections/occult abscesses

*But not sufficiently specific to be of diagnostic value in individual patients.

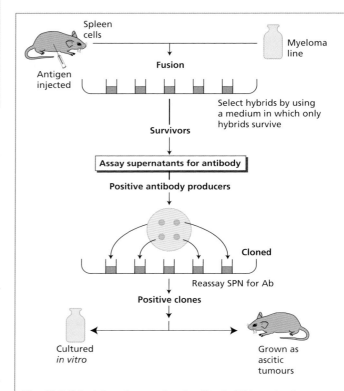

Fig. 19.2 Principles of monoclonal antibody (Ab) production. SPN, supernatants.

a single cell and its progeny and are therefore identical throughout their variable and constant regions; they react only with one determinant (epitope) on a given antigen. Spleen cell suspensions from immunized mice contain numerous secreting B cells from different clones recognizing different epitopes. These B cells are fused with a non-secreting myeloma cell line to form hybrids that have the antibody-producing capacity of the parent B cell and the immortality of the malignant plasma cell. Hybrid cells are then selected and cloned (Fig. 19.2). Large-scale culture can provide considerable quantities of such antibodies, which are pure and precise in their reactivity. The choice of the type of antibody depends on the nature of the assay.

For protein measurements, human serum is mixed with the relevant antiserum for that protein. At low concentrations, the immune complexes remain in suspension as fine particles that can disperse a beam of light. **Light dispersion** can be measured using turbidimetry or nephelometry. So long as the amount of detecting antibody in the assay is in excess of the amount of antigen being added, for a constant antibody concentration, the amount of light scatter is proportional to the concentration of the antigen in the human serum being tested. If patient immunoglobulin levels are very high, the amount of immune complexes decreases with the addition of excessive amounts of antigen ('hook effect'). Therefore, readings may be spuriously low ('prozone effect'. With appropriately diluted patient samples, however, the method is rapid and suitable for automation; precise results can be obtained in 1–2 h from venepuncture.

For some proteins, machine-compatible reagents may not be available. Under these circumstances, laboratories may use the **single** radial immunodiffusion (RID) technique originally described by Mancini. Both RID and centrifugal analysis can be used for **measurement of many proteins** in serum, amniotic fluid, cerebrospinal fluid, saliva and gastrointestinal juice. They include not only human immunoglobulins, but also a range of other immune reactants, acute-phase proteins, transport proteins, coagulation proteins and 'tumour markers'. Standard preparations are used, which have been calibrated against international World Health Organization (WHO) standards. *Each hospital laboratory determines its own reference range for each protein* and this will vary according to the method and antisera used and the ethnic origin of the group. *Reference ranges of most proteins also vary with age, especially in children,* and 95% of the 'normal' population will fall within that range.

19.2.2 Qualitative investigation of immunoglobulins

Serum

It is essential that sera sent for immunoglobulin quantification are screened by serum **protein electrophoresis** for the presence of paraproteins (monoclonal bands), since these abnormal immunoglobulins may react with the standard antisera in a different way due to variable epitopes and structural changes. The principle of the methodology is given here, though most of these assays are now automated.

In protein electrophoresis, a wet membrane or gel is stretched across an electrophoresis tank, and filter-paper wicks provide a continuous buffer phase. Serum samples are applied to the surface on the cathodal side and an electric current is passed through the membrane or gel for about 45 min. It is then removed and the protein bands visualized with an appropriate dye (Fig. 19.3). A normal serum is

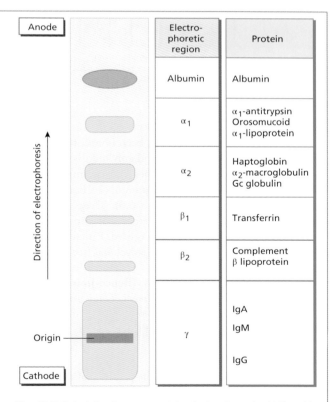

Fig. 19.3 Principle of serum protein electrophoresis. At the pH of routine electrophoresis (pH 8.6), serum proteins carry a net negative charge and migrate towards the anode. Some weakly charged proteins, such as immunoglobulins, are carried back towards the cathode by the flow of buffer.

always run with the test specimens for comparison and quality control. Since this is done by machine now, the electrophoretic strip can be visualized on the computer or printed out. Discrete monoclonal immunoglobulin (M) bands can appear anywhere along the strip and must be investigated further. False-positive bands, which are not due to immunoglobulin, may be caused by haemoglobin (in a haemolysed sample), fibrinogen (in plasma or an incompletely clotted specimen) or aggregated IgG (in a stored specimen). It is therefore important to send fresh clotted blood specimens for this test. An even faster technique is to use capillary zone electrophoresis (CZE), which is highly automated.

When an M band is found on electrophoresis, the nature of the band must be determined by **immunofixation,** also automated. Several samples of the patient's serum are first electrophoresed on agar gel (Fig. 19.4). Specific antisera to IgG, IgA, IgM and κ and λ light chains are then applied to the electrophoresed samples. Precipitation (i.e. immunofixation) of the M protein is achieved by incubating the gel and antisera. Unfixed (non-precipitated) protein is washed from the gel and the 'fixed' bands are stained and visualized. In the absence of a heavy-chain abnormality, an abnormal reaction with antisera specific for light chains alone suggests that the M band is due to free monoclonal light chains or, very rarely, an IgD or IgE paraprotein. An abnormal reaction with a heavy-chain antiserum alone is very unusual. Individual M bands can be quantified by **densitometry** – also automated; this measures the intensity of stain taken up by each band and produces a tracing corresponding to the electrophoretic strip (Fig. 19.5). The proportion attributable to the monoclonal protein is expressed as a percentage of the whole tracing and converted to absolute terms (g/l) by reference to the total serum protein concentration. Scanning densitometry is the most reliable method for measuring paraprotein concentration, particularly for serial monitoring or in samples containing large amounts of non-paraprotein immunoglobulins. Quantitation by comparison of the levels of free κ and λ light chains provides another, faster way to monitor changes in paraprotein levels for clinical management in lymphoproliferative diseases (Chapter 6).

Gross elevations of the immunoglobulin levels indicate the need to measure the relative serum viscosity (RSV); this is the time taken for a given volume of serum to pass through a narrow capillary tube, relative to water. RSV is normally 1.4–1.8. Symptoms of hyperviscosity (see Chapter 6, Case 6.9) usually develop when the RSV value exceeds 4.0.

Provided the serum is fresh, a heavy deposit of protein at the origin in serum electrophoresis may indicate the presence of **cryoglobulins.** Cryoglobulins are immunoglobulins that form precipitates, gels or even crystals in the cold. The severity of the symptoms (see Chapter 11, Case 11.7 and section 11.6.3) depends on the cryoprotein concentration and the temperature at which cryoprecipitation occurs (thermal range). If cryoglobulins are suspected clinically, a fresh specimen of blood must be taken directly into a warmed

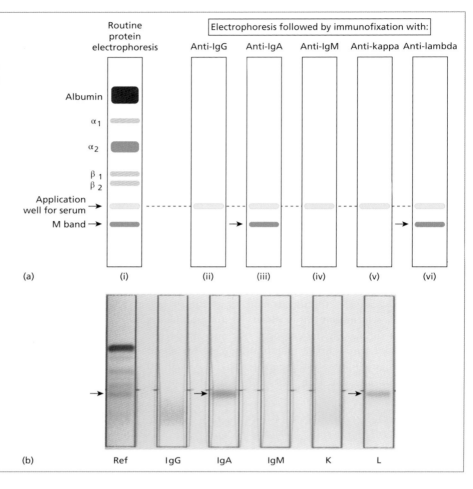

Fig. 19.4 Typing an M band by immunofixation. In this schematic example (a), the M band found on electrophoresis (i) is identified as an IgA (type λ), as shown on the actual fixation gel (b).

Urine

Analysis of urine is essential in suspected myeloma, any condition in which a serum M band has been found, hypogammaglobulinaemia of unknown cause and amyloidosis.

Normal immunoglobulin synthesis is accompanied normally by production of excessive amounts of free polyclonal light chains (see Chapter 6, section 6.6). These are excreted into the urine, where they can be detected in minute amounts in everyone if a really sensitive assay is used. Patients with renal damage excrete larger quantities of polyclonal free light chains in the urine.

Free monoclonal light chains (Bence-Jones proteins) *cannot be detected by routine measurement of total urinary protein or urine dipstick testing.* The only reliable test for suspected 'Bence-Jones proteinuria' consists of three stages:

- Concentration of urine.
- Electrophoresis to demonstrate the presence of an M band.
- Immunofixation to confirm that the monoclonal band is composed of either monoclonal κ or λ free light chains. The excretion of a whole paraprotein by a damaged kidney may give a false-positive result, unless the free light chain nature of the M band is confirmed or the serum paraprotein is run alongside for identification.

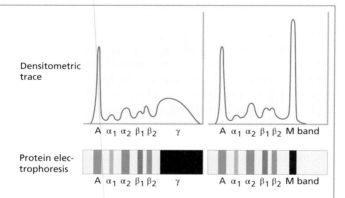

Fig. 19.5 Densitometric analysis of protein electrophoresis for quantification of an M band. A, albumin. Normal trace on left.

container (37 °C) and delivered warm (37 °C) to the laboratory; it is allowed to clot at 37 °C and also separated at 37 °C. Aliquots of separated serum are kept at 4 °C for 24 h or longer. Centrifugation and washing of any resultant precipitate must be done at 4 °C. The precipitate is redissolved by warming back to 37 °C and then analysed for its constituent proteins by immunofixation at 37 °C in order to determine the type of cryoglobulin (Chapter 11).

Urine electrophoresis has largely been replaced by the measurement of serum free light chains. This testing can be automated and is therefore far less labour intensive. It is also quantitative and can thus be used to monitor the response to treatment. In light chain-only myeloma and some plasmacytomas (localized B-cell tumours), measurement of serum free light chains is essential for diagnosis and monitoring.

Cerebrospinal fluid

IgG and albumin concentrations in cerebrospinal fluid (CSF) can be measured. Since albumin is not synthesized in the brain, the relationship between IgG and albumin – the CSF IgG index – gives an indirect indication of how much CSF IgG has been synthesized by lymphocytes inside the brain (Fig. 19.6). The CSF IgG index is given by dividing (IgG CSF/IgG serum) by (Alb CSF/Alb serum) and should be less than 0.72. The index therefore corrects for reductions in the albumin–IgG ratio associated with diseases that alter the permeability of the blood–brain barrier. In contrast to serum, the IgG in CSF is often of a restricted nature and forms **oligoclonal bands**, i.e. there are two or more discrete bands rather than a diffuse increase. Oligoclonal bands cannot be detected by routine electrophoresis of unconcentrated CSF and the degree of concentration needed (80-fold) to make bands visible induces artefacts. The most satisfactory method is isoelectric focusing and immunofixation with an enzyme-labelled antiserum to IgG (Fig. 19.7). CZE can also be used. This is an essential test in the investigation of demyelinating disorders such as multiple sclerosis (see Chapter 17, Case 17.2); each set of bands is unique.

19.3 Investigation of complement and immune-complex disorders

Assays for complement components in the serum are divided into those assays that recognize the antigenic nature of the individual complement components and those that measure functional activity, such as cell lysis.

19.3.1 Assays for individual components

Immunochemical measurements (section 19.2) of C3 and C4 are the most useful assays. International reference preparations and reliable automated methods are widely available. Measurements of other components can be done but are rarely needed, except in patients with suspected genetic deficiencies, atypical haemolytic uraemic syndrome (aHUS) and abnormal functional assays. C1 inhibitor must be measured if hereditary or acquired angioedema is suspected (see Chapter 11, Case 11.5 and section 11.6.1). Low or absent C4 during an attack of angioedema is highly suggestive. A functional assay is required to confirm type II hereditary angioedema.

Low levels of complement components are more relevant clinically than high levels. As complement components are acute-phase

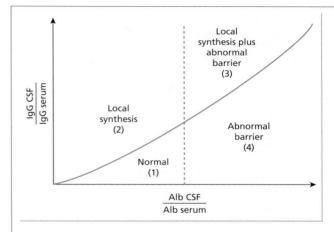

Fig. 19.6 Cerebrospinal fluid (CSF) IgG index. The *y* axis shows increasing values for the quotient of IgG in CSF: IgG in serum, and the *x* axis shows increasing values for the quotient of albumin in CSF: albumin in serum. The four areas signify (1) normal; (2) local synthesis (normal barrier function); (3) local synthesis plus abnormal barrier function; (4) barrier function abnormal (not local synthesis).

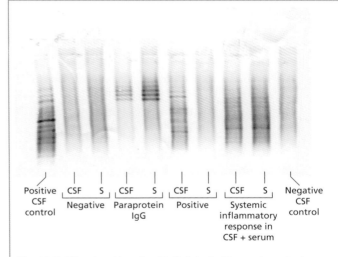

Fig. 19.7 Oligoclonal bands of IgG detected in cerebrospinal fluid (CSF). Isoelectric focusing separates proteins within a pH gradient according to their acidic or basic nature. The proteins are then transferred to a nitrocellulose membrane by blotting and the nitrocellulose immunofixed with an antiserum to IgG to show the IgG-specific bands. The pattern is interpreted by comparing paired samples of CSF and serum (S). A positive test is one where oligoclonal IgG bands are found in CSF but not in serum.

reactants, rates of synthesis rise in any inflammatory condition. To understand complement changes in disease, it is useful to consider complement components in three groups (Fig. 19.8):

- Early components of the classical pathway.
- Early components of the alternate pathway.
- Late components common to both pathways.

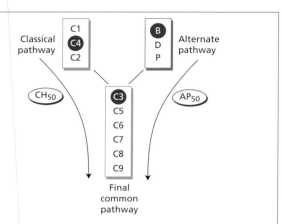

Fig. 19.8 Complement components distributed into three groups (see text). Ringed components are those measured as representatives of the groups. Functional integrity of the classical and alternate pathways is measured by CH_{50} and AP_{50} assays (see text).

Table 19.2 Interpretation of complement changes in disease

Level of component

C4	C3	Factor B	Activation pathway	Examples
↓	↓	N	Classical pathway	Systemic lupus erythematosus (SLE); vasculitis
↓	↓	↓	Classical and alternate pathways	Gram-negative bacteraemia
				Some cases of SLE
N	↓	↓	Alternate pathway	C3 NeF autoantibody
↓	N	N	Classical pathway to C4 and C2 only	Hereditary angioedema (C1⁻ inhibitor deficiency)
↑	↑	↑	Increased synthesis of components	Acute and chronic inflammation

In practice (Table 19.2), low C4 and C3 but normal factor B levels suggest that activation of the classical pathway alone has occurred; if C4, C3 and factor B levels are low, the alternate pathway is probably also activated, either via the feedback loop (see Chapter 1) or by simultaneous activation. Normal C4 levels with low C3 and factor B concentrations provide evidence of activation of the alternate pathway alone.

Serial measurements of C3 and C4 are useful in monitoring disease activity or treatment in patients with some forms of glomerulonephritis, systemic lupus erythematosus (SLE) and vasculitis. If low initially, they often return to normal in remission (see Chapters 9 and 10). *Routine complement tests are of little value in other acute and chronic inflammatory diseases.*

19.3.2 Detection of complement breakdown products

Even if complement levels are normal due to increased synthesis, measuring 'breakdown' or activation products of the pathway may recognize consumption. This may be helpful in unexpected acute shock, where a new material that has been used invasively is suspected to cause alternate pathway activation of C3. The electrophoretic mobility of native C3 and that of its cleavage products (e.g. C3c and C3dg) are different. Other activation products, such as C3a, C5a, C1r/C1s complex and C5b/9 complex, can also be measured. C5bC9 assays are used in the diagnosis of patients with atypical haemolytic uraemic syndrome (aHUS) and in the monitoring of treatment with eculizumab, a monoclonal antibody that blocks the activation of C5 by the C5 convertase. It is used to treat aHUS and paroxysmal nocturnal haemoglobinuria, where there is pH-dependent complement-mediated lysis of red blood cells due to an acquired defect of complement regulatory proteins on the red cell (CD55 and CD59).

19.3.3 C3 nephritic factor

C3 nephritic factor (C3 NeF) is an autoantibody to activated C3 that stabilizes the alternate pathway C3 convertase and allows further C3 breakdown (see Chapter 9). C3 NeF is suspected in renal patients in whom an unexplained low C3 level is found; these are usually patients with kidney disease, lipodystrophy or recurrent infections. It is detected by incubation of the patient's serum with normal serum; this allows the C3 nephritic factor in the patient's serum to break down C3 in the normal serum.

19.3.4 Functional assays

Functional assays are essential if a genetic defect of complement is suspected, but are not helpful in other conditions.

The commonest assay used in routine laboratories is the **CH_{50} assay** (total haemolytic complement; Fig. 19.8). This estimates the quantity of serum required (as a complement source) to produce haemolysis of 50% of a standard quantity of antibody-opsonized red blood cells. Patients' sera are always titrated against a standard serum. A similar functional assay of the alternate complement pathway is also available. Provided that specimens reach the laboratory promptly, these assays are sensitive and reliable. The C5b-C9 assay may give comparable results. Functional assays for C1 inhibitor are required as part of the investigation of suspected hereditary angioedema.

Tests for circulating immune complexes in serum are no longer available, as the tests are unreliable and the results uninterpretable.

19.3.5 Direct immunofluorescence for immune complexes in tissues

In all conditions where an immune-complex aetiology is suspected, **direct analysis of tissue biopsies** should be done. Biopsy specimens for direct immunofluorescent examination must not be fixed, but delivered directly to the laboratory in approved tissue culture medium by arrangement. They are then snap-frozen and sliced; sections are well washed in saline to reduce background staining, before incubation with the appropriate conjugated antiserum. Staining should include immunoglobulin heavy chains and C3. A parallel section is also stained with haematoxylin and eosin to show the morphology of the specimen. The technique is commonly used for renal (Chapter 9) and skin (Chapter 11) biopsies and is very useful in diagnosis. Indications are given in the relevant clinical chapters.

19.4 Antibodies to microbial antigens

The detection of antibodies to microorganisms has been used in the **diagnosis of infection** for many years. The presence of circulating IgG antibody indicates only that the antigen has been met some time previously. For diagnosis of an infection in a given patient, a significant rise in antibody (IgG) titre (usually fourfold) must be demonstrated in paired sera taken 2 weeks apart. If an immediate answer is required, the presence of a high-titre, specific IgM antibody implies a primary response (see Chapter 1), but **rapid polymerase chain reaction (PCR) for viral and bacterial DNA** is now the method of choice. Serology is reserved for large-scale screening, as in blood products or antenatally.

Detection of antimicrobial antibodies is also an essential part of the **investigation of immune deficiency**. The ability to produce specific antibodies against defined antigens is the most sensitive method of detecting abnormalities of antibody production (see Chapter 3, section 3.2). Such antibodies are usually detected by enzyme-linked immunosorbent assays (ELISA; section 19.5.1) and reported in International Units if there is an international standard, or arbitrary units if no standard is available. Antibodies to Streptococcus pneumoniae are found in most normal adult subjects, but not in those individuals with significant primary antibody deficiency (see Chapter 3). Antibodies to common viral antigens are also useful if there is a history of known viral exposure either by infection or immunization. Similarly, if the patient has been immunized, it is useful to look for antibodies to Pneumococcal polysaccharides, tetanus and diphtheria toxoids. If antibody levels are low, the patient is test-immunized with the appropriate killed vaccine and the response reevaluated 3–6 weeks later (Table 19.3 and Chapter 3, Cases 3.2 and 3.3). It is possible to measure the levels of IgG antibodies to Pneumococcal serotypes. Some serotypes are more immunogenic than others, but a failure to respond to multiple serotypes after immunization is suggestive of a defect in humoral immunity.

Table 19.3 The use of test immunization to assess antibody production in a patient with recurrent infections

Antibody specificity	Pre immunization	Post immunization 4 weeks	Reference range
Pneumococcal polysaccharide			
Total IgG	4	8	80–100 U/ml
IgG1	<1	2	30–80 U/ml
IgG2	<1	<1	45–100 U/ml
Tetanus toxoid	<0.01	7.6	>0.85 U/ml

Pneumococcal antibodies are shown in arbitrary units. Tetanus antibodies are shown in International Units per millilitre. The patient, a 38-year-old man, has responded well to test immunization with tetanus toxoid, but shows no response to Pneumovax. He has a defect in specific antibody production (see Chapter 3).

19.5 Detection of autoantibodies

19.5.1 In serum

The detection of circulating autoantibodies commonly involves one of five methods: immunofluorescence, radioimmunoassay (RIA), enzyme-linked immunoassay (EIA), countercurrent electrophoresis and cell-based flow cytometry. Each type of assay system has its own snags. Immunofluorescence is the least sensitive of these techniques, and depends on subjective interpretation by an experienced observer; it is relatively cheap and reliable in trained hands. RIA requires expensive reagents, facilities for β and γ counting of radioisotopes and facilities for handling and disposal of radioactive waste; nowadays non-radioactive markers are used, with the same principles. EIA avoids the problems of radioisotope handling and disposal, but also requires specialized equipment and careful quality control with proven reagents. Countercurrent electrophoresis is easy and cheap, but relatively insensitive and largely phased out now, with a few exceptions. Cell or bead-based flow cytometry has become available, since purified antigens transfected into standard cell lines or coupled to beads have made this a sensitive method. Rapid throughput screening for nuclear and related antibodies is now available using this technique and has been shown to be robust.

Indirect immunofluorescence

This is used for the detection of many serum autoantibodies (Tables 19.4 and 19.5). Animal tissue can be used when the substrate contains antigens common to human and animal tissue, but some autoantigens are restricted to human tissue or human cell lines. Tissues are snap-frozen and the producer, prior to delivery to the clinical laboratory, cuts sections at –20 °C on a cryostat. The patient's serum is incubated with the substrate for 30 min and unbound proteins are then washed off before a second antibody, with a visible tag (usually fluorescein),

Table 19.4 Indirect immunofluorescent tests for commoner non-organ-specific autoantibodies

Autoantibody	Typical substrate	Staining pattern	Main clinical relevance
Antinuclear antibody (ANA)	Human cell line (HEp2) or rat liver	All nuclei	Screening test for systemic lupus erythematosus
Centromere	Human cell line (HEp2)	Centromere of human chromosomes	Limited systemic sclerosis (CREST syndrome) (Case 11.9)
Smooth-muscle antibody (SMA)	Rat stomach, liver and kidney	Smooth muscle, i.e. muscularis mucosa, muscle of intergastric glands and arterial tunica media	Chronic active hepatitis (Case 14.6); non-specific liver damage (weak)
Antimitochondrial antibody (AMA)	Rat kidney, liver and stomach	All mitochondria (esp. distal renal tubules)	Primary biliary cirrhosis (Case 14.7)
Endomysial antibody	Monkey oesophagus	Sarcolemma of smooth-muscle fibrils	Coeliac disease (Case 14.2); dermatitis herpetiformis
Antineutrophil cytoplasmic antibody (ANCA)	Human neutrophils	Cytoplasmic (cANCA)	ANCA-associated necrotizing crescentric glomerulonephritis (Case 9.5); microscopic polyarteritis
		Perinuclear (pANCA)	Many forms of vasculitis

Table 19.5 Indirect immunofluorescent tests for commoner organ-specific autoantibodies

Autoantibody	Typical substrate	Staining pattern	Major clinical relevance
Gastric parietal cell antibody	Rat stomach	Parietal cells only	Pernicious anaemia (Case 14.1)
Adrenal antibody	Human adrenal	Adrenal cortical cells	Idiopathic Addison's disease (Case 15.5)
Pancreatic islet cell antibody	Human pancreas	β cells of pancreatic islet	Insulin-dependent diabetes (Case 15.4)
Skin antibodies	Human skin or guinea-pig lip	Intraepidermal intercellular cement	Pemphigus vulgaris (Case 11.4)
		Epidermal basement membrane	Bullous pemphigoid

is added. This reacts with those serum IgG antibodies that have combined with antigens in the substrate. The site of antibody fixation can then be visualized by fluorescent microscopy (Fig. 19.9).

An autoantibody is defined by the **staining pattern seen on a given substrate** (Tables 19.4 and 19.5); only patterns of proven clinical significance are reported. Where relevant, a positive serum is titrated to determine the strength of the antibody. The results are expressed as a titre or in International Units if a known standard has been used alongside. Most laboratories use an IgG-specific second antibody, because this isotype of autoantibody is clinically significant. The staining pattern for antinuclear antibodies (ANAs) can be clinically useful by suggesting possible diagnoses (Box 19.2), *but is never diagnostic*. Since anti-Ro antibodies can be detected on ANA screening with human cell lines, ANA-negative lupus is rare (about 1%). Although several autoantibodies can be detected simultaneously by using

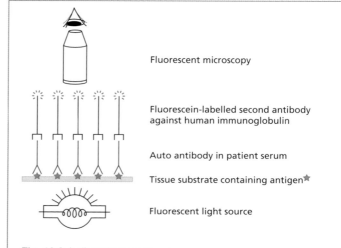

Fluorescent microscopy

Fluorescein-labelled second antibody against human immunoglobulin

Auto antibody in patient serum

Tissue substrate containing antigen★

Fluorescent light source

Fig. 19.9 Indirect immunofluorescence.

Box 19.2 Patterns of nuclear staining for antinuclear antibodies (ANAs) are useful but not diagnostic

Pattern	Appearance	Disease association
Homogeneous (diffuse)		Common pattern
Rim of nucleus (peripheral; annular)		Systemic lupus erythematosus (SLE)
Nucleolar		SLE
Speckled		SLE Sjögren's syndrome Mixed connective tissue disease
Centromere (dividing cells only)		Limited systemic sclerosis (CREST syndrome)

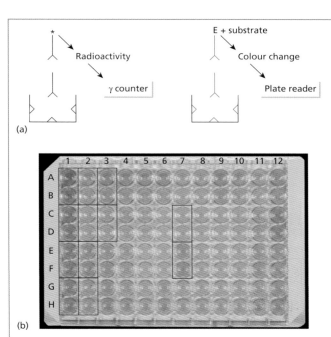

(a)

(b)

Fig. 19.10 (a) Principle of radioimmunoassay vs enzyme-linked immunosorbent assay (ELISA). E, enzyme-labelled antibody that binds to human IgG; * radioisotopically labelled antibody that binds to human IgG. (b) An ELISA assay plate. In this example, anticardiolipin antibodies are being measured. Wells 1AB, 1CD, 1EF, 1GH, 2AB and 2CD contain duplicate samples of standard anticardiolipin antibody activity ranging from highest (1AB) to lowest (2CD). Wells 2EF, 2GH, 3AB and 3CD contain duplicates of known positive and negative quality control samples. Remaining wells contain test sera tested in duplicate. Wells 7CD contain a negative patient serum, while wells 7EF contain a strong positive serum sample.

a composite block of tissues, only tests relevant to the clinical problem should be requested. *Requests for uncritical 'autoantibody screens' are no longer available* (Box 19.1).

Interpretation of the results depends on the class and titre of the antibody and the age and sex of the patient. The elderly, especially women, are prone to develop autoantibodies in the absence of clinical autoimmune disease. ANAs may be triggered by infections (particularly with Gram-negative organisms) and by certain drug treatments. In contrast, high-titre autoantibodies in a child or young adult suggests that overt disease will be evident now or occur later. The ANA test is an example of a test that is sensitive but not specific (see Fig. 19.1) and should only be used for screening patients with appropriate symptoms, as the false-positive rate is about 5–10%.

Radioimmunoassay and enzyme-linked immunosorbent assays

These are extremely sensitive methods of detecting autoantibodies in low concentration (Fig. 19.10). The few RIAs still used for detecting autoantibodies are listed in Table 19.6. The techniques are used in other branches of pathology, for example for hormone assays.

Tests for **antibodies to double-stranded DNA (dsDNA)** are essential if SLE is suspected. They are detected by a variety of methods; those commonly used involve enzyme-labelled DNA or ^{125}I-DNA. Positive results usually indicate SLE or chronic active hepatitis. The dsDNA does gradually dissociate to single-stranded DNA, and it is important to look closely at control binding values for each run to determine the cut-off point for significant positivity. A fluorescent test, using the organism Crithidia luciliae, is specific for dsDNA, but rather insensitive, in that only 60% of SLE patients' sera react. The problem of standardization is helped by the availability of a WHO international standard for anti-dsDNA. While RIA is still recognized as a gold standard for the detection of antibodies to dsDNA, EIA has largely supplanted it in routine use.

Snake venom toxin, α-bungarotoxin, binds strongly to acetylcholine receptors in human skeletal muscle extract. This has been exploited to provide an RIA for **acetylcholine receptor antibodies (AChRAb)**. Purified α-bungarotoxin is labelled with radioiodine and then complexed with human muscle extract. AChRAb react with the antigen and can be precipitated with an antiserum to human immunoglobulin. It is a sensitive assay; about 90% of patients with systemic myasthenia gravis are positive (see Chapter 17, section 17.4), and there are few false positives. This test is essential for diagnosis in myasthenia gravis.

Enzymes can also be used as labels instead of radioisotopes: the tests are then known as **enzyme-linked immunosorbent assays**. In general, they are more sensitive but less

Table 19.6 Some autoantibodies detected by radioimmunoassay

Antibody	Method	Result	Clinical relevance
Double-stranded DNA antibody	^{125}I-DNA – direct binding	Percent of binding or IU/ml	Systemic lupus erythematosus (Cases 10.8 and 10.9)
			Chronic active hepatitis (Case 14.7)
Acetylcholine receptor antibody	Direct binding of ^{125}I α-bungarotoxin complexed with acetylcholine	Binding reported as fmol/l of specific antibody receptors from cultured cell lines	Myasthenia gravis (Case 5.2)

Table 19.7 Some autoantibodies detected by enzyme-linked immunosorbent assay (ELISA)

Antibody	Target autoantigen	Clinical relevance
Thyroid microsomal antibody	Thyroid peroxidase	Autoimmune thyroid disease (Cases 15.1, 15.2 and 15.3)
Mitochondrial (M2) antibody	E2 pyruvate dehydrogenase complex	Primary biliary cirrhosis (Case 14.7)
Glomerular basement membrane antibody	C terminal end of type IV collagen	Antiglomerular basement membrane nephritis (Case 9.5)
Antineutrophil cytoplasmic antibody		
cANCA	Proteinase 3	ANCA-associated necrotizing crescentic glomerulonephritis (Case 9.6)
pANCA	Myeloperoxidase	Microscopic polyarteritis
Double-stranded DNA antibody	dsDNA	Systemic lupus erythematosus (Cases 10.8 and 10.9)
Phospholipid antibody	Cardiolipin	Primary phospholipid antibody syndrome (Case 16.6)
		Systemic lupus erythematosus (Cases 10.8 and 10.9)

specific (see Fig. 19.1) than RIAs. Because the problem of handling and disposal of radioisotopes is avoided, their 'green' credentials mean EIAs are used increasingly in immunoassays (Table 19.7). For example, although countercurrent electrophoresis (see section 19.2.2) was the 'gold standard' for detecting and identifying antibodies to extractable nuclear antigens (Table 19.8), automated EIA assays using pure, recombinant antigens are now the method of choice.

Countercurrent immunoelectrophoresis

Countercurrent immunoelectrophoresis (CIE) involves electrophoresis of antigens and antibodies towards each other. At the appropriate pH, relatively acidic antigens will move rapidly towards the anode and the antibodies towards the cathode, maintaining their original concentrations. If the patient's serum contains a relevant antibody, a precipitin line is formed between the wells (Fig. 19.11). CIE was used for screening test sera for antibodies against 'extractable nuclear antigens' (ENA), but has been superseded by EIA using pure, recombinant antigens as targets.

19.5.2 Biopsy material

Immunohistochemical examination of biopsy specimens of damaged or normal tissue may reveal deposits of immunoglobulins caused by antibodies reacting with an organ or tissue-specific antigens. This approach is especially important in the diagnosis of antiglomerular basement antibody disease (Chapter 9) and the bullous skin disorders (Chapter 11). Biopsies must be handled as outlined in section 19.3.5.

19.6 Tests for allergy and hypersensitivity

Some antibodies to non-invasive extrinsic antigens result in immune damage ('hypersensitivity'). The type of test used depends on whether the damage is predominantly an IgE-mediated (type I) mechanism or an immune-complex-mediated (type III) mechanism involving IgM or IgG antibodies.

In atopic disorders, such as allergic rhinitis or extrinsic asthma (see Chapter 4), skin-prick testing can be useful. Provocation tests, by nasal, bronchial or oral challenge, are the most clinically

Table 19.8 Antibodies to different components of extractable nuclear antigens (ENA)

Antigen	Molecular target	Clinical relevance*
'Smith' (Sm)	Common core proteins of U1, U2, U4, U5, U6 – s RNPs	Alone or with RNP antibody – a subset of SLE (20%)
Ribonucleoprotein (RNP)	U1 – s RNP	High titre – mixed connective tissue disease (Case 10.9) (100%)
Ro (SS-A)	60-kDa small RNP-binding Ro RNAs	Neonatal lupus and congenital heart block
		Subacute cutaneous lupus
La (SS-B)	Transcription terminator of Ro RNAs	Primary Sjögren's syndrome (Case 10.10)
Scl-70	Topoisomerase I	Systemic sclerosis (20%) (Case 11.9)
Jo-1	Histidyl-transfer RNA synthetase	Myositis (Case 10.13), arthritis – often with pulmonary fibrosis

*Figures in parentheses show percentage of patients in disease category who have demonstrable antibody. s RNP, nuclear ribonucleoproteins; SLE, systemic lupus erythematosus; U, uridine rich.

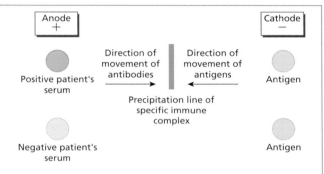

Fig. 19.11 Countercurrent immunoelectrophoresis.

relevant type of test, but are potentially hazardous. These tests are discussed in Chapter 4; this chapter concentrates on laboratory tests only.

19.6.1 Antigen-specific IgE antibodies

The RAST (radioallergosorbent technique) test (Fig. 19.12) enables **antigen-specific IgE antibodies** to be measured. More recently, fluorenzyme immunoassay (FEIA) methods for detection of specific IgE to allergens have come into general usage. These dispense with the need for radioactivity and may be automated to allow faster throughput compared with classical RAST; however, both tests are colloquially known as 'RASTs' or, more accurately, 'specific IgE testing'. The antigen is coupled to a solid phase such as cellulose; only IgE antibodies reactive against this particular antigen are detected by means of an antibody specific for the IgE heavy chain. *RAST results are expensive and should be used only if skin tests are contraindicated or unhelpful.* This includes very young children, those with severe dermatitis, those dependent on medicines that modify skin reactivity, such as antihistamines, and those in whom a severe reaction is possible, such as wasp venom anaphylaxis. Allergen-specific IgE levels are reported quantitatively as arbitrary units/ml or semi-quantitatively as RAST classes 0–6, where 0 is negative, 1 is

borderline, 2 and 3 are positive to a degree, and 4–6 are increasingly strongly positive. The ease with which RASTs can be performed must not be allowed to overexaggerate their value in the assessment of allergic patients. The presence of allergen-specific IgE is a marker of sensitization and does not necessarily equate to disease. Results must be interpreted on the basis of a detailed history, to assess clinical relevance.

19.6.2 Basophil activation test

The basophil activation test (BAT) is a flow cytometry–based functional assay that assesses the degree of cell activation after exposure to type I hypersensitivity stimuli. Cross-linking of the Fc epsilon receptor by an allergen or anti-IgE antibody (positive control) results in a rapid upregulation of intracellular and activation-linked CD63 and CD203c molecules to the cell surface. This is accompanied by mediator (histamine) release. CD63 and CD203c are therefore the target molecules for a flow cytometry–based *in vitro* test to analyse sensitized patients with type I allergy, though there remains some concern about the reproducibility of this assay and, as yet, no quality assessment schemes exist to ensure reproducibility and clinical significance.

19.6.3 Serum tryptase

Total tryptase levels are easily measured using an ELISA, in which a monoclonal antibody is used to capture the tryptase and a second antibody against IgG4 (the IgG subclass of the first monoclonal antibody) coupled to a fluorochrome for detection. This assay system measures both α- and β-tryptase, though the clinical significance of β-tryptase is not yet clear. Tryptase levels in serum are extremely low normally; reference values for healthy individuals give an upper 95th percentile of 13.5 ng/ml in children and adults, so levels above this are considered significant. Since it is essential to investigate sudden unexplained deaths, it is important to know that tryptase levels have been shown to be unaffected at post mortem, although they can be elevated by myocardial infarction. Detecting an

Fig. 19.12 Principle of measurement of antigen-specific IgE antibodies.

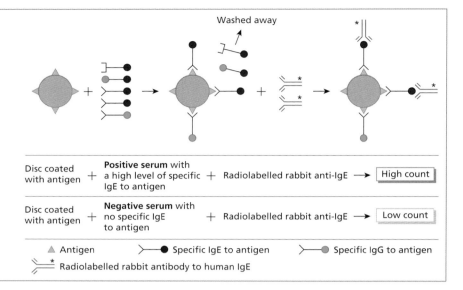

| Disc coated with antigen | + | **Positive serum** with a high level of specific IgE to antigen | + | Radiolabelled rabbit anti-IgE | → | High count |

| Disc coated with antigen | + | **Negative serum** with no specific IgE to antigen | + | Radiolabelled rabbit anti-IgE | → | Low count |

▲ Antigen   ⊶● Specific IgE to antigen   ⊶● Specific IgG to antigen

⫤* Radiolabelled rabbit antibody to human IgE

elevated tryptase in patients presenting to Emergency Departments with allergic symptoms is helpful to confirm the nature of the reaction. Anaphylaxis, particularly to drugs, may not always be accompanied by a rise in tryptase.

A persistent elevation of tryptase is seen in the rare condition mastocytosis, where there are excess mast cells in skin and gut. This may be apparent in the skin as urticaria pigmentosa. These yellowish plaques contain excess mast cells and light stroking of them will lead to histamine release (Darier's sign). Patients with mastocytosis may have severe reactions to some drugs, especially those that are known to degranulate mast cells (opiates and some anaesthetic drugs). They will react badly to insect stings and to immunotherapy. Therefore, patients with venom allergy should have baseline tryptase checked.

19.6.4 Total serum IgE

Measurement of total serum IgE is useful only in patients in whom parasite infestation is suspected, and is of little value in the differentiation between IgE- and non-IgE-mediated disorders (see Chapter 4). This is usually performed by RIA or enzyme immunoassay, since the normal level of IgE in the serum is extremely low (<120 IU/ml). *This test is expensive and of little routine clinical value.* Extremely high levels (50 000 and greater) are seen in the primary immune deficiency hyper-IgE syndrome (see Chapter 3, section 3.4.4); moderate elevations (1000–20 000) are seen in generalized atopic eczema. Normal levels of total IgE do *not* exclude a diagnosis of severe allergic disease.

19.6.5 Precipitating antibodies

Precipitating antibodies to specific antigens are usually IgM or IgG. The investigation of the extrinsic allergic alveolitides (see Chapter 13) requires testing for such antibodies. Precipitation tests are done by the Ouchterlony method; this is insensitive, but cheap compared with immunoassay. Extracts of the

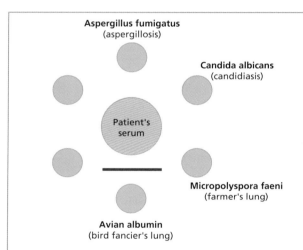

Fig. 19.13 Detection of precipitating antibodies in extrinsic allergic alveolitis. The patient has precipitating antibodies to avian albumin, suggesting possible bird fanciers' lung.

relevant antigens are placed in the outside wells (Fig. 19.13) with the patient's serum in the centre. After several days, the plate is examined for precipitates formed by antibodies complexed with the given antigen. Some of the commonly used antigens (Fig. 19.13) are available commercially and a national external QA scheme is established in the UK. Where an unusual substance is suspected as the cause of a patient's symptoms, a simple extract of that substance can be used as the antigen in a precipitation test.

19.7 Assessment of lymphocytes

Two types of test are used to assess cells:

- Quantification of different types of cells
- *In vitro* assays of their individual functions.

19.7.1 Quantification of lymphocytes

The study of lymphocyte populations was made possible when it was shown that they expressed different cell surface markers. Quantification of T and B lymphocyte subpopulations is essential in immunodeficiency (see Chapter 3) and certain lymphoproliferative diseases (see Chapter 6). The number of circulating CD4⁺ T lymphocytes (Chapter 3) is a strong prognostic factor in human immunodeficiency virus (HIV) infection and is used as one of the surrogate markers for assessing progress of the disease and the need for, and response to, anti-HIV therapy. National and international quality assessment schemes are in operation.

All estimations must be done on fresh anticoagulated blood. Monoclonal antibodies are used to identify human peripheral blood B and T lymphocytes. These antisera recognize CD antigens (see Chapter 1) expressed characteristically, but not uniquely, by cells of a certain lineage and at certain stages of their differentiation. Cells are identified and counted by an automated fluorescence-activated cell scanner – or **flow cytometer** – which measures the fluorescence generated by each labelled cell. Aliquots of whole blood are incubated with appropriately labelled monoclonal antibodies. Cells are aspirated into the machine and surrounded by sheath fluid, which forces the cells to flow through the chamber in single file past a laser beam and light sensors. Light emitted by the excited fluorescent dye on the cell surface is detected by the sensors and analysed by on-board computer software. The instrument can be fitted with detectors for a number of different fluorescent dyes.

Cell populations vary in size and granularity. These properties can be used to define ('gate') the cell population of interest, prior to analysis of the markers (Fig. 19.14). The data can be displayed as a series of profile histograms (Fig. 19.15), with the fluorescent intensity generated by the monoclonal antibody shown on the horizontal axis and the number of cells on the vertical axis; this is important for quality control. If double labelling is used, a dot plot of individual cells shows the intensity of fluorescence of one dye against the intensity of fluorescence of the other (Fig. 19.16) for each cell. The proportions of cells reactive with both antibodies, either one, or neither is shown by the intensity of the dots, and quantitative results are generated by the machine's computer. Results are always expressed in absolute numbers and this is achieved by using a known quantity of marked beads for comparison. Although flow cytometers are expensive, experienced users obtain results quickly and easily, and the results are very accurate due to the vast numbers of cells that are counted (usually 5000–10 000 cells).

It should be noted that values for lymphocyte subsets in children differ significantly from those in normal adults and vary significantly with age, especially in the first 12 months of life.

19.7.2 Functional tests

In vitro tests of lymphocyte function should be performed only if the clinical features suggest abnormal cell-mediated immunity. These assays are therefore only essential in suspected T-cell immunodeficiencies and prior discussion with the laboratory is also essential.

These tests can be done using either whole blood or separated lymphocytes. Either way, fresh anticoagulated blood is required, as viable cells are tested. When lymphocytes are activated by certain substances, a few small resting lymphocytes respond by changing into blast cells over a few days. This process is called **lymphocyte transformation** (see Chapter 1). Stimulating substances are usually of four types (Table 19.9). The proliferative response is measured by using a set quantity of dye (CSFE) incorporated into each cell, which is diluted out by each cell division, or by the expression of cell surface markers, such as CD69, found on activated cells after a few hours. These tests require tissue culture facilities and are time-consuming and expensive. The batch variability and lack of standards make interpretation difficult without rigorous controls.

It is possible to measure a large number of soluble or intracellular cytokines, interleukins, surface adhesion molecules or receptors and their messenger RNAs. Such assays are readily available and non-invasive but, as yet, most must be considered as research investigations.

The exceptions are the interferon production assays. These tests measure the amount of interferon (IFN)-γ produced by lymphocytes in blood in response to incubation with specific extracts of Mycobacterium tuberculosis. Blood from individuals who have been exposed to these specific mycobacteria contains a few circulating CD4 Th1 cells that produce IFN-γ in a secondary immune response to the antigens. Positive controls ensure that the T cells are not suppressed iatrogenically, as many of those tested are patients with rheumatoid arthritis or Crohn's disease receiving immunosuppression or HIV patients. Interferon production can be measured either as the number of cells staining with antisera to IFN-γ

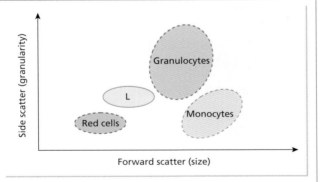

Fig. 19.14 'Gating' of cell populations. A cell population is analysed for forward and side (90%) scatter. Each cell is quantified in this way and represented by a dot on the graph (a dot plot). Each cell population forms a discrete cluster of dots. One such cluster, e.g. lymphocytes (L), can be selected, i.e. 'gated', for further analysis with fluorescent markers, while other cell clusters are ignored. Gating is also commonly performed based on CD45 staining and side scatter.

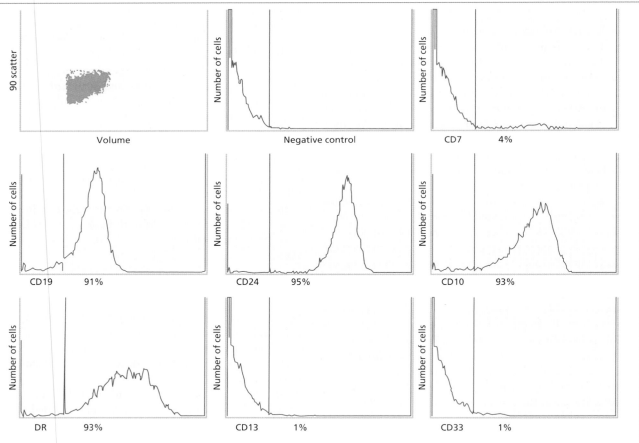

Fig. 19.15 Histograms of immunofluorescent staining of bone marrow cells in a case of acute lymphoblastic leukaemia. The *x* axis represents fluorescence intensity, the *y* axis the number of cells. The percentage of positive cells is based on a cursor set for the negative control. The gated population (blasts) is shown in the dot plot (top left). These blasts are CD19+, CD24+, CD10+ and HLA class II.

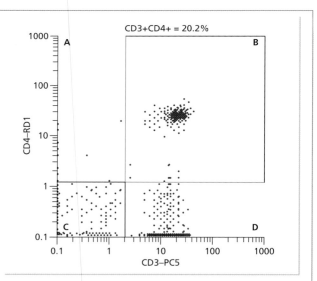

Fig. 19.16 Dual-colour immunofluorescence. A cell preparation has been incubated with two different monoclonal antibodies (MAb) conjugated to different fluorescent dyes (PC5 and RD1): one is anti-CD3; the other is anti-CD4. Lymphocytes in quadrant C stain with neither monoclonal (CD3– CD4–), while those in quadrant B stain with both (CD3+ CD4+). Cells in A stain only with anti-CD4 (very few) and those in D only with CD3.

(ELISPOT) by an ELISPOT reader or by quantitation of secreted IFN-γ in the supernatant of the culture by ELISA. The sensitivity of these assays enables the relatively few specific memory T cells in the blood to be detected easily, even if the patient is immunosuppressed.

19.8 Assessment of neutrophils and monocytes

19.8.1 Neutrophil and monocyte quantification

Absolute numbers of these cells can easily be calculated from the total and differential white blood cell counts.

19.8.2 Functional tests

Tests of neutrophil function are essential in patients with recurrent or severe staphylococcal or fungal infections. Neutrophils can be separated from whole blood using a sedimentation method and their functional properties broken down into a series of key steps (Fig. 19.17).

The **surface proteins that mediate adhesion of neutrophils to vascular endothelium** are the β₂-integrin family (see Chapter 1). These proteins have a common β chain (CD18) that combines with different α chains (CD11a, CD11b and

Table 19.9 Tests of T-lymphocyte activation pathways

Stimulating agent	Example	Activation pathway	Specificity of response	Need for prior exposure
Antigen	Purified protein derivative (PPD) of tuberculosis	TCR	Specific	Yes
Plant mitogen	Phytohaemagglutinin (PHA)		Non-specific	No
Monoclonal antibody	Anti-CD3	TCR/CD3 complex	Non-specific	No
Phorbol ester and calcium ionophore	Phorbol myristate acetate (PMA) and ionomycin	Signal transduction pathway distal to TCR/CD3 complex	Non-specific	No

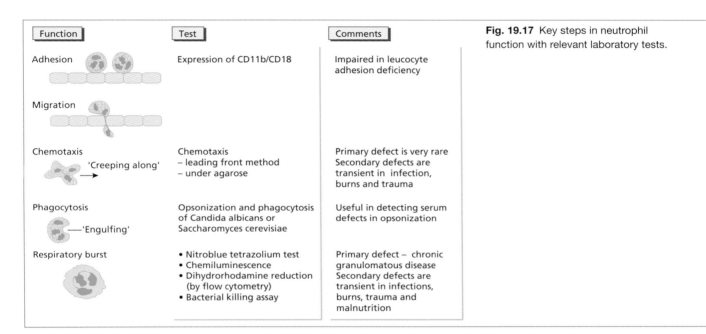

Fig. 19.17 Key steps in neutrophil function with relevant laboratory tests.

CD11c) to form heterodimers including leucocyte function antigen 1 (LFA-1: CD11a/CD18) and complement receptor 3 (CR3: CD11b/CD18). In leucocyte adhesion deficiencies, there are genetic defects resulting in non-functional receptors preventing normal neutrophil adhesion to vascular endothelium. These markers are variably expressed on neutrophils, and can be detected by flow cytometry.

Chemotaxis is the purposeful movement of cells towards an attractant, usually the synthetic peptide f-Met-Leu-Phe. The ability of the patient's serum to generate chemotactic factors can be tested by incubating fresh serum with endotoxin. In the "leading front" type of assay, the cells to be tested are separated from the chemotactic stimulus by a Millipore membrane. After incubation, the filter membrane is removed, fixed and stained. The distance that cells have migrated through the filter towards the stimulus can be measured using a conventional light microscope. *Chemotaxis is not used routinely as the assays are extremely difficult to standardize.*

Phagocytosis is the ingestion of foreign material. Ingestion can be determined by incubation of phagocytic cells with inert particles, such as latex beads, or yeasts or bacteria. Intracellular particles or bacteria can be seen microscopically. Crossover studies using normal controls allow testing of the patient's cells for their ability to phagocytose particles opsonized with normal serum, while the patient's serum is tested for its ability to opsonize particles for ingestion by normal neutrophils. *These are still research assays and are not used routinely.*

Intracellular enzyme activity accompanying the '**respiratory burst**' can be measured by bacterial killing, though this too is a research assay. The **nitroblue tetrazolium (NBT) test** measures the ability of phagocytic cells to ingest and reduce this soluble yellow dye to an intracellular blue crystal. Separated neutrophils are added to a solution containing NBT and stimulated with endotoxin. The cells can be viewed microscopically to count the number of polymorphs containing blue crystals. This is an easy screening test, widely available and essential for the exclusion of chronic granulomatous disease (see Chapter 3, section 3.4 and Case 3.5). More commonly the granulocyte respiratory burst is measured by **dihydrorhodamine (DHR) reduction**. Activation of granulocytes loaded with DHR generates reactive oxygen intermediates that react with DHR, and the resulting increase in fluorescence can be measured by flow cytometry. In the X-linked form of chronic granulomatous disease, carriers demonstrate two cell populations, one reacting with DHR, the other not, whereas neutrophils from affected boys are unable to react with DHR at all (see Chapter 3, section 3.4).

19.9 Recombinant DNA technology in clinical immunology

The huge advances in molecular biology have important implications for the diagnosis and treatment of immunological diseases.

19.9.1 DNA analysis

In molecular pathology, known unique segments of nucleic acid sequences are used as DNA probes to determine the presence of complementary sequences of DNA (or RNA) in patient samples. The target DNA is composed of thousands of nucleotide bases and the reactivity of the probe, a single strand of DNA, with its complementary target – **DNA hybridization** – is the most specific intermolecular interaction known between biological macromolecules.

Nucleic acids remain intact in fresh-frozen as well as formalin-fixed, paraffin-embedded tissues. In the technique of **in situ hybridization**, DNA probes are applied directly to the tissue sections on microscope slides. The principle is essentially similar to other DNA hybridization techniques, except that tissue sections must first undergo deparaffinization and proteolytic digestion to expose intracellular nucleic acid targets.

Restriction endonucleases are enzymes that cleave DNA at sites specifically related to the nucleotide sequences. The use of enzymes of different specificities allows a DNA fragment containing a particular gene to be cut out from the rest of the DNA molecule. In the **Southern blotting technique** (Fig. 19.18), fragments of DNA cleaved by a restriction endonuclease are electrophoresed on agarose gel, smaller fragments migrating further than larger fragments. Among these fragments will be one containing the gene of interest. Alkali denaturation of the DNA fragments uncoils them so that the

resulting single-stranded DNA will hybridize with complementary pieces of DNA after transfer to a special nitrocellulose filter. Blotting the gel with the nitrocellulose filter fixes the DNA fragments at the same positions that they occupied after electrophoresis. A radiolabelled 'probe' containing DNA known to be complementary to the DNA of interest will hybridize to it and the fragment can then be identified by autoradiography of the nitrocellulose filter. The **Northern blotting technique** uses the same principle to transfer RNA, instead of DNA, from gel to blot.

In many genetic disorders, the defect is not known and production of gene-specific probes is not feasible. In these cases, however, the disease-producing gene may be closely linked to the recognition site of a particular restriction endonuclease. Scattered throughout the human genome are harmless variations in DNA sequences that may produce new restriction endonuclease sites or remove preexisting ones. The fragments of DNA produced by a particular restriction enzyme will therefore be of differing lengths in different people. These are called **restriction fragment length polymorphisms (RFLPs)** and are inherited in a simple Mendelian fashion. RFLPs provide a potentially large number of linkage markers for tracing disease-producing genes in families, without knowing anything about the gene itself.

These methods have been largely superseded by a major advance in recombinant DNA technology called the **polymerase chain reaction**, a method for dramatic amplification of target DNA prior to cleavage with a restriction enzyme (Fig. 19.19). Complementary oligonucleotide primers from either end of the target DNA are added to the denatured sample along with a heat-resistant DNA polymerase. If the target sequence is present, the primers anneal to it and provide a starting point for the polymerase to begin the synthesis of second-strand DNA. The newly synthesized double-stranded DNA is then denatured by heating and exposed again to the polymerase enzyme at a lower temperature. In this way, newly synthesized molecules and original DNA can reassociate with the primer and act as templates for further rounds of DNA

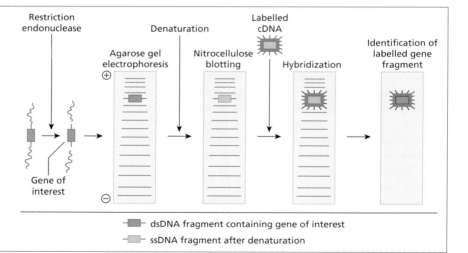

Fig. 19.18 Gene mapping by the Southern blotting technique (see text for explanation).

Restriction endonuclease · Agarose gel electrophoresis · Denaturation · Nitrocellulose blotting · Labelled cDNA · Hybridization · Identification of labelled gene fragment

Gene of interest

–■– dsDNA fragment containing gene of interest
–■– ssDNA fragment after denaturation

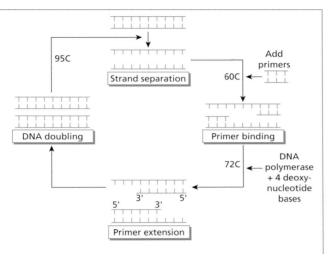

Fig. 19.19 The polymerase chain reaction (see text for explanation).

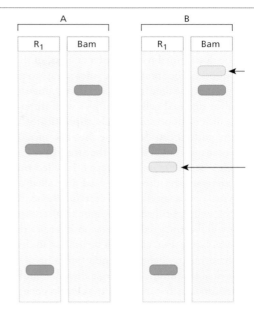

Fig. 19.20 TCR gene rearrangement studies by Southern blotting. DNA was digested with the enzymes Eco R1 (R1) and Bam H1 (Bam). The control (A) shows germline bands for both enzymes, but in a patient with lymphoma (B) the bands are rearranged (arrowed).

synthesis. After completing about 30 cycles, which takes 2–3 h in an automated procedure, the specific target sequence is amplified over 1 million-fold. This powerful and sensitive technique can detect a specific DNA sequence from a single cell (e.g. lymphocyte, sperm), fixed pathological specimens and dried blood spots. The disadvantage is that contamination of the reaction mixture with traces of DNA from another source will lead to false-positive results.

Now that exome and genome sequencing are available in larger institutions, it will not be long before these assays are superseded in turn.

19.9.2 Diagnostic implications

Recombinant DNA technology has led to a major change in methodology for tissue typing (see later) and provides precise **diagnosis of genetic disease**, including prenatally using tissue obtained by chorionic villus sampling, fetoscopy or amniocentesis. It can also detect preclinical cases of autosomal dominant disorders of late onset, and female carriers of X-linked conditions, including some types of congenital immunodeficiency (see Chapter 3). PCR has proved of particular value in the rapid diagnosis of infectious diseases and in immunogenetic studies. One example is the detection of the HIV genome in patients who cannot be determined to be HIV positive by conventional means, such as infants born to HIV-infected mothers. The great sensitivity of PCR and its ease of use with multiple patient samples allow the identification of critical human or viral DNA sequences that would be impossible to detect by other means. Viral loads in blood are now measured routinely for patients with common viruses such as Epstein–Barr virus and cytomegalovirus.

Gene rearrangement studies are used to analyse the origin of potentially malignant lymphocytes that lack conventional T- and B-cell markers. The normal maturation of lymphocytes is associated with somatic gene rearrangements (see Chapter 1) of immunoglobulin heavy and light chain complexes in B cells

and of T-cell receptor (TCR) gene complexes in T cells. Gene rearrangements are random and so the structure of the rearranged genes varies from one cell to another. Clonal expansion of a neoplastic cell results in identical rearrangements for all cells in the clone. By Southern blotting, it is possible to identify a clonal population and distinguish it from a polyclonal proliferation. This technique can detect monoclonality when clonal cells account for 5% or fewer of the cell population, important to determine residual malignant disease in leukaemia.

TCR gene rearrangements are the most definitive, non-morphological approach for the diagnosis of T-cell malignancies (Fig. 19.20). Prior to this approach, diagnosis based on morphology and immunophenotyping with monoclonal antibodies often failed to detect monoclonality.

19.9.3 Genomics and microarrays

Traditional disease classification is based mainly on morphological, histological, biochemical or immunological criteria. However, classification at the level of gene expression provides a potentially more accurate tool for diagnosis and treatment. DNA microarray technology is an extremely powerful tool for analysing the expression of up to 30 000 genes (i.e. the genome) and investigating the underlying disease mechanisms, biomarkers and therapeutic targets of many human diseases. The difficult part is making sense of the vast amounts of data generated. DNA microarrays are small, solid supports, usually glass microscope slides, silicon chips or nylon membranes, onto which DNA sequences from different genes are attached at fixed locations. The microarray exploits the ability of a given mRNA molecule to bind specifically (i.e. hybridize) to the DNA template from which it originated. In a single experiment, the expression level of thousands of genes within tissues or cells can be determined by computer analysis of the amount of mRNA bound to the spots on the microarray, so generating a profile of gene expression in that cell. By tagging the mRNA from control or diseased cells or samples with differently coloured (green or red) fluorescent labels, sophisticated computer analysis of the pattern can determine the ratio of red to green fluorescent intensity at each spot on the array. Determining the level at which a certain gene is expressed is called **microarray expression analysis** and the arrays used are called expression chips. If a gene is overexpressed in a certain disease, then more sample cDNA will hybridize to the spot than control cDNA and the spot will fluoresce red with greater intensity than it will fluoresce green. Expression chips can be used in understanding disease mechanisms by identifying new genes involved in the pathogenesis of autoimmune or allergic disorders and in developing new treatments. For instance, if a certain gene is overexpressed in a disease, expression chips can be used to determine if a new drug reduces this overexpression and modifies progression of the disease. Gene expression patterns can be used as 'fingerprints' to distinguish between different forms of the diseases, most commonly in tumour classification, but with increasing applications elsewhere.

19.10 Histocompatibility testing

There are many histocompatibility antigens on leucocytes and other cells, but those of the human leucocyte antigen (HLA) system are the most important (see Chapter 1). These antigens are present on all tissues of the body, but their availability on peripheral blood lymphocytes enables immunogenetic studies to be carried out easily on these cells. The original test used to detect major histocompatibility complex (**MHC) antigens** was a serological one – the microlymphocytotoxicity test. The application of molecular techniques to tissue typing has led to a fundamental change in methodology for **MHC typing**. These techniques have several advantages over serotyping. Initially, Southern blotting techniques were used to allow identification of RFLPs (see section 19.9.1) that correlated with known serological (HLA-DR/DQ) and cellular (HLA-DW) defined specificities. The development of PCR allowed for the amplification of the polymorphic exons of the MHC class I and class II genes and the analysis of the polymorphic sequence motifs with sequence-specific oligonucleotide hybridization probes. The immobilization of these probes on membranes and later on beads, along with primer sets for sequence-specific priming (SSP), gave rise to the current set of typing reagents. Sanger sequencing provides high-resolution typing and the introduction of next-generation sequencing will reduce the genotyping ambiguity. *These tests are available only in specialized centres where immunogenetic studies are essential for organ and bone marrow transplantation.* They are time-consuming and expensive and require considerable skill and experience to interpret the results. Prior consultation is essential and fresh, anticoagulated whole blood must be sent direct to the laboratory. HLA typing for HLA-B27 is useful in patients with suspected ankylosing spondylitis or HLA-DQ2/DQ8 in excluding patients with suspected coeliac disease. The use of HLA typing in other diseases remains speculative and of research interest only.

The MHC class I and class II loci are the most polymorphic genes in the human genome, with a highly clustered and patchwork pattern of sequence motifs. In the three decades since the first HLA gene was isolated by molecular cloning (a cDNA clone of HLA-B7), thousands of alleles have been identified and the names and sequences of all known alleles have been curated in the IMGT/HLA database. This extensive allelic diversity made and continues to make high-resolution MHC DNA typing very challenging.

APPENDIX

Further Resources

 A list of these useful resources can also be found on the companion website at
www.wiley.com/go/misbah/immunology

Basic science

Immunogenetics

www.ebi.ac.uk/services
   The world's most comprehensive range of freely available and up-to-date molecular databases, including the HLA system, immunoglobulins and T-cell receptors covering nomenclature and sequence information.

CD antigens

www.ebioscience.com/resources/human-cd-chart.htm
   Structured reviews of various protein families including the list of human cell-surface molecules assigned a CD number by international workshops on leucocyte differentiation antigens.

Cytokines

www.copewithcytokines.de/cope.cgi
   Up-to-date survey of literature on cytokines, including potential therapeutic implications. Encyclopaedia of cytokines linked to fully integrated dictionaries on angiogenesis, apoptosis, chemokines, etc.

Macrophage

www.macrophages.com
   Lists freely accessible sources related to macrophages and immunology, for professionals from the Roslin Institute.

Clinical topics

Allergy and Clinical Immunology information and resources

http://journals.lww.com/co-allergy/pages/editorialboard.aspx
   Journal for up-to-date reviews in allergy and clinical immulogoy.

Web page of the Division of Allergy, Immunology and Transplantation of the National Institute of Health, USA

www.niaid.nih.gov/research/daithtm
   Provides succinct summaries of recent workshops and expert reports on a variety of topics in clinical immunology and allergy.

Infection data

www.aidsinfo.nih.gov
   Provides comprehensive coverage of medical aspects of HIV infection, including immunopathogenesis, HIV clinical trials and anti-retroviral drugs; up-to-date guidelines.

Chapel and Haeney's Essentials of Clinical Immunology, Seventh Edition. Edited by Siraj A. Misbah,
Gavin P. Spickett, and Virgil A.S.H. Dalm.
© 2022 John Wiley & Sons Ltd. Published 2022 by John Wiley & Sons Ltd.

www.who.int/hiv/pub/en/
Provides recent publications world-wide and uptodate policies for all countries on HIV.
http://esa.un.org/unpd/wpp/Excel-Data/mortality.htm
United Nations overall mortality figures for all countries.
www.cdc.gov/tb/publications
Useful information about tuberculosis world-wide; teaching and patient information aids.

Cancer

www.cancerresearchuk.org/cancer-help/type/lymphoma/
Cancer Research UK site giving definitions and useful information about lymphoid malignancies as well as all other cancers.

General medical topics

http://emedicine.medscape.com
Covers all medical disciplines.

The Immunology Link

www.immunologylink.com/
Features comprehensive lists of links to immunology associations, journals and databases. The alphabetical list of murine gene knockouts represents excellent value as well as quick access to human gene databases.

Organizations which promote the science and practice of immunology

American Academy of Allergy, Asthma and Immunology

www.aaaai.org

British Society for Immunology

www.immunology.org

British Society for Histocompatibility and Immunogenetics

www.bshi.org.uk/

French Society for Immunology

www.inserm.fr/sfi

British Society for Allergy and Clinical Immunology

www.bsaci.org

European Society for Immunodeficiencies

www.esid.org

Clinical Immunology Society

www.clinimmsoc.org

European Federation of Immunological Societies

www.efis.org

Royal College of Anaesthetists

www.frca.co.uk
Good guidelines about drug anaphylaxis and process of investigation.

Index

Note: Page numbers for figures are in *italics*, tables are in **bold**

Chapel and Haeney's Essentials of Clinical Immunology, Seventh Edition. Edited by Siraj A. Misbah,
Gavin P. Spickett, and Virgil A.S.H. Dalm.
© 2022 John Wiley & Sons Ltd. Published 2022 by John Wiley & Sons Ltd.